Muscle Diseases

Blue Books of Practical Neurology
(Volumes 1–14 published as BIMR Neurology)

Muscle Diseases

Edited by

Anthony H. V. Schapira, D.Sc., M.D., F.R.C.P., F.Med.Sci.
Professor and Chair of Clinical Neurosciences, Royal Free
and University College Medical School, London; Professor of Neurology,
Institute of Neurology, University College London

and

Robert C. Griggs, M.D.
Professor and Chair of Neurology, University of Rochester School of Medicine,
Rochester, New York; Neurologist-in-Chief, Strong Memorial Hospital, Rochester

with 24 Contributors

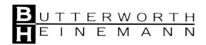

Boston   Oxford   Auckland   Johannesburg   Melbourne   New Delhi

Every effort has been made to ensure that the drug dosage schedules within this text are accurate and conform to standards accepted at time of publication. However, as treatment recommendations vary in the light of continuing research and clinical experience, the reader is advised to verify drug dosage schedules herein with information found on product information sheets. This is especially true in cases of new or infrequently used drugs.

 Recognizing the importance of preserving what has been written, Butterworth–Heinemann prints its books on acid-free paper whenever possible.

 Butterworth–Heinemann supports the efforts of American Forests and the Global ReLeaf program in its campaign for the betterment of trees, forests, and our environment.

Library of Congress Cataloging-in-Publication Data

Muscle diseases / edited by Anthony H.V. Schapira, and Robert C.
  Griggs.
        p.   cm. -- (Blue books of practical neurology ; 24)
    Includes bibliographical references and index.
    ISBN 0-7506-7085-1
    1. Neuromuscular diseases. 2. Muscles--Diseases. I. Schapira,
Anthony H. V. (Anthony Henry Vernon) II. Griggs, Robert C., 1939-
. III. Series.
    [DNLM: 1. Mitochondrial Myopathies. 2. Myositis.
3. Neuromuscular Diseases. W1 BU9749 v.24 1999]
RC925.M84 1999
616.7'44--dc21
DNLM/DLC
for Library of Congress   99-20297
                                                                     CIP

British Library Cataloguing-in-Publication Data
A catalogue record for this book is available from the British Library.

The publisher offers special discounts on bulk orders of this book.
For more information, please contact:
Manager of Special Sales
Butterworth–Heinemann
225 Wildwood Avenue
Woburn, MA 01801-2041
Tel: 781-904-2500
Fax: 781-904-2620

For information on all Butterworth–Heinemann publications available,
contact our World Wide Web home page at: http://www.bh.com

10 9 8 7 6 5 4 3 2 1

Printed in the United States of America

Contents

Contributing Authors

Anthony A. Amato, M.D.
Chief of the Neuromuscular Division and Director of the Clinical Neurophysiology Laboratory, Department of Neurology, Brigham and Women's Hospital, Boston; Associate Professor of Neurology, Harvard Medical School, Boston

Richard J. Barohn, M.D.
Professor and Acting Chair of Neurology, University of Texas Southwestern Medical Center, Dallas

Michael H. Brooke, M.D.
Professor of Neurology, University of Alberta Faculty of Medicine and University of Alberta Hospital, Edmonton, Alberta, Canada

Salvatore DiMauro, M.D.
Lucy G. Moses Professor of Neurology, Columbia University College of Physicians and Surgeons, New York

Robert C. Griggs, M.D.
Professor and Chair of Neurology, University of Rochester School of Medicine, Rochester, New York; Neurologist-in-Chief, Strong Memorial Hospital, Rochester

Ronald G. Haller, M.D.
Professor of Neurology, University of Texas Southwestern Medical Center and Dallas Veterans Affairs Medical Center, Dallas; Director, Neuromuscular Center, Institute for Exercise and Environmental Medicine, Presbyterian Hospital, Dallas

Michael G. Hanna, B.Sc.(Hons), M.D., M.R.C.P.
Consultant Neurologist and Senior Clinical Lecturer, Institute of Neurology, University of London, The National Hospital for Neurology and Neurosurgery, Queen Square and Middlesex Hospital, London

Henry J. Kaminski, M.D.
Associate Professor of Neurology and Neurosciences, Case Western Reserve University School of Medicine, Cleveland; Staff Physician, Department of Neurology, Cleveland Veterans Affairs Medical Center; Director, Myasthenia Gravis Center, University Hospitals of Cleveland

George Karpati, M.D.
Isaac Walton Killam Chair of Neurology, Montreal Neurological Institute, and Professor of Pediatrics, McGill University, Montreal; Senior Neurologist, Montreal Neurological Hospital, Montreal

Sarosh M. Katrak, M.D., D.M.
Honorary Professor and Head, Department of Neurology, Grant Medical College and J. J. Group of Hospitals, Mumbai, India; Consultant Neurologist, Jaslok Hospital and Research Centre, Mumbai

John T. Kissel, M.D.
Professor of Neurology, Division of Neuromuscular Disease, The Ohio State University College of Medicine, Columbus

Frank Lehmann-Horn, M.D.
Professor and Head of Applied Physiology, University of Ulm, Ulm, Germany

Giovanni Meola, M.D.
Associate Professor of Neurology, University of Milan, Milan, Italy; Chairman of Neurology, San Donato Hospital, Milan

Lefkos T. Middleton, M.D.
Chair and Consultant Neurologist, Cyprus Institute of Neurology and Genetics, Nicosia, Cyprus

Robert G. Miller, M.D.
Clinical Professor of Neurology and Neurological Services, Stanford University School of Medicine, Stanford, California; Chairman of Neurology, California Pacific Medical Center, San Francisco

Maria J. Molnar, M.D., Ph.D.
Associate Professor of Neurology, University of Debrecen Medical School, Debrecen, Hungary; Senior Research Physician, National Institute of Neurology and Psychiatry, Budapest, Hungary

Richard T. Moxley III, M.D.
Professor of Neurology and Pediatrics, University of Rochester School of Medicine, Rochester, New York; Director, Neuromuscular Disease Center, University of Rochester Medical Center, Rochester

Richard W. Orrell, B.Sc., M.D., M.R.C.P.
Senior Lecturer, University Department of Clinical Neurosciences, Royal Free Hospital School of Medicine, London; Consultant Neurologist, University Department of Clinical Neurosciences, Royal Free Hospital and Royal Free Hampstead National Health Service Trust, London

Shamima Rahman, M.A., B.M., B.Ch., M.R.C.P.
Medical Research Council Clinical Research Fellow, Institute of Child Health and Royal Free Hospital Medical School, University College London; Honorary Specialist Registrar, Metabolic Unit, Great Ormond Street Hospital for Children, London

Reinhardt Rüdel, Ph.D.
Professor and Head of General Physiology, University of Ulm, Ulm, Germany

Robert L. Ruff, M.D., Ph.D.
Professor and Vice-Chair of Neurology, Case Western Reserve University School of Medicine, Cleveland; Chief of Neurology Service and Acting Chief of Physical Medicine and Rehabilitation Service, Cleveland Veterans Affairs Medical Center, Cleveland

Anthony H. V. Schapira, D.Sc., M.D., F.R.C.P., F.Med.Sci.
Professor and Chair of Clinical Neurosciences, Royal Free and University College Medical School, London; Professor of Neurology, Institute of Neurology, University College London

Noshir H. Wadia, M.D., F.R.C.P. (London), F.A.M.S., F.A.Sc., F.N.A.
Director of Neurology, Jaslok Hospital and Research Centre, Mumbai, India; Former Professor of Neurology, Grant Medical College and J. J. Group of Hospitals, Mumbai

Osama O. Zaidat, M.D.
Chief Resident of Neurology, Case Western Reserve University School of Medicine and Cleveland Veterans Affairs Medical Center, Cleveland

Series Preface

The *Blue Books of Practical Neurology* denotes the series of monographs previously named the *BIMR Neurology* series, which was itself the successor to the *Modern Trends in Neurology* series. As before, the volumes are intended for use by physicians who grapple with the problems of neurologic disorders on a daily basis, be they neurologists, neurologists in training, or those in related fields such as neurosurgery, internal medicine, psychiatry, and rehabilitation medicine.

Our purpose is to produce monographs on topics in clinical neurology in which progress through research has brought about new concepts of patient management. The subject of each book is selected by the Series Editors using two criteria: first, that there has been significant advance in knowledge in that area and, second, that such advances have been incorporated into new ways of managing patients with the disorders in question. This has been the guiding spirit behind each volume, and we expect it to continue. In effect, we emphasize research, both in the clinic and in the experimental laboratory, but principally to the extent that it changes our collective attitudes and practices in caring for those who are neurologically afflicted.

C. David Marsden
Arthur K. Asbury
Series Editors

In Memory of C. David Marsden

David Marsden was the first Series Editor for these monographs; he was asked by Butterworths in 1982 to take on this duty. Shortly thereafter, he recruited one of us (AKA) to join him. The principle that evolved for the Series was that each volume should feature practical aspects of neurology, with emphasis on those areas in which the fruits of research had improved and expanded the management of the neurological disorders in question. This principle is the guiding spirit for the *Blue Books of Practical Neurology* and will remain so for as long as these volumes are published. It is one of the many legacies that David Marsden bequeathed to the fields of neurology and neuroscience, and will serve as a living commemoration of this extraordinary man and his manifold accomplishments.

Arthur K. Asbury
Anthony H. V. Schapira
Series Editors

Preface

Neuromuscular complaints, such as "fatigue," "weakness," and "aching" of muscles, affect a large proportion of the world's population. Specific genetic and other defined, lifelong neuromuscular disorders affect at least 1 in 500 people. This figure is undoubtedly an underestimation in terms of case ascertainment and the identification and characterization of new diseases that fall within the neuromuscular spectrum. Neuromuscular disorders are an important cause of morbidity and mortality with a consequently high economic burden. The clinical evaluation, investigation, diagnosis, and treatment of diseases of muscle and the neuromuscular junction therefore constitute an important area of medicine and, in particular, clinical neurology.

Many people present with complaints that suggest a neuromuscular disease, but a much smaller number actually has a specific disease that must be diagnosed and treated. This challenge confronts the family physician as well as many specialists, including internists, orthopedists, and neurologists—even the most senior expert in neuromuscular disease. With this challenge in mind, Brooke discusses evaluation of the patient with neuromuscular disease in Chapter 1.

Patients with muscle pain and fatigue constitute a large proportion of referrals to physicians and inevitably represent a heterogeneous group of pathologies with different management needs. Kissell and Miller therefore address this issue in the second chapter of the book.

We are privileged to pursue our careers as experts in neuromuscular disease during a period of extraordinary breakthroughs in the discovery of the molecular pathogenesis of nerve and muscle disease. The muscular dystrophies in particular have been at the forefront of the revolution in the molecular neurosciences. The identification, characterization, and development of gene therapy has made Duchenne dystrophy a paradigm for research into other genetic disorders. The emerging molecular classification of the muscular dystrophies provides an opportunity for more accurate diagnosis and genetic counseling and lays the foundation for future treatments. Chapter 3, by Orrell and Griggs, and Chapter 4, by Molnar and Karpati, contain evaluations of the dystrophies and congenital myopathies.

Ion channel disorders underlie many neurologic diseases. The myotonias and other muscle channelopathies are among the first disorders in which the molecular and physiologic abnormalities have been defined and for which treatment is available. Myotonic dystrophy is the most common inherited muscle disease, but it manifests as a systemic disorder. The recognition of a CTG (cytosine-thymidine-guanosine) expansion–negative proximal myopathy as a myotonic variant emphasizes the need to remain alert to new diagnoses and molecular mechanisms in the neuromuscular diseases. The exciting developments in the myotonias and channelopathies are described by Meola and Moxley in Chapter 5 and by Rüdel, Hanna, and Lehmann-Horn in Chapter 6.

Advances in the metabolic myopathies are equally revolutionary. The mitochondrial disorders have been explored by novel molecular biological techniques that have defined both nuclear and mitochondrial DNA etiologies. Rahman and Schapira focus on myopathies and encephalomyopathies caused by mitochondrial dysfunction in Chapter 7. Defects of intermediary and lipid metabolism, and of glycogen and glucose metabolism, are reviewed in Chapter 8 by DiMauro and Haller. Among these, the lipid disorders offer the most opportunity for treatment with the identification of, for instance, carnitine deficiency and riboflavin-responsive acyl-coenzyme A dehydrogenase deficiencies.

Diseases of the neuromuscular junction involve defects of the presynaptic and postsynaptic membranes and include a large spectrum of inherited and acquired disorders. In many of these, the molecular mechanisms and physiologic consequences of neuromuscular transmission defects remain to be defined. Middleton discusses myasthenia gravis and the other neuromuscular junction defects in Chapter 9.

Inflammatory and infective myopathies form an important group of diseases that represents challenges for both diagnosis and treatment. The immunologic abnormalities that characterize and separate polymyositis and dermatomyositis are the targets of drugs that can offer a substantial reduction in morbidity and mortality. In contrast, inclusion body myositis, probably the most common of the "inflammatory" myopathies, remains an enigma in terms of etiology and pathogenesis and is refractory to currently available therapies. Infective myopathies are an important cause of muscle disease worldwide. Their recognition is important, as treatment of them is often effective. The inflammatory and infective myopathies are detailed in Chapter 10 by Amato and Barohn and in Chapter 11 by Wadia and Katrak.

In Chapter 12, Zaidat, Ruff, and Kaminski address endocrine and toxic myopathies. Correction of the underlying endocrine disorder often reverses muscle symptoms. Many widely used drugs are toxic to muscle. Zidovudine, for instance, causes a myopathy through depletion of mitochondrial DNA, whereas certain cholesterol-lowering agents cause a necrotizing, potentially life-threatening myopathy, presumably by their effect on muscle membranes. Prompt recognition of drug-related myopathy is important, as withdrawal usually leads to recovery.

We thank the authors for their contributions; the publishers, particularly Susan Pioli and Leslie Kramer, for their help in the production of this book; and Kieran Price and Shirley Thomas for administrative and secretarial help. Finally, we are grateful to the Series Editors, David Marsden and Arthur Asbury, for inviting us to edit *Muscle Diseases* for their prestigious *Blue Books* collection. David Marsden was a towering figure in neurology throughout the world. His intellect, contribution, and vision will be greatly missed by his many friends and colleagues.

Anthony H. V. Schapira
Robert C. Griggs

Muscle Diseases

1
Clinical Evaluation of Patients with Neuromuscular Disease

Michael H. Brooke

Our knowledge of the various illnesses that affect nerve and muscle has changed markedly since 1990. Even the classification of diseases is different. Known genetic abnormalities have facilitated accurate diagnosis, and the discovery of aberrant proteins provides insight into the basic pathophysiology. Firm scientific principles will likely guide the clinical trials of the future, replacing the inspired and not-so-inspired guesses on which early trials foundered. All of this has altered the face of the specialty, and yet certain aspects remain unchanged. Clinicians still need to assess the patient with weakness. Investigations used in neuromuscular disease have changed, but the accurate diagnosis and assessment of disease is still vital to both the office practice and clinical laboratory. Sometimes, the illness is so characteristic that one can immediately recognize it: the gaunt face of the patient with myotonic dystrophy or the swollen lavender eyelid of the child with dermatomyositis. At other times, the illness defies diagnosis and remains an enigma when the last test results are in. In either case, the process begins with the traditional history-taking and examination.

HISTORY

One of four symptoms or a combination of them usually provokes the visit to the neuromuscular clinic. These are weakness, fatigue, pain, or the referring physician's concern over a raised serum creatine kinase (CK) level.

Weakness

The symptoms of weakness are in many ways the easiest to dissect. Patients who are weak notice specific tasks that are difficult to complete. Initially, it is important to differentiate true weakness from a nonspecific feeling of weakness that is often accompanied by fatigue. The actual reported symptoms will be determined by the groups of muscles involved. The symptoms are stereotyped no matter what the underlying disease is.

Neck Weakness

Neck weakness is often first noticed when the patient struggles to raise his or her head from the pillow, but its most inconvenient manifestation is when an individual rides as a passenger in a vehicle. Braking and acceleration may cause the head to flop uncontrollably back and forth. A simple solution to this is the use of a proper headrest or, failing that, to support the neck with a felt collar, one of the relatively few times that patients find a collar to be useful.

Shoulder and Arm Weakness

The tasks that give difficulty initially for patients with shoulder and arm weakness are those that involve lifting weights above eye level or holding the arms above the head for a prolonged time. Therefore, it is not surprising that the patient reports difficulty in lifting or lowering dishes or blankets from a high shelf, painting the ceiling, or shampooing his or her hair.

Hand Weakness

When grip is weakened, the normal ability to open a tight screw-cap jar or to turn a round doorknob is diminished. This early sign may signify forearm weakness as much as hand weakness. More specific difficulties in using the hands are in gripping and twisting a key and especially in using nail clippers, which is an almost universal problem for patients with intrinsic muscle weakness.

Hip and Leg Weakness

We are so dependent on hip and leg strength to maintain our independence that incipient weakness in these muscles is noted early. Often, increasing difficulty rising from the floor or stepping out of a bathtub heralds the onset. Patients can no longer take the stairs two at a time. The symptoms may be dismissed as the effects of normal aging or being "out of shape." As time passes, the necessity of assistance from the hands (e.g., pushing on one's thighs or gripping railings) increases.

In people with quadriceps weakness, the early difficulty may be noticed in descending stairs or in hiking down hills rather than in impairment of the upward climb. This makes physiologic sense, because the quadriceps muscle is maximally stressed when it is required to lengthen and support the body's weight as the opposite foot steps forward. Difficulty climbing stairs is certainly seen in patients with quadriceps weakness, but weakness of the hip extensors makes climbing stairs more difficult than descending them.

Weakness of the anterior shin muscles causes the patient to catch a toe on small curbs or other objects in his or her path. When the foot evertors are involved, a sprained ankle is a common feature. Weakness of the posterior muscles of the calf provides a separate set of symptoms. The loss of plantar flexion changes the stance and swing phase of walking; the spring to the step is lost. The patient uses various words for this (e.g., "limping" and "shuffling") that are of little help to the clinician, because they may be used for any loss of control in the leg. The patient's family may notice the problem before the patient becomes aware of it.

Cranial Weakness

Double vision, or *diplopia*, is a subject unto itself and is outside the scope of this chapter, other than to point out that one should always ask the patient to which eye he or she ascribes the diplopia on closing one eye. A confident response that it resides in one eye merits a referral to either an ophthalmologist or psychiatrist, even allowing for the rare occurrence of monocular polyopia in some cerebral lesions. Droopy eyelids may be an initial reported symptom in some neuromuscular diseases. Just as frequent is the report that full vision is only possible with the head thrown backward. Surprisingly, patients with neuromuscular disease causing decreased eye movements often do not notice their loss until it is pointed out to them.

Speech abnormalities vary, from the hollow, echoing speech of the patient with lower motor neuron involvement of the palate to the strained, monotonous speech that accompanies upper motor neuron defects. Often, the difficulty is first noticed during a telephone conversation.

When swallowing becomes abnormal, it is immediately noticed and may manifest itself in bouts of choking or in difficulty in getting food down. Nasal regurgitation associated with a loss of the lower motor neurons is a later symptom, except in some patients with myasthenia, in whom it may occur early.

Upper Motor Neuron Symptoms

A parenthetic comment about the symptoms of upper motor neuron involvement is appropriate as it relates to weakness of the limbs. The patient uses a similar set of words to describe the problem. "Limping" and "clumsy" are certainly common to both. The description is more likely to contain words such as "wooden," "heavy," or "leaden" to describe the loss of control and stiffness found in diseases of the pyramidal tracts.

Feeling Weak all Over

One of the prime tasks, and the most difficult task for the clinician, is to separate the patient with true weakness from the patient who simply lacks the energy to do anything. Patients with the latter problem report overwhelming weakness, but when pressed to give examples, they may appear at a loss for an answer. Responses such as "I am just too weak to do any of my housework" are common. If pressed about specific tasks, they reinforce this sense of general exhaustion. When asked about climbing stairs, they not infrequently report that they are just too tired to accomplish it, that they must rest between steps, and so on. So it is with the other tasks listed in the preceding paragraphs. It is not always wise to pose the question too specifically to such patients. Repeated questioning, for example, about whether they have to hang on to the railing when climbing stairs may be answered affirmatively the next time they are asked, either in your office or in the office of the next physician who tries to solve the diagnostic conundrum.

Fatigue

Another difficult set of symptoms to dissect is that of fatigue. The reported symptoms range from exercise intolerance because of a biochemical abnormality to the leaden immobility of the depressed patient. Fatigue, like pain, is real because it is a subjective symptom. It is not helpful to patients to imply that they do not really have fatigue, and if they would only shape up and go about their business the world would be a better place. The only person whose world may be improved by this advice is the physician.

The clinician has to decide whether fatigue is due to an organic muscle disease or something less malign. Fatigue associated with depression may be quite similar to that seen with disease. In many chronic diseases, there is a sense of fatigue. It is the unlovely companion to multiple sclerosis, stroke, and many other illnesses.

Fatigue that is due to neuromuscular transmission failure, as in myasthenia, does not long remain incognito, because the patient describes definite symptoms of weakness during the period of fatigue. Fatigue of which the proximate cause is a defect in the energy supply may also be easier to detect. The symptoms are always associated with exercise and usually start after a predictable length of exercise. Rest relieves the symptoms, usually after a relatively short period of time (10–15 minutes).

Other fatigue states are less well defined. Many patients describe an overwhelming sense of fatigue that prevents them from starting exercise rather than interrupting it. Although exercise may make the symptoms worse, the decline takes place the next day and may last for a week. Such fatigue does not usually occur in isolation. Its companions are pain and depression. It is easy to say that these symptoms are psychosomatic, but there are competitive athletes who have been barely able to shop for groceries in the space of a few months while still trying to hold down their jobs. Invoking the chronic fatigue syndrome as the diagnosis is popular but fails to explain the illness.

Pain

Pain is probably the most common symptom of patients referred to a neuromuscular clinic. Muscle pain is ubiquitous in the population. Fortunately, for most of us it is transient, following a bout of exercise or associated with an acute viral illness. For some, muscle pain is a crippling illness that defies any attempt at treatment. Like fatigue, it is important to try to separate the pain that may accompany known muscle diseases from that which may be associated with anxiety or depression. Like fatigue, it is difficult, and mistakes are easy to make. What follows only provides a guideline.

The patient often finds it difficult to describe the pain associated with the known organic diseases. Often, it is a sense of discomfort or a deep aching in the muscle. The patient refers to the similarity with the pain experienced the morning after exercising the muscle too vigorously. Seldom is the pain severe enough that the patient demands analgesics or opiates. It is poorly localized, other than to the large muscle groups. This is very often the character of the pain seen in the inflammatory myopathies or the aching cramping sensations of the patient with a dystrophinopathy. The exception to this is the pain seen in the acute viral myositis or the rare patient with a muscle abscess. In such patients, the pain may indeed be excruciating and well-localized. The pain in polymyalgia, in addition to an aching feeling, exhibits a sense of stiffness and resistance to movement akin to the muscle running out of oil. The pain of a muscle cramp is distinct, and it is dealt with in the next section of this chapter.

Pain that is more psychosomatic is quite different. It is often precisely described and severe, and it may be quite localized to a part of a muscle. Equally, it may affect every muscle in every limb. Exquisite tenderness to light touch is not a feature of organic pain. Further, the pain is usually unrelenting, 24 hours a day, 7 days a week. As with so many symptoms associated with anxiety or depression, it does not occur in isolation. There is often a history of other pain syndromes or other vague, partially diagnosed disorders. Headaches, gall bladder attacks, gastrointestinal symptoms, and dysmenorrhea are often noted. The patient has often been placed on thyroid medication or cautioned against hypoglycemia without supporting laboratory abnormalities. This is the patient who is likely to find it difficult to work, even though objective findings are nonexistent. When all is said and done, however, this patient presents the greatest challenge of all the problems in neuromuscular disease, and it is seldom that one can be completely certain of the diagnosis of functional pain.

Muscle Cramps

A distinct form of muscle pain is the familiar cramping pain. For the most part, this term is used to denote an intense pain that is associated with an uncontrollable contraction and hardening of the muscle. A palpable lump is found in the area of the contraction. This may occur in healthy individuals and is termed a *physiologic cramp*. An electromyography (EMG) needle placed in the area during a cramp reveals the full interference pattern of normal contraction. Often, the patient volunteers that stretching the muscle brings relief. Conversely, a cramp may be brought about by further contraction of an already shortened muscle. In plain terms, many people can bring on a cramp of the gastrocnemius by pointing the foot down and then forcibly contracting the calf muscles. Leg cramps are particularly prone to occur at night, perhaps because we sleep with feet plantar flexed, and because yawning and stretching are common activities. It appears as if there are individual thresholds for these cramps—some people can produce them readily, whereas others are resistant. Occasionally, the threshold is low enough that the cramps interfere with daily life. Cramps are common in amyotrophic lateral sclerosis, when night cramps are an early harbinger of the disease. Cramps are always indicative of neural activity and never of primary muscle involvement, with one exception: Some patients with a defect in the muscle's energy supply may develop a localized firm contracture of the muscle that is painful. An EMG needle shows it to be electrically silent. Attempts at stretching the affected muscle bring increasing pain and not relief.

Muscle swelling is an unusual symptom, although some patients with inflammatory myopathies or with one of the periodic paralyses experience this. Myoedema, an unusual mounding of the muscle following a brisk percussion, may be seen in hypothyroidism and some other unusual defects in muscle contraction and relaxation.

EXAMINATION

Examination of the patient depends to some extent on the purpose of the examination. In office practice, the information needed may be different from the data needed in a clinical trial. Following the patient's progress in response to treatment is not the same as gathering information for a disability form. There are, however, common features, and the examination in both instances is divided into distinct parts: observation, functional testing, strength testing, and tone and reflexes.

Observation

Much information can be gleaned simply by watching patients from the time they enter the office until the time they leave. Sometimes the information obtained when they are unaware of being watched is more useful than when they are given specific tasks to perform.

Inspection of the limbs may reveal change of muscle bulk: wasting of muscles, which is more common in the denervating diseases, or enlargement of muscles, as is seen in some of the dystrophies. Abnormal twitching of the muscles may be noted at rest. This may be either fasciculation or myokymia. A fasciculation is a brief involuntary contraction of a small area of the muscle, not sufficient to move the joint but noticeable to the naked eye. Profuse fasciculations may accompany amyotrophic lateral sclerosis and some other denervating disorders. Often, they are present in all limbs and are easy to spot. More difficult is knowing how to interpret the isolated fasciculation. The best advice is probably to ignore it.

Fasciculations by themselves may have little significance. Most of us experience these small twitches from time to time. They are exacerbated by fatigue, either physical or mental, and by caffeine or the consumption of other stimulants. Even in the healthy individual, they may become quite widespread and persistent for a period of time. In the context of other signs of neuromuscular involvement, fasciculations do imply a denervating process, particularly anterior horn cell disease. In the absence of any other abnormalities, occasional fasciculations may have no significance.

Myokymia may be very hard to differentiate from fasciculations, and the only reliable way to do it is with the EMG. Myokymic twitches are longer in duration and are often more frequent than fasciculations, giving the muscle surface a roiling, rippling aspect like the wind blowing across a field of grain. Myokymia is an irritative phenomenon in the nerve, producing trains of tetanic activity. Although it may be seen in diabetes, in hypocalcemia, or during recovery from nerve entrapment or a pressure palsy, it may also arise spontaneously.

Functional Testing

Changes in function are noticed by the patient and are the basis of the symptoms. Patients, particularly in the early stages of a disease, are concerned because they notice that something has changed in their ability to carry out ordinary tasks. They do not pay much attention to whether the biceps has lost 30 N of force. For this reason, it is important that the examining physician be able to test function to give us a common language with the patient, who may be baffled by our attempts to explain that he or she has a grade 4 biceps.

The basis for functional testing is to ask the patients to perform tasks that they may encounter in ordinary life. Early in a disease, the individual may experience problems with strenuous tasks that do not occur with simple ones. The clinician should bear this in mind when tailoring the tasks. When the gait of routine walking is normal, it may be instructive to ask the patient to run. The weak subject who has no difficulty stepping onto a low step may struggle when asked to step onto a chair.

Gait

The best time to watch people walk is when they either arrive in the clinic or leave. Patients who are asked to walk for the examiner will seldom walk as they do when seemingly unobserved. This is particularly true of children, and many an exasperated parent has exclaimed, "He never walks like that at home!"

Loss of Shock Absorbers

Normally, the gait is a fluid movement designed to move the torso through space with the least amount of jolting. Loss of muscle strength around the hip disturbs the fluid movement. It is as if one were removing hydraulic shock absorbers: The thud as the heel hits the ground is transmitted unchecked to the pelvis, causing the pelvis to tilt sharply and the gait to assume a waddling character.

Compensatory Lordosis

In the normal standing position of slight flexion, the weight of the body falls on a line slightly in front of the hip joint. Postural muscles have to maintain their tone to prevent flexion of the torso on the hip. As the weakness at the hips becomes more severe, the patient has to throw the shoulders back to compensate for the instability of the extensor muscles. The accentuated lumbar lordosis carries the torso into a position so that the weight of the body falls in a line behind the hip joint, where stability of the back depends on bony and ligamentous structures.

Hyperextension of the Knee

The normal quadriceps exerts enough strength to stabilize the knee under severe mechanical stress. In the average individual, during the phase of walking when the opposite leg is off the ground, the standing knee is flexed slightly as the body's weight swings over it in preparation for the next step. During this critical phase, the knee is prevented from further flexion and collapse by the action of the anterior thigh muscles. If the muscles are weak, the patient feels precarious during this time, because the possibility of the knee giving way and the patient falling is a real one. To compensate for this, a movement develops during the stance phase that hyperextends the knee. Again, the stability of the knee in this position is provided by the locking of the joint and bony structures and not by muscle alone. When such a patient walks, the knee can be seen to hyperextend just before or after the heel hits the ground.

Foot Drop

The well-known slap-footed gait is due to anterior tibial weakness. As the foot is lifted off the ground during the swing phase of walking, the foot cannot be dorsiflexed at the ankle and hangs down. The only way the patient can move the foot upward and avoid a sprained ankle is to throw the foot forward with a quick snapping motion. This must be followed by a rapid placement of the foot on the ground before it has time to fall back into the limp, plantar-flexed position.

Rising from the Floor

The patient is asked to lie supine on the floor and then to stand up in any fashion without hanging onto the furniture. Normally, the individual sits up with perhaps a slight turn and hand support, which becomes more pronounced with age. The feet are then gathered underneath the body, and the individual rises from a squatting position, usually without hand support or with momentary hand support on the floor. Weak patients perform in a different fashion. It is usually described as a Gowers maneuver, but it should be broken down into the individual components as follows.

Turn

The weak patient has to turn his or her body either before or after coming to a sitting position. This is because the support of one or both hands on the floor is needed in the attempt to stand. For most patients, this requires that they turn more or less to face the floor. This initial turn may be as much as 180 degrees in the severely weak patient or 90 degrees or less in the patient with moderate weakness. Other patients, often children with spinal muscular atrophy, do not turn, but after coming to a sitting position, place their hands behind them on the floor and push themselves up.

Hand Support on the Floor

The degree of hand support depends on the amount of hip weakness. The examiner may note whether the hand support is unilateral or bilateral and whether it is momentary or sustained.

"Butt First" Maneuver

I know of no genteel description for this movement. It is most difficult for the patient with hip weakness to come to the upright position from squatting in the normal way. Instead, the patient hikes the hips into the air and straightens from the waist.

Hand Support on the Thigh

Severe hip weakness often necessitates that the patient support the body by placing the hands on the thighs as the body laboriously comes to standing. As with hand support on the floor, it may be noted as unilateral or bilateral, transient or sustained. In addition, there may be repetitive hand support as the body is levered upward.

Stepping on a Stool

The patient is asked to step onto a standard stool, usually approximately 8 in. high. This is a movement easily performed by one with normal strength. The movement is fluid and goes from walking to standing on the stool without breaking step. A considerably more difficult task, but one that is possible for everyone except the elderly, is to step onto a chair. This is a useful test for patients whose mild weakness eludes detection in other tasks.

Hesitation

The patient with hip weakness who is asked to stand on the stool may stop to consider the task in the same way that an individual with normal strength would if asked to step onto a table. This hesitation is often one of the first signs of weakness. It should be recognized that in small children, the height of the usual clinic step may be daunting, and some hesitation is acceptable.

Fast Foot Transfer

The fast foot transfer is one of the most useful signs of weakness and may be noted when the degree of weakness is only moderate. The strong individual places one foot on the stool, with the knee bent, and then the leg is straightened as the other foot is transferred from the floor to the stool. The weight of the body is carried upward on one (the leading) leg. Patients with weakness need both legs under them to be able to carry their weight. This causes them to bring the trailing foot onto the stool before straightening of the leg occurs. They can then carry the body's weight upward by straightening both legs. In this situation, the lead foot is placed on the stool and the trailing foot is rapidly transferred to the stool before the lead leg has a chance to collapse. This is called the *fast foot transfer*.

Throw

When weakness becomes more severe, patients cannot easily get their feet from floor to stool. The legs are weak enough that taking one foot off the floor places the remaining leg in jeopardy of collapse. Patients try to compensate by a quick movement, which makes it appear as if they are trying to throw themselves up onto the step.

A grading form for use in this type of evaluation is illustrated in Appendix 1.1.

Timed Functional Tests

One useful refinement in functional testing is to time the patient's performance with one of the standard tests. There are three common tests related to leg function. The patient is asked to (1) traverse 30 feet as fast as possible, (2) stand from lying supine on the floor, and (3) climb four standard stairs. The timed functional tests are particularly useful in following the progress of the illness in children, in whom strength may be difficult to evaluate. The tests are also useful in following the course of an illness in response to treatment.

Timed functional tests of hand movements are the basis of such tests as the Purdue pegboard test, and bulbar speech function has been measured by having the patient repeat the word "tapaka" and timing 10 repetitions [1].

Pulmonary Function Testing

One of the most useful aspects of functional testing is the evaluation of pulmonary function. It is not only one of the few objective measures of truncal muscles, but it also reflects an activity vital to the patient's well-being. Many muscle clinics have a small portable unit at hand to measure forced vital capacity, maximum voluntary ventilation, and expiratory pressures. If a significant degree of impairment is noted with these tests, more extensive testing in the pulmonary laboratory is indicated.

Strength Testing

Muscle strength has been traditionally evaluated by manual muscle testing. The method works well in the clinic. Quantitative myometry has been introduced in the setting of clinical trials and adds another tool in the measurement of muscle strength. The equipment for the reliable measurement of isometric strength is expensive and time-consuming. Hand-held myometers are designed to be more practical in clinical practice but have some disadvantages.

Manual Muscle Testing

The rating scale for manual muscle testing is based on the Medical Research Council's 1948 brochure. Known as the *MRC scale*, the scoring system originally ran from 0 to 5, but this has not been sufficient in most situations. The problem largely lies in grade 4, which denotes a muscle that is weak but contracts against resistance. This would include a muscle that is minimally weak or one that is more severely involved. The early solution to this was to use the grades 4–, 4, and 4+ to indicate greater and lesser degrees of strength. The full scale, which is often used now, is indicated in Appendix 1.1. Two comments are important: (1) 5– is used to denote a muscle when the examiner cannot decide whether the muscle is weak. It is not used for a minimally weak muscle; (2) 3+ is a muscle that is able to contract against resistance, but after maintaining weak resistance, the muscle involuntarily collapses under the examiner's hand. This is not the same as the sudden collapse of resistance seen in the hysterical patient (sometimes called *sudden give*). In the latter instance, the initial contraction before the collapse is of normal or only slightly reduced force. It is also important to emphasize that the untrained examiner constantly overscores the manual muscle grade. This is due to an underestimation of what is normal. Any parent who has tried to take away a favorite toy from a resistant child is surprised at the normal strength. Although some allowance should be made for age or frailty, most muscles are capable of remaining locked against the examiner's attempt to break them.

The manual muscle test is of only limited use in the evaluation of a single muscle, because the muscle must of necessity spend a long time in grade 4. This stepwise change from one grade to another does not lend itself to the measurement of individual muscles. When many muscles are measured, the change in the total or average score is less steplike, and the changes smooth out as some muscles drop a grade and others stay the same. One of the criticisms of the manual muscle test is that the measurement scale is not interval, and so the data analysis must be nonparametric. On the other hand, when the manual muscle score is used to grade 17 muscles on each side, the resulting composite or average muscle score behaves in every way as interval data [2].

When trying to localize weakness to a particular nerve or root territory, it is important to examine many individual muscles in the distribution of the nerve supply. When dealing with neuromuscular illnesses, such as dystrophies or motor neuron diseases, the physician may not have the time to do such a detailed evaluation. In this case, an abbreviated examination can provide useful information. The key is to test movements at major joints rather than individual muscles. Common practice is to measure the movements listed in Appendix 1.2.

Tone and Reflexes

Assessing tone is very subjective, even though scales, such as the Ashworth scale, have been designed to give some consistency to the process. The simplest system is to grade tone as *normal*, *decreased*, or *increased* and to subdivide increased tone into categories based on how the resistance can be overcome—easily or only with difficulty.

No one completes the first year of a neurology residency without being able to evaluate reflexes. The grading system of 0 = no reflex, 1+ = decreased, 2+ = normal, 3+ = increased, and 4+ = increased with clonus is hallowed by time and use. It is interesting, though, to note how the interpretation is changed by the situation. A brisk reflex may be dismissed as normal in a nervous 20-year-old with an ungrounded fear of dire neurologic disease, when the same reflex would be taken as evidence of upper motor neuron damage in the patient who otherwise has typical amyotrophic lateral sclerosis (ALS).

TESTING USED IN CLINICAL TRIALS

Maximum Voluntary Isometric Contraction

The demands of clinical trial measurements may be very different from those in the office. The need to measure strength in an individual muscle or a few muscles may render manual muscle testing unsuitable, because it is useful only when many different muscle groups are examined. A widely used and well-validated method is *isometric myometry*. The muscle strength is measured in newtons by asking the patient to exert maximal effort against a strain gauge. Proper positioning of the patient is essential, as is ensuring that the limb being tested is appropriately fixed so that accessory muscles cannot be brought into play. The strain gauge must not be allowed to move. To this end, the patient is positioned within an immovable frame to which the strain gauge is attached. This is sometimes known as *fixed myometry* to differentiate it from the use of handheld devices. The handheld myometer is portable and may be useful in certain circumstances. It is difficult to obtain readings that are entirely consistent, however, because the reading depends to some extent on the examiner's strength in resisting the movement made by the patient. It is also more difficult to position the device accurately, and because any force depends on the "lever arm" through which it is exerted, this may influence the reading.

Normal strength varies from subject to subject depending on age, gender, and body build. In measuring manual muscle strength, the trained observer automatically compensates for this. This is one reason why the method is particularly useful in children. If myometry is used as an absolute measure of strength, it is important to be able to establish normal data for the various muscles at various ages—not always an easy task. This has led to the use of transformed scores, or *z scores*, to relate the unknown value to the norm for the particular population being studied [3]. Fortunately, the common use of myometry is to compare the relative measurements of muscle strength in a given muscle on successive occasions as an illness progresses. In this situation, all that is necessary is some estimation of the intrinsic variability of the measurement. Although the readings obtained depend on the positioning of the patient, the patient's motivation, and the normal variability in effort, a trained evaluator can obtain measurements that are reproducible.

Rating Scales

The measurements of a patient's illness that are made by the neurologist usually serve to document muscle strength or other aspects of the disease, but they often give no impression of the impact of the disease on the patient. To this end, a number of functional scales have been developed that may be used to gauge the effect of the disease on the patient's day-to-day life. Three are outlined here: (1) the Schwab and England scale, which was originally designed for people with Parkinson's disease, but which has proved useful in other situations; (2) the ALS functional rating scale (ALSFRS) and the Tufts Quantitative Neuromuscular Examination (TQNE); and (3) the Sickness Impact Profile (SIP). Modifications have been made to the last scale to reduce what is a rather cumbersome tool to a more practical length.

Schwab and England Activities of Daily Living Scale

The Schwab and England scale, which rates the patient's overall ability to function in day-to-day activities, was originally designed for Parkinson's disease [4]. The scale measures activity in a number of different areas. Because it measures disability in general, it has been used in illnesses for which it was not originally designed. It is not always easy to find the original reference in libraries, and the details of the scale are included in Appendix 1.2.

Amyotrophic Lateral Sclerosis Functional Rating Scale

The ALSFRS was specifically designed for ALS and has been validated as a measurement tool in that illness [5]. It shows a close correlation with both the Schwab and England scale and isometric strength testing. It has not been validated as a measurement tool for other illnesses . It may or may not be sensitive to the changes occurring in a particular illness, but it is useful in the clinic to derive some idea of patients' functional abilities. The scale is reproduced in Appendix 1.3.

Sickness Impact Profile and Mini–Sickness Impact Profile

The impact of the illness on the patient is often difficult for the physician to assess. A rating scale known as the *SIP* was designed for this purpose [6]. This is in the form of an exhaustive questionnaire, and the details are not easily found in the literature. The questionnaire may be obtained from the University of Washington in Seattle, according to the instructions in the cited paper. For convenience, the items are included in Appendix 1.4. Because the evaluation is complex and time-consuming, smaller subsets of the questions have been used in specific instances. A 19-item "miniSIP" was found useful in ALS [7]. It may be of use in other illnesses, but it is slanted toward the patient who may be expected to have severe illness (see Appendix 1.4).

Tufts Quantitative Neuromuscular Examination

The TQNE was devised as a rating scale for ALS, as were so many of the scales. The tests are divided into categories to evaluate pulmonary function, oropharyngeal function, timed functional activities, and isometric strength using an electronic strain gauge. It was one of the first widely used scales to incorporate isometric myometry. The scale is valuable in the clinical trial arena, and parts of it can be used in the clinic, but isometric myometry is not easy to carry out in office practice.

SYNTHESIS AND FURTHER TESTING

After the history and the examination, it may be helpful first to decide whether the patient has a definite neuromuscular illness or whether the problem may be psychosomatic, as is sometimes the case in people with nonspecific muscle pains and a normal examination. The next attempted separation is to decide whether the neuromuscular disease is neuropathic, myopathic, or of the neuromuscular junction.

Neurogenic Disease

Disease of the neurons tends to be associated with more wasting than is seen in the myopathies. In addition, the muscle may lose bulk unevenly, giving a stranded appearance. The loss of muscle bulk appears to be more distal than in the myopathies, although this is not always accurate. Spinal muscular atrophies may be proximal, and such illnesses as myotonic dystrophy and Miyoshi myopathy may be distal. Occasionally, with lesions in the nerve roots, paradoxic muscular hypertrophy may be noted early.

Marked fasciculations in the presence of weakness are suggestive of anterior horn cell disease. Any definite sensory abnormality suggests peripheral nerve disease, unless there is a good explanation for its presence from some other cause. Many neurology texts associate the loss of reflexes with neurogenic disease. In the case of peripheral neuropathies, this is often true. The denervating diseases seen in the muscle clinic are different, however, and in both ALS and spinal muscular atrophy, the reflexes are often preserved, or are hyperactive in the case of ALS.

Myopathic Disease

In myopathies, particularly those of recent onset, the degree of weakness is often out of proportion to the preservation of muscle bulk. The archetype of this is the weak hypertrophic muscle of the boy with Duchenne muscular dystrophy. Myopathic muscle may demonstrate severe weakness without any accompanying wasting. Similarly, the reflexes are lost out of proportion to the muscle bulk. The distribution of weakness may also suggest a myopathy. The large proximal muscles of the limbs are commonly affected in the myopathies and are weaker than the more distal muscles.

Disorders of the Neuromuscular Junction

Because disorders of the neuromuscular junction are limited in practical terms to myasthenic syndromes, the familiar hallmarks of these diseases associated with a history of pathologic fatigability place them in a separate category.

At this stage, the patient probably falls into one of two categories. In the first, the precise diagnosis is strongly suspected. This is the case with patients whose illness is recognizable because of a characteristic history and examination. This may include patients with such illnesses as myotonic dystrophy, facioscapulohumeral dystrophy, Emery-Dreifuss muscular dystrophy, and ALS, to name a few among many. In this case, laboratory tests are ordered only to confirm the diagnosis. If one test—for example, an analysis of DNA in myotonic dystrophy—can be used to give indisputable confirmation, there is no need to order tests such as muscle biopsy and EMG, which provide little more than an additional expense. That does not exclude tests that may provide useful information to the family or may change the management. The prognosis of the patient with the clinical appearance of Duchenne or Becker dystrophy and a proven deletion in the gene may be more certain after a muscle biopsy shows a truncated dystrophin, but periodic repetition of CK levels or an EMG adds nothing outside of a research protocol.

The second category consists of those patients who are clearly abnormal but in whom diagnosis is less apparent. These are often patients in need of a diagnostic algorithm. Equally, they are likely to be subjected to a large variety of studies. I know of no foolproof algorithm leading to a certain diagnosis, but the following may be helpful.

Episodic Weakness

Patients may have bouts of weakness with a recognized beginning and end and no symptoms in the interictal period. In this domain lies the patient with periodic paralysis or channelopathies. Patients with alcoholic myopathy may present with painful, weak muscles during or after a binge. Occasionally, patients with myasthenia also fall into this category.

Fluctuating Weakness

The patient with fluctuating weakness notices marked changes in the degree of weakness. This does not refer to the minor fluctuation that is experienced by almost every patient with organic weakness, which I refer to as the "good day/bad day" variation. This is a phenomenon experienced by everyone and is one of the reasons why Olympic athletes with flu and depression do not win gold medals. More severe fluctuation of strength on a day-to-day or week-to-week basis without a return to normal strength is seen in relatively few illnesses. Myasthenia gravis is the most typical example, but it may also occur in some of the inflammatory myopathies. Among the neurogenic illnesses, the autoimmune radiculopathies and multifocal motor neuropathies may sometimes exhibit such fluctuation, although not usually on a day-to-day basis.

Fixed Weakness

Patients with fixed weakness have difficulty that varies little from day to day. They may find that they have more energy from time to time or that they can perform an isolated task less easily today than tomorrow, but in general, their overall level of performance remains the same. The majority of cases fall into this category, and the next step in the diagnostic pathway is to divide them on the basis of progression or nonprogression of the illness and the anatomic distribution of weakness.

Nonprogressive Weakness

Nonprogressive weakness is often the hallmark of the congenital myopathy. *Lack of progression* is a relative term, and there may be widely spaced episodes during which some function is lost, never to be regained. This group of illnesses lacks, however, the steady loss of function that is apparent when the patient with progressive weakness reflects over the last couple of years. When the onset of the nonprogressive illness is in early childhood, accompanied by a history of the same illness in other family members, the diagnosis becomes probable. Congenital myopathies include central core disease, nemaline myopathy with its accompanying respiratory problems, and patients with marked Type I muscle fiber predominance on biopsy. Congenital muscular dystrophies may also be nonprogressive, although the severity of the weakness from the start often obscures the lack of progression. There is some discussion over the progression of weakness in patients with infantile spinal muscular atrophy. The repeated and increasingly severe bouts of respiratory infections are not necessarily evidence of progression of muscle weakness, and many believe that the course in spinal muscular atrophies is a series of plateaus interrupted by short periods of loss of strength.

Progressive Weakness

Progressive weakness characterizes the majority of patients with neuromuscular disease. It is then helpful to consider which part of the body bears the brunt of the illness. It is convenient to consider prominent involvement of the face, neck, and eyes; of the proximal muscles of the limbs; and of the distal muscles of the limbs.

Face, neck, and eyes. This group contains the facioscapulohumeral dystrophies with the attendant typical features of shoulder weakness. Oculopharyngeal dystrophy and mitochondrial disorders, such as Kearns-Sayre syndrome, cause ocular weakness. This is also a feature of myotubular myopathy. Mild facial weakness is seen in a number of different myopathies, but not as the most characteristic feature of the illness. Among the neurogenic disorders causing facial weakness is Möbius syndrome, but in general, face and eye weakness is not a striking finding in the neurogenic disorders. Neck weakness is also seen in a number of conditions, but it may be striking in patients with myasthenia. Neck contractures are often noted in the congenital dystrophies and in some of the congenital myopathies. Again, these are usually part of a larger picture of diffuse weakness.

Proximal limb muscles. Most proximal limb muscle conditions are myopathic. Among the neurogenic causes of proximal weakness, the only common ones are the juvenile spinal muscular atrophies. The infantile variety certainly affects proximal muscles, but the distal muscles are also strikingly weak. Unusual neurogenic conditions, such as porphyria or vascular radiculopathies, may cause proximal weakness, but the diagnosis is usually apparent because of the associated findings, and seldom do these illnesses result in a steady progression of weakness.

Myopathic illnesses include the various limb girdle dystrophies, hence the name. Duchenne and Becker dystrophies are also predominantly proximal. The inflammatory myopathies may present with steadily progressive proximal weakness. Metabolic myopathies that are due to biochemical defects in fatty acid or carbohydrate intolerance usually cause episodic symptoms, but in the late stages of these illnesses, a slow—usually mild—progressive weakness may be found.

Distal limb muscles. Neurogenic disease is a common cause of distal weakness, and the hereditary motor and sensory neuropathies—as well as the more garden variety of neuropathy—are often found. ALS may also begin distally. It is wise not to forget that myopathies may cause distal weakness. Distal myopathies include those described by Miyoshi and Welander, as well as others. The classic example of a distal myopathy is myotonic dystrophy. In the early stages, the patient may present with hand weakness or footdrop, and the diagnosis is elusive. Later, the weakness is more generalized, and the typical facial appearance and the general habitus make the diagnosis obvious. Inclusion body myositis is not really a distal disease, but there is a characteristic involvement of the forearm muscles.

Other Features

Creatine Kinase

When the diagnosis is not easily recognized, a number of ancillary tests may be helpful. The simplest is the serum CK level. The results should be interpreted realizing that the upper limit for CK in the general population is often higher than the stated laboratory standards. CK values in the population conform to a normal distribution only when the log of the value is used. This implies that there are a number of healthy individuals with CK levels higher than the 200–300 level generally accepted as normal. A study of an ambulatory population of healthy people showed that the values varied according to ethnic background (with black people having higher values) and gender (with men having higher values than women) [8, 9]. Exercise, particularly unaccustomed exercise, may elevate CK levels markedly, the peak value usually occurring the day after exercise. Mild elevation of CK may be seen in a number of denervating conditions and myopathies, but when the CK is greater than 1,000 IU, it narrows the diagnosis to myopathic conditions. A CK of this level also implies the need for a biopsy evaluation of the muscle proteins, such as dystrophin and sarcoglycans. In diseases characterized by a deficiency of these structural proteins—such as Duchenne or one of the other dystrophic syndromes—the muscle membrane seems abnormally permeable to CK, and levels of several thousand are noted. Inflammatory myopathies are also associated with marked rise in the level of CK that may be associated with the activity of the disease. Some caution is in order, however, because polymyositis may be active in the presence of a normal CK, and an exacerbation is not always accompanied by a rise in the enzyme level. Biochemical defects and other causes of myoglobinuria are understandable, associated with a brisk rise in CK, often to many thousand IUs. A useful aspect of the CK is that it has a half-life in the blood of 1–2 days. Serial CK may be used to differentiate between a monophasic episode of myoglobinuria, after which the CK declines in linear fashion, and a continuing illness, in which the CK varies more widely.

Contractures

More indicative of myopathic disease than neurogenic illness, contractures of limb muscles are often noted in the muscular dystrophies. They are characteristic of some of the early congenital muscular dystrophies. Contractures of the posterior neck muscles are particularly seen in this group of illnesses. Heel cord contractures and contractures of the iliotibial bands are troublesome in dystrophin deficiency, and contracture of knee extensors or flexors may be seen in other sarcoglycanopathies. A very distinct contracture of the elbows occurs in Emery-Dreifuss muscular dystrophy (Emerin deficiency). This is not to imply that contractures are never seen in denervating diseases. Sometimes, children with the early onset of spinal muscular atrophy may have tight joints, but the phenomenon is more often noted in the dystrophies and in some severe chronic inflammatory myopathies.

Cardiac Abnormalities

A long list of muscle diseases is associated with cardiac abnormalities, from Emery-Dreifuss disease, to myotonic dystrophy, to various muscle protein abnormalities. Because the heart is another muscle, this should not surprise anyone. It is probably helpful to obtain a cardiogram in any patient with a genetic disease of the skeletal muscle, even if it only provides a normal baseline study for the patient.

Pain

Pain may be a part of many neuromuscular illnesses. In some, it is almost incidental, such as the calf pain in the Duchenne patient. In others, it may be the presenting symptom, as in some of the nondystrophic myotonias and other abnormalities of muscle contraction, such as the stiff-man syndrome or in the interictal phase of malignant hyperthermia. Some of the muscle protein deficiencies in adults, such as Becker dystrophy, may actually present with pain, and certainly pain is part of the symptom complex in the illnesses underlying myoglobinuria. Pain is also noted in ALS, in which night cramps may be an early and troublesome problem. Inflammatory myopathies, such as poly- and dermatomyositis, may begin with a deep aching pain; it is worth remembering, however, that in one-half of the patients with poly- and dermatomyositis, pain is absent and weakness is the only symptom. In all of these conditions, the underlying disease is usually obvious.

A more difficult problem is the investigation of the patient in whom pain is the only symptom and when there is no evidence of weakness. As mentioned, there may be clues in the story that cause the physician to suspect a psychosomatic origin, but it is often impossible to decide. The quandary then is to decide whether to risk missing an organic cause for the symptoms by not investigating further or to confirm the hypochondriac's worst suspicions by ordering tests that turn out to be unrevealing. Most of us, I believe, err on the side of overinvestigation, which simply recognizes the vague and uncertain nature of the reported symptoms. Investigating the patient whose pain is unaccompanied by any physical findings is in itself an art form, and I can only outline the studies that are common in our own clinic.

CK levels are essential. An elevated level confirms the need for further investigation. A normal level does not exclude pathology. Because so many of the rheumatologic, collagen vascular, and other autoimmune conditions are associated with muscle pain, a sedimentation rate, protein electrophoresis, and other nonspecific indicators of altered immunity are helpful. Lupus and other collagen vascular diseases may be accompanied by an inflammatory myopathy, and the relevant blood studies are obtained. Uric acid is a by-product of the adenosine triphosphate support pathways and may be elevated in conditions of metabolic stress. Hypothyroidism may cause prominent muscle pain and a marked elevation of CK; it should never be forgotten as a possible cause. If all of these tests are normal, there is no clear history of the symptoms being directly related to exercise, and CK is low, muscle biopsy has generally been unrewarding.

Exercise intolerance may point to the need for exercise testing. This type of study is usually limited to centers with a special interest, but some simple screening tests are easy to obtain. The best known is the forearm lactate test. Any muscle that is working anaerobically—which means any muscle that is performing acute strenuous activity—breaks down glycogen anaerobically and produces lactate, which appears in the venous drainage. The test is carried out with the patient seated and venous access established in the antecubital vein of the arm to be exercised. Traditionally, a cuff is inflated around the upper arm, above systolic pressure. Whether this is necessary is uncertain, because the blood supply has no way of keeping up with the sudden repetitive maximal grip that is demanded. The patient is asked to grip a device repetitively and as strongly as possible for 3 minutes or until fatigue supervenes. There must be some way of measuring the grip strength to determine whether the patient is performing the task realistically. The most common cause of failure of lactate generation is poor effort. Blood is drawn at baseline and every minute thereafter for 5 minutes, and then again at 10 minutes. The normal response is the brisk production of lactate. An absence of lactate production indicates a defect somewhere in the pathway by which carbohydrate is broken down in the muscle. The test may also be used to detect an absence of adenylate deaminase, another putative cause of muscle pain, by measuring hypoxanthine production.

Disorders of fatty acid metabolism may sometimes be detected by the simple expedient of obtaining a respiratory exchange ratio, akin to the old basal metabolic rate. When the body is exclusively using carbohydrates, the amount of oxygen consumed equals the amount of carbon dioxide exhaled: a ratio of 1.0. When fat provides the major source of fuel, the ratio is closer to 0.8. At rest, muscle metabolizes mostly fatty acids and only starts to use carbohydrates under the stress of exercise. Of course, after a period of vigorous exercise, the blood flow increases and muscle once again uses fat as its predominant fuel. Many patients with disorders of fatty acid use in muscle will have a respiratory exchange ratio of close to 1.0 at rest, indicating their dependence on carbohydrate.

Some of the disorders of mitochondrial oxidation of muscle may manifest as pain and fatigue. Such disorders may be suspected in patients because of an abnormally high lactate production in response to exercise, even to the point of having an elevated lactate at rest. Such patients may also be detected by an unusual tachycardia in response to gentle exercise. Having the patient walk the length of the corridor may quicken the pulse to 110 or 120 beats per minute.

The presence of unexplained muscle pain may be an indication for an EMG or a muscle biopsy, as discussed in the following section. Pain in the presence of an elevated CK level demands a muscle biopsy, unless the cause is known from other studies.

Electromyography

EMG may provide an essential part of the diagnosis when it is used intelligently. Used as a routine test on every patient with neuromuscular disease, it can waste the patient's time and resources. However, EMG can provide several types of information.

The use of needle EMG may differentiate neurogenic changes in muscle from primary myopathic involvement. This makes it particularly useful in differentiating proximal myopathies from spinal muscular atrophies or to indicate the direction of further studies in a patient with an enigmatic disease. It is obviously not always useful in patients in whom the diagnosis has already been established. For example, an EMG in a patient with proven dystrophin deficiency provides no additional knowledge and more than a little discomfort to the patient. Yet it is surprising how many times a boy with Duchenne muscular dystrophy shows up in the clinic with a record of multiple EMG studies.

One advantage of needle EMG is that it may be used to sample a wide range of different muscles. In patients with focal neurologic defects, such as disk disease or some other root lesion, it is extremely useful. It is less useful to sample numerous muscles in the neuromuscular diseases, because it is usually not the location of the changes that is important but the type of change—neurogenic or myopathic—that matters. There are obvious exceptions. It may be necessary to sample numerous muscles to increase the certainty of the diagnosis or to hunt for changes such as myotonia, which may not be present in all muscles. In a patient with suspected motor neuron disease, it may be essential to sample many muscles to document the widespread involvement. All of this requires clinical judgment and is one reason why EMG should be performed by those whose qualifications include experience in neuromuscular disease. Equally, it is important to include on the requisition sufficient information to allow the myographer to understand the information that is needed.

EMG can be important in documenting the failure of neuromuscular transmission in the myasthenic diseases. Sometimes this is relatively easy and may be indicated by the abnormal fatigue of the motor unit potential that follows repetitive stimulation. At other times, it may be necessary to use more sophisticated techniques, such as single-fiber EMG.

The evaluation of the nerves' ability to conduct electricity provides information that is unobtainable by any other method. Slowing of electrical conduction in the distal or proximal portion of the nerves may confirm the diagnosis of a neuropathy or radiculopathy and may point the way to a nerve biopsy as a means of establishing a definite etiology. Even more importantly, the demonstration of multiple conduction blocks in the nerve may establish the diagnosis of multifocal motor neuropathy, a treatable condition. Although conduction studies are not indicated when the illness is a demonstrated myopathy, in patients with the lower motor neuron form of ALS, in any patient with a suspected peripheral neuropathy, and in patients with undiagnosed disease with proximal weakness and no clear evidence of a myopathy, conduction studies may be helpful.

Muscle Biopsy

In previous decades, muscle biopsy studies were the only way of differentiating with certainty the various muscular dystrophies, the unique congenital myopathies, and the inflammatory myopathies. Histochemistry opened the window on the multifaceted world of muscle disease. The development of molecular genetics and its related fields has placed muscle biopsy back where it should be: a useful and important, but not preeminent, test. Those of us who regret its demotion are probably of an ilk that also regrets the loss of the proper pronunciation of words beginning with "wh," with the notable exception of "who."

Muscle biopsy, although a simple test that is usually free from complications, is still an invasive procedure and should be done only when the indications are clear. Both open biopsies and needle biopsies are used. Some centers prefer an open biopsy, recognizing that the chance of a sampling error, although small, suggests the need for a larger specimen with better orientation than can be obtained by needle biopsy. Other centers believe that the chance of a sampling error is small enough that needle biopsy is a practical alternative that is quicker and leaves less of a scar. More important are the selection of the muscle and the choice of immunocytochemical and histochemical reactions.

The muscle selection is important. Most biopsies are obtained from the quadriceps or biceps, with the deltoid and gastrocnemius as runners up. The gastrocnemius may suffer from a wide variety of minor abnormalities, even in healthy individuals, and is probably a poor muscle to choose if there is an alternative. Both the deltoid and the gastrocnemius exhibit a predominance of Type 1 fibers, which may make the interpretation of abnormalities a little more difficult. A common mistake in patients with chronic disease is to select a muscle that is severely involved. This may just show the nonspecific "end-stage" changes, which are unhelpful in making the diagnosis. It is better to select a muscle that shows milder changes. Conversely, in an acute recent illness, select the muscle that is more severely involved. When muscle biopsy is used to detect minimal changes, an uninvolved muscle may be chosen, such as when performing biopsy of ALS. Clinical and electrical signs of denervation may be present in the arms, without evidence of such in the legs. It is then useful to biopsy an uninvolved quadriceps to look for the subtlest changes of denervation to prove the existence of widespread disease.

The information gained from a biopsy is of three types. First, the biopsy may reliably differentiate changes of denervation from a myopathy. In the distant days when formal fixed, paraffin-embedded tissue was examined, this was about the only differentiation that could be made. Certainly there is use in this, but an EMG may give similar information more economically. Histochemical studies, which reveal details of fiber types and the internal architecture of the fibers, provide further details. They may differentiate the unique pathology of congenital myopathies, such as central core and nemaline disease. They may identify various dystrophies—such as Duchenne, facioscapulohumeral, or myotonic—or confirm the presence and type of inflammatory cells. In this, they go beyond EMG.

Abnormal storage substances may be detected on biopsy, and stains for fat or carbohydrate are commonly part of the routine battery. Amyloid and ubiquitin may be used to confirm the diagnosis of inclusion body myopathy; vimentin and desmin may be seen in other unusual myopathies. In general, if an unusual structure is seen in the fibers on the routine stains, it is helpful to obtain a battery of these types of tests to identify its composition. They probably do not need to be a routine part of every biopsy.

Muscle biopsy has played an increasingly important role in demonstrating the presence or absence of crucial proteins involved in muscle disease. The technique of immunocytochemistry is relatively simple and depends on the use of a labeled antibody to demonstrate its target. In this manner, dystrophin, the five sarcoglycans, calpain, laminin α2, or merosin may all be evaluated. The studies are not inexpensive and should not be obtained on all biopsies. An absolute indication is the presence of a myopathic disease with a CK level of greater than 1,000. Relative indications include any patient with any unexplained myopathy, particularly if there is a family history of the illness.

Unfortunately, muscle biopsy is not a satisfactory way of following the progress of the patient. Whether a second biopsy looks worse or better than the initial sample may depend as much on the sampling error as on the progress of the patient. This may change in the future, if a technique is devised to replace the missing proteins that are associated with the various dystrophies. Then, a repeat biopsy might be necessary to determine the replenishment of the protein or, possibly, the need for further treatment.

Nerve Biopsy

Nerve biopsy, like muscle biopsy, is an invasive technique. Unlike muscle biopsy, the patient often experiences a sense of numbness, sometimes of dysesthesia, in the territory of the excised nerve. The patient may not consider this to be a minor complication, and an advance warning is important. In spite of this, the procedure is important in any patient with a demonstrated abnormality of conduction in the peripheral nerve to search for the characteristic changes of axonal, demyelinative, or inflammatory neuropathies. The abnormal presence of amyloid or other degradation products may provide a specific biochemical diagnosis. Teased fiber preparations are essential to detect changes in internodal length and other degenerative changes. A nerve biopsy that relies on cross-sectional material or on a longitudinal cut of the entire specimen is inadequate.

The sural nerve is commonly biopsied, but it has the disadvantage of possessing only sensory fibers. A satisfactory alternative is a fascicular biopsy from the distal portion of the anterior tibial, although the loss of function may include weakness of the extensor digitorum brevis.

Genetic Studies

DNA studies are now part and parcel of the investigation of muscle disease. Like all tests, they have strengths and weaknesses. DNA testing is simple from the patient's point of view, because it requires only a blood sample. It cannot, however, be used as a general screening test, because each suspected gene has to be looked at individually. The appropriate use in the clinic is to confirm or refute a suspected diagnosis. If the gene is known and probes are available that detect the gene itself, then gene testing requires only a blood sample from the patient. If the location of the gene is known, but probes are available for DNA sequences in the proximity of the gene, then testing may be a little more complicated. Blood samples may then be required, not only from the patient, but from other members of the family, both with and without the illness. The best that can be expected in this situation is the demonstration that the patient does or does not have the errant part of the chromosome that travels with the illness. The results may not always be easy to interpret. Chromosomal DNA has a tendency to recombine in an unusual fashion. The chance of recombination depends on the distance from the actual DNA sequence responsible for the illness and the DNA sequence identified by the probe. Recombination errors are difficult to rule out. A point mutation may be missed. An identified mutation in the gene sequence may not cause pathology. In spite of all this, gene testing is reliable in a large number of neuromuscular diseases.

It is difficult to keep pace with genes as they are identified. One excellent resource is the journal *Neuromuscular Disorders*, which lists the known genetic disorders and the location of the gene and identifies the gene product when known. Most universities can perform gene testing for a number of illnesses. The Internet is also a good source of information about genetic diseases and molecular laboratories involved in DNA testing. The best-known resource is the On-Line Mendelian Inheritance in Man at http://www3.ncbi.nlm.nih.gov/Omim/. The Canadian College of Medical Genetics maintains a list of known genetic disorders and the corresponding gene abnormalities at http://www.ucalgary.ca/UofC/faculties/medicine/medgenetics/CCMG/lablist.htm. There is a corresponding list of contact addresses at http://www.ucalgary.ca/UofC/faculties/medicine/medgenetics/CCMG/labaddr.htm. The University of Kansas has a list of resources related to human genetics at http://www.kumc.edu/gec/geneinfo.html.

REFERENCES

1. Andres PL, Hedlund W, Finison L, et al. Quantitative motor assessment in amyotrophic lateral sclerosis. Neurology 1986;36:937–941.
2. Brooke MH, Griggs RC, Mendell JR, et al. Clinical trial in Duchenne dystrophy. I. The design of the protocol. Muscle Nerve 1981;4:186–197.
3. Andres PL, Thibodeau LM, Finison LJ, Munsat TL. Quantitative assessment of neuromuscular deficit in ALS. Neurol Clin 1987;5:125–141.

4. Schwab R, England A. Projection Technique for Evaluating Surgery in Parkinson's Disease. In J Gillingham, L Donaldson (eds), Third Symposium on Parkinson's Disease. Edinburgh, UK: Livingstone, 1969;152–157.
5. Cedarbaum JM, Stambler N. Performance of the Amyotrophic Lateral Sclerosis Functional Rating Scale (ALSFRS) in multicenter clinical trials. J Neurol Sci 1997;152(suppl 1):S1–S9.
6. Bergner M, Bobbitt RA, Carter WB, et al. The sickness impact profile: development and final revision of a health status measure. Med Care 1981;19:787–805.
7. McGuire D, Garrison L, Armon C, et al. A brief quality of life measure for ALS clinical trials based on a subset of items from the sickness impact profile. J Neurol Sci 1997;152:S18–S22.
8. Worrall JG, Phongsathorn V, Hooper RJ, Paice EW. Racial variation in serum creatine kinase unrelated to lean body mass. Br J Rheumatol 1990;29:371–373.
9. Black HR, Quallich H, Gareleck CB. Racial differences in serum creatine kinase levels. Am J Med 1986;81:479–487.

Chapter 1 Appendices

APPENDIX 1.1

Functional Testing Tables

Patient: _____ Diagnosis: _____ ID#: _____

Gait	Date / /	Date / /	Date / /	Date / /	Date / /	Date / /	Date / /	Date / /	Date / /
Normal									
Lordosis									
Loss of shock absorbers									
Knee hyper-extension									
Footdrop									
Toe-walking									
Nonambulatory									

L, R = left, right; B = bilateral; + = present; ++ = marked; 0 = absent. Check "Normal" if no abnormality.

Time to walk 10 meters = _____ secs.

Rising from the floor	Date / /	Date / /	Date / /	Date / /	Date / /	Date / /	Date / /	Date / /	Date / /
Initial turn (0, 90, 180 degrees)									
Hand support									
Floor (left, right, both)									
Thigh (left, right, both) (S = sustained)									
Butt-first maneuver									
Unable to do task									

Time to stand from lying supine = ___ secs.

Stepping up on stool/chair	Date / /	Date / /	Date / /	Date / /	Date / /	Date / /	Date / /	Date / /	Date / /
Hesitation									
Fast foot transfer									
"Hip dip"									
Unable to do task									

Time to climb four standard stairs = ___ secs.

Strength Testing

Date: _____ Patient: _____ Diagnosis: _____

Major joint	Movement	Side	
Neck			
	Flexion		
	Extension		
Shoulder		Left	Right
	Abduction		
	External rotation		
	Flexion		
Elbow			
	Flexion		
	Extension		
Wrist			
	Flexion		
	Extension		
Finger			
	Abduction		
Thumb			
	Abduction		
Hip			
	Flexion		
	Abduction		
	Extension		
Knee			
	Flexion		
	Extension		
Ankle			
	Dorsiflexion		
	Plantarflexion		
	Eversion		
Great Toe			
	Extension		

5 Normal strength.
5− Examiner is truly uncertain whether the muscle is weak.
4 Weak; muscle moves the limb against resistance.
4+ Examiner has to exert considerable effort to overcome the muscle. Needs to brace him/herself firmly to accomplish this.
4 Examiner can overcome the muscle without bracing him/herself.
4− Examiner can overcome the muscle easily without gripping the limb firmly.
3 Weak muscle moves the limb through full range against gravity but no resistance.
3+ The muscle exerts an initial small amount of resistance against the examiner's hand, but then collapses. (Not the same as hysterical "give way" weakness.)
2 Weak muscle can only move the joint when gravity is eliminated.
1 Flicker of movement.
0 No contraction visible.

Collaborative Investigation of Duchenne Dystrophy Group Functional Rating Scale, Legs

1   Walks, climbs stairs without assistance
2   Walks, climbs stairs with aid of railing
3   Walks, climbs stairs with aid of railing, takes more than 12 secs for four standard stairs
4   Walks unassisted, arises from chair, cannot climb stairs
5   Walks unassisted, cannot rise from chair, cannot climb stairs
6   Walks only with assistance or independently with braces (calipers)
7   Walks in braces but requires assistance for balance
8   Stands in braces but is unable to walk, even with assistance
9   In wheelchair
10 Confined to bed

(Reprinted with permission from MH Brooke, RC Griggs, JR Mendell, et al. Clinical trial in Duchenne dystrophy. I: The design of the protocol. Muscle Nerve 1981;4:186–197.)

APPENDIX 1.2

Schwab and England Activities of Daily Living Scale

100 Completely independent. Able to do all activities without slowness, difficulty, or impairment. Essentially normal. Unaware of any difficulty.

90 Completely independent. Able to do all activities with some degree of slowness, difficulty, and impairment. Might take twice as long. Beginning to be aware of difficulty.

80 Completely independent in most activities. Takes twice as long. Conscious of difficulty and slowness.

70 Not completely independent. More difficulty with some activities. Three to four times as long in some. Must spend a large part of the day with activities.

60 Some dependency. Can perform most activities, but exceedingly slowly and with much effort. Errors. Some impossible.

50 More dependent. Help with half of activities, slower, etc. Difficulty with everything.

40 Very dependent. Can assist in all activities, but few alone.

30 With effort, now and then does a few activities alone or begins alone. Much help needed.

20 Nothing alone. Can be of slight help with some activities. Severe invalid.

10 Totally dependent, helpless. Complete invalid. Care impossible outside hospital setting.

0 Basic bodily functions only. Bedridden.

APPENDIX 1.3

Amyotrophic Lateral Sclerosis Functional Rating Scale

			Score		
Function	4	3	2	1	0
Speech	Normal	Detectable disturbance	Intelligible with repeating	Speech + nonvocal communication	Loss of useful speech
Salivation	Normal	Slight excess + nighttime drooling	Moderate excess; may have minimal drooling	Marked excess, some drooling	Marked drooling; requires constant tissue or handkerchief
Swallowing	Normal	Early problems, occasional choking	Dietary consistency changes	Supplemental tube feed	Exclusive parenteral or enteral feeding
Handwriting	Normal	Slow, sloppy; all words legible	Not all words legible	Able to grip pen; cannot write	Unable to grip pen
Cutting food, handling utensils, no gastrostomy	Normal	Slow, clumsy; no help needed	Slow, cuts most food; some help needed	Someone must cut food; can feed slowly	Needs to be fed
OR: Gastrostomy patients	Normal	Clumsy, performs all manipulations independently	Some help needed with closure and fasteners	Gives minimal assistance to caregiver	Unable to perform any aspect of task
Dressing and hygiene	Normal	Independent and complete self-care with effort	Intermittent assistance or substitute methods	Needs attendant	Total dependence
Turning in bed, adjusting bedclothes	Normal	Slow, clumsy; no help needed	Turns alone or adjusts sheets, but with great difficulty	Can initiate but not turn alone or adjust sheets	Helpless
Walking	Normal	Early difficulties	Walks with assistance	Cannot walk; can move legs	No purposeful leg movements
Climbing stairs	Normal	Slow	Mild unsteadiness or fatigue	Needs assistance	Unable
Breathing	Normal	Short of breath with minimal exertion (walking, talking)	Short of breath at rest	Intermittent ventilatory assistance	Ventilator-dependent
Subtotal					
Total (maximum = 40)					

(Reprinted with permission from JM Cedarbaum, N Stambler. Performance of the Amyotrophic Lateral Sclerosis Functional Rating Scale [ALSFRS] in multicenter clinical trials. J Neurol Sci 1997;152[suppl 1]:S1–S9.)

APPENDIX 1.4

Sickness Impact Profile/ALS-19

Domain	Question	SIP weight	% of SIP/ALS
Body care and management	I make difficult moves with help—for example, getting in or out of cars, bathtubs.	0.84	4.5
Body care and management	I do not move into or out of bed or chair by myself but am moved by person or mechanical aid.	1.21	6.5
Body care and management	I am in a restricted position all the time.	1.25	6.7
Body care and management	I do not bathe myself at all but am bathed by someone else.	1.15	6.2
Body care and management	I use bedpan with assistance.	1.14	6.1
Body care and management	I get dressed only with someone's help.	0.88	4.7
Home management	I am doing less of the regular daily work around the house than I would usually do.	0.86	4.6
Mobility	I stay within one room.	1.06	5.7
Mobility	I stay home most of the time.	0.66	3.5
Social interaction	I am not going out to visit people at all.	1.01	5.4
Ambulation	I do not walk at all.	1.05	5.6
Communication	I am having trouble writing or typing.	0.7	3.7
Communication	I communicate mostly by gestures—for example, moving my head, pointing, sign language.	1.02	5.5
Communication	My speech is understood only by a few people who know me well.	0.93	5.0
Communication	I am understood with difficulty.	0.87	4.7
Recreation and pastime	I am not doing any of my usual physical recreation or activities.	0.77	4.1
Eating	I feed myself but only by using specially prepared food or utensils.	0.77	4.1
Eating	I do not feed myself at all but must be fed.	1.17	6.3
Eating	I am eating no food at all. Nutrition is taken through tubes or intravenous fluid.	1.33	7.1
Totals		**/18.67**	**/100**

ALS = amyotrophic lateral sclerosis; SIP = Sickness Impact Profile.
(Reprinted with permission from D McGuire, L Garrison, C Armon, et al. A brief quality of life measure for ALS clinical trials based on a subset of items from the sickness impact profile. J Neurol Sci 1997;152:S18–S22.)

2
Muscle Pain and Fatigue

John T. Kissel and Robert G. Miller

Muscle pain and fatigue are among the most common reported symptoms encountered by clinicians. In some population-based studies, as many as 20% of individuals reported persistent localized muscle pain, and 10% reported diffuse and widespread muscle discomfort [1]. Similarly, 20–50% of outpatients in a general medical practice described significant fatigue, and 10–25% of outpatient visits involved fatigue as the predominant reported symptom [2–4]. The overlap of muscle pain and fatigue is also considerable. Approximately 90% of patients with persistent muscle pain also report being fatigued, and as many as 95% of patients diagnosed with chronic fatigue syndrome have prominent myalgia [4].

Despite the prevalence of both symptoms, the evaluation of patients with persistent muscle pain, fatigue, or both can be an extremely frustrating experience for patients and clinicians, especially physicians with a particular interest in muscle disease. Both muscle pain and fatigue are nonspecific symptoms that can arise from a wide variety of general medical, rheumatologic, orthopedic, neurologic, or psychiatric conditions. Even intense muscle pain may be completely unrelated to primary muscle disease and originate instead from a disorder involving the peripheral nerves, anterior horn cells, neuromuscular junction, or even the central nervous system. Evaluation of these patients for muscle disease is difficult because there are few good ways to objectively evaluate patients who report only muscle pain and fatigue at the bedside. Routine diagnostic procedures used by the neuromuscular clinician, such as electromyography (EMG) and muscle biopsy, are also frequently not helpful, and the clinician is often forced to rely totally on the patient's subjective reports as a guide to both the diagnostic evaluation and the effectiveness of treatment. Perhaps most frustrating is that only a minority of patients describing persistent muscle pain, fatigue, or both have a definable muscle disease in the usual sense [3, 5]. Rather, many patients, after long and expensive evaluations, end up with a diagnosis of fibromyalgia or chronic fatigue syndrome—two entities that have remained controversial despite an exponential increase in publications related to both disorders over the last 10 years.

This chapter reviews current concepts of muscle pain and fatigue and discusses the evaluation of such patients. Most of the muscle disorders referred to are discussed in other chapters in this volume, and the focus here is on fibromyalgia and chronic fatigue syndrome.

TERMINOLOGY

Part of the difficulty in evaluating patients with myalgia and fatigue relates to the frequent confusion in the patients' description of their symptoms. Patients frequently use the word *pain* to apply to a wide range of abnormal muscle sensations, including cramping, stiffness, numbness, burning, restlessness, and swelling, to name but a few. All clinicians have had the experience of being misled in their initial diagnostic approach by a misinterpretation of the patient's initial reported symptoms. Although the pain described by many patients cannot be easily classified, it is sometimes useful conceptually to consider four principal types of muscle pain: contracture, cramp, stiffness, and deep muscle aching [6].

The least common type of muscle pain results from a contracture, which represents a state of sustained, active muscle contraction that is electrically silent. This phenomenon usually produces a localized hard nodule in the muscle that may persist for hours. Contractures, which are extremely painful, essentially always occur with exercise and are the hallmark of the glycolytic metabolic myopathies, although contracturelike phenomena related to disordered muscle relaxation can occur in other disorders (Table 2.1). The pathogenesis of contractures in these metabolic muscle conditions is poorly understood and should not be confused with the relatively painless, chronic connective tissue contractures that are common in muscular dystrophy. In the glycolytic disorders, contractures appear to result from elevated free adenosine diphosphate levels and the absence of intracellular acidosis during intense exercise [6, 7].

Cramping is also accompanied by intense muscle pain and can produce a palpable mass in the belly of the muscle. Unlike contractures, however, cramps may occur with the muscle at rest and are explosive in onset and short in duration. EMG study of a cramping muscle reveals high-frequency motor unit discharges similar to a maximal muscle contraction [6]. In contrast to contractures, cramps

Table 2.1   Muscle disorders associated with contractures

Myopathies associated with glycolytic enzyme defects
  Phosphorylase deficiency (McArdle disease)
  Phosphofructokinase deficiency
  Phosphoglycerate kinase deficiency
  Phosphoglycerate mutase deficiency
  Debrancher enzyme deficiency
  Lactate dehydrogenase deficiency
Paramyotonia congenita
Hypothyroid myopathy with myoedema
Rippling muscle syndrome
Brody disease

Table 2.2   Conditions associated with cramps

Idiopathic (normal cramps)
    Exertional and postexertional cramps
    Nocturnal leg cramps
Neurogenic cramps
    Motor neuron disease
    Peripheral neuropathies
    Radiculopathies
Cramps that are due to altered neuronal environment
    Pregnancy
    Metabolic disorders
        Renal failure
        Hepatic failure
        Hypothyroidism
        Adrenal insufficiency
    Electrolyte disturbances/volume depletion

can often be relieved by vigorous passive stretching of the muscle. Cramps, particularly those occurring in the gastrocnemius muscles, occur in essentially all individuals. Although the etiology of cramps is uncertain, most evidence suggests that they are neurogenic, originating in the intramuscular motor nerve terminals [8]. As such, widespread or extensive muscle cramps are usually an indication of neurogenic disease (e.g., amyotrophic lateral sclerosis, peripheral neuropathy) or metabolic disorders that alter the microenvironment of motor nerve terminals (e.g., hypothyroidism, dehydration, uremia, and pregnancy; Table 2.2).

Muscle "stiffness" is another word often used by patients to describe a number of different phenomena. In its most common use, the term *stiffness* is used to describe muscle that feels tight to the patient, is resistant to passive stretch, and does not relax normally. Muscle stiffness can arise from a wide range of neurologic disorders affecting every component of the neuraxis, as well as from a number of general medical conditions that cause metabolic derangements that disrupt muscle relaxation [8]. Although reports of stiffness and pain frequently overlap, many patients with excessive muscle stiffness, particularly those related to central mechanisms (e.g., spasticity or rigidity), do *not* have significant pain. Table 2.3 lists the muscle disorders associated with muscle stiffness.

Table 2.3   Muscle disorders associated with muscle stiffness

Hypothyroidism
Myotonic disorders
    Myotonic dystrophy
    Myotonia congenita
    Paramyotonia congenita
    Proximal myotonic myopathy
    Hyperkalemic periodic paralysis
Brody disease
Polymyalgia rheumatica
Fibromyalgia

Table 2.4   Muscle disorders causing localized or diffuse myalgia

Localized myalgia
    Postexercise myalgia
    Focal pressure necrosis
    Trauma
    Focal infiltrating processes
        Tumor
        Sarcoidosis
        Focal myositis
    Localized infections (bacterial, parasitic)
    Vascular occlusion
        Arterial ischemia (thrombotic or embolic)
        Venous occlusion
    Referred "muscle" pain from neuropathic, orthopedic, rheumatologic causes
Generalized myalgia
    Infectious myalgia (especially viral)
        Diffuse parasitic or bacterial infections
    Inflammatory muscle disease (polymyositis, dermatomyositis)
    Eosinophilia-myalgia syndrome
    Toxic myopathies associated with drugs (e.g., lovastatin, chloroquine)
    Hypothyroidism
    Mitochondrial myopathies
    Myoadenylate deaminase deficiency (association with myalgia controversial)
    Rare myopathies
        Paraspinal vacuolar myopathies with myalgia
        Myalgia with tubular aggregates
        X-linked myalgia and cramps
    Polymyalgia rheumatica
    Fibromyalgia

The most common type of muscle pain is the deep discomfort most often described by patients as a "burning" or "dull ache." This type of pain can be either localized to an individual muscle or group of muscles or experienced as a more generalized phenomenon [6, 7, 9, 10]. Muscle diseases that cause focal pain usually involve either local trauma, an infiltrating process (e.g., a tumor or inflammatory disease, like sarcoidosis), vascular disorders (either arterial ischemia or venous thrombophlebitis), or a localized bacterial or parasitic infection (Table 2.4). Diffuse myalgia is probably most common after viral infections but also may occur in the idiopathic inflammatory myopathies (polymyositis or dermatomyositis), toxic or infectious myopathies, and a few relatively rare endocrine myopathies (see Table 2.4). In most of these disorders, muscle pain is accompanied by weakness, which can range from mild to devastating. Relatively common causes of diffuse myalgia without weakness include polymyalgia rheumatica and fibromyalgia (discussed in the section Fibromyalgia that follows).

Like myalgia, *fatigue* is a word frequently used by patients to refer to a number of possible symptoms that must be clarified by the examiner. Fatigue, strictly defined, refers to a sense of tiredness, lack of energy, weariness, and a tendency to avoid physical (and often mental) activities because of an overwhelming sense of exhaustion [11]. Patients often initially use the term *weakness* when trying to describe a sense of fatigue. For example, many fatigued patients describe an inability to perform some routine activity, such as walking one block, because of "weakness," when in reality they are simply too fatigued and exhausted and could accomplish the activity if strength alone were the issue. It is important for the clinician to elicit a detailed history about exactly why certain activities cannot be performed, particularly in relation to the patient's other reported symptoms. This is particularly important because fatigue is a multifactorial phenomenon, depending on the individual's emotional state, sleep habits, cardiopulmonary status, degree of conditioning, and general medical status [6, 11]. Although the neuromuscular junction disorders and some myopathies (most notably the mitochondrial disorders, some of the metabolic myopathies, and myotonic dystrophy) can be associated with significant fatigue, fatigue in isolation almost never indicates a primary muscle disease. However, many patients with severe muscle disease and advanced weakness report fatigue and decreased endurance because they are having to do more activities with less muscle (overuse syndrome).

PATHOGENESIS

Despite an extensive body of research, knowledge of the pathophysiology of muscle pain and fatigue remains limited. Layzer and others have found it useful to consider muscle pain as arising from one or more of three basic mechanisms: mechanical pain from distention, inflammatory or chemical pain, and ischemic pain [6, 12]. Mechanical pain typically results from physical distention of muscle, such as from an infiltrating mass lesion or excessive muscle tension, as occurs in cramps. Intense physical exercise that results in actual tearing of muscle fibers may also result in mechanical type pain. Pain signals from these stimuli travel predominantly through thinly myelinated group 3 (A-δ fibers) and to a lesser extent through unmyelinated group 4 (type C) fibers. Branch endings from these fibers distribute widely in the endomysium, tendons, and fascia, and respond to a variety of mechanical, thermal, and chemical stimuli [6, 12–18].

Inflammatory or chemical pain is typified by that experienced in patients with inflammatory muscle disease. This type of pain presumably results from damage to the muscle and the secondary release of a wide range of inflammatory and chemical mediators, which stimulate chemically responsive nociceptors in muscle. These chemical substances include serotonin, histamine, bradykinin, various prostaglandins, hydrogen ions, calcium and other electrolytes, and a whole family of lymphokines [12]. Receptor stimulation by these substances results in a firing of predominantly unmyelinated group 4 fibers [16]. In contrast to mechanical pain, chemically mediated pain is slow in onset and persists after muscle damage occurs.

A third type of muscle pain occurs during periods of ischemia. This type of pain is most commonly seen in patients suffering intermittent claudication from severe lower extremity peripheral vascular disease. This pain is also experienced in healthy individuals during sustained, high-intensity exercise involving isometric contractions. The mechanisms underlying ischemic pain are unknown. The pain usually resolves quickly when normal circulation is restored, suggesting that the local production of some toxic metabolite stimulates the nociceptors to produce pain. Despite intensive investigations and exploration of a number of possible candidate substances, most notably lactate and adenosine, none has been identified as the true pain-producing metabolite [6, 12, 18].

It must be stressed that this classification, although conceptually useful, is somewhat artificial in that many, if not most, types of muscle injury result in pain produced by several of these different mechanisms, and it can be impossible to distinguish them clinically. For example, dermatomyositis, although inflammatory in nature, results from a microvasculopathy that results in true ischemic damage to the muscle. The aching pain experienced by some patients with this condition probably results from a combination of inflammatory and ischemic mechanisms.

Another example of the difficulty in determining the pathogenesis of muscle pain is exemplified by the myalgia that follows overly vigorous or sustained, unaccustomed physical activity ("weekend warrior" syndrome). This type of pain, which has been experienced by all individuals, is typically a deep, chronic aching pain accompanied by muscle tenderness and stiffness. Symptoms typically begin within 12–24 hours of the intense activity and persist for periods of 1–7 days [6, 9, 10]. The precise origin of this pain is uncertain and probably depends on a combination of mechanical, chemical, and ischemic factors. Creatine kinase (CK) levels usually rise after the activity, suggesting that actual physical damage to the muscle fiber occurs, a theory supported by histologic studies [19–25]. Eccentric muscle contraction (i.e., contraction during muscle lengthening) is more likely to produce these changes and subsequent muscle pain than are concentric contractions, which occur during muscle shortening [19, 21, 25, 26]. That exercise-induced pain has a delayed onset after exercise, however, suggests that factors other than mechanical damage to the muscle, most likely involving chemical mediators, must be involved in the production of the pain [6, 26].

The pathogenesis of muscle fatigue is an even more complex and poorly understood phenomenon than that of muscle pain. The sensation of fatigue is a complex phenomenon depending on multiple physical and psychological factors involving both the central and peripheral nervous systems. Frequently, a patient's sensation of fatigue has little to do with the physiologic phenomenon of true muscle exhaustion. Under normal circumstances, muscle can maintain its maximal contractive force for only short periods (usually a matter of seconds) before fatigue begins, and the desired force can no longer be maintained. The duration that a muscle can exert a given effort is inversely proportional to the amount of force exerted and directly proportional to the amount of recovery time allowed for the muscle between efforts [27, 28]. Studies have shown that this type of muscle fatigue is associated with marked changes in the metabolic pathways involved in supplying the muscle with adenosine triphosphate and phosphocreatine. Fatigue following intense muscle activities is associated with a fall in phosphocreatine levels and a rise in levels of inorganic phosphate, hydrogen ions, potassium, lactate, hypoxanthine, and uric acid [29–34]. Which of these by-products is most important in serving as a "fatigue chemical" is unclear. With more prolonged, submaximal exercise, such as marathon running, fatigue and exhaustion occur as glycogen is progressively depleted from muscles. The fatigue and exhaustion noted by patients with various metabolic myopathies, including the mitochondrial myopathies and glycolytic defects, probably also depend on such metabolic factors involving glycogen.

In addition to these biochemical factors, multiple other anatomic and physiologic variables help determine the fatigability of a given muscle. The distribution of fiber types within a given muscle, capillary density of the muscle fiber, changes in excitation-contraction coupling, efficiency of neuromuscular transmission, pattern of motor unit recruitment, and level of conditioning all integrate to determine the fatigability, endurance, and efficiency of a given muscle [35–38].

DISORDERS ASSOCIATED WITH MUSCLE PAIN OR FATIGUE

Most of the disorders associated with muscle pain listed in Table 2.4 are discussed in other chapters of this volume. Several primary muscle conditions are notable for having pain, fatigue, or both, as their predominant manifestations.

Vacuolar Myopathies with Myalgia

Petrella and colleagues reported a series of four patients who presented with severe, diffuse myalgia; chronic fatigue; elevated serum CK levels (two to five times normal); and paraspinal muscle biopsies characterized by vacuolar changes and glycogen deposits [39]. Two of the patients developed mild proximal weakness years after the onset of myalgia. All four patients had abnormal EMGs with positive sharp waves, fibrillation potentials, complex repetitive discharges, or myotonia, predominantly in paraspinal muscles. Histochemical and biochemical analyses for other causes of vacuolar myopathy were negative. Whether these individuals have a unique muscle disorder is unclear and can only be determined as other patients are reported. One of the patients was eventually diagnosed with phosphorylase deficiency, suggesting some underlying biochemical defect leading to muscle pain and fatigue.

Myalgia with Tubular Aggregates

Several case reports and retrospective analyses have suggested an association between muscle pain and the finding of tubular aggregates on muscle biopsy. In one retrospective analysis, 63% of patients with tubular aggregates had prominent symptoms of myalgia [40–42]. In many of these patients, myalgia was the only presenting symptom. In some patients, ultrastructural analysis revealed cylindrical, spiral-like structures in communication with the tubular aggregates [40]. Because tubular aggregates are derived from proliferating sarcoplasmic reticulum, which plays a crucial role in muscle contraction and relaxation, these structures may account in some way for the prominent exertional myalgia and cramping in these patients. The biochemical events involved, however, are uncertain.

X-Linked Myalgia and Cramps Due to Dystrophinopathy

A single large family with an X-linked recessive disorder characterized by muscle cramps and myalgia has been reported [43]. Patients typically had CK levels in the thousands and calf hypertrophy, but no muscle weakness. EMG studies revealed myopathic features, and muscle biopsy showed nonspecific myopathic abnormalities. Western blot analysis revealed a normal amount of dystrophin of reduced size, and DNA analysis revealed a deletion in the first third of a dystrophin gene, causing a 15% reduction in the size of the protein. How this reduced-size dystrophin results in such prominent reports of myalgia and cramping in this family is uncertain, but it is compatible with the prominent muscle aching and pain occasionally experienced by other patients with Becker dystrophy.

Polymyalgia Rheumatica

Although not technically a muscle disease, polymyalgia rheumatica is often discussed in association with myopathic illnesses, because its primary manifestation is one of diffuse, aching muscle pain and fatigue. In fact, polymyalgia rheumatica may be one of the more common causes of muscle pain in adults older than age 50, with one study suggesting a prevalence of 600 per 100,000 individuals in this population [44]. The condition affects older individuals, with a mean age at onset of 70 years, and is more common in women by a 3 to 1 ratio [45, 46]. The disorder is characterized by the indolent onset of myalgia, stiffness, aching, and fatigue predominantly affecting the neck, shoulder, and hip regions. Symptoms are typically worse in the morning, when prominent stiffness and "gelling" occur. The pain is worse with movement and can be quite debilitating. Muscle tenderness is unusual. True weakness is distinctly uncommon and suggests underlying vasculitic involvement of muscle. Low-grade fevers, weight loss, depression, and anemia can accompany the muscular manifestations.

Laboratory evaluation typically reveals normal CK levels and marked elevation of the erythrocyte sedimentation rate, often to values greater than 100 mm per hour. It is important to note, however, that approximately 10% of patients with polymyalgia rheumatica have only mildly elevated or even normal sedimentation rates [46, 47]. Muscle biopsies are invariably normal or show only minimal abnormalities. This is not surprising, because the origin of the pain is related more to synovitis than to true muscle involvement.

Although there is an unquestionable relationship between polymyalgia rheumatica and giant cell arteritis, the nature of the association is uncertain and somewhat controversial [46–48]. Polymyalgia rheumatica occurs in approximately 50% of patients with giant cell arteritis, and approximately 15% of patients with polymyalgia eventually develop giant cell arteritis [44]. The muscle symptoms may begin before, during, or after the development of the headache, scalp tenderness, jaw claudication, and vision loss typical of giant cell arteritis. In patients with both syndromes, it is unclear whether the myalgia is due to subclinical vascular involvement of muscle, a concurrent immunologic process directed against muscle, or some other chemical or metabolic factor [49].

The diagnosis of polymyalgia rheumatica is made on the basis of clinical history and the elevated erythrocyte sedimentation rate. Diagnostic temporal artery biopsy is recommended in all patients with symptoms suggesting giant cell arteritis, but it is not indicated in patients with polymyalgia symptoms alone [47]. Although occasional patients with polymyalgia rheumatica respond to nonsteroidal anti-inflammatory drugs, most patients require treatment with prednisone, usually in doses of 5–40 mg per day. This usually results in dramatic improvement of the myalgia and stiffness, and function rapidly improves. Patients with recent or impending vision loss that is due to giant cell arteritis must be treated immediately and more aggressively, usually with higher doses of prednisone (60–80 mg/day) and sometimes intravenous pulse methylprednisolone [46]. In both instances, the dose of prednisone should be increased until the clinical symptoms and erythrocyte sedimentation rate have normalized. The dose can then be gradually reduced while monitoring the sedimentation rate and clinical status. Most patients require treatment for 1–2 years.

Fibromyalgia

The majority of patients who present with muscle pain does not have a definable myopathic disorder in the usual sense, despite intensive evaluation. Currently, most of these individuals are diagnosed with the syndrome of *fibromyalgia*, a condition that has been discussed under a number of different names for approximately a century [1]. The term *fibrositis* was initially applied to the condition by Gowers in 1904, and Kellgren first demonstrated that consistent patterns of pain could be elicited from deep muscle and fascia stimulation in such patients [50, 51]. Over the years, an impressive collection of at times imaginative names—including *myofascial pain syndrome*, *fibrositis*, *fibromyositis*, *myofibrositis*, *muscular rheumatism*, *tension rheumatism*, *aches and pains syndrome*, *generalized rheumatism*, and *nonarticular rheumatism*—have been applied to the same condition, with the term *fibromyalgia* first suggested by Hench in 1976 [52–54]. This profusion of terminology reflected the uncertainties about the underlying pathophysiology of the condition, an uncertainty that has persisted to the present.

Current interest in this condition can be traced principally to the publication in 1981 by Yunus and colleagues of a matched controlled study of *primary fibromyalgia*, which has become the preferred name for this controversial syndrome [55]. Some investigators feel that fibromyalgia does not exist as a definable entity, while others believe it is a strictly psychogenic phenomenon [54, 56, 57]. Still others have hypothesized that fibromyalgia, while a distinct entity, does not fit into a traditional biomedical model of disease and is best considered in a psychosocial conceptualization [53]. Despite continuing controversy, the vast majority of clinicians and investigators who see patients with muscle pain has embraced fibromyalgia as a valid syndrome that is as real as any other condition (e.g., migraine headaches) for which the diagnostic criteria are predominantly clinical and the underlying pathophysiology poorly understood [10, 58]. Although the literature on this subject is at times confusing, the epidemiology, clinical features, diagnostic criteria, laboratory findings, and treatment approaches have all been addressed in well-designed studies.

From this perspective, a diagnosis of fibromyalgia provides a frame of reference for the physician to use in dealing with patients with this condition and helps the physician design a diagnostic and therapeutic approach to the patient who avoids unnecessary testing. From a practical perspective, because the concept of fibromyalgia has been embraced by the vast majority of clinicians, it does no good for the neuromuscular practitioner to deny that it exists, refer to it as a "wastebasket term," or simply assign some other equally vague term (e.g., *pain amplification syndrome* or *aches and pain syndrome*) to the condition [54].

Epidemiology

Fibromyalgia is clearly the most common cause of muscle aches and pains in the general population. Prevalence surveys have found that approximately 2% of individuals fulfilled diagnostic criteria for fibromyalgia [1, 59]. The condition is more common in women; in one population-based study of 3,000 patients, 3.4% of women and 0.5% of men were affected [59]. The condition increases with age and affects approximately 7% of women older than 60 years. In clinic-based studies, fibromyalgia is one of the most common entities seen by rheumatologists, composing 10–20% of new patient consultations. In these referral-based studies, patients are younger, with the median age at onset in the 30s [1, 60].

Clinical Features

By definition, the predominant clinical feature of fibromyalgia is chronic, diffuse muscle pain, aching, and stiffness. Patients usually describe most of their discomfort as arising in the muscle itself, although joint pain is also described. Symptoms tend to be proximal, although predominant symptoms can affect any area of the body. Onset is usually insidious and slowly progressive, and patients frequently have difficulty pinpointing the onset of their difficulties. Most patients have *primary* fibromyalgia, in that the symptoms develop independently of any other medical condition. Some patients develop the classic symptoms and signs of fibromyalgia in the setting of another medical disorder (e.g., diabetes or rheumatoid arthritis); the term *secondary* or *concomitant* fibromyalgia has been applied to these individuals [61]. A minority of patients describe a sudden onset of symptoms after an infectious illness, trauma, or work-related injury, although this entity is controversial [62].

A number of ancillary symptoms are associated with myalgia that often can obscure the nature of the underlying condition. The most common symptoms are fatigue, morning stiffness, and nonrestorative sleep, all of which are found in more than 75% of patients [61, 63]. Paresthesia, headache, anxiety, irritable bowel syndrome, Raynaud-like discoloration of the fingertips, subjective sensations of swelling, dysmenorrhea, and urinary frequency and urgency also occur in many patients. Interestingly, fatigue and not pain is often the most disabling symptom in patients with fibromyalgia, highlighting the overlap between this condition and chronic fatigue syndrome (see the section Chronic Fatigue Syndrome that follows) [60, 64].

The examination of patients with fibromyalgia typically reveals normal strength and range of motion. Although minor weakness has been described in individual muscles, this can almost always be attributed to deconditioning effects. Classically, the examination is most notable for the presence of multiple tender points [55, 61, 65–68]. Perhaps no aspect of fibromyalgia has generated more controversy than the existence and definition of tender points, in large part because of different opinions about the most appropriate method of checking for them (i.e., digitally or with a dolorimeter), the degree of pressure that needs to be exerted when testing, and the number and distribution of areas that need to be assessed. In 1990, the American

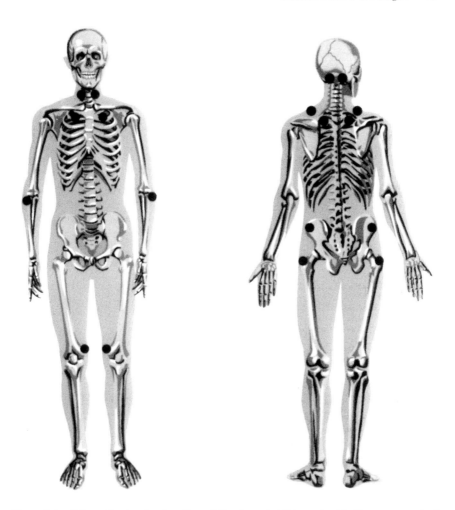

Figure 2.1   Schematic showing location of "tender points" important in the assessment of patients with suspected fibromyalgia. See Table 2.5 for anatomic descriptions of each point. (Adapted from F Wolfe, HA Smythe, MB Yunus, et al. The American College of Rheumatology 1990 criteria for the classification of fibromyalgia—report of the Multicenter Criteria Committee. Arthritis Rheum 1990;33:160–172.)

College of Rheumatology supervised a multicenter study involving 558 patients (293 with fibromyalgia and 265 controls) assessed both through digital palpation and dolorimetry. In this study, a tender point was defined as present or positive if the patient reported distinct pain of mild or greater degree with digital palpation of approximately 4 kg/cm² (the approximate pressure needed to blanch the nail bed). Using these criteria, the presence of tenderness in 11 of 18 stimulus points (nine paired discrete sites; Figure 2.1; Table 2.5) had a sensitivity of 88.4% and a specificity of 81.1% for patients previously diagnosed with fibromyalgia [61, 63]. This study has been criticized for using circular reasoning, because the fibromyalgia

Table 2.5   Diagnostic criteria for fibromyalgia

A. History of widespread pain involving both sides of the body and areas above and below the waist, as well as the axial skeleton
B. Pain on digital palpation in at least 11 of 18 tender points, including bilateral:
   1. Anterior
      a) Anterior aspect of the intertransverse spaces of C5-7 level
      b) Anterior second rib region, near the costochondral junction
      c) Elbow region, 2 cm distal to the lateral epicondyle
      d) Knee, at the medial fat pad proximal to the joint line
   2. Posterior
      e) Occipital area at the suboccipital muscle insertion
      f) Trapezius muscle, midpoint of upper border
      g) Supraspinatous, above the scapular spine near medial border
      h) Upper outer quadrant of the buttock muscle in anterior fold of gluteal muscle
      i) Greater trochanter, just posterior to the trochanteric prominence

Source: Adapted from F Wolfe, HA Smythe, MB Yunus, et al. The American College of Rheumatology 1990 criteria for the classification of fibromyalgia—report of the Multicenter Criteria Committee. Arthritis Rheum 1990;33:160–172.

patients were selected for study on the basis of tender points, but the results have been confirmed and extended in other investigations [66–68].

Based largely on the results of this and similar studies, current diagnostic criteria for fibromyalgia include two major criteria: (1) the presence of widespread diffuse muscle aching and pain for at least 3 months, and (2) the demonstration of pain and tender points on digital palpation in at least 11 of 18 defined sites (see Table 2.5). Using these criteria, the clinician is able to make a positive diagnosis relatively early in the evaluation of the patient, eliminating the need to make a diagnosis of exclusion after a very long and costly evaluation. In addition, the criteria eliminate the need to consider ancillary findings, such as fatigue, headache, and paresthesia, in making a diagnosis. Like all diagnostic criteria, however, the criteria for fibromyalgia were designed mainly for research studies and can be too restrictive for routine clinical use. Many patients, for example, present with diffuse reports of muscle aches and pains and fewer than 11 tender points. Obviously, many of these patients have to be managed for presumed fibromyalgia.

A final point related to the diagnosis of fibromyalgia concerns distinguishing tender points from "trigger points." The latter are defined as areas that, when palpated, cause referred pain in a stereotypical pattern predictable for each trigger point [63, 66]. These trigger points have been classically described as useful in distinguishing myofascial pain syndrome from fibromyalgia. Proponents of this position refer to "taut bands" as palpable tight regions in muscle with characteristic EMG findings that correspond to trigger point areas [66]. Several studies, however, have demonstrated that such distinctions are impossible to make by most clinicians, and the overlap between fibromyalgia and myofascial pain syndrome as typically defined is often so extensive as to make the distinction meaningless [67].

Laboratory Findings

The laboratory evaluation of patients with primary fibromyalgia, including CK levels and other serum studies, typically reveals no abnormalities. Occasional patients fulfill criteria for fibromyalgia in the setting of a concomitant rheumatologic or other medical condition, such as rheumatoid arthritis or Sjögren syndrome. In these individuals with concomitant fibromyalgia, the pattern of serologic abnormalities reflects the underlying disease.

Multiple EMG studies, using both surface and needle electrodes, have been performed in patients with fibromyalgia. Although minor, nonspecific abnormalities have been demonstrated in some patients, no consistent abnormality has been defined, either in relation to muscle function in general or to tender points in particular [69]. Similarly, several muscle biopsy studies, including ultrastructural analyses, have shown predominantly normal or only nonspecific findings [69–73]. Metabolic studies on muscle are also invariably normal, and there is no role at present for muscle biopsy in the diagnostic evaluation of patients with suspected fibromyalgia.

Although sleep studies are occasionally helpful in patients with predominant reports of nonrestorative sleep, they are not helpful in making a diagnosis and are of more interest from a pathophysiologic standpoint. Fibromyalgia patients have a higher number of episodes of oxygen desaturation during sleep than controls, as well as decreased low-frequency bands (delta and theta) on power spectral electroencephalographic analysis during sleep [74, 75]. These findings may explain in part the prominent fatigue experienced by some patients.

Pathophysiology

Despite extensive research, the pathophysiology of fibromyalgia remains completely unknown. Although a detailed discussion of the multiple hypotheses concerning the condition is beyond the scope of this chapter, several conclusions seem valid based on the cumulative scientific investigations performed to date and the extensive experience of clinical investigators. The first conclusion is that although muscle pain and stiffness are the central features of the condition, fibromyalgia is not primarily a muscle disease. Multiple studies have failed to document any convincing evidence of a primary anatomic, physiologic, biochemical, or functional abnormality in muscle to explain the muscle stiffness and pain. The second conclusion is that fibromyalgia is probably not a single disease, but rather a chronic pain syndrome that overlaps with other similar conditions, such as chronic fatigue syndrome (see the section on it that follows), irritable bowel syndrome, migraine headaches, and various psychiatric disorders [1, 4]. This concept leads immediately to the third conclusion: It is extremely unlikely that a single definable cause for fibromyalgia will be found. Multiple immunologic, endocrinologic, virologic, histologic, infectious, sleep, epidemiologic, and cognitive and psychological studies have been performed in patients with fibromyalgia. Although most have documented some minor abnormalities in each parameter examined, none has uncovered a consistent, reproducible change that could cause the condition.

Much current attention has therefore turned to a psychosocial model of fibromyalgia, focusing on the concept that the pain of fibromyalgia may represent up-regulation of abnormal central pain mechanisms, which may result from a number of genetic, biochemical, infectious, or traumatic events [1, 58, 69]. According to this model, fibromyalgia results from a generalized pain intolerance that is due to functional abnormalities in the central nervous system [76]. This hypothesis is supported by a study showing decreased regional cerebral blood flow to the thalami and caudate nuclei in 10 women with fibromyalgia compared with controls [77]. Another recent study supporting this view examined the response of fibromyalgia patients to intravenous morphine, lidocaine, and ketamine [78]. Ketamine, an *N*-methyl-D-aspartic acid receptor antagonist, resulted in significantly decreased pain and tenderness in fibromyalgia patients compared with the other agents, suggesting a central mechanism for pain.

Treatment

The treatment of fibromyalgia is challenging and frequently disappointing for both the patient and clinician. Although numerous studies have examined various therapies in fibromyalgia, there have been relatively few well-designed controlled trials [76, 79]. In addition, most studies have been of relatively brief duration, a problem in assessing treatment for a condition that is usually lifelong. For most patients, a therapeutic approach involving four elements is appropriate: (1) patient reassurance, (2) judicious pharmacologic intervention, (3) graded exercise with muscle stretching and relaxation as tolerated, and (4) psychiatric referral for definable psychiatric conditions.

It is important to begin treatment by reassuring patients that the clinician recognizes their symptoms as "real" and follows patients regularly to assist them in dealing with their illness. Patients should understand that there is no serious, crippling condition to account for their symptoms and that fibromyalgia is a common, manageable disorder that does not evolve into other conditions over time. Patients also should be instructed about treatment options available, sleep hygiene, and avoidance of behaviors that elicit symptoms.

Several studies have documented that at least 20% of fibromyalgia patients have a concurrent psychiatric disorder, and approximately 35% describe a significant history of depression at some time during their lives [4, 80]. The prevalence of psychiatric disorders is particularly high in patients seen at tertiary referral centers [81]. Although there is little data on the effects of psychiatric treatment on the fibromyalgia symptoms, psychiatric referral in patients with definable disorders seems appropriate. Patients with severe disease who are impaired in most activities of daily living merit referral to a multidisciplinary pain management program, preferably one that specializes in fibromyalgia [63, 76].

The cornerstones of pharmacologic therapy involve the tricyclic agents, in particular amitriptyline (10–75 mg/day) and cyclobenzaprine (10–30 mg/day) [82–86]. These drugs are effective at doses lower than those usually used for depression, suggesting that their effect in fibromyalgia is independent of effects on mood. This is also supported by the fact that other antidepressants, such as fluoxetine, have proved ineffective in fibromyalgia [87]. Multiple other medications have been tried, including prednisone, various nonsteroidal anti-inflammatory drugs, various other antidepressants, phenothiazines, different sedative hypnotics, and ondansetron [63, 88, 89]. Although many of these agents provide short-term relief for individual symptoms (such as reducing anxiety with alprazolam or improving sleep with zolpidem), no agents have been shown to provide sustained relief for most symptoms. Graded exercise programs aimed at improving cardiovascular fitness have improved both objective and subjective measures of pain in fibromyalgia. Because symptoms often increase during the initial phases of such regimens, it is important to continue these programs beyond 12 weeks [90, 91].

The limitations of current treatments for fibromyalgia are indicated by the fact that approximately 90% of fibromyalgia patients seek alternative forms of treatment, including dietary regimens, acupuncture, hypnosis, biofeedback, chiropractic manipulations, and massage therapy [63, 92]. There is no good data on the effectiveness of such therapies.

Prognosis

Little information is available on the long-term outcome of patients with fibromyalgia. Anecdotal reports suggest that most patients continue to be symptomatic for years; complete remissions in adults are unusual. In most studies that have examined long-term prognosis, patients describe worsening of symptoms at follow-up times of 3–5 years, whereas studies with follow-up periods of 10 years or more reported improvement in most patients [1, 93]. For example, a study by Kennedy and Felson surveyed 29 patients 10 years after their initial presentations [94]. Sixty-five percent reported significant improvement of their symptoms, and 55% reported feeling "well or very well." Most patients were still working, and 75% were still taking medications for their condition. Approximately 25% of fibromyalgia patients receive some type of disability payment during the course of their illness [69]. The prognosis appears to be better for children [95].

Chronic Fatigue Syndrome

Like fibromyalgia, chronic fatigue syndrome was initially described more than 100 years ago and has been discussed under a wide variety of names, including *neurasthenia, chronic brucellosis, postviral fatigue syndrome, epidemic neuromyasthenia, chronic Epstein-Barr infection, chronic fatigue and immune dysfunction syndrome, yuppie flu*, and *myalgic encephalomyelitis. Chronic fatigue syndrome* is the name coined in 1988 for a chronic illness characterized by debilitating fatigue and a variety of other systemic symptoms, including myalgia, sleep disturbance, and cognitive impairment [96]. Like fibromyalgia, chronic fatigue syndrome is a controversial entity in that the condition is defined by symptoms alone, has no associated diagnostic physical findings or laboratory tests, is of unknown cause, and currently has no specific treatment.

Epidemiology

Fatigue is one of the most common symptoms for which individuals consult physicians and is reported by approximately 20% of patients seeking primary medical care [4]. In most of these individuals, fatigue is transient and easily attributable to another medical or psychiatric condition. Population-based studies have suggested that the prevalence of chronic fatigue syndrome as defined by the Centers for Disease Control and Prevention (CDC) criteria is between 0.1% and 1.5% of the population. Although chronic fatigue syndrome can affect persons of any age, including children, it typically affects individuals in the third and fourth decade and is three to four times more common in women than in men [1, 79, 97].

Clinical Features

As the name suggests, the pathognomonic feature of chronic fatigue syndrome is unremitting, overwhelming fatigue. Unlike fibromyalgia, in which symptom onset is typically indolent and slowly progressive, the onset of fatigue in chronic fatigue syndrome is typically sudden, and patients are often able to date the onset of their disease quite specifically, often attributing it to some minor infectious illness or traumatic event. The fatigue is usually constant, but typically becomes much worse 12–24 hours after even mild activity. Patients therefore often avoid even mild exertion and over time can become progressively disabled, sometimes becoming bedridden and unable to do even simple self-care tasks [98].

Along with fatigue, patients usually have a whole host of other symptoms, including myalgia, neuropsychiatric symptoms (difficulty with concentration, forgetfulness, irritability, and depression), and sleep disturbances [99]. Other less common symptoms include fevers, sore throat, headache, arthralgia, swollen neck or arm glands, paresthesia, nausea, and anorexia. Psychiatric manifestations can also be prominent, and approximately 60% of patients have a concurrent diagnosable psychiatric disorder [100]. Depression, anxiety, and somatization disorders are significantly more frequent in chronic fatigue syndrome patients than controls [4].

Physical examination is normal in the vast majority of patients; pharyngitis, fever, and lymphadenopathy are so rarely present that they have been dropped from current diagnostic criteria [2, 101, 102]. Interestingly, the only consistent abnormality documented on examination is the presence of tender points in up to 70% of patients [103, 104].

In 1994, the CDC revised their 1988 case definition criteria for chronic fatigue syndrome and proposed new diagnostic guidelines (Table 2.6) [102]. The new criteria differ from previous criteria in eliminating physical examination findings as

Table 2.6   Diagnostic criteria for chronic fatigue syndrome

A. Chronic, unexplained, persistent, or relapsing fatigue of new onset (i.e., not lifelong) that is
   1. Not alleviated by rest
   2. Not the result of ongoing exertion
   3. Severe enough to result in substantial reduction of activity
B. Four or more of the following present for ≥6 mos and not predating the fatigue
   1. Memory or concentration impairment severe enough to interfere with activities
   2. Sore throat
   3. Tender cervical or axillary lymph nodes
   4. Muscle pain
   5. Pain in multiple joints without swelling or redness
   6. Headaches of new type, pattern, or severity
   7. Nonrestorative sleep
   8. Postexertional malaise lasting >24 hrs

Source: Adapted from K Fukada, SE Straus, I Hickie, et al. The chronic fatigue syndrome: a comprehensive approach to its definition and study. Ann Intern Med 1994;121:953–959.

minor criteria, reducing the exclusions previously defined on the basis of psychiatric disorders, and reducing the number of minor symptoms required for diagnosis. These criteria are very helpful in establishing a diagnosis and reducing the need for unnecessary evaluations. As in fibromyalgia, however, these criteria were designed mainly for research and cannot be viewed too restrictively in regard to individual patients. They do, however, provide useful guidelines for evaluation. Australian and British investigators have also developed diagnostic criteria, although they do not differ significantly from those of the CDC [105].

Laboratory Features

Although minor laboratory abnormalities are not infrequently documented in patients with chronic fatigue syndrome, no consistent abnormality or pattern of abnormalities has been demonstrated, and no tests have been shown to be of diagnostic or predictive value [2, 106]. Current recommendations are that the laboratory evaluation be restricted to a complete blood cell count with differential, urinalysis, sedimentation rate, electrolytes, creatinine, liver function studies, and thyroid stimulating hormone [102, 107]. Although 10–20% of patients have circulating autoantibodies, they are of low concentration and doubtful clinical significance.

Studies of muscle function have been uniformly unrevealing. Serum CK is essentially always normal, and EMG studies are normal except for suggesting incomplete voluntary effort or lack of central drive [10, 108]. Muscle biopsies in patients with chronic fatigue syndrome have shown no consistent abnormality and are not helpful, either diagnostically or in providing any information about the etiology of the condition [109–111].

The role of autonomic studies, including tilt-table testing, in the evaluation of patients with chronic fatigue syndrome is unclear. One investigation described abnormal responses to upright tilt in 22 of 23 patients with chronic fatigue syndrome compared with similar abnormalities in only 4 of 14 controls [112]. Seventy percent of the chronic fatigue syndrome patients in this study had abnormalities in stage 1 of upright tilt, and nine patients reported marked improvement after treatment of the presumably neurally mediated hypotension. Unfortunately, the tilt-table studies were not repeated (or not reported) in the treated individuals, and similarly deconditioned controls were not studied. If these provocative observations can be confirmed, however, autonomic and tilt-table testing may play an important role in the diagnosis and management of patients with chronic fatigue syndrome.

Pathogenesis

The pathogenesis of chronic fatigue syndrome is unknown. Although patients often link the onset of their disease to some mild infectious illness—and early reports linked the syndrome to a number of different infectious agents, including Epstein-Barr virus, herpes virus type 6, and even Lyme disease—no convincing association between an infectious agent and chronic fatigue syndrome has been identified [4, 101, 113]. Similarly, although multiple subtle abnormalities of immune function have been described in these patients, the significance of these findings is uncertain, and most investigators agree that immunodeficiency is not the primary pathogenic abnormality [101, 114, 115]. Sleep abnormalities have also been described, many similar to those in fibromyalgia, but whether these are primary or secondary is unclear [116].

Studies of muscle function in chronic fatigue syndrome do not support the view that chronic fatigue syndrome is a primary muscle disorder. Although some studies have demonstrated provocative abnormalities of muscle function or biochemistry, it is likely that most of these changes are secondary to prolonged disuse and inactivity, rather than a primary defect. For example, patients with chronic fatigue syndrome have reduced aerobic capacity and reduced maximal heart rate compared with controls, as well as higher plasma lactate concentration with exercise and more rapid development of feelings of exhaustion [114, 117–120]. In some patients, lactate values rise more rapidly than in controls at low work rates, suggesting a subtle abnormality of muscle energy metabolism [119]. Magnetic resonance spectroscopy studies have shown reduced adenosine triphosphate concentrations at peak exercise in these patients, suggesting an impairment in oxidative metabolism [121]. Similar studies, however, have not confirmed these findings [122].

Other studies of muscle function in chronic fatigue syndrome strongly suggest that the fatigue is probably central in origin. Voluntary activation of the tibialis anterior muscle during maximal sustained exercise was significantly lower in chronic fatigue syndrome patients than controls, despite otherwise normal muscle metabolism and function [123]. These findings are in agreement with others that suggest that the main difficulty in chronic fatigue syndrome patients is that they perceive fatigue at levels of activity not associated with true muscle exhaustion.

This concept that the pathogenesis of fatigue in chronic fatigue syndrome may arise from predominantly central mechanisms is an attractive pathogenic hypothesis for a number of reasons. The abnormalities in sleep and autonomic regulation with orthostatic tilt might be manifestations of a primary central regulatory dysfunction. Such a process might also explain the subtle neurocognitive and neuropsychological abnormalities demonstrated in these patients [124–127], as well as the pattern of hypothalamic–pituitary–adrenal axis dysfunction documented in some [4]. Central neuroimaging studies and other data have led some investigators to hypothesize dysfunction in the ascending brain stem reticular activating system or central raphe neurons [114]. At this time, however, the evidence for such an abnormality is circumstantial, and further work is needed in this area.

One difficulty in studying the pathogenesis of chronic fatigue syndrome is that like fibromyalgia, chronic fatigue syndrome might arise from a number of different causes. Significant overlaps exist in the clinical features, examination and laboratory findings, psychosocial features, and predisposing factors between chronic fatigue syndrome and fibromyalgia; the cardinal features of the two syndromes—namely, myalgia, fatigue, and nonrestorative sleep—are the same for both entities. It is possible, therefore, that these two conditions may simply represent different manifestations of a similar underlying pathophysiologic process [4].

Treatment

No treatment has been shown to be effective for patients with chronic fatigue syndrome. Because of the many minor abnormalities discovered in investigations of this syndrome, many treatments have been tried based on a presumed infectious or immunologic pathogenesis. In particular, antiviral therapy with acyclovir; immunologic therapy with immunoglobulin infusions and leukocyte extracts; and supplement therapy with vitamin B_{12}, folic acid, and liver extracts have proven ineffective [101]. In general, treatment follows those guidelines given for fibromyalgia with attention directed toward individual symptoms. The judicious use of tricyclic antidepressants and nonsteroidal anti-inflammatory drugs is appropriate, as is psychiatric referral in patients with overt depression, anxiety, or other psychiatric diagnoses. Patients need to be reassured that there is not some other underlying disease leading to their fatigue. Cognitive-behavioral therapy administered by trained therapists aimed at dealing with the social and psychological aspects of the disease, as well as developing coping strategies other than the avoidance of physical activity, can be useful [128, 129]. This is important because even patients who embrace the diagnosis often look for other diagnoses or treatments. Several studies have shown that chronic fatigue syndrome patients have an average of 15–20 physician visits per year to both primary physicians and specialists, and 14 additional visits to alternative practitioners [130, 131].

Prognosis

Although the symptoms of chronic fatigue syndrome often worsen during the initial months after diagnosis, the longer-term prognosis is somewhat better. One study of 445 patients surveyed an average of 1.5 years after their initial evaluation revealed that 61% reported improvement, although only 2% were symptom-free [132]. Other studies have suggested similar rates of improvement, with good prognostic features being younger age at onset, absence of significant psychiatric comorbidity, and an initial response to therapy [133]. In addition, patients identified in a community setting appear to do better than those followed in tertiary referral centers. An important point is that significant deterioration after the first few years of illness is very unusual [101]. Disability in these individuals, however, remains a significant problem, with as many as one-third of patients in some series reported to be on extended disability from work [4].

Clearly, better treatments for this condition are urgently needed. An intriguing randomized, double-blind crossover trial of hydrocortisone (5–10 mg/day for 1 month) in 32 patients with chronic fatigue syndrome reported by Cleare et al. described significant *short-term* improvement in fatigue scores in the treated group compared with controls, with 28% of treated patients achieving "normal" fatigue scores [134]. Confirmation of these findings with longer periods of follow-up would suggest that effective pharmacotherapy is at least feasible for these patients.

EVALUATION OF THE PATIENT WITH MUSCLE PAIN AND FATIGUE

From the previous discussion and the review of the voluminous literature on muscle pain and fatigue, several conclusions about the evaluation of these patients are apparent. The first is that despite an intensive diagnostic evaluation, most patients

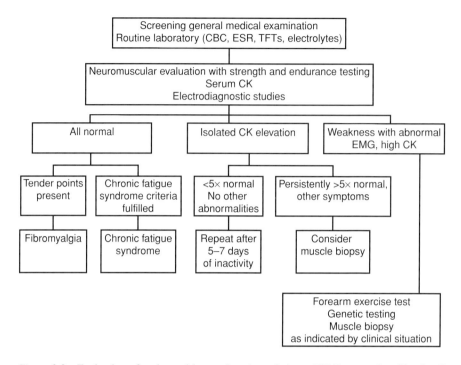

Figure 2.2 Evaluation of patient with muscle pain or fatigue. (CBC = complete blood cell count; ESR = erythrocyte sedimentation rate; TFTs = thyroid function tests; CK = creatine kinase; EMG = electromyography.)

presenting with muscle pain, fatigue, or both do *not* have a definable, specific muscle abnormality. This is particularly true for patients presenting with muscle pain and fatigue alone (i.e., without weakness or demonstrable laboratory abnormality). Indeed, Mills and Edward were able to document a specific diagnosis in only one-third of 109 consecutive patients presenting with myalgia [5]. A second conclusion is that the most common disorders associated with chronic muscle pain and fatigue are fibromyalgia and chronic fatigue syndrome, respectively; many patients, as discussed earlier, will have features of both conditions. Finally, the diagnoses of fibromyalgia and chronic fatigue syndrome generally do not require exhaustive testing or consultation by multiple medical subspecialists.

With these conclusions in mind, an evaluation of the patient with muscle pain and fatigue as outlined in Figure 2.2 has been useful for the authors. All patients should obviously have a detailed history and physical examination that includes strength testing (either manual muscle testing or computerized strength testing) and bedside endurance testing (e.g., determining the time patients can maintain outstretched arms or legs and the number of deep knee bends that can be performed) [10]. Patients suspected of having fibromyalgia should also be evaluated for the presence of tender points. If not already performed, a series of routine blood studies should be obtained, including CK, thyroid studies, sedimentation rate, complete blood cell count, and electrolytes. Electrodiagnostic studies are also indicated in most patients.

Those patients with normal results to these initial studies who generally fulfill the criteria for fibromyalgia, chronic fatigue syndrome, or both are probably best managed symptomatically for these conditions, assuming they have had a general medical evaluation for other systemic disorders. Patients with definite weakness and myopathic electrodiagnostic studies or elevated CK levels deserve further evaluation through forearm exercise testing, muscle biopsy, or genetic testing (e.g., Xp21 deletion analysis), depending on the clinical situation.

Patients with isolated elevations in CK with normal strength and normal EMG represent difficult management problems. Because of the extreme variability in CK levels on the basis of activity, race, and gender, it is important to not overinterpret minor elevations in serum CK [20, 135]. Because even modest exercise can elevate the CK, it is appropriate to repeat the CK after 5–7 days of rest (no athletic activity) before deciding whether the patient needs further evaluation. Even in those individuals, diagnostic evaluation is seldom fruitful unless the level is greater than three to five times normal or muscle weakness is present [10]. Patients with clearly exercise-induced myoglobinuria must therefore be evaluated individually with forearm exercise testing for lactate and ammonia and muscle biopsy, even if the resting CK and electrodiagnostic studies are normal.

Using this approach, most patients with myalgia and fatigue can be appropriately diagnosed early in the evaluation process, including those patients with fibromyalgia and chronic fatigue syndrome. Many patients (and physicians) find these two diagnoses frustrating, in that a "real disease" has not been identified. At the very least, however, patients with these diagnoses can be reassured that there is no "serious" underlying disorder present and are usually gratified that a clinician has approached their problems in an organized, thoughtful fashion. In addition, these diagnoses eliminate the need for further diagnostic testing and reduce the risk that the patient will be treated in an inappropriately aggressive manner.

REFERENCES

1. Goldenberg DL. Fibromyalgia, chronic fatigue syndrome, and myofascial pain. Curr Opin Rheumatol 1996;8:113–123.
2. Lane TJ, Matthews DA, Manu P. The low yield of physical examinations and laboratory investigations of patients with chronic fatigue. Am J Med Sci 1990;299:313–318.
3. Shafran SD. The chronic fatigue syndrome. Am J Med 1991;90:730–739.
4. Buchwald D. Fibromyalgia and chronic fatigue syndrome. Rheum Dis Clin North Am 1996; 22:219–243.
5. Mills KR, Edward RHT. Investigative strategies for muscle pain. J Neurol Sci 1983;58:73–88.
6. Layzer RB. Muscle Pain, Cramps, and Fatigue. In C Franzini-Armstrong, AG Engel (eds), Myology (2nd ed). New York: McGraw-Hill, 1994;1754–1768.
7. Lane RJM, Fuller GN. Clinical Presentation: Symptoms and Signs of Muscle Disease and Their Interpretation. In RJM Lane (ed), Handbook of Muscle Disease. New York: Marcel Dekker, 1996;1–17.
8. Auger RG. Diseases associated with excess motor unit activity. Muscle Nerve 1994;17:1250–1263.
9. Kincaid JC. Muscle pain, fatigue, and fasciculations. Neurol Clin 1997;15:697–709.
10. Griggs RC, Mendell JR, Miller RG. Muscle Pain and Fatigue. In Evaluation and Treatment of Myopathies. Philadelphia: FA Davis, 1995;389–407.
11. Krupp LB, Pollina DA. Mechanisms and management of fatigue in progressive neurological disorders. Curr Opin Neurol 1996;9:456–460.

12. Newham DF, Edwards RHT, Mills KR. Skeletal Muscle Pain. In PD Wall, R Melzack (eds), Textbook of Pain. Edinburgh, UK: Churchill Livingston, 1994;423–439.
13. Kumazawa T, Mizumura K. Thin-fiber receptors responding to mechanical, chemical and thermal stimulations in the skeletal muscle of the dog. J Physiol 1977;273:179–194.
14. Mense S. Sensitization of group IV muscle receptors of bradykinin by 5-hydroxytryptamine and prostaglandin E_2. Brain Res 1981;225:95–105.
15. Mense S, Stahnke M. Responses in muscle afferent fibers of slow conduction velocity to contractions and ischemia in the cat. J Physiol 1983;342:383–397.
16. Hiss E, Mense S. Evidence for the existence of different receptor sites for algesic agents at the endings of muscular group IV afferent units. Pflugers Arch 1976;362:141–146.
17. Graven-Nielsen T, McArdle A, Phoenix J, et al. In vivo model of muscle pain: quantification of intramuscular chemical, electrical, and pressure changes associated with saline-induced muscle pain in humans. Pain 1997;69:137–143.
18. Sylven C, Jonzon B, Fredholm BB, Kaijser L. Adenosine injection into the brachial artery produces ischaemia like pain or discomfort in the forearm. Cardiovasc Res 1988;22:674–678.
19. Newham DJ, Mills KR, Quigley BM, Edwards RHT. Pain and fatigue after concentric and eccentric muscle contractions. Clin Sci 1983;64:55–62.
20. Newham DJ, Jones DA, Edwards RHT. Large delayed plasma creatine kinase changes after stepping exercise. Muscle Nerve 1983;6:380–385.
21. Armstrong RB, Ogilvie RW, Schwane JA. Eccentric exercise-induced injury to rat skeletal muscle. J Appl Physiol 1983;54:80–93.
22. Armstrong RB. Initial events in exercise-induced muscular injury. Med Sci Sports Exerc 1990; 22:429–435.
23. Friden J. Muscle soreness after exercise: implications of morphological changes. Int J Sports Med 1984;5:57–66.
24. Schwane JA, Johnson SR, Vandenakker CB, Armstrong RB. Delayed-onset muscular soreness and plasma CPK and LDH activities after downhill running. Med Sci Sports Exerc 1983;15:51–56.
25. Newham DJ, McPhail G, Mills KR, Edwards RHT. Ultrastructural changes after concentric and eccentric contractions of human muscle. J Neurol Sci 1983;61:109–122.
26. Teague BN, Schwane JA. Effect of intermittent eccentric contractions on symptoms of muscle microinjury. Med Sci Sports Exerc 1995;27:1378–1384.
27. Jorgensen K, Fallentin N, Krogh-Lund C, Jensen B. Electromyography and fatigue during prolonged, low-level static contractions. Eur J Appl Physiol 1988;57:316–321.
28. Boska MD, Moussavi RS, Carson PJ, et al. The metabolic basis of recovery after fatiguing exercise of human muscle. Neurology 1990;40:240–244.
29. Miller RG, Boska MD, Moussavi RS, et al. 31P nuclear magnetic resonance studies of high energy phosphages and pH in human muscle fatigue. J Clin Invest 1988;81:1190–1196.
30. Miller RG, Giannini D, Milner-Brown HS, et al. Effects of fatiguing exercise on high-energy phosphates, force, and EMG: evidence for three phases of recovery. Muscle Nerve 1987;10:810–821.
31. Majumdar R, Cwik VA, Solonynko G, Brooke MH. Relationship of oxypurine release to contractile failure in dinitrophenol treated muscle. Acta Physiol Scand 1993;149:249–255.
32. Sjogaard G. Role of exercise-induced potassium fluxes underlying muscle fatigue: brief review. Can J Physiol Pharmacol 1991;69:238–255.
33. Bigland-Ritchie B, Woods JJ. Changes in muscle contractile properties and neural control during human muscular fatigue. Muscle Nerve 1984;7:691–699.
34. Nosek TM, Fender KY, Godt RE. It is diprotonated inorganic phosphage that depresses muscle force in skinned skeletal muscle fibers. Science 1987;236:191–193.
35. Bystrom S, Kilbom A. Electrical stimulation of human forearm extensor muscles as an indicator of handgrip fatigue and recovery. Eur J Appl Physiol 1991;62:363–368.
36. Tesch PA, Wright JE. Recovery from short term intense exercise; its relation to capillary supply and blood lactate concentration. Eur J Appl Physiol 1983;52:98–103.
37. Moussavi RS, Carson BA, Boska MD, et al. Nonmetabolic fatigue in exercising human muscle. Neurology 1989;39:1222–1226.
38. Tesch PA, Thorsson A, Fujitsuka N. Creatine phosphate in fiber types of skeletal muscle before and after exhaustive exercise. J Appl Physiol 1989;66:1756–1759.
39. Petrella JT, Giuliani MJ, Lacomis D. Vacuolar myopathies in adults with myalgias: value of paraspinal muscle investigation. Muscle Nerve 1997;20:1321–1323.
40. Danon MJ, Carpenter S, Harati Y. Muscle pain associated with tubular aggregates and structures resembling cylindrical spirals. Muscle Nerve 1989;12:265–272.

41. Niakan E, Harati Y, Danon MJ. Tubular aggregates: their association with myalgia. J Neurol Neurosurg Psychiatry 1985;48:882–886.
42. Beyenburg S, Zierz S. Chronic progressive external ophthalmoplegia and myalgia associated with tubular aggregates. Acta Neurol Scand 1993;87:397–402.
43. Ghospe SM, Lazaro RP, Lava NS, et al. Familial X-linked myalgia and cramps: a nonprogressive myopathy associated with a deletion in the dystrophin gene. Neurology 1989;39:1277–1280.
44. Salvarani C, Gabriel SE, O'Fallon WM, Hunder GG. Epidemiology of polymyalgia rheumatica in Olmstead County, Minnesota. Arthritis Rheum 1995;38:369–373.
45. Brooks RC, McGee SR. Diagnostic dilemmas in polymyalgia rheumatica [see comments]. Arch Intern Med 1997;157:162–168.
46. Hunder GG. Giant Cell Arteritis and Polymyalgia Rheumatica. In WN Kelley, S Ruddy, ED Harris, CB Sledge (eds), Textbook of Rheumatology (5th ed). Philadelphia: Saunders, 1997;1123–1132.
47. Salvarani C, Macchioni P, Boiardi L. Polymyalgia rheumatica. Lancet 1997;350:43–47
48. Turnbull J. Temporal arteritis and polymyalgia rheumatica: nosographic and nosologic considerations. Neurology 1996;46:901–906.
49. Kojima S, Takagi A, Ida M, Schiozawa R. Muscle pathology in polymyalgia rheumatica: histochemical and immunohistochemical study. Jpn J Med Sci Biol 1991;30:516–523.
50. Gowers WR. Lumbago: its lessons and analogues. BMJ 1904;1:117–121.
51. Kellgren JH. Observations on referred pain arising from muscle. Clin Sci 1938;3:175–190.
52. Hench PK. Nonarticular rheumatism, twenty-second rheumatism review: review of the American and English literature for the years 1973 and 1974. Arthritis Rheum 1976;19(suppl):1081–1089.
53. Goldenberg DL. What is the future of fibromyalgia? Rheum Dis Clin North Am 1996;22:393–406.
54. Bohr T. Problems with myofascial pain syndrome and fibromyalgia syndrome. Neurology 1996;46:593–597.
55. Yunus M, Masi AT, Calabro JJ, et al. Primary fibromyalgia (fibrositis): clinical study of 50 patients with matched normal controls. Semin Arthritis Rheum 1981;11:151–171.
56. Cohen ML. Fibromyalgia syndrome, a problem of tautology. Lancet 1993;342:906–909.
57. Bennett RM. Fibromyalgia and the facts. Sense or nonsense. Rheum Dis Clin North Am 1993;19:45–59.
58. Yunus MB. Towards a model pathophysiology of fibromyalgia: aberrant central pain mechanisms with peripheral modulation. J Rheumatol 1992;19:846–850.
59. Wolfe F, Ross K, Anderson J, et al. The prevalence and characteristics of fibromyalgia in the general population. Arthritis Rheum 1995;38:19–28.
60. Schochat T, Croft P, Raspe H. The epidemiology of fibromyalgia. Br J Rheumatol 1994;33:783–786.
61. Wolfe F, Smythe HA, Yunus MB, et al. The American College of Rheumatology 1990 criteria for the classification of fibromyalgia: report of the Multicenter Criteria Committee. Arthritis Rheum 1990;33:160–172.
62. Wolfe F, Potter J. Is fibromyalgia a disabling disorder? Rheum Dis Clin North Am 1996;22:369–391.
63. McCain GA. A cost-effective approach to the diagnosis and treatment of fibromyalgia. Rheum Dis Clin North Am 1996;22:323–349.
64. Wolfe F, Hawley DJ, Wilson K. The prevalence and meaning of fatigue in rheumatic disease. J Rheumatol 1996;23:1407–1417.
65. Simms RW, Goldenberg DL, Felson DT, Mason JH. Tenderness in 75 anatomic sites: distinguishing fibromyalgia patients from controls. Arthritis Rheum 1988;31:182–187.
66. Borg-Stein J, Stein J. Trigger points and tender points. One and the same? Does injection treatment help? Rheum Dis Clin North Am 1996;22:305–321.
67. Wolfe F, Simons DG, Fricton J, et al. The fibromyalgia and myofascial pain syndromes: a preliminary study of tender points and trigger points in persons with fibromyalgia, myofascial pain syndrome and no disease. J Rheumatol 1992;19:944–951.
68. Jacobs JWG, Greenen R, van der Heide A, et al. Are tender point scores assessed by manual palpation in fibromyalgia reliable? Scand J Rheumatol 1995;24:243–247.
69. Simms RW. Is there muscle pathology in fibromyalgia? Rheum Dis Clin North Am 1996;22:245–266.
70. Drewes AM, Andreasen A, Schroder HD, et al. Pathology of skeletal muscle in fibromyalgia: a histo-immuno-chemical and ultrastructural study. Br J Rheumatol 1993;32:479–483.
71. Bengtsson A, Henriksson KG, Larsson J. Muscle biopsy in primary fibromyalgia. Scand J Rheumatol 1986;15:1–6.
72. Lindh M, Johansson G, Hedberg M, et al. Muscle fiber characteristics, capillaries and enzymes in patients with fibromyalgia and controls. Scand J Rheumatol 1995;24:34–37.

73. Yunus MB, Kalayan-Raman UP. Muscle biopsy findings in primary fibromyalgia and other forms of nonarticular rheumatism. Rheum Dis Clin North Am 1989;15:115–134.
74. Lario BA, Valdivielso LA, Lopez JA, et al. Fibromyalgia syndrome: overnight falls in arterial oxygen saturation. Am J Med 1996;101:54–60.
75. Drewes AM, Nielsen KD, Taagholt SJ, et al. Sleep intensity in fibromyalgia: focus on the microstructure of the sleep process. Br J Rheumatol 1995;34:629–635.
76. Bennett RM. Multidisciplinary group programs to treat fibromyalgia patients. Rheum Dis Clin North Am 1996;22:351–367.
77. Mountz JM, Bradley LA, Modell JG, et al. Fibromyalgia in women. Abnormalities of regional cerebral blood flow in the thalamus and the caudate nucleus are associated with low pain threshold levels. Arthritis Rheum 1995;38:926–938.
78. Sorensen J, Bengtsson A, Backman E, et al. Pain analysis in patients with fibromyalgia. Scand J Rheumatol 1995;24:360–365.
79. Goldenberg DL. Fibromyalgia, chronic fatigue syndrome, and myofascial pain syndrome. Curr Opin Rheumatol 1997;9:135–143.
80. Katz RS, Kravitz HM. Fibromyalgia, depression, and alcoholism: a family history study. J Rheumatol 1996;23:149–154.
81. Aaron LA, Bradley LA, Alarcon GS, et al. Psychiatric diagnoses in patients with fibromyalgia are related to health care–seeking behavior rather than to illness. Arthritis Rheum 1996;39:436–445.
82. Carette S, McCain GA, Bell DA, et al. Evaluation of amitriptyline in primary fibrositis. Arthritis Rheum 1986;29:655–659.
83. Goldenberg DL, Felson DT, Dinerman H. A randomized, controlled trial of amitriptyline and naproxen in the treatment of patients with fibromyalgia. Arthritis Rheum 1986;29:1371–1377.
84. Jaeschke R, Adachi J, Guyatt C, et al. Clinical usefulness of amitriptyline in fibromyalgia: the results of 23 N-of-1 randomized controlled trials. J Rheumatol 1991;18:447–451.
85. Santandrea S, Montrone F, Sarzi-Puttini P, et al. A double-blind crossover study of two cyclobenzaprine regimens in primary fibromyalgia syndrome. J Int Med Res 1993;21:74–80.
86. Godfrey RG. A guide to the understanding and use of tricyclic antidepressants in the overall management of fibromyalgia and other chronic pain syndromes. Arch Intern Med 1996;156:1047–1052.
87. Cortet B, Houvenagel E, Forzy GE. Evaluation of the effectiveness of serotonin (fluoxetine hydrochloride) treatment: open study in fibromyalgia. Rev Rhum Mal Osteoartic 1992;59:497–500.
88. Hrycaj P, Stratz T, Mennet P, Muller W. Pathogenetic aspects of responsiveness to ondansetron (5-hydroxytryptamine type 3 receptor antagonist) in patients with primary fibromyalgia syndrome—a preliminary study. J Rheumatol 1996;23:1418–1423.
89. Moldofsky H, Lue FA, Mously C, et al. The effect of zolpidem in patients with fibromyalgia: a dose ranging, double blind, placebo controlled, modified crossover study. J Rheumatol 1996;23:529–533.
90. McCain GA, Bell DA, Mai FM, et al. A controlled study of the effects of a supervised cardiovascular fitness program on the manifestations of the primary fibromyalgia syndrome. Arthritis Rheum 1988;31:1135–1141.
91. Nichols DS, Glenn TM. Effects of aerobic exercise on pain perception, affect, and level of disability in individuals with fibromyalgia. Phys Ther 1994;74:327–332.
92. Pioro-Boisset M, Esdaile JM, Fitzcharles M-A. Alternative medicine use in fibromyalgia syndrome. Arthritis Care Res 1996;9:13–17.
93. Ledingham J, Doherty S, Doherty M. Primary fibromyalgia syndrome: an outcome study. Br J Rheumatol 1992;32:139–142.
94. Kennedy M, Felson DT. A prospective long-term study of fibromyalgia syndrome. Arthritis Rheum 1996;39:682–685.
95. Buskila D, Neumann L, Hershman E, et al. Fibromyalgia syndrome in children: an outcome study. J Rheumatol 1995;22:525–528.
96. Holmes GP, Kaplan J, Grantz N, et al. Chronic fatigue syndrome: a working case definition. Ann Intern Med 1988;108:387–389.
97. Bates D, Schmitt W, Buchwald D, et al. Prevalence of fatigue and chronic fatigue syndrome in a primary care practice. Arch Intern Med 1993;153:2759–2765.
98. Buchwald D, Pearlman T, Umali J, et al. Functional status in patients with chronic fatigue syndrome, other fatiguing illnesses, and healthy individuals. Am J Med 1996;171:364–370.
99. Komaroff AL, Fagioli LR, Geiger AM, et al. An examination of the working case definition of chronic fatigue syndrome. Am J Med 1996;100:56–64.
100. Wessely S, Chalder T, Hirsch S, et al. Psychological symptoms, somatic symptoms, and psychiatric disorder in chronic fatigue and chronic fatigue syndrome: a prospective study in the primary care setting. Am J Psychiatry 1996;153:1050–1059.

101. Salit IE. The chronic fatigue syndrome: a position paper. J Rheumatol 1996;23:540–544.
102. Fukada K, Straus SE, Hickie I, et al. The chronic fatigue syndrome: a comprehensive approach to its definition and study. Ann Intern Med 1994;121:953–959.
103. Buchwald D, Garrity D. Comparison of patients with chronic fatigue syndrome, fibromyalgia and multiple chemical sensitivities. Arch Intern Med 1994;154:2049–2053.
104. Goldenberg DL, Simms RW, Geiger A, et al. High frequency of fibromyalgia in patients with chronic fatigue seen in a primary care practice. Arthritis Rheum 1990;33:381–387.
105. Bates DW, Buchwald D, Lee J, et al. A comparison of case definitions of chronic fatigue syndrome. Clin Infect Dis 1994;18:S11–S15.
106. Bates DW, Buchwald D, Lee J, et al. Clinical laboratory test findings in patients with chronic fatigue syndrome. Arch Intern Med 1995;155:97–103.
107. Wessely S, Chalder T, Hirsch S, et al. Postinfectious fatigue: prospective cohort study in primary care. Lancet 1995;345:1333–1338.
108. Lloyd AR, Gandevia SC, Hales JP. Muscle performance, voluntary activation, twitch properties and perceived effort in normal subjects and patients with the chronic fatigue syndrome. Brain 1991; 114:85–98.
109. Edwards RH, Gibson H, Clague JE, Helliwell T. Muscle histopathology and physiology in chronic fatigue syndrome. Ciba Found Symp 1993;173:102–117.
110. Connolly S, Smith DG, Doyle D, Fowler CJ. Chronic fatigue: electromyographic and neuropathological evaluation. J Neurol 1993;240:435–438.
111. Behan WMH, More IAR, Behan PO. Mitochondrial abnormalities in the postviral fatigue syndrome. Acta Neuropathol (Berl)1991;83:61–65.
112. Bou-Holaigah I, Rowe PC, Kan J, Calkins H. The relationship between neurally medicated hypotension and the chronic fatigue syndrome. JAMA 1995;274:961–967.
113. Mawle AC, Nisenbaum R, Dobbins JG, et al. Seroepidemiology of chronic fatigue syndrome: a case-control study. Clin Infect Dis 1995;21:1386–1389.
114. Dickinson DJ. Chronic fatigue syndrome-aetiological aspects. Eur J Clin Invest 1997;27:257–267.
115. Buchwald D, Wener MH, Pearlman T, Kith P. Markers of inflammation and immune activation in chronic fatigue and chronic fatigue syndrome. J Rheumatol 1997;24:372–376.
116. Moldofsky H. Fibromyalgia, sleep disorder and chronic fatigue syndrome. Ciba Found Symp 1993;173:262–279.
117. Riley MS, O'Brien CJ, McCluskey DR, et al. Aerobic work capacity in patients with chronic fatigue syndrome. BMJ 1990;301:953–956.
118. Lane RJM, Woodrow D, Archard L. Lactate responses to exercise in chronic fatigue syndrome. J Neurol Neurosurg Psychiatry 1994;54:662–663.
119. Lane RJM, Burgess AP, Flint J, et al. Lactate responses to exercise and psychiatric disorder in the chronic fatigue syndrome. BMJ 1995;311:544–545.
120. Gibson H, Carroll N, Clague JE, Edwards RHT. Exercise performance and fatigability in patients with chronic fatigue syndrome. J Neurol Neurosurg Psychiatry 1993;56:993–998.
121. Wong R, Lopaschuk G, Zhu G, et al. Skeletal muscle metabolism in the chronic fatigue syndrome. In vivo assessment by 31P nuclear magnetic resonance spectroscopy. Chest 1992;102:1716–1722.
122. Barnes PRN, Taylor DJ, Kemp GO, Rada CK. Skeletal muscle bioenergetics in the chronic fatigue syndrome. J Neurol Neurosurg Psychiatry 1993;56:679–683.
123. Kent-Braun JA, Sharma KR, Weiner MW, et al. Central basis of muscle fatigue in chronic fatigue syndrome. Neurology 1993;43:125–131.
124. Joyce E, Blumenthal S, Wessely S. Memory, attention, and executive function in chronic fatigue syndrome. J Neurol Neurosurg Psychiatry 1996;60:495–503.
125. Moss-Morris R, Petrie KJ, Large RG, Kydd RR. Neuropsychological deficits in chronic fatigue syndrome: artifact or reality? J Neurol Neurosurg Psychiatry 1996;60:474–477.
126. Prasher D, Smith A, Findley L. Sensory and cognitive event-related potentials in myalgic encephalomyelitis. J Neurol Neurosurg Psychiatry 1990;53:247–253.
127. DeLuca J, Johnson SK, Ellis SP, Natelson BH. Cognitive functioning is impaired in patients with chronic fatigue syndrome devoid psychiatric disease. J Neurol Neurosurg Psychiatry 1997;62: 151–155.
128. Deale A, Chalder T, Marks I, Wessely S. Cognitive behavior therapy for chronic fatigue syndrome: a randomized controlled trial. Am J Psychiatry 1997;154:408–414.
129. Sharpe M, Hawton K, Simkin S, et al. Cognitive behaviour therapy for the chronic fatigue syndrome: a randomised controlled trial. BMJ 1996;312:22–26.
130. Lloyd AR, Pender H. The economic impact of chronic fatigue syndrome. Med J Aust 1992;157: 599–601.

131. Bombardier CH, Buchwald D. Chronic fatigue syndrome, and fibromyalgia disability and health care use. Med Care 1996;34:924–930.
132. Bombardier CH, Buchwald D. Outcome and prognosis of patients with chronic fatigue vs. chronic fatigue syndrome. Arch Intern Med 1995;155:2105–2110.
133. Bonner D, Ron M, Chalder T, et al. Chronic fatigue syndrome: a follow up study. J Neurol Neurosurg Psychiatry 1994;57:617–621.
134. Cleare AJ, Heap E, Malhi GS, et al. Low-dose hydrocortisone in chronic fatigue syndrome: a randomised crossover trial. Lancet 1999;353:455–488.
135. Wong ET, Cobb C, Umhara MK, et al. Heterogeneity of serum creatine kinase activity among racial and gender groups of the population. Am J Clin Pathol 1983;79:582–586.

3
Muscular Dystrophies: Overview of Clinical and Molecular Approaches

Richard W. Orrell and Robert C. Griggs

The muscular dystrophies are genetically determined myopathies characterized by progressive weakness. They comprise a wide range of disorders, from severe childhood-onset forms that lead to early death, to more benign adult forms that do not affect total life span and may cause minimal disability. Until recently, it has only been possible to classify these disorders on the basis of their clinical presentation—for example, limb-girdle, facioscapulohumeral, Duchenne/Becker, and myotonic. Identification of the molecular basis of the muscular dystrophies now allows a classification and understanding based on the genetic or pathologic process, as determined by DNA or protein analysis or testing. Table 3.1 presents a classification based on genes and proteins that have been identified. Table 3.2 presents a classification for which the genetic cause has been identified but not fully defined; the protein abnormality at the time of writing is unknown [1].

In this chapter, we deal with facioscapulohumeral dystrophy (FSHD) and some of the less common muscular dystrophies. Other chapters deal specifically with diseases of the muscle membrane proteins (including dystrophinopathies, sarcoglycanopathies, calpainopathies, and congenital myopathies), and the myotonic dystrophies (myotonic dystrophy and proximal myotonic myopathy).

FSHD is a relatively common muscular dystrophy for which the genetic locus and abnormality have been defined, but the gene or genes causing the disease are not defined. The distal myopathies have recently been linked to chromosomal regions, but the genetic abnormality has not yet been described. Oculopharyngeal muscular dystrophy has recently been recognized to be due to a small trinucleotide repeat expansion in the PABP2 (polyadenyl binding protein) gene. Other genetically defined dystrophies include Type VI collagen in Bethlem myopathy, emerin in Emery-Dreifuss muscular dystrophy, tafazzins in Barth syndrome, and plectin in epidermolysis bullosa simplex with late-onset muscular dystrophy. We expect that further molecular, genetic, biochemical, and clinicopathologic studies will further define the pathogenesis of these disorders. Understanding some of the rarer muscular dystrophies will contribute to our understanding and management of muscular dystrophies and the wider spectrum of neurodegenerative disorders.

Table 3.1 A classification of muscular dystrophies based on identified gene and protein abnormalities

Group/disease	Inheritance	Gene	Gene product
Calpainopathies			
Limb-girdle	AR	LGMD2A (CAPN3)	Calpain-3
Caveolin			
Limb-girdle	AD	LGMD1C (CAV3)	Caveolin-3
Collagen			
Bethlem myopathy	AD	COL6A1, COL6A2	Collagen type VI subunit (α1 or α2)
Dysferlin			
Miyoshi myopathy	AR	MM	Dysferlin
Limb-girdle myopathy	AR	LGMD2B	Dysferlin
Dystrophinopathies			
Duchenne/Becker	XR	DMD (DYS)	Dystrophin
Emerin			
Emery-Dreifuss	XR	EMD	Emerin
Fukutin			
Fukuyama congenital muscular dystrophy	AR	FCMD	Fukutin
Merosin			
Congenital muscular dystrophy with merosin deficiency	AR	LAMA2	Merosin, or laminin α2 chain
Myotubularin			
Myotubular myopathy	XR	MTMX	Myotubularin
Plectin			
Epidermolysis bullosa simplex associated with late-onset muscular dystrophy	AR	MD-EBS	Plectin
Polyadenyl binding protein			
Oculopharyngeal	AD	OPMD (PABP2)	Polyadenyl binding protein 2
Protein kinase			
Myotonic dystrophy	AD	DM	Myotonin protein kinase
Ryanodine receptor			
Central core disease	AD	CCD (RYR1)	Ryanodine receptor
α-Tropomyosin			
Nemaline myopathy	AD	NEM1 (TPM3)	α-Tropomyosin
Sarcoglycanopathies			
Limb-girdle	AR	LGMD2D (SGCA)	α-Sarcoglycan, or adhalin
	AR	LGMD2E (SGCB)	β-Sarcoglycan
	AR	LGMD2C (SGCG)	γ-Sarcoglycan
	AR	LGMD2F (SGCD)	δ-Sarcoglycan
Tafazzin			
Barth syndrome	XR		Tafazzin

XR = X-linked recessive; AR = autosomal recessive; AD = autosomal dominant.

Source: Adapted from JC Kaplan, B Fontaine. Neuromuscular disorders: gene location. Neuromuscul Disord 1999;9:I–XIV.

Table 3.2   A classification of muscular dystrophies in which the gene and protein abnormality have not yet been identified

Disease	Inheritance	Gene	Gene location
Facioscapulohumeral	AD	FSHD	4q35
Limb-girdle	AD	LGMD1A	5q22-34
	AD	LGMD1B	1q11-21
	AR	LGMD2G	17q11-12
Distal myopathies			
Nonaka-hereditary inclusion body myopathy	AR	DMRV	9
Markesbery-Griggs-Udd	AD	TMD	2q31-33
ADDM-Welander	AD	MPD1	14q11.2-13
Myotonic			
Proximal myotonic myopathy	AD	DM2	3q
Myotonic dystrophy type 2	AD	DM2	3q
Congenital myopathies			
Nemaline	AR	NEM2	2q21.1-22

AR = autosomal recessive; AD = autosomal dominant.

Source: Adapted from JC Kaplan, B Fontaine. Neuromuscular disorders: gene location. Neuromuscul Disord 1998;8:I–VII.

FACIOSCAPULOHUMERAL DYSTROPHY

FSHD is an autosomal dominant disorder. The prevalence is approximately 1 in 20,000, it being the third most common muscular dystrophy. There is a distinctive pattern of progressive muscular weakness involving the face, scapular stabilizer, proximal arm, and peroneal muscles (Figure 3.1). The clinical pattern of weakness has defined the condition until recently, when the identification of a specific genetic abnormality—truncation of the number of 3.3 kb repeats in the telomeric region of chromosome 4q—has allowed a molecular genetic classification. Historically, two clinical patterns of FSHD were identified [2]. A gradually descending autosomal dominant form identified by Duchenne de Boulogne in 1855–1872, and a "jump" form—in which the progressive descent of weakness jumps from the upper body to the peroneal muscles—identified by Erb in 1882–1884 (the autosomal dominant inheritance of this form was recognized by Landouzy and Dejerine in 1885).

Age at onset is from infancy to middle age. The initial weakness typically affects the facial muscles, especially orbicularis oculi and oris. Masseter, temporalis, extraocular, and pharyngeal muscles are usually unaffected. Initially, the patient is unable to bury the eyelashes on tight eye closure, and the eyelids may be easily prized apart. In later stages, the sclera may remain exposed.

Clinical signs are present in more than 95% of those affected—or predicted to be affected in multigenerational families—by age 20 years [3]. Shoulder weakness is the most common presenting symptom, with facial weakness being ignored or overlooked. Involvement of the scapular fixator muscles—latissimus dorsi, trapezius, rhomboids, and serratus anterior—gives a typical appearance (see Figure 3.1). Scapular winging may be prominent (Figure 3.2). The deltoid muscle is char-

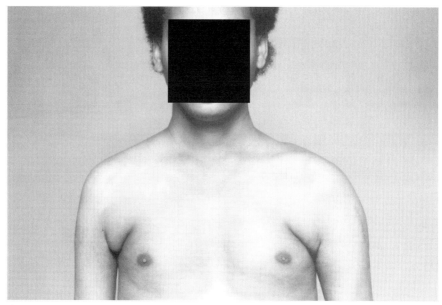

A

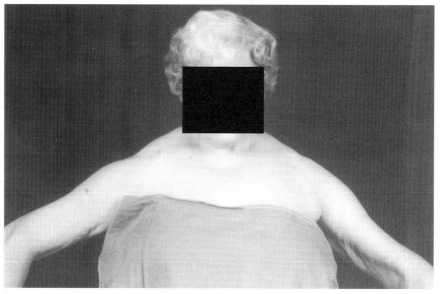

B

Figure 3.1   Facioscapulohumeral dystrophy. (**A**) The bilateral axillary creases and the horizontal position of the clavicles are characteristic. (**B**) Characteristic appearance on attempting shoulder abduction.

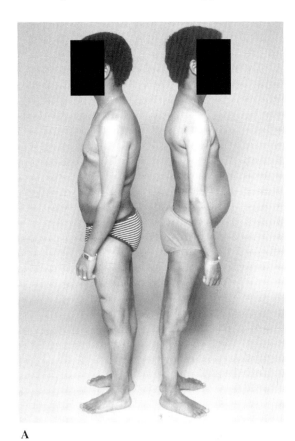

Figure 3.2 Facioscapulo-humeral dystrophy (FSHD). (**A**) Monozygotic twins: Only one is affected with FSHD. The brother on the right has accentuated lordosis. (**B**) View of affected twin showing scapular winging.

A

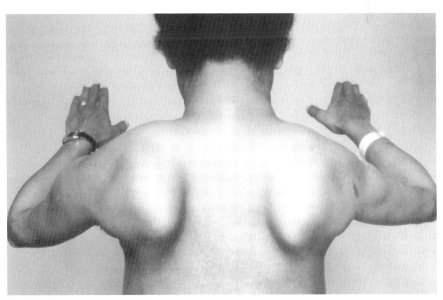

B

Table 3.3   Diagnostic criteria for facioscapulohumeral dystrophy (FSHD)

Inclusion
    Weakness of face or scapular stabilizers (in familial cases, facial weakness is present in >90% of affected individuals)
    Scapular stabilizer weakness greater than hip-girdle weakness (applicable in mild to moderate FSHD)
    Autosomal dominant inheritance in familial cases
Exclusion
    Extraocular or pharyngeal muscle weakness
    Prominent and diffuse elbow contractures
    Cardiomyopathy
    Distal symmetric sensory loss
    Dermatomyositic rash or signs of a systemic connective tissue disease
    Muscle biopsy findings suggestive of an alternative diagnosis
    Electromyographic evidence of myotonia or neurogenic potentials
Supportive features
    Asymmetry of muscle weakness
    Descending sequence of involvement
    Early, often partial, abdominal muscle weakness (positive Beevor sign)
    Sparing of deltoid muscles
    Typical shoulder profile: straight clavicles, forward sloping of shoulders
    Relative sparing of neck flexors
    Selective weakness of wrist extensors in distal upper extremities
    Sparing of calf muscles
    High-frequency hearing loss
    Retinal vasculopathy

Source: Produced by the Facioscapulohumeral Consortium at the International Conference on the Cause and Treatment of FSHD, Boston, 1997.

acteristically not affected. Involvement of the pectoralis major gives a characteristic appearance of the axillary folds and flattened chest wall (see Figure 3.1). In the lower limb, the tibialis anterior is particularly affected, leading to footdrop. The involvement is usually bilateral and is typically asymmetric in quantitative terms; strictly symmetric involvement makes the diagnosis suspect.

The establishment of clinical defining features has developed and been refined with the establishment of molecular diagnostic criteria. These have been proposed by members of the Facioscapulohumeral Consortium, an international group of physicians and scientists interested in FSHD. The current clinical diagnostic criteria are shown in Table 3.3 [4]. The extent of muscle involvement among patients is variable and may range from minimal weakness of the face to disability requiring a wheelchair, which eventually occurs in approximately 20% of patients. Life span is not significantly affected. The condition is slowly progressive, and there is an undocumented impression that a stepwise course may be observed.

Most clinical descriptions have been based on cross-sectional studies. Because of the slow progression of the disease over many years, longitudinal studies have only recently been initiated. Baseline measurements compared with a large cohort of control subjects for a prospective natural history study by the FSHD Group demonstrated weakness in muscles not previously considered to be affected in FSHD, including knee extensors and flexors [5]; a major difference in strength between the right and left side of the body, unrelated to handedness, was also demonstrated. (Previous clinical observations had suggested greater involvement of the dominant side in FSHD, attributing the more rapid progression of the disease to mechanical stress on the limb [6].)

FSHD may be associated with retinal abnormalities, in particular retinal telangiectasia, exudation, and detachment (Coats disease) [7], and with sensorineural hearing loss. Coats disease is very rare, but a mild to moderate retinal vasculopathy and high-frequency hearing loss may be found in a higher proportion of FSHD patients [8, 9]. Cardiac muscle is generally considered to be unaffected, but atrial tachyarrhythmias have been reported [10, 11], as have asymptomatic abnormalities on cardiac single photon emission computed tomography [12].

Muscle biopsy shows dystrophic changes, but inflammatory changes have been observed in 40–80% of biopsies. It appears that although the mononuclear cell infiltrates may enhance the muscle fiber damage, T-cell mediated myonecrosis is unlikely, and the inflammatory response observed is different from that in inflammatory myopathies and Duchenne muscular dystrophy [13]. The differential diagnosis includes conditions excluded by other investigations as indicated in Table 3.3; for example, desmin myopathy, polymyositis, inclusion body myositis, mitochondrial myopathy, and congenital myopathies are generally excluded by characteristic histopathologic changes. More difficult are the limb-girdle dystrophies and scapuloperoneal myopathies, which have less specific histologic features and may have mild facial weakness. Sporadic cases of these disorders may be impossible to distinguish from FSHD on clinical and histologic criteria.

Molecular Genetics

The full pathogenic mechanism of disease causation in FSHD is not known, but there has been progress in determining the genetic mechanism. Genetic linkage studies located the genetic defect to the terminal region of chromosome 4 at 4q35 (Figure 3.3) [14]. A subclone, p13E-11, of a cosmid (13E) that hybridized to a homeobox gene in this region was used as a probe. Probe p13E-11 detected small EcoRI digestion fragments in patients with FSHD [15]. The fragments ranged in size from 14 to 28 kb, with the size in control subjects being 30–300 kb. However, these short fragments could also be found in controls, and a family with FSHD and linkage to 4q35 had no small fragment segregating with the disease [16].

The polymorphic EcoRI fragment detected by p13E-11 predominantly comprises a 3.3-kb tandem repeat sequence termed D4Z4, defined by KpnI restriction sites (see Figure 3.3). The variability in fragment size was demonstrated to be due to deletion of an integral number of D4Z4 repeats [17]. Each 3.3-kb D4Z4 repeat contains two homeoboxes (i.e., DNA binding protein domains that regulate developmental gene expression) and two repetitive sequences—LSau and hhspm3—but does not appear to encode a protein [18, 19].

The p13E-11 probe identified two nonallelic loci and a 9.5-kb fragment on the Y chromosome. The nonchromosome 4q35 fragment was assigned to 10qter by linkage analysis [20]. Both alleles give similar fragments with EcoRI digestion. The 4q35 and 10qter fragments sometimes overlap in size and compromise the utility of this as a diagnostic test for FSHD. However, the 10q repeat sequences contain a restriction site for BlnI that is not present on the 4q35 repeat [21]. This leads to complete digestion of the 10q allele on double digestion with EcoRI and BlnI to give fragments of 3.3 kb, but persistence of the 4q allele, allowing a dis-

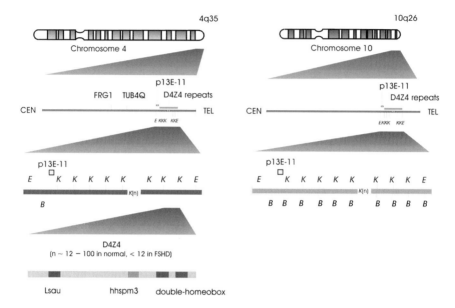

Figure 3.3   Diagrammatic representation of the hierarchical genetic organization of the telomeric regions of chromosomes 4q and 10q. The FRG1 and TUB4Q genes, D4Z4 repeats, and p13E-11 probe are described in the text. In healthy individuals, there are approximately 12–100 copies of D4Z4 on chromosome 4, and fewer than 12 copies in patients with facioscapulohumeral dystrophy. (B = BlnI; E = EcoRI; K = KpnI restriction sites; CEN = centromere; TEL = telomere.) (Reprinted with permission from RW Orrell, R Tawil, J Forrester, et al. Definitive molecular diagnosis of facioscapulohumeral dystrophy. Neurology 1999; 153:1822–1826.)

tinction between these two fragments and an improvement in the diagnostic potential of this technique. There is a single BlnI site on the proximal portion of the chromosome 4 EcoRI fragment proximal to the D4Z4 repeat, leading to a reduction in size of this fragment by approximately 3 kb [21].

These techniques have been applied to FSHD patient populations in several countries. Originally, the size range for the EcoRI fragment in FSHD was reported as 14–28 kb [15, 22], but subsequent refinements of technique, especially the use of pulsed field gel electrophoresis, have shown that larger sizes are associated with FSHD. In our experience, the affected individuals have EcoRI fragments 38 kb or smaller [23, 24], although it appears that occasional patients with clinical appearance of FSHD do not have the small fragment size. In 130 British patients, 94.6% had fragments sized smaller than 34 kb, but 10 patients with presumed or possible FSHD were found to have fragments larger than 48 kb. Four hundred controls had sizes larger than 38 kb [25]. In Taiwan, affected individuals had sizes from 10.5 to 28.0 kb [26]. The present consensus appears to be that a fragment size of 38 kb or smaller is likely to represent FSHD, but a few patients do appear to fall outside this range. Preliminary evidence suggests that a small number of patients with a clinical appearance of FSHD do not have the identified genetic linkage on chromosome 4q, raising the possibility of other genetic loci [27].

In genotyping individuals and families, some individuals appear to be monosomic or trisomic for the 4q35-linked p13E-11 fragment. This has been attributed to subtelomeric exchange of 4q35 and 10q26 regions in affected and unaffected individuals [28]. This is a relatively frequent finding, present in 20% of the general Dutch population. It may lead to some initial confusion in the interpretation of the genotype, but it can be clarified by studying other family members.

As many as 30% of individuals with 4q-linked FSHD have de novo mutations, both parents being unaffected [23, 29]. There is evidence for germ line mosaicism contributing to apparent new mutations [30–32]. In a study of eight patients with FSHD who had unaffected parents, two affected sisters had FSHD [30]. This high rate of de novo mutations is balanced by a reduction in reproductive fitness of FSHD patients. In 34 Brazilian families, one-third with new mutations, biological fitness was reduced to between 0.6 and 0.8, with no difference between males and females [29]. Tawil et al. found the relative fitness of FSHD males was 0.66 when compared with FSHD females [33].

We and other groups have observed that the group of patients with sporadic FSHD—cases in which both parents have been examined and do not have any clinical evidence of the disease and have normal D4Z4 repeat size—have a smaller D4Z4 repeat size than those with a family history of FSHD [29]. A more severe disease progression is associated with a shorter D4Z4 repeat fragment [33, 34].

A careful study of disease progression using quantitative isometric myometry suggested anticipation, with more severe disease in successive generations. However, the D4Z4 repeat number remains stable from generation to generation, and this clinical observation cannot yet be explained at a molecular level [22, 29, 33]. The genetic influence appears to affect disease severity, but not the relative affection of individual muscles, as illustrated by a study of three monozygotic twins with FSHD [35]. Two of the twin pairs had similar degrees of disability and age at onset of symptoms, but there was asymmetry in the involvement of specific muscles. The other pair was discordant in that one of the twins did not exhibit clinical features of FSHD (see Figure 3.2).

The mechanism by which the truncation of the number of D4Z4 repeats causes disease and the responsible gene or genes remain unknown at present. A patient with monosomy of distal 4q, and hence with no D4Z4 repeats, but also missing neighboring genetic components, did not have clinical features of FSHD [36], suggesting that the D4Z4 repeats may be exerting their influence on more proximal regions of the chromosome. Genetic studies suggest that the gene is not within the repeats. It has been proposed that the truncation of the D4Z4 repeats may lead to a phenomenon called *position effect variegation* (PEV), which is observed in heterochromatic regions [37]. PEV is the variable expression of a gene placed adjacent to a junction between euchromatin and heterochromatin, such as the telomeric site of the D4Z4 repeats. Heterochromatinization is the spreading of the heterochromatin into euchromatin to affect the gene expression [37– 40]. It is possible that in FSHD, the D4Z4 repeats act as a barrier to this spread, with truncation of the repeats allowing heterochromatization of proximal chromatin. PEV may exert its effect up to 1 megabase from the site of the genetic mutation, and the search for genes has so far yielded two candidates. There do not appear to be any genes distal to the repeats. FSHD Region Gene 1 (FRG1) is 100 kb proximal to the D4Z4 repeats, but no evidence for PEV-induced alteration of the RNA transcript levels was observed in lymphocytes or muscle biopsies of patients or controls [41]. Tubulin 4q gene (TUB4q) is 80 kb proximal to D4Z4, with 88% homology to β2-tubulin. The β tubulins are subunits of microtubules and potential candidates for FSHD, but the sequence variability and other observations suggest that TUB4q is a pseudogene [42]. Much effort is now being focused on identifying the responsible gene or genes. Additional strategies include studies of the spontaneous mutant myd (myodystrophy) mouse, in which the mutation maps to mouse chromosome 8, which is syntenic with human chromosome 4q [43].

Treatment

No treatment has proved to halt or reverse the progression of muscle wasting and weakness in FSHD. Until the molecular genetic approaches reveal the pathogenesis of the disease—and, we hope, indicate possible therapeutic options—treatment will be based on that of a myopathy. Prednisone has been used in small groups of patients, but a carefully designed pilot study in eight patients for 12 weeks indicated no significant benefit for patients with FSHD [44]. Physical aids may be used, and it has recently been suggested that upper eyelid loading with 24-karat gold implants may correct the eyelid deformity and prevent exposure keratitis [45].

In designing clinical therapeutic trials for a slowly progressive disease, studying the natural history of the disease and determining appropriate measurements for use in carefully designed trials have been necessary. A prospective longitudinal study of the natural history of FSHD by the FSHD Group used quantitative muscle testing (QMT), manual muscle testing (i.e., maximum voluntary isometric contraction testing), and functional testing [46]. The QMT was used to develop regression models relating strength to age, gender, and height in healthy individuals. The QMT in FSHD patients was then expressed as a deviation from this average normal performance. Using a control group as a reference has the advantages of providing a clinically meaningful interpretation, allowing for loss of muscle strength as a result of aging, and being able to use the normative data to study other neuromuscular diseases. Assessment of nine muscle groups, on both sides, takes approximately 1 hour to perform for each patient.

The FSHD Group concluded that using these techniques, a two-armed clinical trial involving 160 patients per group, and a 1-year follow-up would have 80% power to detect complete arrest of the progression of the disease. These strategies were used in a pilot trial of a β-agonist (albuterol) in the treatment of FHSD. Previous evidence suggests an anabolic effect of β-agonists, including muscle hypertrophy. A slow-release preparation of albuterol, 8 mg twice a day, was given for 3 months. A significant increase in lean body mass and muscle strength occurred [47]. A larger, 1-year, double-blind, placebo-controlled trial is being performed in the United States; a similar trial is planned in Holland.

SCAPULOPERONEAL SYNDROME

The status of scapuloperoneal syndrome is not fully defined. Clinical features overlap with FSHD and limb-girdle muscular dystrophies, both of which may include weakness of scapular and peroneal muscles and may now be defined at a molecular level. Historically, some patients with scapuloperoneal syndrome appear to have had a predominant neurogenic cause for the muscle weakness, whereas others have primary myopathy. Davidenkow described patients with scapuloperoneal syndrome and clinical sensory loss [48]. This has since been referred to as *Davidenkow syndrome* [49]. The patients may have pes cavus and depressed reflexes. The sensory and motor nerve conduction is abnormal, indicating a neuropathic disease.

The clinical presentation of scapuloperoneal syndrome is shoulder weakness or footdrop at any time from early childhood to middle age. The pelvic girdle muscles may be affected, and there may be mild facial weakness. Inheritance is usually autosomal dominant, with cases that are autosomal recessive and sporadic being more often neuropathic. The serum creatine kinase (CK) may be normal or mildly elevated. The pathologic findings reflect the variability of primary myopathic or neuropathic disease. The availability of molecular diagnostic testing for FSHD has led to the reclassification of some patients previously diagnosed with scapuloperoneal syndrome as having FSHD. Some of these patients have the milder phenotypes of FSHD, and it will be of interest to determine how many patients presently diagnosed clinically with FSHD but not fulfilling currently agreed-on molecular diagnostic criteria are subsequently shown to have another molecular basis to their myopathy—especially those with only mild facial weakness or scapuloperoneal syndrome.

DISTAL MYOPATHIES

The distal myopathies are clinically defined as primary muscle disorders with progressive muscular weakness and wasting commencing in the hands or feet; usually without abnormalities of cranial nerve innervated muscles, sensory loss, or central nervous system involvement; and with pathologic features of a myopathy [50]. They may be sporadic or hereditary. The distal myopathies are rare, and earlier reports were often insufficient to classify, especially to exclude a neuropathic cause such as one of the hereditary and sensory motor neuropathies, often called *Charcot-Marie-Tooth disease*. At least four distinct syndromes have been defined by clinical, pathologic, and genetic criteria (Table 3.4). The genetic loci are now emerging, and the genes will follow in due course.

Table 3.4 Distal myopathies

Possible entities
    Infantile onset
    Juvenile onset
Definite entities
    Early-adult onset, onset in legs, autosomal recessive
        Type I: Onset in posterior compartment: autosomal recessive distal myopathy;
            (Miyoshi): 2p13 (dysferlin)
        Type II: Onset in anterior compartment: distal myopathy with rimmed vacuole
            formation; (Nonaka): 9
    Late-adult onset, autosomal dominant
        Onset in hands: (Welander)
    Late-adult onset, autosomal dominant
        Onset in legs: tibial muscular dystrophy (TMD; Markesbery-Griggs-Udd): 2q31-33
    MPD1
        Autosomal dominant distal myopathy MPD1;14q11.2-13

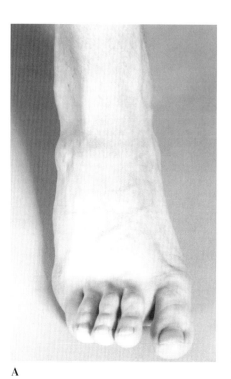
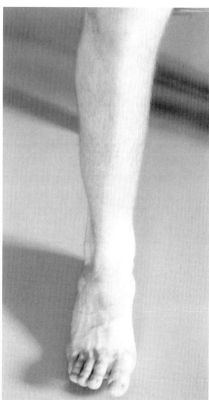

A   B

Figure 3.4   Miyoshi myopathy. (**A**) Distal wasting, posterior greater than anterior compartment. (**B**) Preservation of extensor digitorum brevis bulk and preserved ability to spread the toes.

Autosomal Recessive Distal Muscular Dystrophy (Miyoshi Myopathy)

A number of patients with sporadic or autosomal recessive distal myopathy have been described. Originally, many of the families originated in Japan, and the disease has been termed *Miyoshi myopathy* [51]. An increasing number of patients are being diagnosed in Western countries, many of these being sporadic [52]. The muscle weakness commences in the distal leg, usually in the gastrocnemius muscles, with difficulty climbing stairs or running (Figure 3.4). The most sensitive test is asking the subject to hop on one leg [50]. Hand muscles may also be affected. The lower limb reflexes are usually intact but may be absent in some patients. The weakness may be asymmetric in approximately 50% of patients [52]. The disease is progressive and may later involve knee extensors and shoulder and upper arm muscles (Figure 3.5). In a study of 24 Dutch patients, one-third of the patients were dependent on a wheelchair for transport out of the house at 10 years of disease duration [52].

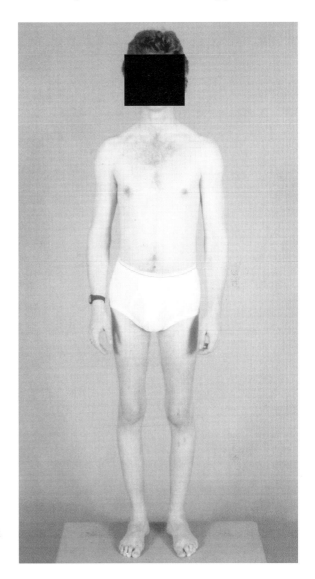

Figure 3.5 Miyoshi myopathy: Patient has severe posterior compartment leg and moderate proximal arm weakness.

Serum CK is strikingly elevated (10–150 times normal), and some asymptomatic patients have initially been diagnosed as idiopathic hyperCKemia [52]. Muscle biopsy shows dystrophic features, but features suggestive of active denervation may also be observed. Electromyography (EMG) findings supportive of active denervation may also be present.

The gene for ARDMD (Miyoshi myopathy) is mapped to chromosome 2p13 [53]. A form of autosomal recessive limb girdle muscular dystrophy, LGMD2B, also maps to this region, and the conditions are allelic. Limb-girdle muscular dystrophy and Miyoshi myopathy mapping to LGMD2B have been reported to occur in the same family [54]. Mutations of a gene in this region have been identified in both Miyoshi myopathy and LGMD2B. This gene has been termed *dysferlin*, as the predicted protein dysferlin, expressed in skeletal muscle, is homologous to the *Caenorhabditis elegans* protein fer-1 [55, 56].

Distal Myopathy with Rimmed Vacuole Formation (Nonaka Myopathy)

Nonaka et al. described an autosomal recessive familial distal myopathy with rimmed vacuole and lamellar body formation (DMRV) [57]. The onset is in the distal legs, affecting the tibialis anterior muscle and presenting with footdrop. (In Miyoshi myopathy—ARDMD—the onset is usually, but not invariably, in the gastrocnemius muscle.) The intrinsic foot muscles may be involved.

Serum CK is normal or slightly elevated. The muscle biopsy features are characteristic, including rimmed vacuoles on Gomori trichrome staining and eosinophilic inclusion bodies in muscle fibers. The vacuolated muscle fibers contain accumulations of amyloid beta protein and hyperphosphorylated tau protein. There is no evidence of inflammatory changes. However, similar pathologic features are present in inclusion body myositis—even though inflammatory changes are present here—the familial forms of which may be termed hereditary inclusion body myopathies (HIBM). An autosomal recessive myopathy in Persian Jews—with progressive distal and proximal muscle weakness but sparing the quadriceps—which shows these histopathologic features has been considered to be an HIBM, and the gene was mapped to chromosome 9p1-q1 [58]. Studies in seven families with DMRV have demonstrated linkage to a similar region on chromosome 9, suggesting that DMRV is allelic to HIBM in Persian Jews [59].

Welander Distal Myopathy

Welander described an autosomal dominant myopathy in patients of Scandinavian descent, especially Swedish [60]. This is the most common distal myopathy. Initial presentation is weakness and wasting of the small muscles of the hands causing difficulty with fine hand movements—fastening buttons, for example—often beginning in the thumb and index finger. The distal leg extensors may be affected next (the distal flexors may also be affected), with difficulty walking, inability to stand on the heels, or footdrop. Proximal limb muscle weakness may be present in some patients. Onset is generally from age 20 years to old age.

Muscle biopsy and EMG show myopathic features, but more recent studies have demonstrated distal sensory disturbance [61] and muscle biopsy and EMG features suggestive of a neurogenic component. Rimmed vacuoles and cytoplasmic (13–17 nm) and intranuclear (16–21 nm) tubulofilamentous inclusions may be found. The gene has not yet been identified, but loci of other distal myopathies on chromosomes 2, 9, and 14 have been excluded [62]. There is work suggesting that the exclusion of chromosome 14 was in error and that the disorder is at the locus assigned to Gowers distal myopathy (T. Voit, M.D., personal communication, 1998).

Tibial Muscular Dystrophy

Udd et al. described 66 patients with an autosomal dominant, late adult–onset distal myopathy concentrated in two regions of Finland [63]. The weakness selectively involves the tibialis anterior and later the long toe extensor muscles (but extensor digitorum brevis is spared), with onset from age 35 years. Life span is generally not affected, and patients remain independently mobile, although they may require a walking aid.

Serum CK is normal or mildly elevated. Muscle biopsy shows dystrophic changes, and rimmed vacuoles containing occasional tubulofilamentous inclusions may be seen.

A similar late adult–onset distal myopathy was described by Markesbery et al. in a single family [64]. In these patients, the weakness spread to involve intrinsic hand and wrist extensors and, eventually, proximal limb and trunk muscles.

Linkage has been demonstrated in families from Finland at chromosome 2q31-33 [65]. The haplotyping suggests one common ancestor for the mutation in Finland. In a family with consanguinity, the homozygous individuals had a more severe muscular dystrophy [65]. The family described by Markesbery et al. appears to be allelic [66].

Autosomal Dominant Distal Myopathy, MPD1

A single family with autosomal dominant distal myopathy of British ancestry is reported by Laing et al. [67]. Patients have selective weakness of toe and ankle extensor, and sternomastoids, followed by progressive weakness of finger extensors. Otherwise, there is relative sparing of hand and forearm muscles. Proximal muscles may be mildly affected. Age at onset is 4–25 years. Serum CK is mildly elevated, and muscle biopsy and EMG show myopathic features. Linkage for the MPD1 locus has been demonstrated at chromosome 14q11.2-13 [67, 68]. Initially considered distinct from the other four distal myopathies, this disorder appears to be allelic with Welander distal myopathy (T. Voit, M.D., personal communication, 1998).

BETHLEM MYOPATHY

Bethlem myopathy is a rare autosomal dominant myopathy [69]. The clinical features include slowly progressive limb-girdle weakness from childhood onward, with periods of arrest for several decades; flexion contractures of fingers, elbows, and ankles; and absence of cardiac involvement (Figure 3.6). The muscle weakness and atrophy are generally mild, with extensors weaker than flexors and facial muscles unaffected. The flexion contractures especially affect the interphalangeal joints of the index to little fingers, the elbows, and the ankles, but may also affect metacarpophalangeal joints, wrists, knees, hips, shoulders, and neck. The condition is generally benign. It was first described in three unrelated Dutch families in 1976 [70]; subsequently, similar features have been recognized in many families in other parts of the world. It differs from other myopathies with contractures in that Bethlem myopathy does not have the cardiac involvement found

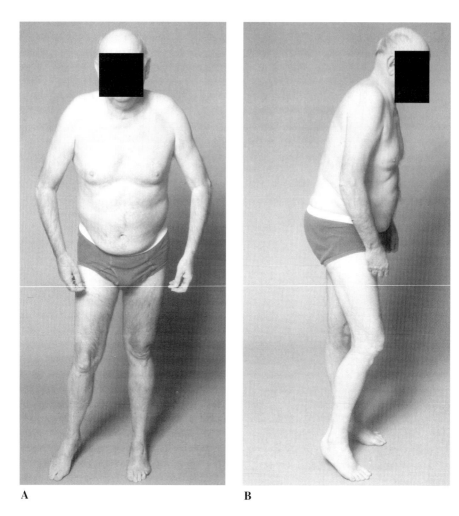

A   B

Figure 3.6   Bethlem myopathy. (**A**) Front view of patient showing elbow contractures. (**B**) Lateral view showing the typical posture and knee contractures.

in Emery-Dreifuss muscular dystrophy. Also, Bethlem myopathy is autosomal dominant, whereas the inheritance of Emery-Dreifuss is generally X-linked. The rigid spine syndrome also has contractures but seldom has a family history.

Serum CK is normal or slightly elevated in Bethlem myopathy. EMG shows myopathic features. Muscle biopsy, including electronmicroscopy, shows only nonspecific myopathic features without the extensive necrosis and regeneration of muscle fibers seen in most muscular dystrophies.

Bethlem myopathy has been demonstrated to be due to a type VI collagen disorder in several families [71]. Nine Dutch families were linked to 21q22.3, the site of COL6A1 and COL6A2, and one French Canadian family to 2q37, the site of COL6A3. COL6A1–3 are the genes for the α1–3 subunits of type VI collagen. In the Dutch families, a heterozygous missense mutation was present in one family in COL6A1, and a similar type of mutation present in two families in COL6A2. Both mutations disrupt the Gly-X-Y motif of the triple helical domain by substitution of Gly for Val or Ser. Disruption of the triple helix motif is also found in other collagen disorders (i.e., osteogenesis imperfecta [COL1A1, COL1A2], Ehlers-Danlos syndrome [COL1A1, COL1A2, COL3A1], X-linked Alport syndrome [COL4A5], and autosomal recessive Alport syndrome [COL4A3, COL4A4]). Type VI collagen is present in most tissues, including skeletal muscle endomysium and perimysium. The disruption of the triple helix motif may affect proteolytic cleavage, post-translational processing, collagen monomer formation, and assembly of large multimers. Jobsis et al. propose that the disease mechanism involves either abnormal myoblast differentiation or disturbed extracellular matrix organization [71]. In a family of French Canadian origin, the disease was not linked to 21q but to 2q, where the COL6A3 (α3 subunit of Type IV collagen gene) is located [72].

EMERY-DREIFUSS MUSCULAR DYSTROPHY

Emery-Dreifuss muscular dystrophy (EDMD) is an X-linked disorder, characterized by slowly progressive wasting and weakness of the scapulohumeral and anterior tibial and peroneal muscle groups [73]. A similar syndrome may occasionally be inherited in autosomal dominant or recessive forms. There is no pseudohypertrophy. Muscle contractures develop early—before significant muscle weakness—in the elbows, Achilles tendons, and posterior cervical muscles, resulting in a typical appearance of elbow flexion, equinovarus ankle deformity, and limited neck flexion (Figure 3.7). Cardiomyopathy with conduction defects is common. Unlike Duchenne dystrophy, there is no intellectual impairment. Onset is usually at approximately age 4 years, with variable severity within a family.

Serum CK is variable, ranging from normal to elevated 10-fold. EMG and muscle biopsy show myopathic features. Carrier females may manifest clinical features of myopathy and may also develop cardiac arrhythmias with sudden death when skeletal muscle weakness is not yet apparent. Carrier detection is therefore important, providing opportunity for detection and treatment of cardiac disorders. Heart block is a common cause of death, and regular cardiac assessment allows appropriate insertion of a cardiac pacemaker. Active and passive muscle stretching may delay the development of muscle contractures.

The gene was mapped to Xq28 [74]. Lack of emerin in cardiac and skeletal muscle has been shown to cause a significant proportion of EDMD. The EDMD gene is approximately 2,100 base pairs with 6 small exons [75, 76]. It encodes the protein emerin, which comprises 254 amino acids, with a 20 amino acid hydrophobic domain at the carboxy terminus (which is similar to that found in other membrane proteins of the secretory pathway involved in vesicular transport). Mutations in the EDMD gene have been demonstrated in patients and families with EDMD [76–78]. These mutations are generally unique. They include point mutations, small deletions or insertions, or are in the region of splice junctions interfering with messenger RNA (mRNA) splicing, all of which

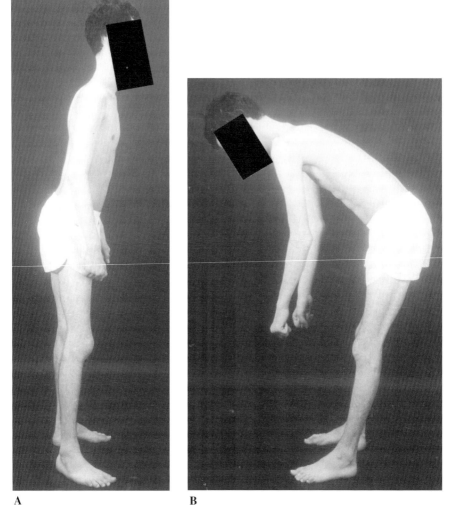

A   B

Figure 3.7   (**A**) A young man with Emery-Dreifuss muscular dystrophy (emerin negative on immunostaining) demonstrating fixed flexion posture, especially at the elbows. (**B**) There is limited flexion of the spine, with contractures especially of the posterior cervical muscles. (Courtesy of Professor Francesco Muntoni, Hammersmith Hospital, London, England.)

create premature stop codons and result in a truncated protein. Emerin is ubiquitously expressed. It is normally localized to the nuclear membrane; in its mutant form, it appears to have a more random distribution in the cell and is abnormally phosphorylated by cell cycle mediated events [79]. Mutations have not been found in all patients—familial and sporadic—and possibly other genes cause a similar phenotype [76–78]. Some patients previously described as having scapuloperoneal syndrome or rigid spine syndrome may in fact have EDMD.

OCULOPHARYNGEAL MUSCULAR DYSTROPHY

Oculopharyngeal muscular dystrophy (OPMD) affects ocular and pharyngeal muscles, causing ptosis, dysphagia, and dysarthria, but may also affect other limb-girdle and distal limb muscles [80, 81]. Levator palpebrae muscles are usually affected first, with onset in middle age, but may occur earlier. Inheritance is autosomal dominant with complete penetrance, but with variable expression. The muscle weakness progresses slowly and is rarely disabling, although ptosis may obstruct vision, and dysphagia may lead to weight loss, inanition, and death unless treated [82].

Muscle biopsy shows myopathic features with rimmed vacuoles frequently seen; these vacuoles contain myelin figures and cell debris. Intranuclear filaments may be seen on electronmicroscopy [83]. OPMD was first recognized in French Canadians, in whom the frequency of the mutation is estimated at 1 in 8,000 individuals in the Province of Quebec. The frequency in France is estimated to be much lower, at 1 in 200,000. A single founder chromosome is proposed to have been introduced to the French Canadians in 1648 [84].

Linkage for OPMD was demonstrated on chromosome 14q11 [80]. A short GCG repeat expansion has been demonstrated in the PABP2 gene (poly[A] binding protein 2) in 144 families studied [84]. In a control population of French Canadians, 98% had six GCG repeats ([GCG]6), and 2% had a polymorphism (GCG)7. The expanded alleles in OPMD ranged from eight to 13 repeats. When the severity of OPMD was assessed by the time taken to swallow 80 ml of ice-cold water, patients who were homozygous for (GCG)9 and compound heterozygotes (GCG)9 (GCG)7 had a more severe phenotype. Patients homozygote for (GCG)7 may also have a mild phenotype, presenting as apparent autosomal recessive inheritance. Unlike the previous repeat expansions recognized in neurologic disorders, these expansions are short and stable, with only a single increase from (GCG)9 to (GCG)12 observed in 70 French Canadian families.

The PABP2 gene has six exons and 6,002 base pairs, the GCG repeat being in the N terminal region of exon 1. PABP2 mRNA is highly expressed in skeletal muscle, and PABP2 protein is found exclusively in the nucleus, where it is involved in mRNA polyadenylation. The normal (GCG)6 repeat encodes the first six alanine residues of a homopolymeric stretch of 10 alanine residues (i.e., there are 10 alanine in [GCG]6 and 13 in [GCG]9).

The function of the polyalanine tract is not known, but attempts will be made to reconcile this with the observation of nuclear filament inclusions in three of the CAG repeat diseases (Huntington Disease, SCA1, and SCA2). The polyalanine may play a role in polymerization, possibly forming β sheet structures and being resistant to degradation [84].

BARTH SYNDROME

Barth syndrome is an X-linked disorder with features of skeletal myopathy and cardiomyopathy, short stature, and neutropenia [85]. Most patients have increased 3-methylglutaconicaciduria and low blood cholesterol levels. There is weakness of skeletal muscles, but sparing of extraocular and bulbar muscles. Abnormal mitochondria are found in many tissues, including muscle. It presents in infants (boys) and is often fatal in childhood because of cardiac failure or sepsis. Linkage studies in two large families localized the gene to distal Xq28 [86, 87].

Mutations in the G4.5 gene were found in patients with Barth syndrome [88]. The G4.5 gene comprises 11 exons. There is differential splicing of exons 5, 6, and 7, producing five different mRNAs, and there are two different 5' ends, giving up to 10 mRNAs. The translated proteins have been called *tafazzins*, which may be present in different amounts in different tissues and have no known similarity to other proteins. The proteins range from 129 to 292 amino acids. The mutations found in Barth syndrome, segregating with the disease and not found in the general population, are single base changes (substitution, deletion, or insertion) at the splice junction or generating stop codons; they interrupt translation of the tafazzins [88]. A study of patients from 14 families with Barth syndrome did not demonstrate a correlation between the type or site of mutation and clinical features [89].

EPIDERMOLYSIS BULLOSA SIMPLEX WITH LATE-ONSET MUSCULAR DYSTROPHY

Epidermolysis bullosa simplex with late-onset muscular dystrophy (EB-MD) is an autosomal recessive variant of epidermolysis bullosa, in which chronic skin blistering is associated with progressive muscular dystrophy. The blistering is usually present at birth, and the muscular dystrophy may manifest from early childhood to adult life. The muscle weakness usually presents in adult life, and there may be widespread muscular atrophy and ptosis. There may be possibly more extensive neurodegeneration in later life, with extensive cerebral and cerebellar atrophy documented in a 33-year-old patient [90]. The limb weakness is progressive and may lead to disability requiring a wheelchair.

The muscle biopsy shows myopathic features, the most striking finding being ultrastructural disorganization of myofibrils and sarcomeres (and absent staining with antibodies to plectin). In the skin, tissue separation—epidermis from underlying dermis—occurs within the basal keratinocytes at the level of the hemidesmosomal inner plaque, where the high–molecular weight cytomatrix protein plectin is expressed [91].

Deficiency of plectin is the cause of EB-MD [90]. The PLEC1 gene is on chromosome 8q24.13ter. Homozygous mutations have been described in a number of patients with EB-MD, including small insertion and deletion mutations leading to premature stop codons. Compound heterozygous mutations are also found [92]. PLEC1 encodes the cytoskeletal plectin protein, which is widely distributed through stratified squamous epithelium, muscle, and brain. Plectin is a hemidesmosome (i.e., the complexes that anchor the basal cells of squamous and transitional epithelia to the underlying mesenchyme). Plectin and HD1 immunofluorescence staining of skin and muscle is absent in affected patients. Plectin, desmin, and HD1 colocalize to the Z disks of myofibrils. Plectin and HD1 are probably the same or closely related proteins. HD1 is absent from the Z disks in EB-MD. Impaired plectin expression in muscle correlates with altered expression of muscle intermediate filament protein desmin, and desmin is abnormally located at the periphery of muscle fibers, suggesting a defective anchorage of the intermediate filament cytoskeleton. It is proposed that plectin could function as a cytoskeletal membrane attachment protein in muscle, possibly mediating the binding of muscle proteins, such as actin, to membrane complexes, similar to its function in skin. The deficiency of plectin may therefore lead to impaired anchorage of the cytoskeleton to the plasma membrane and result in cell fragility or myopathy [93].

REFERENCES

1. Kaplan JC, Fontaine B. Neuromuscular disorders: gene location. Neuromuscul Disord 1998;8:I–VII.
2. Kazakov VM. History of the recognition and description of the facioscapulohumeral muscular dystrophy (FSHD) and on the priorities of Duchenne, Erb, Landouzy and Dejerine. Acta Cardiomiologica 1995;7:79–94.
3. Lunt PW, Compston DAS, Harper PS. Estimation of age dependent penetrance in facioscapulohumeral muscular dystrophy by minimising ascertainment bias. J Med Genet 1989;26:755–760.
4. Tawil R, Figlewicz DA, Griggs RC, et al. Facioscapulohumeral muscular dystrophy: a distinct regional myopathy with a novel molecular pathogenesis. Ann Neurol 1998;43:279–282.
5. Tawil R, McDermott MP, Mendell JR, et al. Facioscapulohumeral muscular dystrophy (FSHD): design of natural history study and results of baseline testing. Neurology 1994;44:442–446.
6. Brouwer OF, Padberg GW, van der Ploeg RJO, et al. The influence of handedness on the distribution of muscular weakness of the arm in facioscapulohumeral muscular dystrophy. Brain 1992;115:1587–1598.
7. Taylor DA, Carroll JE, Smith ME, et al. Facioscapulohumeral dystrophy associated with hearing loss and Coats syndrome. Ann Neurol 1982;12:395–398.
8. Padberg GW, Brouwer OF, deKeizer RJW, et al. On the significance of retinal vascular disease and hearing loss in facioscapulohumeral muscular dystrophy. Muscle Nerve 1995;(suppl 2):S73–S80.
9. Brouwer OF, Padberg GW, Ruys CJM, et al. Hearing loss in facioscapulohumeral muscular dystrophy. Neurology 1991;41:1878–1881.
10. Stevenson WG, Perloff JK, Weiss JN, Anderson TL. Facioscapulohumeral dystrophy: evidence for selective genetic electrophysiologic cardiac involvement. J Am Coll Cardiol 1990;15:292–299.
11. DeVisser M, DeVoogt GW, La Riviere GV. The heart in Becker muscular dystrophy, facioscapulohumeral muscular dystrophy and Bethlem myopathy. Muscle Nerve 1992;15:591–596.
12. Faustmann PM, Farahati J, Rupilius B, et al. Cardiac involvement in facio-scapulo-humeral muscular dystrophy: a family study using Thallium-201 single-photon-emission-computed tomography. J Neurol Sci 1996;144:59–63.
13. Arahata K, Ishihara T, Fukunaga H, et al. Inflammatory response in facioscapulohumeral muscular dystrophy (FSHD): immunocytochemical and genetic analyses. Muscle Nerve 1995;(suppl 2):S56–S66.
14. Wijmenga C, Frants RR, Brouwer OF, et al. Location of facioscapulohumeral muscular dystrophy gene on chromosome 4. Lancet 1990;336:651–653.
15. Wijmenga C, Hewitt JE, Sandkuijl LA, et al. Chromosome 4q DNA rearrangements associated with facioscapulohumeral muscular dystrophy. Nat Genet 1992;2:26–30.
16. Weiffenbach B, Dubois J, Storvick D, et al. Mapping the facioscapulohumeral muscular dystrophy gene is complicated by chromosome 4q35 recombination events. Nat Genet 1993;4:165–169.
17. van Deutekom JCT, Wijmenta C, van Tienhoven EAE, et al. FSHD associated DNA rearrangements are due to deletions of integral copies of a 3.2 kb tandemly repeated unit. Hum Mol Genet 1993;2:2037–2042.
18. Hewitt JE, Lyle R, Clark LN, et al. Analysis of the tandem repeat locus D4Z4 associated with facioscapulohumeral muscular dystrophy. Hum Mol Genet 1994;3:1287–1295.
19. Lyle R, Wright TJ, Clark LN, Hewitt JE. The FSHD-associated repeat, D4Z4, is a member of a dispersed family of homeobox-containing repeats, subsets of which are clustered on the short arms of the acrocentric chromosomes. Genomics 1995;28:389–397.
20. Bakker E, Wijmenga C, Vossen RHAM, et al. The FSHD-linked locus D4F104S1 (p13E-11) on 4q35 has a homologue on 10qter. Muscle Nerve 1995;(suppl 2):S39–S44.
21. Deidda G, Cacurri S, Piazzo N, Felicetti L. Direct detection of 4q35 rearrangements implicated in facioscapulohumeral muscular dystrophy (FSHD). J Med Genet 1996;33:361–365.
22 Goto K, Lee JH, Matsuda, et al. DNA rearrangements in Japanese facioscapulohumeral muscular dystrophy patients: clinical correlations. Neuromuscul Disord 1995;5:201 208.

23. Orrell RW, Forrester JD, Tawil R, et al. Application of definitive molecular diagnostic criteria in facioscapulohumeral dystrophy: clinical implications of position effect variegation (abstract). Ann Neurol 1997;42:986.
24. Orrell RW, Tawil R, Forrester J, et al. Definitive molecular diagnosis of facioscapulohumeral dystrophy. Neurology 1999;153:1822–1826.
25. Upadhyaya M, Maynard J, Rogers MT, et al. Improved molecular diagnosis of facioscapulohumeral muscular dystrophy (FSHD): validation of the differential double digestion for FSHD. J Med Genet 1997;34:476–479.
26. Hsu YD, Kao MC, Shyu WC, et al. Application of chromosome 4q35qter marker (pFR-1) for DNA rearrangement of facioscapulohumeral muscular dystrophy patients in Taiwan. J Neurol Sci 1997;149:73–79.
27. Gilbert JR, Stajich JM, Wall S, et al. Evidence for heterogeneity in facioscapulohumeral muscular dystrophy (FSHD). Am J Hum Genet 1993;53:401–408.
28. van Deutekom JCT, Bakker E, Lemmers RJLF, et al. Evidence for subtelomeric exchange of 3.3 kb tandemly repeated units between chromosomes 4q35 and 10q26: implications for genetic counselling and etiology of FSHD1. Hum Mol Genet 1996;5:1997–2003.
29. Zatz M, Marie SK, Passos-Bueno MR, et al. High proportion of new mutations and possible anticipation in Brazilian facioscapulohumeral muscular dystrophy families. Am J Hum Genet 1995;56:99–105.
30. Griggs RC, Tawil R, Storvick D, et al. Genetics of facioscapulohumeral muscular dystrophy: new mutations in sporadic cases. Neurology 1993;43:2369–2372.
31. Upadhaya M, Maynard J, Osborn M, et al. Germinal mosaicism in facioscapulohumeral muscular dystrophy (FSHD). Muscle Nerve 1995;(suppl 2):S45–S49.
32. Kohler J, Rupilius B, Otto M, et al. Germline mosaicism in 4q35 facioscapulohumeral muscular dystrophy occurring predominantly in oogenesis. Hum Genet 1996;98:485–490.
33. Tawil R, Forrester J, Griggs RC, et al. Evidence for anticipation and association of deletion size with severity in facioscapulohumeral muscular dystrophy. Ann Neurol 1996;39:744–748.
34. Lunt PW, Jardine PE, Koch M, et al. Phenotypic-genotypic correlation will assist genetic counseling in 4q35-facioscapulohumeral muscular dystrophy. Muscle Nerve 1995;(suppl 2):S103–S109.
35. Griggs RC, Tawil R, McDermott M, et al. Monozygotic twins with facioscapulohumeral dystrophy (FSHD): implications for genotype/phenotype correlation. Muscle Nerve 1995;(suppl 2):S50–S55.
36. Tupler R, Berardinelli A, Barbierato L, et al. Monosomy of distal 4q does not cause facioscapulohumeral muscular dystrophy. J Med Genet 1996;33:366–370.
37. Winokur ST, Bengtsson U, Feddersen J, et al. The DNA rearrangement associated with facioscapulohumeral muscular dystrophy involves a heterochromatin-associated repetitive element: implications for a role of chromatin structure in the pathogenesis of the disease. Chromosome Res 1994;2:225–234.
38. Henikoff S. Position-effect variegation after 60 years. Trends Genet 1990;6:422–426.
39. Henikoff S. A reconsideration of the mechanism of position effect. Genetics 1994;138:15.
40. Wakimoto BT. Beyond the nucleosome: epigenetic aspects of position-effect variegation in Drosophila. Cell 1998;93:321–324.
41. van Deutekom JCT, Lemmers RJLF, Grewal PK, et al. Identification of the first gene (FRG1) from the FSHD region on human chromosome 4q35. Hum Mol Genet 1996;5:581–590.
42. van Deutekom J. Towards the molecular mechanism of facioscapulohumeral muscular dystrophy [thesis]. Leiden, the Netherlands: University of Leiden, 1996.
43. Grewal PK, van Deutekom JCT, Mills KA, et al. The mouse homolog of FRG1, a candidate gene for FSHD, maps proximal to the myodystrophy mutation on Chromosome 8. Mamm Genome 1997;8:394–398.
44. Tawil R, McDermott MP, Pandya S, et al. A pilot trial of prednisone in facioscapulohumeral muscular dystrophy. Neurology 1997;48:46–49.
45. Sansone V, Boynton J, Palenski C. Use of gold weights to correct lagophthalmos in neuromuscular disease. Neurology 1997;48:1500–1503.
46. The FSH-DY Group. A prospective, quantitative study of the natural history of facioscapulohumeral muscular dystrophy (FSHD): implications for therapeutic trials. Neurology 1997;48:3846.
47. Kissel JT, McDermott MP, Natarajan R, et al. Pilot trial of albuterol in facioscapulohumeral muscular dystrophy. Neurology 1998;50:1402–1406.
48. Davidenkow S. Scapuloperoneal amyotrophy. Arch Neurol 1939;41:694–701.
49. Schwartz MS, Swash M. Scapuloperoneal atrophy with sensory involvement: Davidenkow's syndrome. J Neurol Neurosurg Psychiatry 1975;38:1063–1067.

50. Griggs RC, Markesbery WR. Distal Myopathies. In AG Engel, C Franzini-Armstrong (eds), Myology. New York: McGraw-Hill, 1994;1246–1257.
51. Miyoshi K, Iwasa M, Kawai H, et al. Autosomal recessive distal muscular dystrophy: a new variety of distal muscular dystrophy predominantly seen in Japan. Nippon Rinsho 1977;35:3922–3928.
52. Linssen WHJP, Notermans NC, Van der Graaf Y, et al. Miyoshi-type distal muscular dystrophy. Clinical spectrum in 24 Dutch patients. Brain 1997;120:1989–1996.
53. Illarioshkin SN, Ivanova-Smolenskaya IA, Tanaka H, et al. Refined genetic location of the chromosome 2p-linked progressive muscular dystrophy gene. Genomics 1997;42:345–348.
54. Weiler T, Greenberg CR, Nylen E, et al. Limb-girdle muscular dystrophy and Miyoshi myopathy in an aboriginal Canadian kindred map to LGMD2B and segregate with the same haplotype. Am J Hum Genet 1996;59:872–878.
55. Liu J, Aoki M, Illa I, et al. Dysferlin, a novel skeletal muscle gene, is mutated in Miyoshi myopathy and limb girdle dystrophy. Nat Genet 1998;20:31–36.
56. Bashir R, Britton S, Strachan T, et al. A gene related to *Caenorhabditis elegans* spermatogenesis factor fer-1 is mutated in limb-girdle muscular dystrophy type 2B. Nat Genet 1998;20:37–42.
57. Nonaka I, Sunohara N, Ihiura S, Satoyoshi E. Familial distal myopathy with rimmed vacuole and lamellar (myeloid) body formation. J Neurol Sci 1981;51:141–155.
58. Mitrani-Rosenbaum S, Argov Z, Blumenfeld A, et al. Hereditary inclusion body myopathy maps to chromosome 9p1-q1. Hum Mol Genet 1996;5:159–163.
59. Ikeuchi T, Asaka T, Saito M, et al. Gene locus for autosomal recessive distal myopathy with rimmed vacuoles maps to chromosome 9. Ann Neurol 1997;41:432–437.
60. Welander L. Myopathia distalis tarda hereditaria. Acta Med Scand 1951;141(suppl 265):1124.
61. Borg K, Ahlberg G, Borg J, Edstrom L. Welander's distal myopathy: clinical, neurophysiological and muscle biopsy observations in young and middle aged adults with early symptoms. J Neurol Neurosurg Psychiatry 1991;54:494–498.
62. Ahlberg G, Norg K, Edstrom L, Anvert M. Welander distal myopathy is not linked to other defined distal myopathy gene loci. Neuromuscul Disord 1997;7:256–260.
63. Udd B, Partanen J, Halonen P, et al. Tibial muscular dystrophy. Late adult-onset distal myopathy in 66 Finnish patients. Arch Neurol 1993;50:604–608.
64. Markesbery WR, Griggs RC, Leach RP, Lapham LW. Late onset hereditary distal myopathy. Neurology 1974;23:127.
65. Haravuori H, Makela-Bengs P, Udd B, et al. Linkage in tibial muscular dystrophy (TMD) on chromosome 2q31-33 [abstract]. Neuromuscul Disord 1997;7:459.
66. Haravuori H, Makela-Bengs P, Figlewicz DA, et al. Tibial muscular dystrophy and late-onset dital myopathy are linked to the same locus on chromosome 2q. Neurology 1998;40:A186.
67. Laing NG, Laing BA, Meredith C, et al. Autosomal dominant distal myopathy: linkage to chromosome 14. Am J Hum Genet 1995;56:422–427.
68. Binz N, Nowak K, Butler A, et al. Refinement of the distal myopathy MPD1 and exclusion of candidate genes [abstract]. Neuromuscul Disord 1997;7:460.
69. Jobsis GJ, Visser M. Bethlem Myopathy. In RJM Lane (ed), Handbook of Muscle Disease. New York: Marcel Dekker, 1996;159–163.
70. Bethlem J, van Wijngaarden GK. Benign myopathy, with autosomal dominant inheritance: a report on three pedigrees. Brain 1976;99:91–100.
71. Jobsis GJ, Keizers H, Vreijling, et al. Type VI collagen mutations in Bethlem myopathy, an autosomal dominant myopathy with contractures. Nat Genet 1996;113–115.
72. Speer MC, Tandan R, Rao PN, et al. Evidence for locus heterogeneity in the Bethlem myopathy and linkage to 2q37. Hum Mol Genet 1996;5:1043–1046.
73. Mastaglia FL, Kakulas BA. X-linked dystrophies: clinical and pathological features. In RJM Lane (ed), Handbook of Muscle Disease. New York: Marcel Dekker, 1996;201–221.
74. Gonzales GG, Thomas NST, Stayton CL, et al. Assignment of Emery-Dreifuss muscular dystrophy to the distal region of Xq28: the results of a collaborative study. Am J Hum Genet 1991;48:468–480.
75. Bione S, Maestrini E, Rivella S, et al. Identification of a novel X-linked gene responsible for Emery-Dreifuss muscular dystrophy. Nat Genet 1994;8:323–327.
76. Bione S, Small K, Aksamonvic VMA, et al. Identification of new mutations in the Emery-Dreifuss muscular dystrophy gene and evidence for genetic heterogeneity of the disease. Hum Mol Genet 1995;4:1859–1863.
77. Klauck SM, Wilgenbus P, Yates JRW, et al. Identification of novel mutations in three families with Emery-Dreifuss muscular dystrophy. Hum Mol Genet 1995;4:1853–1857.

78. Nigro V, Bruni P, Ciccodicola A, et al. SSCP detection of novel mutations in patients with Emery-Dreifuss muscular dystrophy: definition of a small C-terminal region required for emerin function. Hum Mol Genet 1995;4:2003–2004.
79. Ellis J, Craxton M, Yates J, Kendrick-Jones J. Aberrant intracellular targeting and cell cycle-dependent phosphorylation of emerin contribute to the Emery-Dreifuss muscular dystrophy phenotype. J Cell Sci 1998;111:781–792.
80. Brais B, Xie YG, Sanson M, et al. The oculopharyngeal muscular dystrophy locus maps to the region of the cardiac α and β myosin heavy chain genes on chromosome 14q11.2-q13. Hum Mol Genet 1995;4:429–434.
81. Schmalbruch H. Other Dystrophies with Autosomal Dominant Inheritance. In RJM Lane (ed), Handbook of Muscle Disease. New York: Marcel Dekker, 1996;297–309.
82. Victor M, Hayes R, Adams RD. Oculopharyngeal muscular dystrophy: familial disease of late life characterized by dysphagia and progressive ptosis of the eyelids. N Engl J Med 1962;267:1267–1272.
83. Tome F, Fardeau M. Nuclear inclusions in oculopharyngeal muscular dystrophy. Acta Neuropathol (Berl) 1980;49:85–87.
84. Brais B, Bouchard J, Xie Y, et al. Short GCG expansions in the PABP2 gene cause oculopharyngeal muscular dystrophy. Nat Genet 1998;18:164–167.
85. Barth PG, Scholte HR, Berden JA, et al. An X-linked mitochondrial disease affecting cardiac muscle, skeletal muscle and neutrophil leucocytes. J Neurol Sci 1983;62:327–355.
86. Bolhuis PA, Hensels PA, Hulsebos TJM, et al. Mapping of the locus for X-linked cardioskeletal myopathy with neutropenia and abnormal mitochondria (Barth syndrome) to distal Xq28. Am J Hum Genet 1991;48:481–485.
87. Ades LC, Gedeon AK, Wilson MJ, et al. Barth syndrome: clinical features and confirmation of gene localisation to distal Xq28. Am J Med Genet 1993;45:327–334.
88. Bione S, D'Adamo P, Maestrini E, et al. A novel X-linked gene, G4.5 is responsible for Barth syndrome. Nat Genet 1996;12:385–389.
89. Johnston J, Kelley RI, Feigenbaum A, et al. Mutation characterization and genotype-phenotype correlation in Barth syndrome. Am J Hum Genet 1997;61:1053–1058.
90. Smith FJD, Eady RAJ, Leigh IM, et al. Plectin deficiency results in muscular dystrophy with epidermolysis bullosa. Nat Genet 1996;13:450–457.
91. Pulkkinen L, Smith FJD, Shimizu, et al. Homozygous deletion mutations in the plectin gene (PLEC1) in patients with epidermolysis bullosa simplex associated with late-onset muscular dystrophy. Hum Mol Genet 1996;5:1539–1546.
92. Dang M, Pulkkinen L, Smith FJD, et al. Novel compound heterozygous mutations in the plectin gene in epidermolysis bullosa with muscular dystrophy and the use of protein truncation test for detection of premature termination codon mutations. Lab Invest 1998;78:195–204.
93. Gache Y, Chavanas S, Lacour JP, et al. Defective expression of plectin/HD1 in epidermolysis bullosa simplex with muscular dystrophy. J Clin Invest 1996;10:2289–2298.

4

Muscular Dystrophies Related to Deficiency of Sarcolemmal Proteins

Maria J. Molnar and George Karpati

The discovery of dystrophin and related molecules has revolutionized our understanding and the diagnosis of a large group of muscular dystrophies [1] and signaled the dawning of a new era in the molecular biology of the muscular dystrophies [2]. Dystrophin and its molecular associates are tightly associated [3] and form an essential cytoskeletal system at the muscle fiber surface membrane [4–7]. The normalcy of this system is critical for maintaining the integrity of the sarcolemma and the muscle fiber [8].

The clinically relevant molecules of the sarcolemma-related cytoskeleton include dystrophin; α- and β-dystroglycans; α-, β-, γ-, and δ-sarcoglycans; laminin α2 (merosin); utrophin; and syntrophins [9, 10]. These molecules form a complex system that connects the intracellular cytoskeletal actin to the extracellular matrix [11] (Figures 4.1 and 4.2).

In this chapter, we review the three major clinical syndromes [8, 12] (dystrophinopathies, sarcoglycanopathies, and merosin-deficient muscular dystrophy) related to the genetic deficiencies of these proteins (Table 4.1). We consider historical aspects, molecular-biochemical background, clinical phenotype, genetics, muscle pathology and histochemistry, prognosis, and treatment.

DYSTROPHINOPATHIES

Historical Aspects

The first description of Duchenne muscular dystrophy (DMD) by Duchenne de Boulogne dates back to 1881, but apparently, Edward Meryon had already recognized the disease in 1851 [13].

The progress of accumulating knowledge about DMD can be divided into three periods. During the *classical period* (1881–1950s), many of the basic clinical and some myopathologic phenotypic features were identified. In the

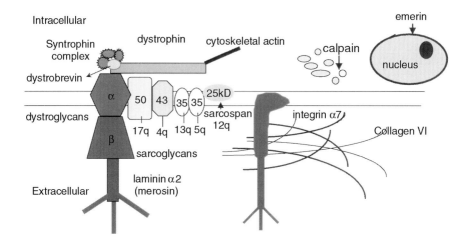

Figure 4.1   Schematic illustration of the principal extrajunctional sarcolemmal molecules that are relevant to muscular dystrophy.

modern period (1950s–1980s), more refined genetic and biochemical information accrued, including the recognition of markedly increased creatine kinase (CK) activity in the blood. The *molecular period,* starting in the early 1980s, brought with it an avalanche of invaluable new information that led to the discovery of the culprit gene (and its mutations), as well as its protein product, dystrophin—the deficiency of which is the basic biochemical defect in DMD. Because the main discoveries in this period of DMD research are particularly illustrative of the practical dividends that creative applications of

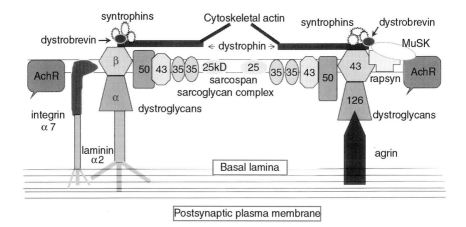

Figure 4.2   Schematic illustration of the principal junctional sarcolemmal molecules. (AchR = acetylcholine receptor; MuSK = muscle-specific receptor tyrosine kinase.)

Table 4.1   Salient features of the principal sarcolemma-related muscular dystrophies.

Disease	Gene	Mutation	Deficient protein	Animal model
Duchenne dystrophy	Dystrophin Xp21	Deletion Duplication Point mutation	Dystrophin 427 kd	mdx Mouse Golden retriever dog
Becker dystrophy	Dystrophin Xp21	Deletion Duplication Point mutation	Dystrophin 427 kd	—
α-Sarcoglycanopathy	α-Sarcoglycan 17q	Point mutation Small deletion Duplication	α-Sarcoglycan 50 kd	—
β-Sarcoglycanopathy	β-Sarcoglycan 4q12	Point mutation Small deletion Duplication	β-Sarcoglycan 43 kd	—
γ-Sarcoglycanopathy	γ-Sarcoglycan 13q12	Point mutation Small deletion	γ-Sarcoglycan 32 kd	—
δ-Sarcoglycanopathy	δ-Sarcoglycan 5q	Point mutation Small deletion	δ-Sarcoglycan 35 kd	Dystrophic hamster
Congenital muscular dystrophy	Laminin α2 6q22	Point mutation	Laminin α2 (merosin) 90 kd	dy/dy Mouse

the modern tools of science can bring about, highlights of the major achievements are listed below:

- Cytogenic localization of DMD gene to the short arm of the X chromosome on the basis of occurrence of DMD in a girl with an X-autosomal translocation involving a breakpoint at Xp21 [14].
- Description of the first linkage of a cloned cDNA sequence on the short arm of the X chromosome to DMD, opening up the restriction fragment length polymorphism analysis in DMD [15, 16].
- Discovery that in a male patient ("BB"), a microscopically observable deletion at Xp21 on the short arm of the X chromosome caused not only DMD, but chronic granulomatous disease, retinitis pigmentosa, and McLeod syndrome [17].
- With use of the technique of subtraction hybridization, the cloning of specific DNA fragments absent from the genome of patient "BB," these DNA fragments being candidates for parts of the DMD gene [18].
- Isolation of candidate cDNAs for portions of the DMD gene [19].
- Localization and cloning of DNA sequences at the Xp21 deletion breakpoints in patient "BB" [20].
- Isolation of a cDNA clone corresponding to a portion of the DMD gene using material from a female DMD patient with an X-autosomal translocation [21].
- Complete cloning of DMD cDNA (coding sequence of gene) and a preliminary account of DMD gene [22].
- Identification of the protein product of DMD gene (23) and determination of the complete sequence of dystrophin [24].

- Identification of expression characteristics of the DMD gene in different cell types and tissues in vivo and in vitro [25–28].
- Localization of dystrophin to the sarcolemma of skeletal muscle fibers by microscopic immunocytochemistry [29–32] and demonstration of its absence in DMD and in mdx muscle fibers.
- Discovery that deletion in the dystrophin gene accounts for a large percentage of DMD and BMD cases [22, 33–36] and the identification of deletional "hot spots" [37].
- Identification of exon reduplication in the dystrophin gene [38].
- "In-frame" and "out-of-frame" deletions in BMD and DMD, respectively [20, 39–41], and differences in dystrophin size in DMD versus BMD [42].
- Dystrophin profile in DMD and mdx heterozygotes [43–45].
- Discovery of a dystrophin-deficient myopathy in a strain of golden retriever dogs [46].
- Discovery of differences between brain and muscle dystrophin genes and proteins [47].
- Conversion of dystrophin-negative to -positive muscle fibers by intramuscular normal myoblast transfer in mdx mice [48, 49].
- Discovery that point mutation in the dystrophin gene is the cause of mdx dystrophy [50].
- Discovery of C-terminal portion of an autosomal analogue of dystrophin mRNA [51]. This later led to the discovery of utrophin.
- Discovery that small-caliber dystrophin-deficient muscle fibers are resistant to necrosis [52].
- Discovery that dystrophin at its C-terminus is associated with an integral membrane glycoprotein complex, presumably for membrane anchorage [53]. The dystrophin-associated glycoprotein complex is deficient in Duchenne muscle [54]. These proteins were later called *sarcoglycans*.
- Discovery that dystrophin probably forms a hexagonal lattice beneath the plasma membrane because of two hinge regions in the rod domain [55].
- Discovery that dystrophin-positive muscle fiber segments may occur in DMD or mdx muscle, possibly because of "reverse mutation(s)" that can restore the competency of the dystrophin gene in some myonuclei [56, 57].
- Identification of a variety of isoforms of dystrophin [58].
- Discovery that dystrophin-deficient mdx muscle fibers show heightened vulnerability to lengthening contractions [59].
- Discovery that in mdx mice made transgenic by dystrophin, the dystrophic phenotype is corrected [60, 61].
- Discovery that dystrophinopathy can be a frequent cause of Duchenne-like dystrophy in females [62].
- Identification of sarcoglycan deficiencies as a possible cause of Duchenne or limb-girdle dystrophies [63–67].
- Characterization of another class of dystrophin-associated proteins: syntrophins [68].
- Discovery of merosin deficiency as a cause of congenital muscular dystrophy because of its gene mutation [69].
- Partial correction of dystrophic phenotype in mdx mice by a truncated utrophin transgene [70].
- Discovery that prednisone improves and stabilizes muscle strength in DMD [71].

- Discovery that myoblast transfer is not effective for the treatment of DMD [72, 73].
- Discovery that adenovirus vector-mediated dystrophin minigene transfer to muscles of mdx mice creates short-term sarcolemmal dystrophin with beneficial effects [74, 75].
- Discovery that immunosuppression of the host markedly improves the longevity of dystrophin created by adenovirus-mediated gene transfer [76].
- Discovery that a new generation of adenovirus vector ("gutted vector") improves the efficiency of full-length dystrophin gene transfer [77].
- Discovery that abundant utrophin—created by adenovirus-mediated gene transfer—in mdx muscle markedly improves the dystrophic phenotype [78].
- Announcement by the Muscular Dystrophy Association (USA) of plans for a single-muscle phase I gene therapy trial in Duchenne patients (fashioned after the first myoblast transfer study) using the "gutted" adenovirus vector [79].

Molecular-Biochemical Background

The DMD Gene

The DMD gene is by far the largest among the known genes, containing approximately 2.4 million base pairs [80, 81]. It is localized at the short arm of the X chromosome (Xp21.1), and it can be displayed by in situ hybridization with fluorescent DNA probes [82]. The coding sequence of the gene, including the untranslated regions of the mRNA, is approximately 13.9 thousand base pairs [22]. The gene contains 79 exons.

The dystrophin gene produces several isoforms of dystrophin [81, 83, 84]. Seven distinct promoters have been identified [81], each driving a tissue-specific dystrophin as shown in Table 4.2. For DMD, the three large (full-length) molecular weight (427 kd) dystrophins are important. They are controlled by three dif-

Table 4.2   Salient features of the major dystrophin isoforms

Name and molecular weight (kd)	Promoter location	Transcript size (kb)	Principal tissue occurrence	Relevant to Duchenne muscular dystrophy?
Muscle type, 427	Exon 1	13.9	Skeletal muscle Smooth muscle	Yes
Brain type, 427	Exon 1	13.9	Cerebral cortex and hippocampus	Yes
Purkinje, 427	Exon 1	13.9	Purkinje cells	?
Dp 260	Intron 29	?	Retina	?
Dp 140	Intron 44	7.5	Kidney/brain	No
Dp 116 (Apo-dystrophin I)	Intron 55	5.2	Schwann cells	No
Dp 71 (Apo-dystrophin II)	Intron 62	4.5	Ubiquitous except mature muscle (highest in brain and heart)	
			Also occurs in fetal muscle	No

ferent promoters in exon 1: the muscle promoter [85], the brain promoter, and the Purkinje promoter [86–88].

The three full-length isoforms only differ in the first exons. Their approximate transcription time is 16 hours [89]. Although Dp260, the retinal isoform [90], is also absent in DMD, clinically manifest visual impairment does not occur.

In addition to the major isoforms cited above, dystrophin also has splice variants affecting the C-terminus [91]. The best studied is the one from which exon 78 is excluded. This variant is detectable mainly in embryonic tissues, implying some developmental regulation. Another splice variation involves exons 71–74, producing 10 different in-frame splice variants. The functional significance of the splice variant is unknown.

Dystrophin

Dystrophin is a muscle isoform that is a rod-shaped molecule of 427 kd, approximately 175 nm long, containing 3,685 amino acids [23, 81, 92, 93]. There are four functional domains:

- NH_2 globular domain (500 amino acids), with three distinct actin-binding sites (Abs 1,2,3) [94].
- The rod domain (2,840 amino acids), with 24 tandem α helical spectrinlike repeats with four proline-rich hinge regions, where the molecule is believed to be bent in vivo to assume a hexagonal configuration [55]. In the fourth hinge, there is a short domain consisting of two tryptophans (WW/WNP).
- Cystine-rich domain (150 amino acids), with probable calcium-binding capacity attached to the intramembranous protein β-dystroglycan, and its 3' end probably attached to α-syntrophin and possibly to AO protein (see Figure 4.1).
- Carboxy terminus domain (420 amino acids), with its 5' half linked to β-dystroglycans and its 3' half probably attached to α-syntrophin and possibly to the AO (87 kd) protein [95, 96].

In muscle, dystrophin constitutes approximately 5% of the membrane-associated cytoskeletal protein [97]. Dystrophin is situated at the cytoplasmic aspect of the plasma membrane [98, 99]. The association of dystrophin with other sarcolemmal proteins is depicted in Figure 4.1 and further discussed under Sarcoglycanopathies.

It has been suggested that in situ dystrophin forms antiparallel homologous multimers [100]. Proof of this, however, is still lacking.

On immunostaining, dystrophin shows a costameric pattern [101] being localized at the cell surface at the I band level only [102]. This distribution coincides with that of spectrin, ankyrin, vinculin, α_3/β_1 integrin, talin, and desmin [103]. Thus, at the I band level, there is a complex subplasmalemmal cytoskeletal meshwork.

Dystrophin is particularly abundant at the neuromuscular junction and may contribute to the stabilization of endplate-specific molecules, along with utrophin [104, 105]. Dystrophin is also abundant at the myotendinous junction [106, 107]. The various isoforms of dystrophin are discussed above and shown in Table 4.2.

The functions of dystrophin are not fully defined [100]. It probably has multiple physiological roles that vary according to the different isoforms in different cell types. In skeletal muscle, the probable main role is mechanical reinforcement of the sarcolemma. Dystrophin-deficient fibers are particularly vulnerable to lengthening contractions [59, 108]. Dystrophin may also enable the sarcolemma to assume the normal folding and plication or festooning configuration in the relaxed state, so that it can remain intact when muscle fibers are stretched [109, 110]. Dystrophin may also serve as an anchor or stabilizer of intramembranous molecules, such as the sarcoglycans, the function of which is still obscure. Thus, some consequences of dystrophin deficiency may reflect the loss of sarcoglycan functions.

Another tantalizing role of dystrophin was recently suggested. The finding of a peculiar domain of two tryptophans near the β-dystroglycan binding site is consistent with a hypothesis that dystrophin may also have a role in signal transduction [111]. The cognate ligand for this domain is still unknown. The possible signaling function of dystrophin is consistent with a scenario that in dystrophin deficiency states, a defective cell signaling leads to an abnormal control of muscle fiber caliber (hypertrophy or smallness) [112].

The functional role of dystrophin in the brain is undetermined. Its predominant localization at the synaptic membrane [113] is consistent with a function of stabilization of receptors or ion channels or synaptic vesicles. The function of the short dystrophins is also completely obscure, although DP116 may contribute to the stabilization of sodium channels at nodes of Ranvier in peripheral nerves [114].

Utrophin

Utrophin is a 395-kd protein that is encoded by a one million base pair gene at chromosome 6q24 [51, 116–119]. The amino acid sequence and domain characteristics are very similar to that of dystrophin [115, 120]. In normal muscle, utrophin is expressed only at the neuromuscular postjunctional sarcolemma at the crest of the junctional folds [121, 122], blood vessels, intramuscular nerves, and myotendinous junction [51, 118, 119, 123, 124]. It is anchored to the same dystrophin-associated proteins as dystrophin in muscle [125]. It is expressed in most mature tissues and in embryonic myoblasts and myotubes. In regenerating muscle fibers of mature muscle, as well as in dystrophin-deficient fibers and fibers in inflammatory myopathies, utrophin is upregulated and expressed throughout the extrajunctional sarcolemma [126]. It is hypothesized that this is a mitigating factor in DMD, and without this apparent compensation, DMD could lead to a faster rate of muscle cell destruction and loss. In fact, in a dystrophin-deficient boy who was suspected to have utrophin deficiency, the dystrophic process was particularly rapid [127].

In mdx animals, "knock-out" of the utrophin gene aggravates the phenotype [128]. In transgenic mdx mice, utrophin overexpression eliminated the dystrophic phenotype, implying that utrophin can serve as a functional surrogate of dystrophin [72]. This has potentially important therapeutic implications.

Clinical Phenotypes

The following clinical phenotypes are relevant to dystrophin deficiency [129]:

- Typical severe DMD cases with or without mental subnormality
- Preclinical (postnatal) cases and Duchenne fetuses
- Milder DMD ("outliers")
- Manifesting DMD heterozygotes and DMD in females

- Becker dystrophy
- Quadriceps myopathy
- Cramps with myoglobinuria
- Phenotypically normal individuals (?idiopathic hyperCKemia)

The typical severe Duchenne cases occur at a frequency of 1 per 3,500 live births [13]. The child appears healthy at birth, but early motor milestones are usually somewhat delayed. However, until age 3–5 years, usually neither the parent nor the pediatrician recognizes any abnormality.

The initial symptoms include clumsy gait, slow running, difficulty getting up from a deep position, difficulty climbing steps, and a waddling gait. In some cases, the initial suspicion arises because of slow learning. In still other rare instances, the first attention is drawn to the diagnosis when, after a general anesthesia, the child develops an unexplained cardiac arrest or an episode of myoglobinuria and some features of malignant hyperthermia [130]. Examination reveals muscle weakness that is most prominent in the pelvic and shoulder girdles, as well as in the proximal lower and upper limbs and trunk erectors, particularly at the lumbar and thoracic regions [129]. This is responsible for the exaggerated lumbar lordosis and thoracolumbar scoliosis. Distally, muscles are less affected. The pelvic girdle and proximal leg muscle weakness is responsible for the Gowers sign. Respiratory muscle involvement is relatively late, beginning at the end of the second decade. Craniobulbar muscles, particularly those serving extraocular movements, are spared throughout.

Initially, certain muscles, particularly those of the calves, show hypertrophy, whereas all other muscles eventually atrophy. In the hypertrophied muscles, initially there is true increase of muscle fiber caliber (true hypertrophy) rather than increased muscle bulk that is due to excessive adipose replacement of lost muscle fibers (pseudohypertrophy). The cause of true muscle hypertrophy of DMD muscle fibers is not fully explained. However, the loss of dystrophin as a possible mediator of cell-volume regulation may play a role in this process [112].

The progression of muscle weakness and loss of function for the activities of daily living is relentless and takes place at a more or less predictable rate [131]. In some patients ("outliers"), the rate of progression is somewhat slower. In the typical situation, the child loses the ability of independent ambulation by age 9–11 years. By the end of the first or beginning of the second decade, respiratory insufficiency may necessitate at least intermittent respiratory assistance, particularly at night. Despite all therapeutic efforts, a fatal outcome is expected to occur during the third decade, by which time symptomatic cardiomyopathy usually develops. Throughout the course of the disease, complications may arise, which include contractures at various locations, particularly in the lower extremities; thoracic scoliosis that can aggravate respiratory insufficiency; and mental subnormality. The last is not progressive, but it can significantly aggravate the motor disability [132]. It is presumed to be due to the lack of brain dystrophin [133].

Duchenne Muscular Dystrophy in Females

Cells of females have two X chromosomes, derived 50% paternally and 50% maternally. During early embryonic development, one of the X chromosomes becomes inactivated in a random fashion, leaving 50% of the remaining chromosomes paternal and 50% maternal (Lyon hypothesis) [134]. Thus, the daughters of DMD carrier females have at least 50% of the myonuclei containing a normal dystrophin gene. This is sufficient to generate enough dystrophin to prevent muscle fiber necrosis and loss, as long as the normal genes are evenly distributed throughout the muscle fibers [135]. An exception to this rule occurs when a bias of X chromosome inactivation is present [136]. In such instances, less than 50% of the myonuclei may contain a wild-type dystrophin gene, and there is a chance of significant dystrophin deficiency with a variably severe dystrophic phenotype. This is particularly prone to occur as a result of twinning, when one of the identical twin heterozygotes has a biased X chromosome inactivation resulting in a dystrophic clinical phenotype [137].

In some cases, isolated females may present with dystrophin-deficient myopathy indistinguishable from DMD [62]. These cases may represent unknown carriers in whom a biased X chromosome inactivation created dystrophin deficiency. Such patients, in fact, may be one of identical twins whose embryonic sibling was unknowingly lost during pregnancy. Other genetic alterations (i.e., OX phenotype [Turner's syndrome]) often interferes with the random X inactivation and can produce symptomatic DMD [138, 139].

Becker Muscular Dystrophy

Becker muscular dystrophy (BMD) is an allelic variant of DMD in which the mutation of the dystrophin gene produces a reduced amount of truncated dystrophin that is not capable of maintaining the integrity of the sarcolemma [140–142]. However, the pace of muscle fiber damage or loss is considerably slower than in DMD, and this is also reflected in a more benign clinical phenotype, recognized by Becker in 1955. Although the incidence of BMD is one-fifth to one-tenth that of DMD, its prevalence is higher because of its more benign natural history and because BMD men are capable of procreating offsprings. It is of particular importance that all daughters of BMD fathers are obligate carriers.

Initial symptoms of BMD are similar to those of DMD, but age at onset is usually later (3–20 years). Loss of independent ambulation happens between 12 and 40 years. Death from respiratory insufficiency or cardiomyopathy usually occurs between 30 and 60 years.

Other Dystrophin-Deficient Phenotypes

Other dystrophin-deficient phenotypes include rarer, relatively mild syndromes, such as myopathy localized to the quadriceps muscles [143] and a syndrome of muscle cramps and myoglobinuria [144]. In some asymptomatic people, a mild to moderate but consistently elevated serum CK activity is found for which there is no obvious explanation. In such persons, a minor defect in the rod region of the dystrophin gene has been postulated but rarely proven [145].

Laboratory Investigation

The activity of serum CK (mainly the muscle [MM] isoform) and of other muscle enzymes is markedly elevated (up to 200-fold), even in the preclinical state. In fact, high serum CK activity is present in umbilical cord blood; percutaneous umbilical cord blood testing has been suggested as a neonatal screening method [146]. With the progression of the disease, serum CK activity tends to decline, which reflects the diminishing muscle mass.

Electromyography (EMG) shows typical features with an unusual abundance of single fiber activity. Electrocardiography, in advanced cases, shows increased R/S amplitude in lead V_1 and deep compressed Q waves in the precordial leads [147].

Myopathology and Pathogenesis

The cardinal myopathologic lesion in a proximal limb muscle biopsy is segmental necrosis of muscle fibers and subsequent regeneration of this segment [148, 149]. For still-unknown reasons, necrotic fibers in DMD tend to occur in small groups of 3–10. Regeneration is vigorous in early stages of the disease, but as the disease progresses, regeneration becomes more and more suboptimal and produces muscle fiber segments with reduced caliber. Eventually, regeneration completely fails in individual necrotic muscle fiber segments, leading to loss of muscle fibers and adipose cell replacement. The progressively impaired regenerative capacity of DMD muscle fibers may be explained by the "exhaustion" of satellite cells after having undergone many cycles of cell divisions that are entailed in previous regenerative activity. This "exhaustion" produces loss of proliferative capacity or myogenicity.

The initial fine structural change that occurs in the subsequently necrotic segment is a focal breach of the plasma membrane [148, 150]. Before that event, there is focal separation of the plasma membrane and basal lamina [148], which can be explained by the loss of the appropriate linkage molecules. Such breaches can be repaired by rapid apposition of flat, cisternlike membrane configurations to the gap. Such repaired sites are marked focal depression of the muscle fiber surface and the duplication or triplication of the basal lamina over the site of the repair. The repair also entails the exteriorization of superficial segments of muscle fibers.

If such rapid repair fails to materialize, the massive Ca^{2+} influx initiates necrosis that spreads laterally along the axis of muscle fibers until the necrotic segment is isolated from the surviving stumps by a newly formed demarcating membrane. The time course of these events can be studied precisely in the experimental micropuncture model of muscle fibers in vivo in rats [151].

The massive extracellular calcium influx activates proteosomal proteases of muscle fibers, which is an important part of the necrotic process.

The currently prevailing thought is that the lack of dystrophin in muscle fibers creates a mechanically weakened sarcolemma [152, 153], which becomes susceptible to focal tears on contractile activity [108]. In small-caliber muscle fibers, relative mechanical stress per unit surface-membrane area is less than in larger fibers. This could explain why small-diameter fibers (i.e., those of the extraocular muscles or cranial muscles) are relatively spared from necrosis and its consequences in DMD and its animal model mdx [52].

DMD muscle contains many abnormally small- and large-diameter muscle fibers. The small-caliber fibers may arise as result of the following processes: impaired regeneration to reduced girth, failure of fiber volume homeostasis because of dystrophin deficiency, and loss of cell volume caused by the above-described repair of the surface membrane. Hypertrophic fibers may arise as a result of a compensatory process or may also be a reflection of failed volume homeostasis of dystrophin-deficient muscle fibers [112].

The connective tissue excess in DMD muscles is a relatively early event and may not simply represent a "replacement" phenomenon of lost muscle fibers. It has been suggested that certain fibrogenic cytokines, such as transforming growth factor–β derived from tissue macrophages, stimulate fibroblasts to excessive collagen production [154].

Hypercontracted muscle fiber segments are relatively common in DMD muscle. Some believe that these arise in vivo in the tissue and represent an early phase of muscle fiber necrosis. However, it is much more likely that they are produced at the time of the biopsy removal, when the excessively fragile sarcolemma suffers focal breaches on removal of the tissue. This concept is supported by the fact that hypercontracted muscle fibers are also frequently found in normal biopsies of children.

Mononuclear inflammatory cell infiltrates (including CD8+ cells) may be present, but confusion with a primary inflammatory myopathy should not arise [155].

Histochemistry and Cytochemistry

Immunostaining reveals lack of dystrophin at the surface of muscle fibers. The exception is in rare isolated or small groups of fibers, in which full or partial immunostaining is present (Color Plate 1) [42, 156, 157]. These are the so-called revertant fibers, in which, segmentally, the dystrophin gene in some myonuclei becomes competent, presumably because of a second "corrective" mutation in a myogenic stem cell during early myogenesis [56, 57]. There are currently three useful monoclonal antibodies commercially available for dystrophin immunostaining. These antibodies (Novocastra 1, 2, 3) recognize epitopes in the mid-rod NH_2-terminus and COOH-terminus, respectively. In BMD, immunostaining can be patchy, and a given antibody may give completely negative results if the target epitopes are missing on account of the protein truncation (in-frame deletion; Color Plate 2).

In most DMD muscle fibers, particularly the regenerating ones, variable intensity of extrajunctional sarcolemmal utrophin immunostaining is present (see Color Plate 1) [126, 158]. This is not due to an enhanced transcription, but is probably related to a saturation of orphaned dystrophin receptors by utrophin at the cell surface [159].

There is a markedly attenuated immunostaining for α- and β-dystroglycans and all sarcoglycans [160], but not of merosin. The dystroglycan and sarcoglycan depletion is secondary to the dystrophin deficiency [161], because replacement of dystrophin in transgenic mdx mice or after gene transfer by adenovirus vector brings about normalization of the dystrophin-associated molecules and down-regulates utrophin [61, 78]. By contrast, in primary sarcoglycan deficiency, dystrophin immunostaining is normal [162].

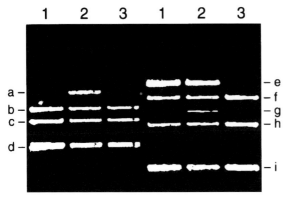

Figure 4.3   Products of multi-plex polymerase chain reaction from blood cells are displayed on agarose gel. The amplified exons are as follows: a = 48; b = 17; c = 8; d = 44; e = 45; f = 19; g = 52; h = 12; i = 4. In patient 1, a and g are missing, implying a deletion of at least exons 48–52; in patient 3, a, e, and g are missing, implying a deletion of at least exons 45–52. In patient 2, no deletions are present.

Total (DMD) or partial (BMD) dystrophin deficiency can be verified by Western blot analysis. This is particularly important in the diagnosis of BMD, because in this case, the dystrophin molecular weight is less than the normal 427 kd (Color Plate 2).

Phenotype/Genotype Correlation

In approximately 65% of the patients, an out-of-frame deletion—detectable by multiplex PCR [35]—is present [163, 164, 165]. There are two regions of deletion hot spots. One is centered just at the 3' end of the N-terminus; the other is around exons 44–45. A deletion may take only one exon or many exons (Figure 4.3). Out-of-frame deletions invariably create a stop codon downstream and produce an unstable, truncated dystrophin transcript and usually no detectable dystrophin protein. In approximately 5% of the cases, there is a reduplication of one or more exons leading to a subverted reading frame [166]. In the remainder of cases, there are presumed point mutations, causing splicing errors or other abnormalities [167–169]. In Becker dystrophy, the deletions are in-frame, which causes a trans-latable but truncated transcript leading to a truncated protein of smaller-than-nor-mal quantity [170] (see Color Plate 2).

As a rule of thumb, deletion in the N-terminus or C-terminus region [171] causes moderate to severe phenotypes, whereas deletion in the rod regions tends to cause milder phenotypes. Several exceptions to this rule have been reported but not fully explained [172–174]. Ultimately, four natural factors seem to determine the sever-ity of the phenotype: the amount of dystrophin, the quality of dystrophin, the even-ness of its distribution along the muscle fibers, and the possible compensating mechanisms for dystrophin deficiency. Perhaps the degree of utrophin up-regula-tion may play a role in that respect. The prevalence of revertant fibers probably does not have a significant compensating role for the overall dystrophin deficiency.

Genetic Counseling and Prenatal Diagnosis

In approximately two-thirds of cases, the dystrophin gene defect is transmitted to DMD boys by carrier females conforming to the patterns of mendelian X-linked recessive inheritance. However, in one-third of cases, the defect arises as a result of a new mutation in the germ cells of parents or during very early embryogenesis. Thus, DMD could not be eradicated even by a perfect carrier detection and absolute control of DMD birth to carriers. Nevertheless, the diagnosis of new DMD cases always demands provision of proper genetic counseling to all female family members at potential risk of having a DMD (or carrier) offspring. This includes the proband's mother, sisters, maternal female cousins, and maternal aunts.

If the DMD mutation diagnosed in the proband is a specific gene rearrangement, the same mutation is sought in somatic cells of the females at risk [175]. However, this may be difficult, in view of the presence of a normal allele in addition to the mutant one. The mutational analysis therefore requires special techniques (quantitative fluorescent polymerase chain reaction) [176–178]. Some carriers show a mosaic pattern of dystrophin immunostaining [179] (Color Plate 3), but it is not a sufficiently consistent finding for reliable diagnosis. If the proband does not have an identifiable dystrophin gene rearrangement, an attempt at linking the mutant dystrophin allele to a polymorphic DNA segment (that is close enough to the dystrophin gene to be assumed to be coinherited) may provide information regarding a possible carrier state [180]. If the investigation indicated a lack of mutation of the dystrophin gene in a somatic cell, the risk of the birth of a DMD boy still remains at approximately 10% because of germ line mosaicism (i.e., the presence of mutated dystrophin gene in some germ cells [181]). Detection of germ line mosaicism requires extraordinary efforts not usually performed in routine clinical work.

If the investigation determines that a woman is a carrier for DMD, half of her sons will have DMD, and half of her daughters will be carriers. The options that a carrier can follow for the prevention of the birth of a DMD boy include prevention of all future pregnancies or prenatal diagnosis. Prenatal diagnosis may simply determine the sex of the fetus, and the carrier may terminate all male pregnancies. Alternatively, DNA from amniocytes or from a chorionic villus biopsy is analyzed for the known mutation [182]. In the case of a positive outcome in a male fetus, termination could be chosen. More sophisticated approaches to diagnosis include preimplantation genetic analysis of the embryo, which is practically feasible but is rarely used in routine practice. This includes the determination of whether a given gene defect is present in a single cell derived from a few-cell-stage embryo produced by in vitro fertilization. In such cases, the embryo remains viable and may be implanted into the uterus if there is no dystrophin gene defect found. The moral issues surrounding such a protocol in the complex field of reproductive technology have not been defined in most countries [183].

Treatment and Management

In general terms, definitive treatment of DMD could theoretically be brought about by three types of strategies: (1) pharmacologic agents that reduce or eliminate the vulnerability of dystrophin-deficient muscle fibers to necrosis; (2) molecular treatment (i.e., replacing the defective dystrophin gene with a wild-type one [or at least a functionally adequate one] or upregulating the expression of the surrogate molecule utrophin); or (3) protein replacement (i.e., dystrophin administration, which is not practical or feasible).

Steroids are the only pharmacologic agents that showed a beneficial effect in DMD in controlled studies [71]. The mechanism of action for this effect is still obscure. Steroids do not work by up-regulating utrophin transcription [159]. Stabilization of the lipid bilayer by steroids of the plasma membrane has been suggested as a possible mechanism. Immunosuppressive action of corticosteroids is unlikely to be important, because other immunosuppressive drugs are not generally useful.

Gene replacement therapy is a promising avenue for the treatment of DMD. Initially, cell-mediated normal dystrophin gene transfer (myoblast transfer) was expected to be useful, but after several trials in DMD boys, the procedure was found to be practically ineffective [73, 184]. After success with transgenic mdx mice [61, 185, 186], the attention turned to direct dystrophin gene transfer [187]. In muscles of animal models of dystrophin deficiency (mdx mice and golden retriever dogs), abundant, functionally useful dystrophin was generated by adenovirus-mediated dystrophin gene transfer even with a truncated (Becker type) "minigene" [74–76]. Overexpression of Dp71, however, was not useful in mitigating the dystrophic phenotype in transgenic mdx mice [188, 189]. With the advent of an improved adenovirus vector (in which all viral genes had been deleted), the full-length dystrophin cDNA can be introduced into muscle fibers [190]. This vector evokes little deleterious immunologic reaction in the host and can generate, for extended periods, full-length dystrophin that prevents necrosis of muscle fibers [191].

Overexpression of utrophin in mdx mice after utrophin gene transfer has a similar beneficial effect on the dystrophic phenotype [78].

Before dystrophin gene transfer becomes ready for human trials, a safe and cost-effective systemic route of administration of the vector must be worked out in preclinical experiments. Additionally, cost-effective and safe, large-scale therapeutic vector production in a good manufacturing practice mode should be established [191].

Palliative measures for the management of DMD include various methods of bracing, tendon lengthening and transfer, proper wheelchair seating, physiotherapy, and assisted respiration in the late stages of the disease [131]. Attention to the educational, social, cultural, and psychological needs of the patient is of paramount importance.

SARCOGLYCANOPATHIES

The discovery of several dystrophin-associated molecules at the skeletal muscle surface membrane allowed for a new molecular classification of the limb-girdle dystrophies (LGMD) [192, 193]. The autosomal recessive LGMD—previously designated as LGMD 2A, 2D, 2E, 2C, and 2F—arise from mutations in genes encoding calpain and four different dystrophin-associated proteins, α-, β-, γ-, and δ-sarcoglycans, respectively [63–67, 162, 194–207]. An autosomal dominant variety of LGMD has also been described as type I [208, 209].

Molecular-Biochemical Background

Dystrophin is associated with several sarcolemmal proteins that are presumed to stabilize the surface membrane during contraction-relaxation [210]. These are called *dystrophin-associated proteins* (DAPs; see Figures 4.1 and 4.2) [152]. A part of this cytoskeleton is responsible for attaching the intracellular actin to the extracellular basal lamina. Some studies have classified that DAPs fall into three groups [210], as shown in Figure 4.1.

1. Dystroglycan complex
   α-Dystroglycan (156 kd)
   β-Dystroglycan (43 kd)
2. Sarcoglycan complex
   α-Sarcoglycan (or adhalin; 50 kd) [211]
   β-Sarcoglycan (43 kd)
   γ-Sarcoglycan (35 kd)
   δ-Sarcoglycan (35 kd)
   Sarcospan (25 kd)
3. Syntrophin complex [68, 212, 213]
   α-Syntrophin (60 kd)
   β1-Syntrophin (60 kd)
   β2-Syntrophin (60 kd)

The extracellular matrix around the muscle fibers is a complex network with a composition that includes collagen, fibronectin, laminin, and proteoglycans. It is a specialized extracellular matrix with relatively static structure. This is thought to contribute to the proper migration, proliferation, and regeneration of myogenic cells during development or after injury or grafting.

The components of the basal lamina include a variety of laminins. Laminins are heterotrimer molecules, each composed of one heavy (α) chain, and two light chains (β and γ) [214]. Currently, five α chains, three β chains, and two γ chains are known. The various combinations of heavy and light chains give rise to several types of laminin [215]. The laminin of muscle fibers is composed of α2 heavy chain and β1 or β2 and γ1 light chains. Merosin is the collective term of laminins that contain α2 heavy chain (laminins 2 and 4). Merosin is situated in the basal lamina of muscle fibers [216]. Laminin binds directly to specific molecules of the basal lamina, such as entactin/nidogen and heparan sulfate proteoglycan/perlecan [214]. Several molecules have been suggested as cell-surface receptors for laminin, including dystroglycans, integrins, and lectins [217]. The dystroglycans link laminin 2 to the dystrophin-actin complex [5]. The role of integrins as a laminin receptor is based on a deficiency of α7/β1 integrin in muscle in the merosin-deficient congenital muscular dystrophy [218]. Mice homozygous for α7 integrin deficiency show signs of muscular dystrophy, confirming the notion that a link between the subsarcolemmal cytoskeleton and the extracellular matrix is essential for the integrity of the sarcolemma [219].

The dystroglycan complex is a receptor of the extracellular matrix proteins. It is distributed ubiquitously in various tissues and identified as a 156 kd, large α-dystroglycan and 43 kd β-dystroglycan in skeletal muscle. α-Dystroglycan is an extracellular protein that binds to laminin α2 and to β-dystroglycan, as a transmembranous protein. β-Dystroglycan binds intracellularly to the cysteine-rich region and to the first half of the C-terminus domain of dystrophin [9, 95, 220]. N-terminus of dystrophin binds to actin filaments in the subsarcolemmal cytoskeletal networks [221]. This "dystrophin axis"—comprising actin-dystrophin-dystroglycan-laminin [206]—appears to play an important role in creating a cell-matrix adhesion junction between the plasmalemma to the mechanically strong basal lamina. This could mechanically stabilize the sarcolemma during contraction and relaxation of muscle fibers.

The sarcoglycan complex is a group of membrane-integrated proteins. It is considered to be the "side arm" of the "dystrophin axis" because it is linked by lateral association with dystrophin (directly binding to the cysteine-rich domain of dystrophin or to the first half of the C-terminus) [96]. However, the exact microtopographic relationship between the sarcoglycan complex and the dystrophin-dystroglycan complex is not well understood.

The sarcoglycan complex contains at least five components: 50-kd α, 43-kd β, and 35-kd γ/δ subunits, and the 25-kd sarcospan [222]. The α-sarcoglycan was originally named *adhalin* after the arabic word for muscle, *adhal* [102]. It is oriented with its carboxy terminus, projecting inside the muscle cell. It has alternatively spliced isoforms [223]. The extracellular domain of this protein has some homology to the nerve growth-factor receptor, raising the possibility that it may interact with ligands in the extracellular matrix [10]. The β-, γ-, and δ-sarcoglycans are oriented with the N-termini toward the cytoplasm.

All four sarcoglycans share some common characteristics: All are N-glycosylated and have a similar structure, consisting of a short intracellular domain, a single transmembrane domain, and a larger extracellular domain [64, 66, 67, 202]. α- And γ-sarcoglycans are expressed exclusively in skeletal, cardiac, and smooth muscle cells [65, 102]. β-Sarcoglycan is expressed in multiple tissues, but most abundantly in skeletal and cardiac muscle [202]. The sarcoglycan complex spans the muscle membrane and interacts with dystrophin at the membrane's cytoplasmic face [9]. The molar ratio of the α-, β-, γ-, and δ-sarcoglycans is 1 to 1 to 1 to 1.

An abnormality of this complex plays a crucial role in the pathogenesis of the muscular dystrophies. It is likely that when any one of the components of the sarcoglycan complex is absent, the complex may not be formed, and the loss of the entire complex may ensue. Therefore, the severe childhood autosomal recessive muscular dystrophy (SCARMD) phenotype may develop, irrespective of which sarcoglycan gene is primarily mutated. This is the reason that SCARMD is considered the "model" sarcoglycanopathy. The sarcoglycanopathies compose approximately 10% of the autosomal recessive LGMDs [224, 225].

The syntrophin complex is also associated with dystrophin. It consists of three proteins. Each of these is slightly less than 60 kd encoded by three separate genes [1, 212, 226]. α-Syntrophin is expressed only in skeletal muscle, whereas the other two (β1 and β2) have a wide tissue distribution. α-Syntrophin is present along the length of muscle cells located at the inner membrane surface. The syntrophin proteins bind to the distal C-terminus regions of dystrophin [95]. Syntrophin deficiency has not been reported as a cause of the muscular dystrophy.

Dystrobrevin is encoded on chromosome 2p22-23 [227]. It is considered an important protein in the formation and maintenance of neuromuscular junction. Dystrobrevin binds directly to the syntrophin; its C-terminus binds to the C-terminus of dystrophin [228]. Positive dystrobrevin immunostain of the sarcolemma in normal skeletal muscle indicates that it colocalizes with dystrophin and the DAP complex. By contrast, dystrobrevin membrane staining is severely reduced in DMD muscles. Interestingly, dystrobrevin staining at the sarcolemma is also markedly reduced in patients with LGMD arising from the loss of sarcoglycan components. Dystrobrevin depletion thus is a general feature of dystrophies linked to both dystrophin and DAP deficiencies. It suggests that a perturbation of the cytoplasmic moieties of the DAP complex may be involved in the pathogenesis of LGMD [229].

Other proteins (not shown in Figure 4.1)—such as vinculin and talin—appear to bind to the dystrophin complex [210]. The association of a neuronal nitric oxide synthetase homologue protein with dystrophin has also been described [230].

Other intracellular proteins, such as the soluble enzyme calpain 3 (calcium activated neutral protease; CANP3) also have an important role in the etiopathogenesis of some muscular dystrophies [195, 198, 231]. Mutation in its gene can result in a subtype of LGMD [194, 198, 220]. Calpain 3 (previously known as *p94*) is a muscle-specific member of the calpain family of nonlysosomal cysteine proteases, which includes ubiquitin and μ- and m-calpain (now called *calpain-1* and *-2*) [232]. The function or substrates of calpain 3 are not yet known, but recently, a specific binding site for titin was identified [233].

At the neuromuscular junction, agrin, acetylcholine receptor, muscle-specific receptor tyrosine kinase (MuSK), rapsyn, β-dystroglycan, utrophin, and laminin β2 probably play an important role in its differentiation (see Figure 4.2) [234]. Agrin is a large multidomain heparan sulfate proteoglycan of the postsynaptic membrane, which is localized to the extracellular matrix that controls neuromuscular junction formation and induces the clustering of acetylcholine receptors (AChRs) in the muscle membrane beneath the nerve terminals. Agrin acts through a specific receptor, which is thought to have an MuSK as one of its components [235]. On the cytoplasmic face of the postsynaptic membrane, another protein—the rapsyn—is receptor-associated and essential for clustering AChRs at the neuromuscular junction. Rapsyn also acts through activity of the synapse-specific receptor tyrosine kinase MuSK [236].

Clinical Phenotypes

Some patients with primary sarcoglycanopathy or calpainopathy are clinically indistinguishable from those with primary dystrophinopathies [192, 193]. These cases are usually diagnosed as having SCARMD, DMD-like muscular dystrophy, or LGMD. The age at onset and severity of the myopathy is heterogeneous. The clinical signs usually appear between 2 and 20 years of age. The patients have normal early milestones. The initial symptoms are waddling gait, toe-walking, exercise intolerance, and painful muscle swelling, without myoglobinuria. The most common findings include increased lumbar lordosis, tight Achilles tendon, winged scapulae, and calf hypertrophy. The patients have progressive proximal muscle weakness (hip girdle more affected than shoulder girdle). Weakness of the neck and trunk flexors is also an early feature. The Gowers sign is usually present. Involvement of the distal muscles occurs later. There is no cardiac dysfunction. The degree of the adhalin deficiency is proportionate to the clinical severity [12, 207, 224]. Five to ten percent of dystrophin-positive muscular dystrophies prove to be α-sarcoglycanopathy [225, 237].

Clinically, calpainopathy—which has critical symptoms that may appear between 2 and 40 years of age—is very similar. Patients have increased serum CK, calf hypertrophy, and weakness predominantly in the pelvic-girdle muscles.

In some cases, scapuloperoneal weakness is observed. These patients are able to walk until they are in their 40s [238].

Laboratory Investigation

Serum CK is elevated 10–120 times above the upper limit of normal. No correlation exists between CK levels and age or functional stage. EMG shows typical myopathic abnormalities.

Muscle Pathology and Histochemistry

Muscle biopsies show dystrophic features similar to those described in DMD, including a wide variation in fiber size, fiber hypertrophy, and an increase of endomysial connective tissue [239]. Necrosis and regeneration are intense, particularly in young, severely affected patients. Type 1 fiber predominance is common.

Immunohistochemistry

In most cases of sarcoglycanopathies, calpainopathies, and merosin deficiencies, the dystrophin staining is normal. The immunostaining with antibodies against α-, β-, γ-, and δ-sarcoglycans is variable [240]. In most cases, the adhalin immunostaining is markedly deficient, which can be used as a screening procedure to detect any sarcoglycanopathies (Color Plate 4). Adhalin deficiency can therefore be secondary to loss of other sarcoglycans and vice versa [202, 241]. Duchenne and Becker dystrophies usually show secondary sarcoglycan deficiency. This is why dystrophinopathy must always be excluded before making a diagnosis of primary sarcoglycanopathy [12].

The immunohistochemical analysis of the α-, β-, γ-, and δ-sarcoglycans confirms that loss of any one sarcoglycan leads to the secondary reduction or absence of others [202, 241]. In severely affected patients, the onset of disease was before age 10 years, and all four sarcoglycans were absent from muscle. Western blot and gene analyses are necessary to identify the primary gene defect.

Genetics

Sarcoglycanopathies are due to mutations in any one of the α-, β-, γ-, and δ-sarcoglycan genes. The chromosomal localization of these genes is shown in Figure 4.1 and Table 4.1. In the genetic analysis of sarcoglycanopathies, defects must be found in both alleles of a particular sarcoglycan gene. The mutations (missense and nonsense point mutations, small deletions, and duplications) are the most frequent in the gene of α-sarcoglycan (34%) [237], less frequent in the β-sarcoglycan (16%), and less in the γ- and δ-sarcoglycan genes [225]. No mutations have been found in 42% of the patients [225]. The prevalence of sarcoglycan gene mutations was the highest among the patients with severe muscular dystrophy beginning in childhood. A pathogenic single-base mutation must be differentiated from neutral polymorphisms, which are the most frequent in the α- and γ-sarcoglycan genes [211, 242]. A highly penetrating single-base substitution has not been identified. Recently, the ε-sarcoglycan gene has been described, which has a high homology to α-sarcoglycan [243]. Its mutation has not been identified as a cause of muscular dystrophy.

Treatment

The same general principles for treatment apply as for DMD, but our personal experience suggests that steroids are not effective. The efficacy of δ-dystroglycan gene replacement by adenovirus-mediated gene transfer into muscle of the δ-dystroglycan-deficient hamsters bodes well for the treatment [244]. Because most of the sarcoglycan cDNAs are relatively small, the highly desirable adeno-associated virus vector could be the delivery vehicle of choice.

MEROSIN-DEFICIENT CONGENITAL MUSCULAR DYSTROPHY

Congenital muscular dystrophy (CMD) represents heterogeneous disorders characterized clinically by hypotonia, wasting, and weakness affecting facial and limb muscles and joint contractures [245]. Various phenotypes have been defined. CMD may be limited to skeletal muscle, but it can involve the central nervous system as well. CMD with the absence of the laminin α2 chain in the skeletal muscle is referred to as *merosin-deficient CMD* [246]. In 1994, Tome et al. demonstrated that laminin α2-deficient patients show striking cerebral white matter abnormalities, but most are intellectually normal [69]. From 30% to 40% of neonatal-onset CMD was shown to be due to laminin α2 (merosin) deficiency [157, 247]. The merosin-deficient muscular dystrophy must be distinguished from the Fukuyama type, which is another autosomal recessive congenital muscular dystrophy [248]. The Fukuyama type is prevalent in Japan and is associated with severe mental retardation and structural changes in the central nervous system, such as lissencephaly and hydrocephalus [248]. Its incidence is approximately one-half that of DMD, but it is rarely observed in other countries, in contrast with laminin α2 (merosin) deficient CMD. In Fukuyama congenital muscular dystrophy, the gene locus 9q31.3-33 is different from that of merosin 6q22-23, and for unknown reasons, merosin immunostaining reveals partial deficiency. In the dy dystrophic mouse, there is merosin deficiency that is due to a mutation of its gene [249–251].

Clinical Phenotypes

The patients with merosin deficiency are usually hypotonic at birth. Some display multiple joint contractures. There is generalized muscle weakness. The facial, neck, and chest musculature is variably involved; the limb muscles are more severely affected proximally than distally. The tendon reflexes are decreased or absent. The mental development is usually normal. Many patients will never ambulate.

An abnormal expression of the laminin β1 chain was described in an adult-onset LGMD [252].

Investigations

The serum CK and aldolase are usually normal or mildly increased. The EMG reveals a myopathic pattern, although peripheral nerve involvement may be present [253]. Magnetic resonance imaging of the brain reveals high-intensity signals in the white matter.

Muscle Pathology and Histochemistry

Muscle biopsy shows striking pathologic changes consistent with a dystrophic process. An increased variation in fiber diameter, replacement of muscle by adipose tissue, and connective tissue proliferation are the characteristic features. Some patients showed marked interstitial inflammation in their muscle. Pegoraro et al. [246] reported that CMD with primary laminin α2 chain deficiency may present microscopically as an inflammatory myopathy. Immunostaining for dystrophin α-, β-, γ-, and δ-sarcoglycans and β-dystroglycan is positive in all fibers. The laminin α2 chain was completely deficient in most cases, but there are some with only partial merosin deficiency (Color Plate 5). There appears to be a compensatory increase of the laminin α1 immunostaining.

Merosin is normally detectable in Schwann cell basal lamina of cutaneous nerves and in the basal lamina of the corium. In CMD, there is no immunoreactivity in these structures [247, 254]. Thus, in merosin-negative CMD patients, skin biopsy may provide an alternative possibility for definitive diagnosis.

Genetics

Merosin-deficient congenital muscular dystrophy is transmitted as an autosomal recessive trait. The gene of laminin α2 (merosin) is localized on chromosome 6q2 (255). The laminin α2 gene and protein are very large; therefore, it is difficult to screen for mutations responsible for the disease. Several nonsense and splice-site mutations in the LAMA2 gene were identified in CMD patients, resulting in truncated protein affecting either the short arm domains or the C-terminal globular domain [256, 257]. LAMA2 missense mutation of the laminin α2 gene was identified in cases with partial deficiency of merosin [257, 258].

Prenatal diagnosis can be performed by linkage analysis or by immunocytochemical analysis of laminin α2 in chorionic villus samples [259].

Treatment

The principles for treatment are similar to those applicable to DMD. The large size of merosin cDNA (approximately 9 kb) poses the same problems for merosin gene transfer by adenovirus vector.

DEFICIENCIES OF OTHER PROTEINS RESULTING IN MUSCLE DYSTROPHY

The muscle form of the cytoplasmic soluble enzyme calpain 3 (CANP3) [260] has a role in the etiopathogenesis of the muscular dystrophies [195, 198, 233]. The deficiency of this protein, which is due to mutations in its gene, can result in a form of LGMD [198, 220, 231]. The CANP3 gene is localized on chromosome 15q15.1-21.1. Its mutations lead to deficiency or absence of the muscle-specific calpain [198].

In some patients with adult-onset pelvifemoral muscle weakness, an abnormal expression of the laminin β1 chain was described [252]. The laminin β1 chain is a part of the laminin 2 heterotrimer.

Integrins (α7/β1) may show an abnormal expression and localization in myofibers of merosin-deficient human patients [218].

Recently, genetic deficiency of two other sarcolemmal proteins have been discovered as causes of limb-girdle dystrophy. Caveolin-3 deficiency causes LGMD-1B [261], and dysferlin deficiency causes LGMD-2B [262].

CONCLUSION

The development of molecular science has greatly improved our understanding of the muscular dystrophies. By a systematic approach, a precise molecular diagnosis can be established in the majority of cases (Figure 4.4). In particular, the differentiation of primary versus secondary deficiencies is possible. However, there are still instances in which the genetic defect and its consequences have not yet been uncovered. The in-depth understanding of the molecular pathology and pathogenesis of the dystrophies have paved the way for the eventual development of definitive molecular therapy.

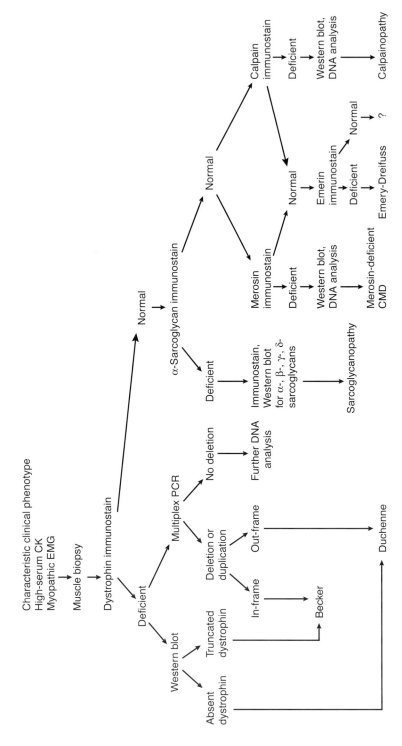

Figure 4.4   A flow diagram depicts a diagnostic strategy in the investigation of patients who present with a dystrophic clinical phenotype. (CK = creatine kinase; EMG = electromyography; PCR = polymerase chain reaction; CMD = congenital muscular dystrophy.)

REFERENCES

1. Worton, R. Muscular dystrophies: diseases of the dystrophin-glycoprotein complex. Science 1995;270:755–756.
2. Karpati G, Brown R Jr. The dawning of a new era in the molecular biology of the muscular dystrophies. Brain Pathol 1996;6:17.
3. Zubrzycka-Gaarn EE, Hutter OF, Karpati G. Dystrophin is tightly associated with the sarcolemma of mammalian skeletal muscle fibers. Exp Cell Res 1991;192:278–288.
4. Ervasti JM, Campbell KP. Membrane organization of the dystrophin-glycoprotein complex. Cell 1991;66:1121–1131.
5. Ervasti JM, Campbell KP. A role for the dystrophin-glycoprotein complex as a transmembrane linker between laminin and actin. J Cell Biol 1993;122:809–823.
6. Ibraghimov-Beskrovnaya O, Ervasti JM, Leveille CJ, et al. Primary structure dystrophin-associated glycoproteins linking dystrophin to the extracellular matrix. Nature 1992;355:696–702.
7. Lindenbaum MH, Carbonetto S. Dystrophin and partners at the cell surface. Curr Opin Biol 1993;3:109–111.
8. Campbell KP. Three muscular dystrophies: loss of cytoskeletal-extracellular matrix linkage. Cell 1995;80:675–679.
9. Sunada Y, Campbell K. Dystrophin-glycoprotein complex: molecular organization and critical roles in skeletal muscle. Curr Opin Neurol 1995;8:379–384.
10. Brown HR. Dystrophin-associated proteins and muscular dystrophies: a glossary. Brain Pathol 1996;6:19–24.
11. Beckmann JS. Genetic studies and molecular structures: the dystrophin associated complex. Hum Mol Genet 1996;5:865–867.
12. Hoffman EP, Clemens PR. HyperCKemic, proximal muscular dystrophies and the dystrophin membrane cytoskeleton, including dystrophinopathies, sarcoglycanopthies, and merosinopathies. Curr Opin Rheumatol 1996;8:528–538.
13. Emery AEH. Duchenne Muscular Dystrophy. Oxford Monographs on Medical Genetics (2nd ed). Oxford, UK: Oxford University Press, 1993.
14. Greenstein RM, Reardon MP, Chan TS. An X-autosome translocation in a girl with Duchenne muscular dystrophy (DMD): evidence for DMD gene localization. Pediatr Res 1977;11:457.
15. Murray JM, Davis KE, Harper PS, et al. Linkage relationship of a cloned DNA sequence on the short arm of the X-chromosome to Duchenne muscular dystrophy. Nature 1982;300:69–71.
16. Davies KE, Pearson PL, Harper PS, et al. Linkage analysis of two cloned DNA sequences flanking the Duchenne muscular dystrophy locus on the short arm of the human X-chromosome. Nucleic Acids Res 1983;11:2302–2312.
17. Francke U, Ochs HD, de Martinville B, et al. Minor X-21 chromosome deletion in a male associated with expression of Duchenne muscular dystrophy, chronic granulomatous disease, retinitis pigmentosa and McLeod syndrome. Am J Hum Genet 1985;37:250–267.
18. Kunkel LM, Monaco AB, Biddlesworth W, et al. Specific cloning of DNA fragments absent from the DNA of a male patients with an X-chromosome deletion. Proc Natl Acad Sci U S A 1985;82:4778–4782.
19. Monaco AB, Neve RL, Colletti-Feener C, et al. Isolation of candidate DNAs for portions of the Duchenne muscular dystrophy gene. Nature 1986;323:646–650.
20. Monaco AB, Bertelson CK, Colletti-Feener C, et al. Localization and cloning of Xp21 deletion break points involved in muscular dystrophy. Hum Genet 1987;75:221–227.
21. Burghes AHM, Logan C, Hu X, et al. A cDNA clone from the Duchenne/Becker muscular dystrophy gene. Nature 1987;328:424–437.
22. Koenig M, Hoffman EP, Bertelson CJ, et al. Complete cloning of the Duchenne muscular dystrophy (DMD) cDNA and preliminary genomic organization of the DMD gene in normal and affected individuals. Cell 1987;50:509–517.
23. Hoffman EP, Brown RH, Kunkel LM. Dystrophin: the protein product of the Duchenne muscular dystrophy locus. Cell 1987;51:919–928.
24. Koenig M, Monaco AB, Kunkel LM. The complete sequence of dystrophin predicts a rod-shaped cytoskeletal protein. Cell 1988;53:219–228.
25. Chelly J, Caplan JC, Maire P, et al. Transcription of the dystrophin gene in human muscle and non-muscle tissues. Nature 1988;333:858–860.
26. Nudel U, Robzyk K, Yaffe D. Expression of the putative Duchenne muscular dystrophy gene in different myogenic cell cultures and in the brain. Nature 1988;333:635–638.

27. Lev AA, Feener CC, Kunkel LM, et al. Expression of the Duchenne's muscular dystrophy gene in cultured muscle cells. J Biochem 1988;262:15817–15820.
28. Miranda AF, Bonilla E, Martucci G, et al. An immunocytochemical study of dystrophin in muscle cultures from patients with Duchenne muscular dystrophy and unaffected controls. Am J Pathol 1988;132:410–416.
29. Zubrzycka-Gaarn EE, Bulman DE, Karpati G, et al. The Duchenne muscular gene product is localized in sarcolemma of human skeletal muscle. Nature 1988;333:466–469.
30. Arahata K, Ishiuwa S, Ishiguro T, et al. Immunostaining of skeletal and cardiac muscle surface membrane with antibody against Duchenne muscular dystrophy peptide. Nature 1988;333:861–863.
31. Bonilla E, Samitt CE, Miranda AF, et al. Duchenne muscular dystrophy: deficiency of dystrophin at the muscle cell surface. Cell 1988;54:447–452.
32. Carpenter S, Karpati G, Zubrzycka-Gaarn E, et al. Dystrophin is localized to the plasma membrane of human skeletal muscle fibers by electron-microscopic cytochemical study. Muscle Nerve 1990;13:376–380.
33. Bartlett RJ, Percak-Vance J, Koh LH, et al. Duchenne muscular dystrophy: high frequency of deletions. Neurology 1988;38:1–4.
34. Malhotra SB, Hart KA, Klamut HJ, et al. Frame-shift deletions in patients with Duchenne and Becker muscular dystrophy. Science 1988;242:755–759.
35. Chamberlain JS, Gibbs RA, Rainier JE, et al. Deletion screening of the Duchenne muscular dystrophy locus via multiplex DNA amplification. Nucleic Acids Res 1988;16:11131–11156.
36. Hoffman EP, Kunkel LM. Dystrophin abnormalities in Duchenne/Becker muscular dystrophy. Neuron 1989;2:1019–1029.
37. Forrest SM, Cross GS, Speer A, et al. Preferential deletion of exons in Duchenne and Becker muscular dystrophies. Nature 1987;329:638–640.
38. Hu Y, Burghes AHM, Ray PN, et al. Partial gene duplication in Duchenne and Becker muscular dystrophies. J Med Genet 1988;25:369–376.
39. Medori R, Brooke MH, Waterston RAH. Genetic abnormalities in Duchenne and Becker dystrophies: clinical correlation. Neurology 1989;39:461–465.
40. Forrest SM, Cross GS, Flint T, et al. Further studies of gene deletions that cause Duchenne and Becker muscular dystrophies. Genomics 1988;2:109–114.
41. Baumbach LL, Chamberlain JS, Ward PA. Molecular and clinical correlations of deletions leading to Duchenne and Becker muscular dystrophies. Neurology 1989;39:465–474.
42. Hoffman EP, Fischbeck KH, Brown RH, et al. Characterization of dystrophin in muscle-biopsy specimens from patients with Duchenne's or Becker's muscular dystrophy. N Engl J Med 1988;318:1363–1368.
43. Arahata KM, Ishihara T, Kamakura K. Mosaic expression of dystrophin in symptomatic carriers of Duchenne's muscular dystrophy. N Engl J Med 1989b;320:138–142.
44. Watkins SC, Hoffman EP, Slater HS, et al. Dystrophin distribution in heterozygote mdx mice. Muscle Nerve 1989;12:861–868.
45. Karpati G, Zubrzycka-Gaarn EE, Carpenter S, et al. Age-related conversion of dystrophin-negative to -positive fibre segments of skeletal but no cardiac muscle fibres in heterozygote mdx mice. J Neuropathol Exp Neurol 1990;49:96–105.
46. Cooper BJ, Winnard NJ, Stedman H, et al. The homologue of Duchenne locus is defective in X-linked muscle dystrophy in dogs. Nature 1988;334:154–156.
47. Nudel U, Zuk D, Einat P, et al. Duchenne muscular dystrophy gene product is not identical in muscle and brain. Nature 1989;337:76–78.
48. Partridge TA, Morgan JE, Coulton GR. Conversion of mdx myofibers from dystrophin-negative to -positive by injection of normal myoblasts. Nature 1989;337:176–179.
49. Karpati G, Pouliot Y, Zubrzycka-Gaarn EE, et al. Dystrophin is expressed in mdx skeletal muscle fibers after normal myoblast implantation. Am J Pathol 1989;135:27–32.
50. Sicinski P, Geng Y, Ryder-Cook AS, et al. The molecular basis of muscular dystrophy in the mdx mouse: a point mutation. Science 1989;244:1578–1580.
51. Love DR, Dickson G, Spurr NK, et al. An autosomal transcript in skeletal muscle with homology to dystrophin. Nature 1989;339:55–58.
52. Karpati G, Carpenter S. Small-caliber skeletal muscle fibers do not suffer deleterious consequences of dystrophic gene expression. Am J Med Genet 1986;25:653–658.
53. Campbell KP, Kahl SD. Association of dystrophin and an integral membrane glycoprotein. Nature 1989;338:259–262.
54. Ervasti JM, Ohlendieck K, Kahl SD, et al. Deficiency of a glycoprotein component of the dystrophin complex in dystrophic muscle. Nature 1990;345:315–319.

55. Koenig M, Kunkel LM. Detailed analysis of the repeat domain of dystrophin reveals four potential hinge segments that may confer flexibility. J Biol Chem 1990;265:4560–4566.
56. Nicholson LVB. The "rescue" of dystrophin synthesis in boys with Duchenne muscular dystrophy. Neuromuscul Disord 1993;3:525–531.
57. Nicholson LVB, Johnson MA, Bushby KMD, et al. The functional significance of dystrophin positive fibers in Duchenne muscular dystrophy. Arch Dis Child 1993;68:632–636.
58. Bar S, Barnea E, Levy Z, et al. A novel product of the DMD gene which greatly differs from the known isoforms in its structure and tissue distribution. Biochem J 1990;272:557–560.
59. Weller B, Karpati G, Carpenter S. Dystrophin-deficient mdx muscle fibers are preferentially vulnerable to necrosis induced by experimental lengthening contractions. J Neurol Sci 1990;100:9–13.
60. Wells JW, Wells KE, Walsh FS, et al. Human dystrophin expression corrects myopathic phenotype on transgenic mdx mice. Hum Mol Genet 1992;1:35–40.
61. Cox GA, Cole NM, Matsumara K, et al. Overexpression of dystrophin in transgenic mdx mice eliminated dystrophic symptoms without toxicity. Nature 1993;364:725–729.
62. Hoffman EP, Arahata K, Minetti C, et al. Dystrophinopathy in isolated cases of myopathy in females. Neurology 1992;42:967–975.
63. Roberds SL, Letrucq F, Allamand V, et al. Missense mutations in the adhalin gene linked to autosomal recessive muscular dystrophy. Cell 1994;78:625–633.
64. Lim LE, Duchlos F, Broux O, et al. Beta-sarcoglycan: characterization and role in limb-girdle muscular dystrophy linked to 4q12. Nat Genet 1995;11:257–285.
65. Noguchi S, McNally EM, Ben Othmane K, et al. Mutations in the dystrophin-associated protein gamma-sarcoglycan in chromosome 13 muscular dystrophy. Science 1995;270:819–822.
66. Nigro V, Moreira E, Piluso G, et al. Autosomal recessive limb-girdle muscular dystrophy, LGMD2F is caused by a mutation in the delta-sarcoglycan gene. Nat Genet 1996a;14:195–198.
67. Nigro V, Piluso G, Belsito A, et al. Identification of a novel sarcoglycan gene at 5q33 encoding a sarcolemmal 35 kDa glycoprotein. Hum Mol Genet 1996b;5:1179–1186.
68. Ahn AH, Kunkel LM. Syntrophin binds to an alternatively spliced exon of dystrophin. J Cell Biol 1995;128:363–371.
69. Tome FM, Evangelista T, Leclerc A, et al. Congenital muscular dystrophy with merosin deficiency. C R Acad Sci III 1994;317:351–357.
70. Tinsley JM, Potter AC, Phelps SR, et al. Amelioration of dystrophin phenotype of mdx mice using a truncated dystrophin transgene. Nature 1996;384:349–359.
71. Griggs RC, Moxley RT, Mendel JR, et al. Prednisone in Duchenne dystrophy. A randomized controlled trial defining the time course and dose response. Arch Neurol 1991;48:383–388.
72. Karpati G, Acsadi G. The potential for gene therapy in muscular dystrophy and other genetic muscle diseases. Muscle Nerve 1993;16:1141–1143.
73. Mendell JR, Kissel JT, Amato AA, et al. Myoblast transfer in the treatment of Duchenne's muscular dystrophy. N Engl J Med 1995;333:832–838.
74. Ragot T, Vincent N, Chafey P, et al. Efficient adenovirus-mediated transfer of a human minidystrophin gene to skeletal muscle of mdx mice. Nature 1993;361:647–650.
75. Acsadi G, Lochmüller H, Jani A, et al. Dystrophin expression in muscles of mdx mice after adenovirus-mediated in vivo gene transfer. Hum Gene Ther 1996;7:129–140.
76. Lochmüller H, Petrof BJ, Pari G. Transient immunosuppression by FK506 permits a sustained high level dystrophin expression after adenovirus-mediated dystrophin minigene transfer to skeletal muscles of adult dystrophic (mdx) mice. Gene Ther 1996;3:706–716.
77. Kochanek S, Clemens P, Mitanik, et al. A new adenoviral vector: replacement of all viral coding sequences with 28 Kb of DNA independently expressing full length dystrophin and β-galactosidase. Proc Natl Acad Sci U S A 1996;93:5731–5736.
78. Gilbert R, Nalbantoglu J, Tinsley JM, et al. Efficient utrophin expression following adenovirus gene transfer in dystrophic muscle. Biochem Biophys Res Commun 1998;242:244–247.
79. Wahl M. Human trials set for DMD. Quest 1998;1:9.
80. Mandel JG. The gene and its product. Nature 1989;339:154–156.
81. Sadoulet-Puccio HM, Kunkel LM. Dystrophin and its isoforms. Brain Pathol 1996;6:25–35.
82. Gussoni E, Blau HM, Kunkel LM. The fate of individual myoblasts after transplantation into muscles of DMD patients. Nat Med 1997;3:970–977.
83. Lederfein D, Levy S, Augier N, et al. A 71-kilodalton protein is a major product of the Duchenne muscular dystrophy gene in brain and other nonmuscular tissues. Proc Natl Acad Sci U S A 1992;89:5346–5350.
84. Makover A, Zuk D, Breakston E, et al. Brain-type and muscle-type promoters of the dystrophin gene differ greatly in structure. Neuromuscul Disord 1991;1:39–45.

85. Klamut HJ, Ganagopadhyay SB, Worton RG, et al. Molecular and functional analysis of the muscle-specific promoter region of the Duchenne muscular dystrophy gene. Mol Cell Biol 1990;10:193–205.
86. Chelly J, et al. Dystrophin gene transcribed from different promoters in neuronal and glial cells. Neuron 1990;344:64–65.
87. Boyce FM, Beggs AH, Feener C, Kunkel LM. Dystrophin is transcribed in brain from a distant upstream promoter. Proc Natl Acad Sci U S A 1991;88:1276–1280.
88. Gorecki DC, Monaco AP, Derry JM, et al. Expression of four alternative dystrophin transcripts in brain regions regulated by different promoters. Hum Mol Genet 1992;1:505–510.
89. Tennyson CN, Klamut HJ, Worton RG. The human dystrophin gene requires 16 hours to be transcribed and is co-transcriptionally spliced. Nat Genet 1995;19:184–190.
90. Pillers DM, Bulman DE, Weleber RG, et al. Dystrophin expression in the human retina is required for normal function as defined by retinography. Nat Genet 1993;4:82–86.
91. Feener CA, Koenig M, Kunkel LM. Alternative splicing of human dystrophin mRNA generates isoforms at the carboxy terminus. Nature 1989;338:509–511.
92. Hoffman EP, Kahl SD. Improved diagnosis of Becker muscular dystrophy by dystrophin testing. Neurology 1989;39:1011–1017.
93. Ahn AH, Kunkel LM. The structural and functional diversity of dystrophin. Nat Genet 1993;3: 283–291.
94. Levine BA, Moir AJG, Patchell VB, Berry SC. The interaction of actin with dystrophin. FEBS Lett 1990;263:159–162.
95. Suzuki JM, Yoshida M, Hayashi K, et al. Molecular organization at the glycoprotein-complex-binding site of dystrophin. Three dystrophin-associated proteins bind directly to the carboxy-terminal portion of the dystrophin. Eur J Biochem 1994a;220:283–292.
96. Suzuki A, Yoshida M, Yamamoto H. Ozawa E. Glycoprotein-binding site of dystrophin is confined to the cysteine-rich domain and the first half of the carboxy-terminal domain. FEBS Lett 1994b;308:154–160.
97. Ohlendieck K, Campbell KP. Dystrophin constitutes 5% of membrane cytoskeleton in skeletal muscle. FEBS Lett 1991a;283:230–234.
98. Cullen MJ, Walsh J, Nicholson LVB, et al. Ultrastructural localization of dystrophin in human muscle by using gold immunolabeling. Proc R Soc Lond B Biol Sci 1990;240:197–210.
99. Cullen MJ, Walsh J, Nicholson LVB, et al. Immunogold labelling of dystrophin in human muscle, using an antibody to the last 17 amino acids of the C-terminus. Neuromuscul Disord 1991;1:113–119.
100. Karpati G. Recent developments in the biology of dystrophin and related molecules. Curr Opin Neurol Neurosurg 1992;5:615–621.
101. Minetti C, Beltrame F, Marcenaro G, et al. Dystrophin at the plasma membrane of human muscle fibers shows a costameric localization. Neuromuscul Disord 1992;2:99–109.
102. Porter GA, Dmytrenko GM, Winkelmann JC, Block RJ. Dystrophin colocalizes with β-spectrin in distinct subsarcolemmal domains in mammalian skeletal muscle. J Cell Biol 1992;117:997–1005.
103. Craig SW, Pardo JV. Gamma actin, spectrin, and intermediate filament proteins colocalize with vinculin at costameres, myofibril-to-sarcolemma attachment sites. Cell Motil Cytoskeleton 1983;3:449–462.
104. Byers TJ, Junkel LM, Watkins SC. The subcellular distribution of dystrophin in mouse skeletal, cardiac, and smooth muscle. J Cell Biol 1991;115:411–421.
105. Zhao J, Yoshioka K, Miyatake M, et al. Dystrophin and a dystrophin-related protein in intrafusal muscle fibers, and neuromuscular and myotendinous junctions. Acta Neuropathol (Berl) 1992;84: 141–146.
106. Samitt CE, Bonilla E. Immunocytochemical study of dystrophin at the myotendinous junction. Muscle Nerve 1990;13:493–500.
107. Tidball JG, Law DJ. Dystrophin is required for normal thin filament-membrane association at myotendinous junctions. Am J Pathol 1992;138:17–21.
108. Petrof BJ, Shrager JB, Stedman HH, et al. Dystrophin protects the sarcolemma from stresses developed during muscle contraction. Proc Natl Acad Sci U S A 1993;90:3710–3714.
109. Hutter OF, Burton FL, Bovell DK. Mechanical properties of normal and mdx mouse sarcolemma: bearing on the function of dystrophin. J Muscle Res Cell Motil 1991;12:585–589.
110. Hutter OF. The membrane hypothesis of Duchenne muscular dystrophy: quest for functional evidence. J Inherit Metab Dis 1992;15:565–577.
111. Bork P, Sudol M. The WW domain: a signalling site in dystrophin? Trends Biochem Sci 1994;19: 531–533.

112. Hardiman O. Dystrophin deficiency, altered cell signalling and fiber hypertrophy. Neuromuscul Disord 1994;4:305–315.
113. Lidov HGW, Byers TJ, Watkins SC, Kunkel LM. Localization of dystrophin to postsynaptic regions of central nervous system cortical neurons. Nature 1990;348:725–728.
114. Byers TJ, Lidov HGW, Kunkel LM. An alternative dystrophin transcript specific to peripheral nerve. Nat Genet 1993;4:77–81.
115. Blake DJ, Tinsley JM, Davies KE. Utrophin: a structural and functional comparison to dystrophin. Brain Pathol 1996;61:37–47.
116. Love DR, Morris GE, Ellis JM, et al. Tissue distribution of the dystrophin-related gene product and expression in the mdx and dy mouse. Proc Natl Acad Sci U S A 1991;88:3243–3247.
117. Buckle VJ, Guenet JL, Simon-Chazottes D. Localisation of a dystrophin-related autosomal gene to 6q24 in man, and mouse chromosome 10 in the region of the dystrophia muscularis (dy) locus. Hum Genet 1990;85:324–326.
118. Kuhrana TS, Hoffman AP, Kunkel LM. Identification of a chromosome 6-encoded dystrophin-related protein. J Biol Chem 1991a;265:16717–16720.
119. Kuhrana TS, Watkins SC, Chagey P. Immunolocalization and developmental expression of dystrophin-related protein in skeletal muscle. Neuromuscul Disord 1991b;1:185–194.
120. Tinsley JM, Blake DJ, Roche A, et al. Primary structure of dystrophin-related protein. Nature 1992;360:591–592.
121. Ohlendieck K, Ervasti JM, Matsumura K, et al. Dystrophin-related protein is localized to neuromuscular junctions of adult skeletal muscle. Neuron 1991;7:499–508.
122. Pons F, Augier N, Leger JOC, et al. A homologue of dystrophin is expressed at the neuromuscular junctions of normal individuals and DMD patients and of normal and mdx mice. FEBS Lett 1991;282:161–165.
123. Nguyen TM, Elli JM, Loe DR. Localization of the DMDL-gene-encoded dystrophin-related protein using a panel of nineteen monoclonal antibodies. J Cell Biol 1991;115:1695–1700.
124. Man N, Ellis JM, Love DR, et al. Localization of the DMDL gene-encoded dystrophin-related protein using a panel of nineteen monoclonal antibodies: presence at the neuromuscular junctions in the sarcolemma of dystrophic skeletal muscle, in vascular and other smooth muscles, and in proliferating brain cell lines. J Cell Biol 1991;115:1695–1700.
125. Matsumura K, Ervasti JM, Ohlendieck K, et al. Association of dystrophin-related protein with dystrophin-associated proteins in mdx mouse muscle. Nature 1992b;360:588–591.
126. Karpati G, Carpenter S, Morris G, et al. Localization and quantitation of chromosome 6-encoded dystrophin-related protein in normal and pathological muscle. J Neuropathol Exp Neurol 1993;52:119–128.
127. Chevron M-P, Echenne B, Damaille J. Absence of dystrophin and utrophin in a boy with severe muscular dystrophy. N Engl J Med 1994;331:1162–1163.
128. Grady RM, Teng H, Nichol MC, et al. Skeletal and cardiac myopathies in mice lacking utrophin and dystrophin: a model for Duchenne muscular dystrophy. Cell 1997;90:729–738.
129. Brooke MH. A Clinicians' View of Neuromuscular Disease. Baltimore: Williams & Wilkins, 1977.
130. Farell PT. Anaesthesia-induced rhabdomyolysis causing cardiac arrest: case report and review of anaesthesia and the dystrophinopathies. Anaesth Intensive Care 1994;22:597–601.
131. Brooke MH, Fenichel GM, Griggs R, et al. Duchenne muscular dystrophy: pattern of clinical progression and the effects of supportive therapy. Neurology 1989;39:475–481.
132. Dubowitz V. Intellectual impairment in muscular dystrophy. Arch Dis Child 1965;40:296–301.
133. Lidov HGW. Dystrophin in the nervous system. Brain Pathol 1996;6:63–77.
134. Matthews PM, Benjamin D, Van Bakel I, et al. Muscle x-inactivation patterns and dystrophin expression in Duchenne muscular dystrophy carriers. Neuromuscul Disord 1995;5:209–220.
135. Matthews PM, Karpati G. The pattern of X chromosome inactivation is a key determinant of the clinicopathological phenotype of Duchenne muscular dystrophy carriers. Neurology 1995;45:689–690.
136. Pegoraro E, Schimke RN, Garcia C, et al. Genetic and biochemical normalization in female carriers of Duchenne muscular dystrophy: evidence for failure of dystrophin production in dystrophin-competent myonuclei. Neurol 1995;45:677–690.
137. Pena SDJ, Karpati G, Carpenter S, et al. The clinical consequences of X-chromosome inactivation: Duchenne muscular dystrophy in one of monozygotic twins. J Neurol Sci 1987;79:337–344.
138. Ferrier P, Bamatter F, Klein D. Muscular dystrophy (Duchenne) in a girl with Turner's syndrome. J Med Genet 1965;2:38.
139. Baiget M, Tizzano E, Volpini V, et al. DMD carrier detection in a female with mosaic Turner's syndrome. J Med Genet 1991;28:209–210.
140. Becker PE, Kiener F. Eine neue X-chromosomale muskeldystrophie. Arch Psychiat-Z Neurol 1955;193:427–448.

141. Koenig M, Beggs AH, Moyer M, et al. The molecular basis for Duchenne versus Becker muscular dystrophy: correlation of severity with type of deletion. Am J Hum Genet 1989;45:498–506.
142. Beggs AH, Hoffman EP, Snyder JR, et al. Exploring the molecular basis for variability among patients with Becker muscular dystrophy: dystrophin gene and protein studies. Am J Hum Genet 1991;49:54–67.
143. Sunohara N, Arahata K, Hoffman EP. Quadriceps myopathy: forme fruste of Becker muscular dystrophy. Ann Neurol 1990;28:634–639.
144. Gospe SM Jr, Lazaro JP, Lava NS, et al. Familial X-linked myalgia and cramps: a nonprogressive myopathy associated with a deletion in the dystrophin gene. Neurology 1989;39:1277–1280.
145. Bushby K, Goodship AH, Haggerty D, et al. Duchenne muscular dystrophy and idiopathic hyperCKemia in a family causing confusion in genetic counselling. Am J Med Genet 1996;66:237–238.
146. Jacobs HK, Wrogeman K, Greenberg CR, et al. Neonatal Screening for Duchenne Muscular Dystrophy. The Canadian Experience In BJ Schmid, Diamont AJ, Loghin-Grosso NS (eds), Current Trends in Infant Screening. Amsterdam, the Netherlands: Elsevier, 1989;361–366.
147. Farrah MG, Evans EB, Vignos JP. Electrocardiographic evaluation of left ventricular function in Duchenne's muscular dystrophy. Am J Med 1980;69:248–254.
148. Carpenter S, Karpati G. Duchenne muscular dystrophy: plasma membrane loss initiates muscle cell necrosis unless it is repaired. Brain 1979;102:147–161.
149. Schmalbruch J. Segmental fiber breakdown and defects of the plasmalemma in diseased human muscles. Acta Neuropathol (Berl) 1975;33:129–141.
150. Mokri B, Engel AG. Duchenne dystrophy: electron microscopic findings pointing to a basic or early abnormality in the plasma membrane of the muscle fibers. Neurology 1975;25:1111–1120.
151. Carpenter S, Karpati G. Segmental necrosis and its demarcation in experimental micropuncture injury of skeletal muscle fibers. J Neuropathol Exp Neurol 1989;48:154–170.
152. Matsumura K, Campbell KP. Dystrophin-glycoprotein complex: its role in the molecular pathogenesis of muscular dystrophies. Muscle Nerve 1994;17:2–15.
153. Menke A, Jokusch H. Decreased osmotic stability of dystrophin-less muscle cells from the mdx mouse. Nature 1991;349:69–71.
154. Bernasconi P, Toschiana E, Confalonieri P, et al. Expression of transforming growth factor beta 1 in dystrophic patient muscles correlates with fibrosis. Pathogenic role of a fibrogenic cytokine. J Clin Invest 1995;96:1137–1144.
155. Arahata K, Engel AG. Monoclonal antibody analysis of mononuclear cells in myopathies. I: Quantitation of subsets according to diagnosis and sites of accumulation and demonstration and counts of muscle fibers invaded by T cells. Ann Neurol 1984;16:193–208.
156. Arahata KM, Hoffman EP, Kunkel LM, et al. Dystrophin diagnosis: comparison of dystrophin abnormalities by immunofluorescence and immunoblot analyses. Proc Natl Acad Sci U S A 1989a;86:7154–7158.
157. Hoffman EP. Clinical and histopathological features of abnormalities of the dystrophin-based membrane cytoskeleton. Brain Pathol 1996;6:49–61.
158. Taylor J, Muntoni F, Dubowitz V, et al. The abnormal expression of utrophin in Duchenne and Becker muscular dystrophy is age related. Neuropathol Appl Neurobiol 1997;23:399–405.
159. Pasquini F, Guerin C, Blake D, et al. The effect of glucocorticoids on the accumulation of utrophin by cultured normal and dystrophic human skeletal muscle satellite cells. Neuromuscul Disord 1995; 5:105–114.
160. Ohlendieck K, Matsumura K, Ionasescu VV, et al. Duchenne muscular dystrophy: deficiency of dystrophin-associated proteins in the sarcolemma. Neurology 1993;43:795–800.
161. Ohlendieck K, Campbell KP. Dystrophin-associated proteins are greatly reduced in skeletal muscle from mdx mice. J Cell Biol 1991;115:1685–1694.
162. Ljunggren A, Duggan D, McNally EM, et al. Primary adhalin deficiency as a cause of muscular dystrophy in patients with normal dystrophin. Ann Neurol 1995;38:367–372.
163. Gillard EF, Chamberlain JS, Murphy EG, et al. Molecular and phenotypic analysis of patients with deletions within the deletion-rich region of the Duchenne muscular dystrophy (DMD) gene. Am J Hum Genet 1989;45:507–520.
164. Bushby KM. Genetic and clinical correlations of Xp21 muscular dystrophy. J Inherit Metab Dis 1992;15:551–564.
165. Abbs S, Bobrow M. Analysis of quantitative PCR for the diagnosis of deletion and duplications carriers in the dystrophin gene. J Med Genet 1992;29:191–196.
166. Hu XY, Ray PN, Murphy EG, et al. Duplicational mutation at the Duchenne muscular dystrophy locus: its frequency, distribution, origin, and phenotype genotype correlation. Am J Hum Genet 1990; 46:682–695.

167. Bulman DE, Gangopadhyay SM, Bebchuck KG. Point mutation in the human dystrophin gene: identification through western blot analysis. Genomics 1991;10:457–560.

168. Roberts RG, Bobrow M, Bentley DR. Point mutations in the dystrophin gene. Proc Natl Acad Sci U S A 1992;89:2331–2335.

169. Yau SC, Roberts RG, Bobrow M, et al. Direct diagnosis of carriers of point mutations in Duchenne muscular dystrophy. Lancet 1993;341:273–275.

170. England SB, Nicholson LVB, Johnson MA, et al. Very mild muscular dystrophy associated with the deletion of 46% of dystrophin. Nature 1990;343:180–181.

171. Bies RD, Caskey CT, Fenwick R. An intact cysteine-rich domain is required for dystrophin function. J Clin Invest 1992;90:666–672.

172. Hoffman EP, Garcia CA, Chamberlain JS, et al. Is the carboxyl-terminus of dystrophin required for membrane association? A novel, severe case of Duchenne muscular dystrophy. Ann Neurol 1991;30:605–610.

173. Gangopadhyay SB, Sherratt TG, Heckmatt JZ, et al. Dystrophin in frameshift deletion patients with Becker muscular dystrophy. Am J Hum Genet 1992;51:562–570.

174. Helliwell TR, Ellis JM, Mountford RC, et al. A truncated dystrophin lacking C-terminal domain is localized at the muscle membrane. Am J Hum Genet 1992;50:508–514.

175. Bushby KMD, Emery AMH. Genetic Aspects of Neuromuscular Disease. In J Walton, G Karpati, D Hilton-Jones (eds), Disorders of Voluntary Muscle. Edinburgh, UK: Churchill Livingstone, 1994;924–947.

176. Prior TW, Papp AC, Snyder PJ, et al. Determination of carrier status in Duchenne and Becker muscular dystrophies by quantitative polymerase chain reaction and allele-specific oligonucleotides. Clin Chem 1990;36:2113–2117.

177. Schwartz LS, Tarleton J, Popvich B, et al. Fluorescent multiplex linkage analysis and carrier detection for Duchenne/Becker muscular dystrophy. Am J Hum Genet 1992;51:721–729.

178. Mansfield ES, Robertson JM, Lebo RV, et al. Duchenne/Becker muscular dystrophy carrier detection using quantitative PCR and fluorescence-based strategies. Am J Med Genet 1993;48:200–208.

179. Vainzof M, Favanello RCM, Pavanello I, et al. Dystrophin immunofluorescence pattern in manifesting and symptomatic carriers of Duchenne's and Becker muscular dystrophies in different ages. Neuromuscul Disord 1991;1:177–204.

180. Clemens PR, Fenwick RG, Chamberlain JS, et al. Carrier detection and prenatal diagnosis in Duchenne and Becker muscular dystrophy families, using dinucleotide repeat polymorphisms. Am J Hum Genet 1991;49:951–960.

181. Van Essen AJ, Abbs S, Bauget M, et al. Parental origin and germline mosaicism of deletions and duplications of the dystrophin gene: a European study. Hum Genet 1992;8:249–257.

182. Simard L, Gingras F, Labuda D. Direct analysis of amniotic fluid cells by multiplex PCR provides rapid prenatal diagnosis for Duchenne muscular dystrophy. Nucleic Acids Res 1991;19:2501.

183. Royal Commission on Reproductive Technologies. Proceed With Care. Ottawa: Canadian Communications Group, 1993;921–933.

184. Karpati G, Ajdukovic G, Arnold D, et al. Myoblast transfer in Duchenne muscular dystrophy. Ann Neurol 1993;34:8–17.

185. Matsumara K, Lee CL, Caskey CT, Campbell KD. Restoration of dystrophin-associated proteins in skeletal muscle of mdx mice for dystrophin gene. FEBS Lett 1993;320:276–280.

186. Hauser MS, Phelps SF, Chamberlain JS. Expression of dystrophin minigenes in the muscles of mdx mice partially prevents the development of dystrophic symptoms [abstract]. Am J Hum Genet 1994;55:A47.

187. Karpati G, Acsadi G. The principles of gene therapy in Duchenne dystrophy. Clin Invest Med 1994;17:499–509.

188. Greenberg DS, Sunada Y, Campbell KT, et al. Exogenous Dp71 restores the levels of dystrophin associated proteins but does not alleviate muscle damage in mdx mice. Nat Genet 1994;8:340–344.

189. Cox GA, Sunada Y, Campbell AKP, et al. Dp71 can restore the dystrophin-associated glycoprotein complex in muscle but fails to prevent dystrophy. Nat Genet 1994;8:333–339.

190. Clemens PR, Kochanek S, Sunada Y, et al. In vivo muscle gene transfer of full length dystrophin with an adenoviral vector that lacks all viral genes. Gene Ther 1996;3:965–972.

191. Karpati G, Gilbert R, Petrof B, Nalbantaoglu J. Gene therapy research for Duchenne and Becker muscular dystrophies. Curr Opin Neurol 1997;10:430–435.

192. Bushby KM, Beckmann JS. The limb-girdle muscular dystrophies. Proposal for a new nomenclature. Neuromuscul Disord 1995;5:337–343.

193. Duggan DJ, Hoffman EP. Autosomal recessive muscular dystrophy and mutations of the sarcoglycan complex. Neuromuscul Disord 1996;6:475–482.

194. Beckmann JS, Richard I, Hillaire D, et al. A gene for limb girdle muscular dystrophy maps to chromosome 15 by linkage. C R Acad Sci III 1991;111:141–148.
195. Young K, Foroud T, Williams P, et al. Confirmation of linkage of limb-girdle muscular dystrophy, type 2, to chromosome 15. Genomics 1992;13:1370.
196. Matsumura K, Tome FMS, Collin H, et al. Deficiency of the 50K dystrophin-associated glycoprotein in severe childhood autosomal recessive muscular dystrophy. Nature 1992;359:320–322.
197. Azibi K, Bachner L, Beckmann JS, et al. Severe childhood autosomal recessive muscular dystrophy with the deficiency of the 50 kDa dystrophin-associated glycoprotein maps to chromosome 13q12. Hum Mol Genet 1993;2:1423–1428.
198. Richard I, Boux O, Allamand V, et al. Mutations in the proteolytic enzyme calpain 3 cause limb-girdle muscular dystrophy type 2A. Cell 1995;81:1–20.
199. Kaplan J-C, Campbell KP. Missense mutations in the adhalin gene linked to autosomal recessive muscular dystrophy. Cell 1994;78:625–633.
200. Piccolo F, Roberds SL, Jeanpierre M, et al. Primary adhalinopathy: a common cause or autosomal recessive muscular dystrophy of variable severity. Nat Genet 1995;10:243–245.
201. Passos-Bueno MR, Moreira E, Vainzof M, et al. A common missense mutation in the adhalin gene in three unrelated Brazilian families with a relatively mild form of autosomal recessive limb-girdle muscular dystrophy. Hum Mol Genet 1995;4:1163–1167.
202. Bönnemann CG, Modi R, Noguchi S, et al. Beta-sarcoglycan (A3b) mutations cause autosomal recessive muscular dystrophy with loss of the sarcoglycan complex. Nat Genet 1995;11:266–276.
203. Bönnemann CG, Passos-Bueno MR, McNally EM, et al. Genomic screening for beta-sarcoglycan gene mutations: missense mutations may cause severe limb-girdle muscular dystrophy type 2E (LGMD 2E). Hum Mol Genet 1996;5:1953–1961.
204. Ben Othmane K, Ben Hamida M, Pericak-Vance MA, et al. Linkage of Tunisian autosomal recessive Duchenne-like muscular dystrophy to the pericentromeric region of chromosome 13q. Nat Genet 1992;2:315–317.
205. Piccolo F, Jeanpierre M, Leturcq F, et al. A founder mutation in the gamma-sarcoglycan gene of Gypsies possibly predating their migration out of India. Hum Mol Genet 1996;5:2019–2022.
206. Passos-Bueno MR, Moreira E, Vainzof, et al. Linkage analysis in autosomal recessive limb-girdle muscular dystrophy (AR LGMD) maps a sixth form to 5q33-34 (LGMD2F) and indicates that there is at least one more subtype of AR LGMD. Hum Mol Genet 1996;5:815–820.
207. Eymar B, Romero NB, Leturcq F. Primary adhalinopathy (α-sarcoglycanopathy): clinical, pathologic and genetic correlation in 20 patients with autosomal recessive muscular dystrophy. Neurology 1997;48:1227–1234.
208. Speer MC, Yamaoka LH, Gilchrist JM, et al. Confirmation of genetic heterogeneity of limb girdle muscular dystrophy: linkage of an autosomal dominant form to chromosome 5q. Am J Hum Genet 1992;50:1211–1217.
209. Van der Kooi AJ, Van Meegan M, Ledderhof TM, et al. Genetic localization of a newly recognized autosomal dominant limb girdle muscular dystrophy with cardiac involvement (LGMD 1B) to chromosome 1q11-21. Am J Hum Genet 1997;60:891–895.
210. Ozawa E, Yoshida M, Suzuki A, et al. Dystrophin-associated proteins in muscular dystrophy. Hum Mol Genet 1995;4:11711–11715.
211. McNally EM, Passos-Bueno R, Bönnemann CG, et al. Mild and severe muscular dystrophy caused by a single gamma-sarcoglycan mutation. Am J Hum Genet 1996;59:1040–1047.
212. Adams M, Butler M, Deyer T, et al. Two forms of mouse syntrophin a 58 kD dystrophin-associated protein, differ in a primary structure and tissue distribution. Neuron 1992;11:531–540.
213. Yang B, Jung D, Rafael JA, et al. Identification of α-syntrophin binding to syntrophin triplet, dystrophin and utrophin. J Biol Chem 1995;270:1–4.
214. Wewer UM, Engwall E. Merosin/laminin-2 and muscular dystrophy. Neuromuscul Disord 1996;6:409–418.
215. Burgson RE, Chiquet M, Deutzmann R, et al. A new nomenclature for the laminins. Matrix Biol 1994;13:209–211.
216. Engvall E. Laminin variants: why, where and when? Kidney Int 1993;43:2–6.
217. Mercurio AM. Laminin receptors: achieving specificity through cooperation. Trends Cell Biol 1995;5:419–423.
218. Vachon PH, Zu H, Lui L, et al. Integrins (alpha7beta1) in muscle function and survival. Disrupted expression in merosin-deficient congenital muscular dystrophy. J Clin Invest 1997;110:1870–1881.
219. Mayer U, Saher G, Fassier R, et al. Absence of integrin alpha7 causes a novel form of muscular dystrophy. Nat Genet 1997;17:318–323.

220. Jung D, Yang B, Meyer J, et al. Identification and characterization of dystrophin anchoring site of β dystroglycan. J Biol Chem 1995;270:27305–27310.
221. Cullen MJ, Watkins SC. Ultrastructure of muscular dystrophy: new aspects. Micron 1993;24: 287–307.
222. Crosbie RH, Heighway J, Venzke DK, et al. Sarcospan, the 25-kDa transmembrane component of the dystrophin-glycoprotein. J Biol Chem 1997;50:31221–31224.
223. McNally EM, Yoshida M, Mizuno Y, et al. Human adhalin is alternatively spliced and the gene is located on chromosome 17q21. Proc Natl Acad Sci U S A 1994;91:9690–9694.
224. Duggan DJ, Fanin M, Pegoraro E, et al. α-Sarcoglycan (adhalin) deficiency: complete deficiency patients are 5% of childhood-onset dystrophin normal muscular dystrophy and most partial deficiency patients do not have gene mutations. J Neurol Sci 1996;140:30–39.
225. Duggan DJ, Gorospe JR, Fanin M, et al. Mutations in the sarcoglycan genes in patients with myopathy. N Engl J Med 1997;336:618–624.
226. Ahn A, Yoshida M, Anderson M, et al. A distinct 59 kDa dystrophin associated protein encoded on chromosome 8q23-24. Proc Natl Acad Sci U S A 1994;91:4446–4450.
227. Blake DJ, Nawrotski R, Peters MF, et al. Isoform diversity of dystrobrevin, the murine 87-dKa postsynaptic protein. J Biol Chem 1996;271:7802–7810.
228. Sadoulet-Puccio HM, Rajaka M, Kunkel LM. Dystrobrevin and dystrophin: an interaction through coiled-coil motifs. Proc Natl Acad Sci U S A 1997;94:12413–12418.
229. Metzinger L, Blake DJ, Squier MV, et al. Dystrobrevin deficiency at the sarcolemma of patients with muscular dystrophy. Hum Mol Genet 1997;6:1185–1191.
230. Grozdanovic Z, Christova T, Gosztonyi G, et al. Absence of nitric oxide synthetase 1 despite the presence of the dystrophin complex in human striated muscle. Histochem J 1997;29:97–104.
231. Spencer MJ, Tidball JG, Anderson LVB, et al. Absence of calpain 3 in a form of limb-girdle muscular dystrophy (LGMD2A). J Neurol Sci 1997;146:173–178.
232. Sorimachi H, Imajoh-Ohmi S, Emori Y, et al. Molecular cloning of a novel mammalian calcium dependent protease distinct from m- and μ-types. Specific expression of the mRNA in skeletal muscle. J Biol Chem 1989;264:20106–20111.
233. Sorimachi H, Kinbara K, Kimura S, et al. Muscle-specific calpain, p94, responsible for limb girdle muscular dystrophy type 2A associates with connectin through ISZ, a p94-specific sequence. J Biol Chem 1995;270:31158–31162.
234. Meier T, Hauser DM, Chiquet M, et al. Neural agrin induces ectopic postsynaptic specializations in innervated muscle fibers. J Neurosci 1997;17:6534–6544.
235. Fuhrer C, Sugiyama JE, Tylor RG, Hall ZW. Association of muscle-specific kinase MuSK with the acetylcholine receptor in mammalian muscle. EMBO J 1997;16:4951–4969.
236. Gillespie SK, Balasubramanian S, Fum ET, Huganir RL. Rapsyn clusters and activates the synapse-specific receptor tyrosine kinase MuSK. Neuron 1996;16:953–962.
237. Hayashi YK, Arahata K. The frequency of patients with adhalin deficiency in a muscular dystrophy patient population. Nippon Rinsho 1997;55:3165–3168.
238. Richard I, Brenguier L, Dincer P, et al. Multiple independent molecular etiology for limb-girdle muscular dystrophy type 2A patients from various geographical origins. Am J Hum Genet 1997;60: 1128–1138.
239. Van der Kooi AJ, Ginjaar HB, Busch HFM et al. Limb girdle muscular dystrophy: a pathological and immunohistochemical evaluation. Muscle Nerve 1998;21:584–590.
240. Sewry CA, Taylor J, Anderson LVB. Abnormalities in α-, β-, and γ-sarcoglycan in patients with limb-girdle muscular dystrophy. Neuromuscul Disord 1996;6:467–474.
241. Barresi R, Congalonieri V, Lanfossi M, et al. Concomitant deficiency of β- and δ-sarcoglycans in 20 α-sarcoglycan (adhalin)-deficient patients: immunohistochemical analysis and clinical aspects. Acta Neuropathol (Berl) 1997;94:28–35.
242. Allamand V, Leturcq F, Piccolo F, et al. Adhalin gene polymorphism. Hum Mol Genet 1994;3:2269.
243. McNally EM, Ly CT, Kunkel LM. Human epsilon-sarcoglycan is highly related to alpha-sarcoglycan (adhalin), the limb girdle muscular dystrophy 2D gene. FEBS Lett 1998;422:27–32.
244. Holt KH, Lim LE, Straub V et al. Functional rescue of the sarcoglycan complex in the BI0 14.6 hamster using δ-sarcoglycan gene transfer. Mol Cell 1998;1:841–848.
245. Dubowitz V, Fardeau M. Workshop report on congenital muscular dystrophy. Neuromuscul Disord 1995;5:253–258.
246. Pegoraro E, Mancias P, Swerdlow SH, et al. Congenital muscular dystrophy (CMD) with primary laminin α2 deficiency presenting as inflammatory myopathy. Ann Neurol 1996;46:810–814.
247. Sewry CA, Philot J, Mahoney D, et al. Expression of laminin subunits is congenital muscular dystrophy. Neuromuscul Disord 1995;5:307–316.

248. Fukuyama Y, Osawa M, Suzuki H. Congenital progressive muscular dystrophy of the Fukuyama type. Brain Dev 1981;33:1–29.
249. Sunada Y, Bernier SM, Kozak CA, et al. Deficiency of merosin in dystrophic dy mice and genetic linkage of laminin M chain gene to dy locus. J Biol Chem 1994;269:13729–13732.
250. Xu H, Christmas P, Wu XR, et al. Defective muscle basement membrane and lack of M laminin in the dystrophic dy/dy mouse. Proc Natl Acad Sci U S A 1994;91:5572–5576.
251. Arahata KM, Hayashi YK, Koga R. Laminin in animal models for muscular dystrophy: defect of Laminin M in skeletal and cardiac muscle and peripheral nerve of the homozygous dystrophic dy/dy mice. Proc Japan Acad Sci 1993;69B:259–264.
252. Li M, Dickson DW, Spiro JA. Abnormal expression of laminin beta 1 chain in skeletal muscle of adult onset limb-girdle muscular dystrophy. Arch Neurol 1997;54:1457–1461.
253. Matsumura K, Yamada H, Sailo F, et al. Peripheral nerve involvement in merosin-deficient congenital muscular dystrophy and dy mouse. Neuromuscul Disord 1997;7:7–12.
254. Marbini A, Bellanova MF, Ferrari A, et al. Immunohistochemical study of merosin-negative congenital muscular dystrophy: laminin alpha 2 deficiency in skin biopsy. Acta Neuropathol (Berl) 1997;94:103–108.
255. Hillaire D, Leclerc A, Faure S, et al. Localization of merosin-negative congenital muscular dystrophy to chromosome 6q2 by homozygosity mapping. Hum Mol Genet 1994;3:1657–1661.
256. Helbing-Leclerc A, Zhang X, Topolaglu H, et al. Mutations in the laminin a 2-chain gene (LAMA2) cause merosin-deficient congenital muscular dystrophy. Nat Genet 1995;11:216–218.
257. Guicheney P, Vignier N, Helbing-Leclerc A, et al. Genetics of laminin alpha 2 chain (or merosin) deficient congenital muscular dystrophy from identification of mutations to prenatal diagnosis. Neuromuscul Disord 1997;7:180–186.
258. Nissinen M, Helbing-Leclerc A, Zhang X, et al. Substitution of a conserved cysteine-996 in a cysteine rich motif of the laminin α 2-chain in congenital muscular dystrophy with partial deficiency of the protein. Am J Hum Genet 1996;58:1177–1184.
259. Voit T, Fardeau M, Tomé FM. Prenatal detection of merosin expression in human placenta. Neuropediatrics 1994;25:332–333.
260. Sorimachi H, Saido TC, Allamand V, et al. New era of calpain research: discovery of tissue-specific calpains. FEBS Lett 1994;343:1–5.
261. McNally EM, de Sa Moreira E, Duggan DJ, et al. Caveolin-3 in muscular dystrophy. Hum Mol Genet 1998;7:871–877.
262. Liu J, Aoki M, Illa I, et al. Dysferlin, a novel skeletal muscle gene, is mutated in Miyoshi myopathy and limb-girdle muscular dystrophy. Nat Genet 1998;20:31–36.

5
Myotonic Disorders: Myotonic Dystrophy and Proximal Myotonic Myopathy

Giovanni Meola and Richard T. Moxley III

MYOTONIC DISORDERS

Identification of the gene mutations that are responsible for specific forms of inherited myotonia has helped to clarify the once confusing classification of the myotonic disorders. Thus far, all the diseases appear to result either from specific mutations in genes encoding the skeletal muscle chloride or sodium channels or from a protein kinase that may act on an ion channel. A tentative classification can be based on the specific channel abnormality (Table 5.1).

For some of these disorders, such as dominantly inherited myotonia congenita (chloride channel myotonia, Thomsen disease) and hyperkalemic periodic paralysis (sodium channel disease), genetic discoveries combined with physiologic studies give us a reasonably complete view of their pathophysiology. The decrease in chloride conductance, previously shown to account for the delayed relaxation of muscle in dominantly inherited myotonia congenita of Thomsen, has now been shown to result from an alteration in charge in the ion pore formed by the dimerization of the mutated plus the normal chloride channel units [1]. The increase in sodium conductance provoked by elevation of plasma potassium, which has been shown to cause depolarization paralysis of the muscle fibers in attacks of hyperkalemic periodic paralysis, now appears to result from a disruption of fast inactivation of the channel [2].

It has long been noted that the diseases associated with myotonia and periodic paralysis overlap. It is now clear that disorders with either myotonia or periodic paralysis can be allelic disorders of the same ion channel. Thus, in most instances, myotonia congenitas are diseases of the chloride channel but in at least one form can be associated with episodic weakness (i.e., Becker autosomal recessive generalized myotonia). Similarly, most of the potassium-sensitive periodic paralyses result from mutations of the sodium channel, but a number of distinctive or fluctuating myotonias without episodic or fixed paralyses result from allelic mutations of the same sodium channel [3–5]. The myotonias associated with dystrophic features are also likely to result from channel dysfunction [6]. How-

115

Table 5.1   Classification of myotonias

Disease	Mode of inheritance	Gene location	Symbol (gene product)	MIM*
Myotonic dystrophy (Steinert)	Autosomal dominant	19_{q13}	DM (myotonin-protein kinase)	160900
Chloride channel				
Myotonia dominant (Thomsen)	Autosomal dominant	7_{q35}	ClC-1 (muscle chloride channel)	160800
Myotonia recessive (Becker)	Autosomal recessive	7_{q35}	ClC-1 (muscle chloride channel)	255700
Sodium channel				
Hyperkalemic periodic paralysis	Autosomal dominant	$17_{q13.1-13.3}$	SCN4A (sodium channel α-subunit)	170500
Paramyotonia congenita	Autosomal dominant	$17_{q13.1-13.3}$	SCN4A (sodium channel α-subunit)	168300
Potassium-aggravated myotonia	Autosomal dominant	$17_{q13.1-13.3}$	SCN4A (sodium channel α-subunit)	168300
Unknown gene location and defect				
Chondrodystrophic myotonia (Schwartz-Jampel Syndrome)	Autosomal dominant	—	—	—
Proximal myotonic myopathy	Autosomal dominant	—	—	600109

MIM = Mendelian Inheritance in Man.

* From VA McKusick. Mendelian Inheritance in Man. Catalogs of Autosomal Dominant, Autosomal Recessive, and X-linked Phenotypes (11th ed). Baltimore: Johns Hopkins University Press, 1994.

Source: Adapted from Neuromuscular disorders: gene location. Neuromuscul Disord 1997;7:I–XII.

ever, for myotonic dystrophy (DM), the pathophysiology remains very unclear despite a considerable number of human, animal, and tissue culture studies of the gene defect in DM.

One of the important discoveries that has emerged from the extensive genetic investigations of DM is the identification of another disorder that has features similar to but distinct from DM. With the discovery of the gene defect in DM [7–9] and the development of a highly specific gene probe to identify affected individuals [10], a second group of patients without an abnormal expansion of the trinucleotide repeat cytosine-thymidine-guanosine ([CTG]n) in the DM gene has been delineated. These patients have primarily proximal muscle weakness and a less severe clinical course. This newly described disorder is called *proximal myotonic myopathy* (*PROMM*). Myotonia and cataracts are present in PROMM, and both PROMM and DM are multisystem disorders. The pathophysiology underlying both PROMM and DM remains a mystery, and the gene defect is unknown in PROMM. Despite these limitations in our knowledge of these two dystrophic forms of myotonia, there is a significant body of clinical and laboratory information that deserves review. In the sections that follow, we discuss both DM and PROMM.

DEFINITION OF MYOTONIC SIGNS

The literal translation of the Greek word *myotonia* is *muscle stiffness*. Myotonia is the phenomenon of slowed muscle relaxation after vigorous contraction whether by voluntary effort or through mechanical or electrical stimulation. The stiffness may decrease with repeated muscle contractions, a phenomenon termed *warm-up*. Myotonia may increase with muscle activity in some patients, primarily those with sodium channel myotonia. This phenomenon is termed *paradoxical myotonia*. Myotonic muscle reacts to being struck with the percussion hammer by contracting for a period of time, and the muscle also becomes indented transiently. This is the phenomenon of *percussion myotonia*.

Myotonia results from inherited or acquired abnormalities of the electrical properties of the sarcolemma. These alterations typically predispose the muscle membranes to become easily depolarized and result in repetitive discharges that give a characteristic electromyographic (EMG) signal (myotonic runs, or "dive bomber" potentials). The combination of these mechanical and electrical abnormalities is called the *myotonic reaction*. In very mild cases, clinical signs of myotonic stiffness may not be seen; however, EMG study reveals runs of myotonic discharges. This is termed *latent myotonia*. Myotonia is by definition myogenic as opposed to neurogenic, and isolated muscle fibers in vitro show spontaneous myotonic contractions and electrical myotonia.

MYOTONIC DYSTROPHY

Myotonic dystrophy (myotonia atrophica, dystrophia myotonica [DM], myotonic muscular dystrophy, and Steinert disease) is "a genetically determined disorder in which a characteristic pattern of dystrophic muscle disease is accompanied by myotonia and by specific abnormalities of other systems" [11].

This definition, from Harper's outstanding monograph on the subject [11], encompasses the broad spectrum of manifestations of DM that typify this multisystem disease. DM has an extraordinarily wide variation in its symptoms and signs. Persons with DM range from asymptomatic individuals, to those with minimal features (e.g., cataract and asymptomatic myotonia), to those with moderately severe facial and distal limb muscle wasting and weakness, to those with the most severe congenital cases (with hypotonia, respiratory insufficiency, dysphagia, talipes, and mental retardation; Table 5.2) [11, 12].

Epidemiology

DM is a worldwide disease with an estimated frequency of 1 in 8,000 [12] and an estimated heterozygote frequency of approximately 13 per 100,000 [13]. However, "hot spots" of higher frequency have been noted, such as in Saguenay, Province of Northeast Quebec, where the prevalence is 200 per 100,000 [13].

Genealogic studies have subsequently shown that the disease in this region developed in 10–14 generations from a couple that settled there in 1657 [14]. In contrast, population studies indicate that a very low prevalence of DM exists

Table 5.2   Clinical and laboratory features of myotonic dystrophy

	Clinical features	Laboratory tests
Neuromuscular	Myotonia Weakness Reduced deep tendon reflexes	Myotonic runs on electromyography Axonal neuropathy in some cases
Eye	Cataract Ptosis Ophthalmoparesis Retinal pigmentation	Slit lamp
Endocrine	Testicular atrophy Diabetes Pituitary dysfunction Hyperparathyroidism	Follicle-stimulating hormone, testosterone Insulin resistance Growth hormone, prolactin Impaired TRH response Parathormone assay
Skin	Frontal balding Pilomatrixoma	
Cardiovascular	Hypotension Syncope, palpitations Sudden death Mitral valve prolapse	Low blood pressure Electrocardiogram Ecocardiograph
Gastrointestinal	Dysphagia Pseudo-obstruction	Volvulus, megacolon
Central nervous system	Mental retardation	Neuropsychometry Atrophy on CT, white matter lesions on MRI Hypometabolism on SPECT, PET
Immune system	—	Reduced immunoglobulins T-cell function, reduced C3, C4

TRH = thyrotropin-releasing hormone; CT = computed tomography; MRI = magnetic resonance imaging; SPECT = single photon emission computed tomography; PET = positron emission tomography.

Source: Reprinted with permission from RJ Lane, P Shelbourne, KJ Johnson. Myotonic Dystrophy. In JM Lane Russell (ed), Handbook of Muscle Disease. New York: Marcel Dekker, 1996;311–328.

among ethnic Africans (especially central and southern Africans), Chinese (especially southern Chinese), Cantonese, Thai, and Oceanians [15].

Clinical Features

Table 5.2 summarizes the principle clinical and laboratory features of DM. DM is an autosomal dominant, multisystem disease with highly variable clinical manifestations (Table 5.3) [11, 12]. An abnormal, unstable expansion of a trinucleotide repeat in the DM gene on chromosome 19 causes the disease [7–9], and the degree of abnormal expansion correlates reasonably closely with the severity of muscle weakness [16–19]. Discovery of the gene has permitted direct genetic testing of at-risk individuals and has provided new opportunities for genetic counseling and prenatal screening [10, 19].

Table 5.3 Classification of myotonic dystrophy: correlations of clinical signs with age of onset

	Onset	Signs
Mildest	Middle to old age	Cataracts, minimal or no muscle abnormality
Classic	Adolescent and early adult life	Myotonia, muscle weakness (face, forearms, foot dorsiflexors)
Congenital	At birth, frequent history of hydramnios and reduced fetal movements	Neonatal respiratory distress, hypotonia, bilateral facial weakness, feeding difficulty, talipes, mental retardation

Source: Adapted from PR Dyken and PS Harper. Congenital dystrophy myotonica. Neurology 1973;23:465–473; and A Jaspert, R Fahsold, H Grehl, et al. Myotonic dystrophy: correlation of clinical symptoms with the size of the CTG trinucleotide repeat. J Neurol 1995;242:99–104.

It is common to find in living members of a single family some individuals who are minimally affected late in life, others who are severely affected at birth, and a range of intermediate phenotypes. DM combines features of maldevelopment, which are prominent in congenital cases, with those of premature aging and degeneration, which predominate in adult-onset cases.

The tissues that are commonly involved in addition to skeletal muscle include the heart (conduction defect, arrhythmia) [20–26], smooth muscle (impaired intestinal motility and uterine contractility) [11, 12], lens (e.g., cataracts) [11, 12], brain (mental retardation in congenital cases, hypersomnolence and neuropsychiatric manifestations in adult cases) [11, 12, 27–33], and endocrine regulation (testicular atrophy, insulin resistance, abnormal growth hormone release) (see Table 5.2) [11, 12, 34–38].

A cardinal sign of adult DM is myotonia. Myotonia is absent in congenital DM and gradually appears during childhood. DM patients often do not report this symptom or seek treatment for it. Myotonia can be absent in mild cases. In some mild cases, however, it is troublesome and leads to the diagnosis of muscle strain or fibromyalgia, especially when the patient's doctor has not yet established that the patient has DM. It is often described as stiffness and may be attributed to arthritis.

Grip myotonia is demonstrated by asking the patient to relax the hand rapidly after a forceful grip (Figure 5.1). This phenomenon may be less marked after repeated contraction and relaxation (warm-up phenomenon) and is usually worse in the cold. Percussion myotonia is usually demonstrable even if grip myotonia is absent. Striking the thenar eminence with a percussion hammer results in the thumb being drawn across the palm, followed by slow relaxation and return to initial position. Percussion myotonia in other muscles, such as the forearm and tongue, may also be demonstrable and may be accompanied by the production of indentation or grooving of the muscle belly after percussion.

Even when such clinical signs are absent or difficult to elicit, as when muscle wasting and weakness are very severe, myotonia can be demonstrated by EMG, which demonstrates the characteristic "dive bomber" potentials (myotonic runs). There is growing evidence that the apamin-sensitive potassium channel (SK channel), which is overexpressed in DM muscle, may be involved in the generation of myotonia [39]. The alteration in SK channel expression is presumably a

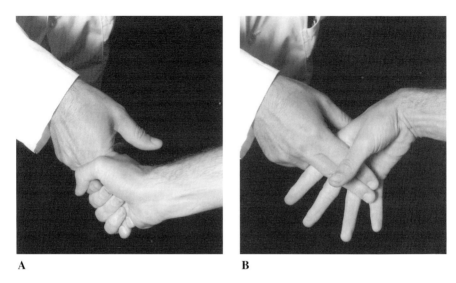

A   **B**

Figure 5.1 Myotonia of grip. (**A**) Shows forceful grip. (**B**) Shows delayed relaxation and myotonia.

secondary effect of the DM mutation. The mechanism responsible for these effects is not understood.

The most severe and disabling feature of DM is progressive muscular weakness and wasting. Wasting is most prominent in the cranial musculature and distal limb muscles. The deep tendon reflexes are usually reduced or absent. Patients typically show bilateral ptosis, weakness of muscles of facial expression, and jaw muscle weakness, which can lead to temporomandibular joint dysfunction. Facial muscle wasting may produce a hatchetlike facies (Figure 5.2). Palatal, tongue, and laryngeal weakness may result in nasal speech and eventually aspiration pneumonia. Sternocleidomastoid weakness and wasting is prominent even in the early stage of disease (Figure 5.3). In the limbs, weaknesses of grip (especially long flexors), wrist function (especially flexors), and footdrop are early signs.

Although there are no widely used scales to determine the severity of muscle weakness and function in DM, some useful approaches are already available to assess phenotype and to correlate the findings with the genotype (e.g., degree of [CTG]n repeat expansion). One group has developed a five-point muscular disability rating scale for DM, based on distal to proximal progression of muscular involvement in the condition (Table 5.4) [40]. Other scales are under development and will complement previously published techniques for quantitating muscle mass and strength in DM [12, 35].

Muscle Pathology

Skeletal muscle in DM may have normal histology. The muscle biopsy is not essential to establish the diagnosis, and a normal biopsy does not rule out the diagnosis. When the biopsy is abnormal, the changes are relatively nonspecific. The

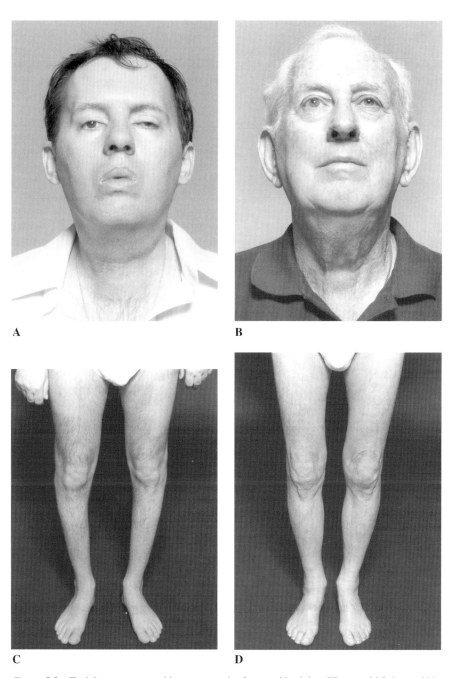

Figure 5.2 Facial appearance and lower extremity front and back in a 77-year-old father and his 41-year-old son, both of whom have myotonic dystrophy. (**A**) and (**B**) contrast the degree of ptosis, facial weakness, wasting masseter temporalis, and sternocleidomastoid muscles. (**C**) and (**D**) contrast the degree of distal lower extremity wasting between the father and son. Overall, the comparison between the father and son emphasizes the phenomenon of anticipation (i.e., the earlier onset of more severe clinical manifestations in successive generations).

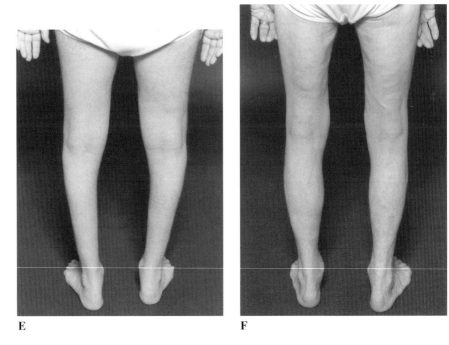

E   **F**

Figure 5.2 (continued)   The degree of distal lower extremity wasting between the father and son are further contrasted in (**E**) and (**F**).

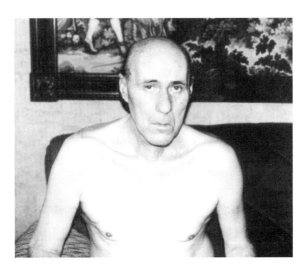

Figure 5.3   Facial features of myotonic dystrophy. The photograph shows the characteristic hatchet-shaped face resulting from facial weakness and weakness and wasting of the jaw muscles. There is also wasting of the sternocleidomastoid muscles. The patient is unable to raise his head against gravity while supine.

Table 5.4 Classification of disease severity in myotonic dystrophy

Grade	Clinical severity
1	No clinical neuromuscular impairment (diagnosed by laboratory tests)
2	Minimal signs (myotonia and cranial signs such as jaw and temporal wasting, sternocleidomastoid wasting/weakness, ptosis, and nasal speech)
	No significant distal weakness
3	Distal weakness (no proximal weakness, except triceps)
4	Mild to moderate proximal weakness
5	Severe proximal weakness

Source: Reprinted with permission from J Mathieu, M De Braeckeleer, C Prevost, et al. Myotonic dystrophy: clinical assessment of muscular disability in an isolated population with presumed homogenous mutation. Neurology 1992;42:203–208.

most common finding—best appreciated on longitudinal sections—is an increase in internal nuclei, frequently arranged in long chains down the center of the fibers. Ring fibers are also seen occasionally. Other features—such as sarcoplasmic masses, small angular fibers, and changes in fiber diameter and architecture—are inconstant and too nonspecific to be of diagnostic value [41]. In the congenital form of DM, a number of rather distinctive changes have been noted, including marked muscle hypoplasia, particularly of type I fibers, and fibers with an unusual peripheral ring, devoid of mitochondria, seen in transverse section [42]. The persistence of chains of central nuclei is reminiscent of fetal myotubes, and the poor histochemical differentiation of fibers in congenital DM suggests that the myopathy of DM may represent a defect in muscle maturation [43].

Genetics and Pathophysiology

In 1992, three groups simultaneously discovered the gene defect in DM [7–9]. The defect results from an unstable, abnormal expansion of the trinucleotide repeat (CTG)n in the 3 noncoding region of a gene on chromosome 19, which codes for serine/threonine kinase [7–9]. Researchers have called this kinase the *DM protein kinase* (*DMPK*) or *myotonin*.

The unstable (CTG)n repeat expansion is the only genetic defect that occurs in patients with DM. No point mutations, deletions, or duplications have been identified in the DMPK gene.

The role of the DMPK in the pathomechanism of DM is still unknown. Such serine/threonine kinases are usually involved in regulating phosphorylation-dephosphorylation reactions. At present, there is no definite substrate that is specifically associated with DMPK and no overall agreement as to the most appropriate assays for DMPK in various tissues. It is not clear whether the levels of DMPK are normal, decreased, or increased in tissues of DM patients. The DMPK gene is expressed mainly in muscle, heart, brain, and lens, but its functions in these tissues are unknown. Current evidence suggests that there is a modest (as much as 50%) reduction of DMPK protein levels in DM muscle. However, knockout mice that are completely lacking in DMPK protein develop normally and show only slight abnormalities in skeletal muscle [44, 45]. It seems unlikely that low levels of DMPK can provide a unitary explanation for the disease.

Two other possible explanations for pathomechanism have been suggested: (1) that the unusual nature and extreme length of the triplet repeat sequence in DM may somehow shut off neighboring genes, perhaps by changing the way in which the DNA is packaged into chromatin [46]; and (2) that messenger RNA molecules synthesized from the mutant copy of the DMPK gene may accumulate in the nucleus and have a toxic effect [47]. These putative disease mechanisms are not mutually exclusive, and the clinical signs may depend on an interaction between them. The relationship between the function of DMPK and the recent observations of abnormal sodium [48] and potassium [39] channel function in muscle from DM patients requires further investigation.

When inheritance of the (CTG)n repeat region is traced through individual families, it usually increases in size in successive generations. Within families, there is a strong tendency for the abnormal expansion of the (CTG)n repeat to become even larger [7–9, 16–19]. This provides a genetic explanation for *anticipation,* the tendency for DM to be more severe in the offspring of successive generations [7–9, 16–19]. Rarely, however, the reverse phenomenon may be observed, with inheritance of a smaller copy number or, exceptionally, a sequence size within the normal range [49]. This intergenerational contraction of repeat size appears to result in individuals who are minimally affected or have no stigmata of the disease and probably accounts for instances of incomplete penetrance in DM families. Table 5.5 summarizes the genetic features of DM.

The size of the DM gene varies within the general population and within patients with DM. In normal alleles, (CTG)5 (5 refers to number of repeats) is the most common, at 35–40% frequency [7, 9, 50]; the normal alleles $(CTG)_{11}$, $(CTG)_{12}$, and $(CTG)_{13}$ each occur at frequencies ranging from 10% to 19%, depending on the population investigated. The DM allele shows CTG repeats greater than 50 and ranging to expansions greater than 2,000 repeats in congenital DM [16–19]. The cause for the unstable expansion of the trinucleotide repeat remains a mystery, but it appears to have resulted from one or two ancient mutations that occurred on a specifically predisposed allele containing an insertion close to the DM gene [50–52].

Diagnosis

Table 5.6 outlines the diagnostic tests that are useful to identify patients with DM. The discovery of the DM gene [7–9] led to the development of specific probes that permit performance of direct molecular diagnostic testing of at-risk individuals [10, 16]. Detailed knowledge of the structure of the DM gene is now available [51–53]. The combination of Southern blot to detect abnormally large DNA fragments with the expanded DM gene and polymerase chain reaction (PCR) to detect small expansions is highly accurate in identifying individuals with DM. Because patients with DM have variable expansion of the CTG repeat that often exceeds 500 base pairs, Southern blot analysis is used as the initial diagnostic test. PCR methods do not reliably amplify CTG repeat expansions exceeding 500 base pairs. However, it is essential to use PCR to search for a slight expansion of the DM gene, such as the small expansions that occur in mildly symptomatic carriers.

Table 5.5 Overview of genetics of myotonic dystrophy

Frequency	Inheritance	Sex bias for transmission of the severe form	Protein/ expression	Disease-causing mechanism	Repeat/ location	Size of repeat in normal alleles	Predisposing normal alleles (frequency)	Linkage disequilibrium
1/8,000 (likely to be a significant underestimate; new calculations in the future will use data obtained by using specific gene probes)	Autosomal dominant with anticipation	Female (almost all cases of congenital myotonic dystrophy result from female transmission of the myotonic dystrophy allele)	Serine/threonine kinase	Unknown Speculation (see text)	CTG/3' untranslated region	(CTG)5–37	Predisposed normal alleles have repeat size of (CTG)19–30 (approximately 0.10)	Yes (absolute)

Notes: Founder effect from only a few ancient mutations. All patients have a specific insertion allele.

Source: Reprinted with permission from RT Moxley III, RC Griggs, R Tawil. Myotonic Disorders. In SH Appel (ed), Current Neurology. St. Louis: Mosby–Year Book, 1995:1–27.

Table 5.6   Useful diagnostic tests in identifying individuals with myotonic dystrophy

Primary value
 Analysis for gene lesions in DNA isolated from white blood cells
 Clinical examination focused towards detection of early muscular and nonmuscular
  alteration
 Electromyography
 Slit-lamp examinations
Secondary value
 Serum creatine kinase
 Muscle biopsy

Source: Reprinted with permission from RT Moxley III, RC Griggs, R Tawil. Myotonic Disorders. In SH Appel (ed), Current Neurology. St. Louis: Mosby–Year Book, 1995;1–27.

Direct molecular testing has exerted a major impact on genetic counseling. DNA analysis is now able to play a critical role in establishing a prenatal diagnosis of DM and in predicting the delivery of a baby with congenital DM [16, 19]. In one study involving 44 families referred for prenatal testing, the investigators used cultured amniocytes or chorionic villus samples and found the analysis of CTG repeat size to be accurate in excluding and identifying the presence of DM in the fetus and in predicting the severity of symptoms [16].

Treatment

The review by Moxley [12, 54] and Tables 5.7 and 5.8 outline important elements of treatment in patients with DM. The primary measures of treatment include supportive therapy for muscle weakness, careful monitoring for cardiac arrhythmias and respiratory insufficiency, and consistent preoperative and postoperative monitoring of patients. Pregnancy and delivery pose special risks for mothers with DM and their offspring (see Table 5.7).

Table 5.7   Maternal-obstetric complications in myotonic dystrophy

Maternal complications
 Increased muscle weakness, especially respiratory
 Increased rate of spontaneous abortion
 Reduced fetal movements and hydramnios
 Prolonged and often ineffective labor
 Sensitivity to general anesthesia (arrhythmias, apnea following cesarean section)
Obstetric complications (all of these complications are several times more frequent than
  in normal women)
 Retained placenta
 Placenta previa
 Neonatal deaths

Source: Reprinted with permission from RT Moxley III, RC Griggs, R Tawil. Myotonic Disorders. In SH Appel (ed), Current Neurology. St. Louis: Mosby–Year Book, 1995;15:1–27.

Table 5.8   Preoperative and postoperative care and complications of anesthesia in patients with myotonic dystrophy

Preoperative evaluation
  Electrocardiogram
  Pulmonary function testing (including supine and upright forced vital capacity)
  Arterial blood gas measurements
Intraoperative monitoring
  Monitor electrocardiogram
  Measure arterial blood pressure
  Use a peripheral nerve stimulator to monitor blockade of peripheral muscle
  Monitor temperature
  Warm the mattress
  Warm intravenous fluids
  Maintain humidification of anesthetic gases
Postoperative care
  Retain the endotracheal tube in place and ventilate if necessary in an intensive care unit
  Monitor respiratory efficiency with checks of oxygen saturation and Pco_2 for at least
    24 hrs postoperatively to avoid overlooking delayed-onset apnea
  Use controlled-flow oxygen therapy with close monitoring of ventilation in patients rely-
    ing on hypoxic drive because of chronic respiratory insufficiency
  Provide early physiotherapy
  Monitor electrocardiogram
  Keep the patient warm
  Monitor swallowing closely to check for sign of aspiration
  Treat all infections vigorously
Anesthetic agents
  When possible, use local or regional anesthesia, such as an epidural block
  Avoid suxamethonium and other depolarizing muscle relaxants
  Avoid or use only minimal doses of thiopental; for muscle relaxation, use short-acting
    agents such as atracurium or vecuronium
  Avoid or use only minimal doses of opiates to avoid respiratory depression
  When possible, avoid general anesthesia; if necessary, use a combination of nitrous
    oxide/oxygen and an agent such as 0.8% enflurane or 1.0% isoflurane
  Use an anticholinesterase such as neostigmine with care; it may be preferable to ventilate
    the patient until the residual curarization wears off

Source: Reprinted with permission from RT Moxley III, RC Griggs, R Tawil. Myotonic Disorders. In SH Appel (ed), Current Neurology. St. Louis: Mosby–Year Book, 1995;15:1–27.

Endocrine disturbances, such as hypogonadism (decreased testosterone levels and testicular atrophy) and postprandial hyperinsulinemia with tissue-specific insulin resistance, commonly occur in patients with DM [11, 12, 38]. Occasionally, testosterone replacement is useful, and therapeutic trials are in progress to determine the potential value of troglitazone in reversing the insulin resistance that frequently occurs [12, 38]. In an attempt to correct a possible defect in muscle anabolism that may occur with the deficiencies of testosterone and insulin action, therapeutic trials with testosterone [35] and recombinant human growth hormone [55] have been carried out. Both treatments led to an increase in muscle mass but did not improve muscle function or strength. A small pilot study of IGF-1, the product hormone of growth hormone, produced an increase in protein synthesis, an increase in insulin response, and an increase in muscle function in five DM patients [56]. These encouraging results require verification, and further research is necessary to establish whether other growth factors have a role in the treatment of DM.

Ultimately, the pathomechanism underlying DM will become clearer. It may be that the serine-threonine kinase coded for by the DM gene fails to phosphorylate an intracellular or membrane-associated substrate that is critical in maintaining protein anabolism. It may be that the insulin resistance in DM results from a failure of the DMPK to regulate the phosphorylation cascade involved in intracellular signaling by the insulin receptor. It is interesting to note that the receptor for insulin is itself a tyrosine kinase that is regulated not only by its degree of phosphorylation on its tyrosine kinase but also by phosphorylation of its serine moieties [38]. It is conceivable that an alteration in the DMPK might lead to its different clinical findings by influencing various kinases, such as the insulin receptor tyrosine kinase, which has a controlling effect in certain specific target tissues for insulin. More research into the pathomechanism of DM is necessary, but most investigators are optimistic that important insights will occur soon and aid in the development of new approaches to treatment.

PROXIMAL MYOTONIC MYOPATHY

The delineation in 1994 of PROMM syndrome, a newly recognized, dominantly inherited myotonic disorder, was a by-product of the discovery of the DM gene and direct genetic testing of the patients. Genetic testing for the abnormal (CTG)n repeat expansion in a subgroup of families with myotonia, weakness, and cataract, but who had other features that were atypical for DM, revealed that affected individuals had no abnormal expansion of the (CTG)n repeat in the DM gene and that there was no genetic link to the skeletal muscle sodium or chloride channel genes. The description of these families led to the recognition of PROMM as a genetically distinct disorder [57]. A detailed history of the discovery of PROMM and an update of information is available in a recent workshop report [58]. Prevalence data are not yet available, but PROMM is probably the second most common inherited myotonic disorder after DM.

Clinical Features

The initial descriptions of patients with PROMM [57, 59–67] have established the clinical and genetic features of this disorder. The core features that lead to the diagnosis of PROMM are autosomal dominant inheritance, proximal muscle weakness, myotonia, cataracts, and a normal size of the (CTG)n repeat in the DM gene. The onset of symptoms is usually in the patient's 30s or 40s. No infantile form of PROMM is apparent that is comparable to the severe form of congenital DM observed in DM related to transmission, almost always by an affected DM mother.

The common presenting symptoms in PROMM are leg stiffness when climbing stairs, difficulty rising from a chair, intermittent locking of grip, and vision impairment because of cataracts.

The earliest signs of weakness appear in the limb-girdle muscles. However, some patients develop weakness in the finger flexors and ankle dorsiflexors, as

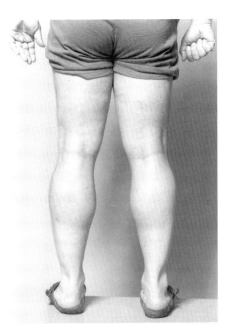

Figure 5.4   Calf hypertrophy in proximal myotonic myopathy patient. (Reprinted with permission from CA Thornton, RC Griggs, RT Moxley. Myotonic dystrophy with no trinucleotide repeat expansion. Ann Neurol 1994;35:269–272.)

well as in the proximal thigh muscles. Infrequently, some families have associated distal weakness as a prominent feature [65]. Although the distribution of weakness in PROMM is definitely greater in proximal muscles, the clinical manifestations of the disease vary widely [65–67]. Weakness may be hard to detect, and often there may be no underlying muscle wasting (Figure 5.4) [67]. Patients often describe myotonia in a very specific and reproducible manner, describing "locking" of the hand and reduced finger dexterity, as in arthritis. However, these symptoms are often intermittent and can be totally absent on clinical testing, with no evidence of percussion or grip myotonia. Similarly, EMG study may fail to detect any myotonic discharges, even after cooling. Cataracts are not easily detectable on routine ophthalmoscopic examination, and a slit-lamp test is often required. In brief, very careful clinical and laboratory assessment is necessary to identify patients with PROMM. In the early stages (younger than age 40 years) or in mild cases, it may be impossible to detect all the core clinical features. This poses a special challenge to those attempting to localize the gene(s) responsible for this disorder. A consortium of experts met in 1997 and have proposed diagnostic criteria as a result of this workshop (Table 5.9) [58].

Genetics

The specific gene defect in PROMM is unknown. All patients have a normal size of (CTG)n repeat expansion in the DM gene. There appears to be no link to chromosomes 19, 7, and 17 [60–62], suggesting genetic homogeneity and indicating that PROMM is a disorder similar to but distinct from DM.

Table 5.9   The diagnostic criteria of proximal myotonic myopathies

Core features
1. Autosomal dominant inheritance: at least two generations
2. Absence of the myotonic dystrophy cytosine-thymidine-guanosine triplet expansion
3. Weakness, predominantly proximal
4. Cataracts: slit-lamp examination shows typical myotonic dystrophy–like polychromatic changes with onset before age 50 yrs
5. Electromyographic myotonia

Supportive findings
6. Myalgia or painful muscle cramps
7. Fluctuating weakness and fluctuating stiffness (myotonia)
8. Calf pseudohypertrophy
9. Hypogonadism: primary
10. Diabetes mellitus/insulin resistance
11. Hypothyroidism
12. Cardiac: conduction defects
13. Chest pain: intermittent noncardiac episodes
14. Deafness: sensorineural
15. Central nervous symptoms: cognitive impairment, hypersomnia, seizures, tremor
16. Gastrointestinal symptoms: dysphagia, constipation
17. Hyperhidrosis
18. Deep tendon reflexes usually preserved
19. Intermittent muscle fasciculations

Notes: As delineated at the 54th European Neuromuscular Centre International Workshop (ENMC), Naarden, The Netherlands, October 1997. Exclusion criteria and laboratory findings are described in the workshop report.
Source: Reprinted with permission from RT Moxley III, F Udd, K Ricker. 54th ENMC International Workshop: PROMM (proximal myotonic myopathies) and other proximal myotonic syndromes. Neuromuscul Disord 1998;8:508–518.

Genetic studies of large informative families are currently under way to identify the gene.

Diagnostic Workup

No single, specific diagnostic test for PROMM exists. Careful clinical assessment, laboratory testing, and genetic analysis are necessary to evaluate patients. Clinical patient assessment is by far the most important single measure. No relative should be considered unaffected unless a careful search has been made for myotonia and muscle weakness.

EMG should always be done in at-risk individuals. Myotonic discharges are variable and sometimes difficult to detect. Cooling and heating [63] of the muscle may help to enhance myotonia. It is useful to repeat the EMG at several points in time in different muscles before concluding that there is no myotonia.

Cataracts occur early in life and are iridescent, posterior capsular opacities that are indistinguishable from the cataracts in DM. Slit-lamp examination is extremely valuable, especially in the elderly, to distinguish these characteristic cataracts of PROMM from those changes commonly seen in the elderly. It is not uncommon for nonspecific whitish opacities to be the only finding in at-risk individuals. It is wise to regard this finding as equivocal and to repeat the test in 1 or 2 years.

Molecular analysis in the absence of CTG expansion is mandatory to rule out in at least one affected member of each family linkage to the DM gene on chromosome 19. Other predictive tests have limited value, such as creatine kinase determination. Creatine kinase levels are frequently elevated two- to 10-fold; however, a significant number of patients have normal levels. The same applies for γ-GT elevation. Serum follicle-stimulating hormone, luteinizing hormone, testosterone, and insulin response to oral or intravenous glucose are still of uncertain value.

Muscle biopsy is of limited value in PROMM. The muscle histologic findings of marked increase in internal nuclei and nuclear chains are very similar to DM. Selective atrophy of type I fibers and sarcolemmal masses are not seen in PROMM, but they help to exclude other myopathies, such as polymyositis, inclusion body myositis, and mitochondrial myopathy. Mild to moderate increases in central nuclei and scattered, angulated, atrophic fibers in the absence of signs of chronic denervation (i.e., type grouping) occur in the majority of PROMM patients.

Diagnosis

The differential diagnosis is mainly concerned with separating PROMM from DM (Table 5.10) or recessive generalized myotonia. Sodium channel myotonic disorders, toxic and inflammatory myopathies, mitochondrial disease, and neuromuscular transmission disorders sometimes mimic certain symptoms in PROMM, but the clinical evaluation, electrodiagnostic testing, and muscle biopsy findings usually exclude these illnesses from serious consideration. Distinguishing PROMM from DM with DNA analysis is important for diagnosis and prognosis. There is no clear evidence that anticipation (the phenomenon of earlier onset and more severe disease in successive generations, discussed previously) or congenital cases occur in PROMM.

Table 5.10   Differential diagnosis: myotonic dystrophy versus proximal myotonic myopathy

	Myotonic dystrophy	*Proximal myotonic myopathy*
Distribution of weakness		
Facial, extraocular	++	+
Distal limbs	++	+
Proximal limbs	+	++
Muscle atrophy	++	+
Muscle pain	–	+
Central nervous system		
Mental retardation	+	–
Hypersomnolence	++	–
Brain atrophy on magnetic resonance imaging	+	–
White matter lesions	+	?
Congenital disease	+	–
Genetic anticipation	++	–

+ = the finding is present; ++ = the finding is present and very prominent; – = the finding is not present; ? = it is not yet known whether the finding occurs.

Prognosis

In general, because of the less frequent involvement of cardiac and respiratory muscle function in patients with PROMM, they have been considered to have a better prognosis compared with patients with DM. Moreover, no congenital form of PROMM has been described, although central nervous system involvement has been suggested [68]. Cardiac arrhythmia may occur in PROMM and requires serial monitoring.

Treatment

At present, no specific treatment exists for the muscle weakness or muscle pain in patients with PROMM. The myotonic stiffness and grip myotonia occasionally become so persistent that a trial of antimyotonia therapy seems appropriate. Insufficient data are available to permit recommendation of a specific drug. Cataracts may at some point require surgical treatment. Cardiac status should be monitored. Careful monitoring of patients with PROMM during surgery and postoperatively with a protocol similar to that outlined for DM (see Table 5.8) seems prudent.

   More specific guidelines for treatment in PROMM will develop as more patients are identified and a more detailed picture of the range of clinical manifestation is established.

REFERENCES

  1. Cannon SC. From mutation to myotonia in sodium channel disorders. Neuromuscul Disord 1997;7:241–249.
  2. Fahlke C, Beck CL, George ALJ. A mutation in autosomal dominant myotonia congenita affects pore properties of the muscle chloride channel. Proc Natl Acad Sci U S A 1997;94:2729–2734.
  3. Trudell RG, Kaiser KK, Griggs RC. Acetazolamide responsive myotonia congenita. Neurology 1987;37:488–491.
  4. Ptácek LJ, Tawil R, Griggs RC, et al. Sodium channel mutations in acetazolamide-responsive myotonia congenita, paramyotonia congenita, and hyperkalemic periodic paralysis. Neurology 1994;44:1500–1503.
  5. Lerche H, Heine R, Pika U, et al. Human sodium channel myotonia: slowed channel inactivation due to substitutions for a glycine within the III-IV linker. J Physiol 1993;470:13–22.
  6. Ptácek LJ, Johnson KJ, Griggs RC. Genetics and physiology of the myotonic muscle disorders. N Engl J Med 1993;328:482–489.
  7. Brook JD, McCurrach ME, Harley HG, et al. Molecular basis of myotonic dystrophy: expansion of a trinucleotide (CTG) repeat at the 3' end of a transcript encoding a protein kinase family member. Cell 1992;68:799–808.
  8. Fu YH, Pizzuti A, Fenwick RG Jr, et al. An unstable triplet repeat in a gene related to myotonic muscular dystrophy. Science 1992;255:1256–1258.
  9. Mahadevan M, Tsilfidis C, Sabourin L, et al. Myotonic dystrophy mutation: an unstable CTG repeat in the 3' untranslated region of the gene. Science 1992;255:1253–1255.
  10. Shelbourne P, Davies J, Buxton J, et al. Direct diagnosis of myotonic dystrophy with a disease-specific DNA marker. N Engl J Med 1993;328:471–475.
  11. Harper PS. Myotonic Dystrophy (2nd ed). Philadelphia: WB Saunders, 1989.
  12. Moxley RT III. Myotonic Muscular Dystrophy. In LP Rowland and S Di Mauro (eds), Handbook of Clinical Neurology. Vol 18. New York: Elsevier; 1992:209–259.
  13. Bouchard G, Roy R, Declos M, et al. Spreading of the gene for myotonic dystrophy in Saguenay (Quebec). J Genet Hum 1988;36:221–237.

14. Mathieu J, De Braekleer M, Prevost C. Genealogical reconstruction of myotonic dystrophy in the Saguenay-Lac-Saint-Jean area. Neurology 1990;40:839–842.
15. Ashizawa T, Epstein HF. Ethnic distribution of the myotonic dystrophy gene. Lancet 1991;338: 642–643.
16. Redman JB, Fenwick RG, Fu YH, et al. Relationship between parental trinucleotide CTG repeat length and severity of myotonic dystrophy in offspring. JAMA 1993;269:1960–1965.
17. Harley HG, Rundel SA, MacMillan JC, et al. Size of the unstable CTG repeat sequence in relation to phenotype and parental transmission in myotonic dystrophy. Am J Hum Genet 1993;52: 1164–1174.
18. Lavedan C, Hofmann-Radvanyi H, Shelbourne P, et al. Myotonic dystrophy: size and sex-dependent dynamics of CTG meiotic instability, and somatic mosaicism. Am J Hum Genet 1993;52:873–883.
19. Tsilfidis C, MacKenzie AE, Mettler G, et al. Correlation between CTG trinucleotide repeat length and frequency of severe congenital myotonic dystrophy. Nat Genet 1992;1:192–195.
20. Church SC. The heart in myotonia atrophica. Arch Intern Med 1967;119:176–181.
21. Forsberg H, Olofsson BO, Andersson S, et al. 24-hour electrocardiography study in myotonic dystrophy. Cardiology 1988;75:241–249.
22. Hawley RJ, Milner MR, Gottdiener JS, et al. Myotonic heart disease: a clinical follow-up. Neurology 1991;41:259–262.
23. The heart in myotonic dystrophy [editorial]. Lancet 1992;339:528–529.
24. Melacini P, Buja G, Fasoli G, et al. The natural history of cardiac involvement in myotonic dystrophy: an eight year follow-up in 17 patients. Clin Cardiol 1988;11:231–238.
25. Morgenlander JC, Nohiria V, Saba Z. EKG abnormalities in pediatric patients with myotonic dystrophy. Pediatr Neurol 1993;9:124–126.
26. De Ambroggi L, Raisaro A, Marchianò V, et al. Cardiac involvement in patients with myotonic dystrophy: characteristic features of magnetic resonance imaging. Eur Heart J 1995;16:1007–1010.
27. Brumback RA. Magnetic resonance imaging and clinical correlates of intellectual impairment in myotonic dystrophy. Arch Neurol 1990;47:253.
28. Glantz RH, Wright RB, Huckman MS, et al. Central nervous system magnetic resonance imaging findings in myotonic dystrophy. Arch Neurol 1988;45:36–37.
29. Huber SJ, Kissel JT, Shuttleworth EC, et al. Magnetic resonance imaging and clinical correlates of intellectual impairment in myotonic dystrophy. Arch Neurol 1989;46:536–540.
30. Damian MS, Bachmann G, Herrmann D, et al. Magnetic resonance imaging of muscle and brain in myotonic dystrophy. J Neurol 1993;240:8–12.
31. Bachmann G, Damian MS, Schilling G. The clinical significance of "white-matter-lesions" in myotonic dystrophy. Radiol J CEPUR 1993;13:15–20.
32. Fiorelli M, Duboc D, Mazoyer BM, et al. Decreased cerebral glucose utilisation in myotonic dystrophy. Neurology 1992;42:91–94.
33. Mielke R, Herholz K, Fink G, et al. Positron emission tomography in myotonic dystrophy. Psychiatry Res 1993;50:93–99.
34. Harper P, Penney R, Foley TP Jr, et al. Gonadal function in males with myotonic dystrophy. J Clin Endocrinol Metab 1972;35:852–856.
35. Griggs RC, Pandya S, Florence JM, et al. Randomised control trial of testosterone in myotonic dystrophy. Neurology 1989;39:219–222.
36. Piccardo MG, Pacini G, Rosa M, et al. Insulin resistance in myotonic dystrophy. Enzyme 1991;45:14–22.
37. Krentz AJ, Clark PM, Cox L, et al. Hyperproinsulinaemia in patients with myotonic dystrophy. Diabetologia 1992;35:1170–1172.
38. Livingston JN, Moxley RT III. Phenotype, genotype and insulin resistance in myotonic dystrophy. Diabetes Rev 1994;2:29–42.
39. Behrens MI, Jahl P, Serani A, et al. Possible role of apamin-sensitive K$^+$ channels in myotonic dystrophy. Muscle Nerve 1994;17:1264–1270.
40. Mathieu J, De Braekleer M, Prevost C, et al. Myotonic dystrophy: clinical assessment of muscular disability in an isolated population with presumed homogenous mutation. Neurology 1992;42:203–208.
41. Casanova G, Jerusalem F. Myopathology of myotonic dystrophy: a morphometric study. Acta Neuropathol (Berl) 1979;4:231–240.
42. Farkas E, Tomé FMS, Fardeau M, et al. Histochemical and ultrastructural study of muscle biopsies in 3 cases of dystrophia myotonica in the newborn child. J Neurol Sci 1974;21:273–288.
43. Argov Z, Gardner-Medwin D, Johnson MA, et al. Congenital myotonic dystrophy: fibre type abnormalities in two cases. Arch Neurol 1980;18:693–696.
44. Reddy S, Smith DB, Rich MM, et al. Mice lacking the myotonic dystrophy protein kinase develop a late onset progressive myopathy. Nat Genet 1996;13:325–334.

45. Jansen G, Groenen PJ, Bachner D, et al. Abnormal myotonic dystrophy protein kinase levels produce only mild myopathy in mice. Nat Genet 1996;13:316–324.
46. Thornton CA, Wymer JP, Simmons Z, et al. Expansion of the myotonic dystrophy CTG repeat reduces expression of the flanking DMAHP gene. Nat Genet 1997;16:407–409.
47. Klesert TR, Otten AD, Bird TD, et al. Trinucleotide repeat expansion at the myotonic dystrophy locus reduces expression of DMAHP. Nat Genet 1997;16:402–406.
48. Rudel R, Ruppersberg JP, Spittelmeister W. Abnormalities of the fast sodium current in myotonic dystrophy, recessive generalised myotonia, and adynamia episodica. Muscle Nerve 1989;12:281–287.
49. Shelbourne P, Winqvist E, Kunert E, et al. Unstable DNA may be responsible for the incomplete penetrance of the myotonic dystrophy phenotype. Hum Mol Genet 1992;1:467–473.
50. Imbert G, Kretz C, Johnson K, et al. Origin of the expansion mutation in myotonic dystrophy. Nat Genet 1993;4:72–76.
51. Neville CE, Mahadevan MS, Barcelo JM, et al. High resolution genetic analysis suggests one ancestral predisposing haplotype for the origin of the myotonic dystrophy mutation. Hum Mol Genet 1994;3:45–51.
52. Lavedan C, Hofmann-Radvanyi H, Boileau C, et al. French myotonic dystrophy families show expansion of a CTG repeat in complete linkage disequilibrium with an intragenic 1kb insertion. J Med Genet 1994;31:33–36.
53. Shaw DJ, McCurrach M, Rundle SA, et al. Genomic organization and transcriptional units at the myotonic dystrophy locus. Genomics 1993;18:673–679.
54. Moxley RT III. Myotonic disorders in childhood: diagnosis and treatment. J Child Neurol 1997;12:116–129.
55. Thornton CA, Griggs RC, Welle S, et al. Recombinant human growth hormone (rHGH) treatment increases lean body mass in patients with myotonic dystrophy [abstract]. Neurology 1993;43:280.
56. Vlachopapadopoulou E, Zachwieja JJ, Gertner JM, et al. Metabolic and clinical response to recombinant human insulin-like growth factor I in myotonic dystrophy—a clinical research center study. J Clin Endocrinol Metab 1995;80:3715–3723.
57. Ricker K, Koch MC, Lehmann-Horn F, et al. Proximal myotonic myopathy: a new dominant disorder with myotonia, muscle weakness, and cataracts. Neurology 1994;44:1448–1452.
58. Moxley RT III, Udd B, Ricker K. 54th ENMC International Workshop: PROMM (proximal myotonic myopathy) and other proximal myotonic syndromes. Neuromuscul Disord 1998;8:508–518.
59. Thornton CA, Griggs RC, Moxley RT III. Myotonic dystrophy with no trinucleotide repeat expansion. Ann Neurol 1994;35:269–272.
60. Ricker K, Koch MC, Lehmann-Horn F, et al. Proximal myotonic myopathy. Clinical features of a multisystem disorder similar to myotonic dystrophy. Arch Neurol 1995;52:25–31.
61. Meola G, Sansone V, Radice S, et al. A family with an unusual myotonic and myopathic phenotype and no CTG expansion (Proximal Myotonic Myopathy, PROMM syndrome): a challenge for future molecular studies. Neuromuscul Disord 1996;6:143–150.
62. Meola G, Sansone V. A newly-described myotonic disorder (proximal myotonic myopathy-PROMM): personal experience and review of the literature. Ital J Neurol Sci 1996;17:347–353.
63. Sander HW, Tavoulareas G, Chokroverty S. Heat sensitive myotonia in proximal myotonic myopathy. Neurology 1996;47:956–962.
64. Moxley RT III. Proximal myotonic myopathy: mini-review of a recently delineated clinical disorder. Neuromuscul Disord 1996;6:87–93.
65. Udd B, Krahe R, Wallgren-Pettersson C, et al. Proximal myotonic dystrophy—a family with autosomal dominant muscular dystrophy, cataracts, hearing loss and hypogonadism: heterogeneity of proximal myotonic syndromes? Neuromuscul Disord 1997;7:217–228.
66. Schuitevoerder K, Ansved T, Solders G, et al. Proximal myotonic myopathy. Analysis of 3 Swedish cases. Acta Neurol Scand 1997;96:266–270.
67. Meola G, Sansone V, Jabbour A, et al. Muscle imaging in proximal myotonic myopathy (PROMM): correlation to muscle atrophy and weakness [abstract]. J Neurol 1997;244:S43.
68. Hund E, Jansen O, Koch MC, et al. Proximal myotonic myopathy with MRI white matter abnormalities of the brain. Neurology 1997;48:33–37.

6
Muscle Channelopathies: Malignant Hyperthermia, Periodic Paralyses, Paramyotonia, and Myotonia

Reinhardt Rüdel, Michael G. Hanna,
and Frank Lehmann-Horn

Since the early 1990s, the molecular basis of a large number of diseases has been demonstrated to be impaired ion-channel function [1, 2, 3]. Collectively, these disorders have become known as the *channelopathies*. Such ion-channel dysfunction has now provided a molecular explanation for a number of well-recognized disorders, which span a number of different tissues and, therefore, medical disciplines. We now refer to *cardiac channelopathies,* such as the long QT syndromes, and *renal channelopathies,* such as Dent disease [1].

However, ion channels are especially important in the excitable tissues of the nervous system, and this is perhaps why the most striking advances have been made in relation to the *neurologic channelopathies.* There are now at least 10 separate genetic neurologic disorders for which the genes have been cloned and shown to code for ion channels, and it seems likely that more will follow [4]. These include central nervous system disorders, such as the episodic ataxias, hemiplegic migraine, and some forms of epilepsy; disorders of the neuromuscular junction, such as congenital myasthenia; and primary disorders of skeletal muscle, which are the subject of this chapter.

The primary skeletal muscle channelopathies include malignant hyperthermia, the periodic paralyses, paramyotonia congenita, and the nondystrophic myotonias. These disorders are now known to be due to mutations in four different voltage-gated skeletal muscle ion channels. In this chapter, we review the clinical features of each of these disorders and describe how molecular genetic advances have led to improvements not only in the classification and diagnosis of these conditions, but also in our understanding of their precise molecular pathogenesis, which should lead to more effective therapies.

MALIGNANT HYPERTHERMIA

Clinical Features, Pathogenesis, and Therapy

Malignant hyperthermia (MH) was originally described in 1960 by Michael Denborough while he was still a medical student [5]. It is the most common cause of

135

death during anesthesia. The international incidence is estimated to be between 1 in 7,000 and 1 in 50,000 anesthesias, with a higher incidence in pediatric anesthesia [6, 7]. In its fulminant form, this is a rapidly fatal disorder. Patients develop generalized muscle rigidity, rhabdomyolysis with elevated creatine kinase (CK), hypercarbia, acidosis, and hyperkalemia after exposure to inhalation narcotics or depolarizing muscle relaxants. There is usually coexistent hyperthermia, but this may be a late sign [8]. In some cases, the symptoms may be localized to individual muscles or muscle groups, such as the masseter causing jaw spasms. Of the inhaled anesthetic agents, all halogenated ethers (isoflurane, desflurane, enflurane, and sevoflurane), as well as halothane, are potential triggers. The most commonly responsible depolarizing muscle relaxant is succinylcholine.

MH is primarily a disorder of skeletal muscle calcium regulation. The triggering substances lead to an increase in the myoplasmic calcium concentration, which is released from the sarcoplasmic reticulum calcium stores via the voltage-dependent muscle ryanodine receptor channel. This leads to a rise in body temperature because of increased muscle metabolism and ultimately to muscle contracture and necrosis with the severe metabolic consequences described.

In addition to withdrawing the triggering agents and instituting supporting measures, dantrolene is a specific and effective therapy—if given early. Dantrolene acts by inhibiting the release of calcium from the sarcoplasmic reticulum. A specific protein receptor for dantrolene located in the skeletal muscle triad has been described [9]. Early administration of this drug has successfully aborted numerous fulminant crises [10] and reduced the mortality rate from approximately 70% to 10%. A further reduction in deaths may be achieved with earlier recognition of the disorder by anesthetists and perhaps in the future by the development of more effective therapies.

Diagnosis and Prevention

Currently, the susceptibility to MH can only be determined by means of the pharmacologic in vitro contracture test [11]. This test requires a large fresh muscle biopsy. It is not ideal, especially for young children. Strips of biopsied muscle are suspended in a bath and electrically stimulated. With halothane and caffeine added to the bath, abnormally high levels of muscle tension develop in muscle from individuals susceptible to MH. In view of its invasive nature, the test is only performed in people suspected to be at risk. It is possible that DNA-based testing for known gene mutations (described later) may facilitate the assessment of at-risk cases in the future. Individuals are considered to be at risk if there has been a suspected MH-like event during previous anesthesia or if they have an immediate relative with established MH. There is also a proven association between certain muscle diseases and a susceptibility to MH. These include central core disease, the King-Denborough syndrome, and familial elevation of CK. Although the in vitro contracture test is invasive, it is specific and has a sensitivity approaching 100%. In contrast to this in vitro test, it is recognized that only 50% of MH-susceptible patients develop an attack on their first exposure to triggering agents in vivo [12].

Genetics

Chromosomal mapping of MH susceptibility was facilitated by the existence of an animal model. In certain breeds of pigs, MH crises can be triggered when the

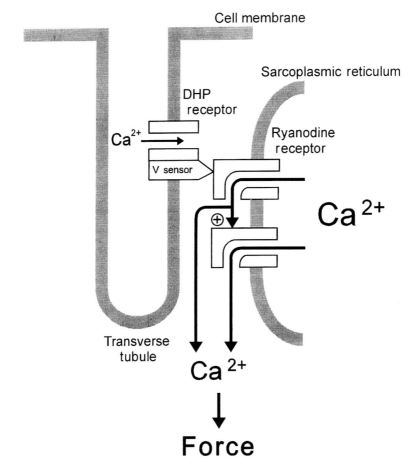

Cell membrane

Sarcoplasmic reticulum

DHP
receptor

Ca^{2+}

Ryanodine
receptor

V sensor

Ca^{2+}

Transverse
tubule

Ca^{2+}

Force

Figure 6.1 The triadic junction between a transverse tubule and the sarcoplasmic reticulum: position of the two calcium (Ca^{2+}) channels of skeletal muscle, the dihydropyridine (DHP) receptor, and the ryanodine receptor. The coupling between the two channels is not fully elucidated. Mutations in the respective genes may cause hypokalemic periodic paralysis, malignant hyperthermia, or central core disease.

animals are stressed (porcine stress syndrome) [13]. This pig model was linked to porcine chromosome 6 [14]. Subsequently, the corresponding cluster of genes was found on human chromosome 19q12-13.2, and linkage was established in some, but not all, MH families [15]. At the same time, the gene encoding the skeletal muscle ryanodine receptor (RYR1) was mapped to the same region, and linkage of some MH families to this locus was reported [16]. The RYR1 is one of the two types of calcium channels expressed in skeletal muscle; the other is the so-called dihydropyridine (DHP) receptor (Figure 6.1).

In some families, linkage of MH susceptibility to RYR1 was excluded [17, 18, 19]. In one pedigree, MH susceptibility was linked to a gene locus on chromosome 7q that contains the gene for the α_2/δ subunit of the DHP receptor of skeletal muscle [20]. In another MH family, linkage was demonstrated to the gene encoding the α_1 subunit of this channel [21].

It was in the recessively inherited porcine stress model that the first point mutation Arg-615-Cys in the RYR1 gene was detected in homozygous form [22, 23]. Subsequently, the homologous point mutation was identified in several MH families linked to the RYR1 gene [24]. In keeping with the dominant mode of inheritance in man, the mutation was found on only one of the two alleles. Seven further point mutations have been identified (Figure 6.2 and Table 6.1). The mutations Gly-248-Arg, Tyr-522-Ser, Gly-2434-Arg, and Arg-2435-His have been detected in a few families, and Cys-35-Arg and Arg-552-Trp in only one family each. In contrast, the mutations Arg-163-Cys, Ile-403-Met, and Arg-614-Cys (porcine homologue) make up 2–5% of the investigated cases. Most common seems to be the mutation Gly-341-Arg in the amino terminal region of the protein that also contains five of the rare human mutations [25].

Mutations in the gene encoding the α_1 subunit of the DHP receptor have been identified in two families with MH (Figure 6.3). They result in an Arg-1086-His or an Arg-1086-Cys substitution in the loop connecting repeats III and IV of the channel [8, 26]. Further study of the pathophysiology caused by this mutation should improve our knowledge of electromechanical coupling.

Pathophysiology of the Ryanodine Receptor, RYR1

The skeletal muscle RYR1 channel is activated by micromolar concentrations of calcium and is inhibited by calcium concentrations greater than 10 μM and by millimolar magnesium concentrations [27, 28]. The channel is regulated by various endogenous and exogenous ligands: Adenosine triphosphate (ATP), calmodulin (only in the absence of calcium), caffeine, and ryanodine activate the channel when at nanomolar concentrations (for review, see reference 29).

The increased sensitivity of MH-susceptible muscle to caffeine is considered to be caused by an altered RYR1 function. Functional tests performed with mutant porcine RYR1 in isolated sarcoplasmic reticulum vesicles have shown that calcium regulation is disturbed. Lower calcium concentrations activate the channel to a higher-than-normal level, and higher-than-normal calcium concentrations are required to inhibit the channel [30]. Calmodulin plays an important role in the regulation of RYR1. Calmodulin activates the channel in the absence of calcium but strongly inhibits it in the presence of activating calcium concentrations [31]. The inhibiting properties of calmodulin were not found altered in mutant RYR1, but its activating properties in the absence of calcium were drastically increased [32].

Investigations of reconstituted mutant RYR1 designed to determine the cause of the increased caffeine sensitivity of MH-susceptible muscle have led to controversial results. Electrophysiologic single-channel measurements on mutant RYR1 did not show increased caffeine sensitivity [33], whereas pharmacologic binding studies showed increased affinity [34].

Muscle Diseases with Malignant Hyperthermia Susceptibility

There has been some debate in the literature regarding the existence of increased MH susceptibility in association with a wide variety of neuromuscular diseases.

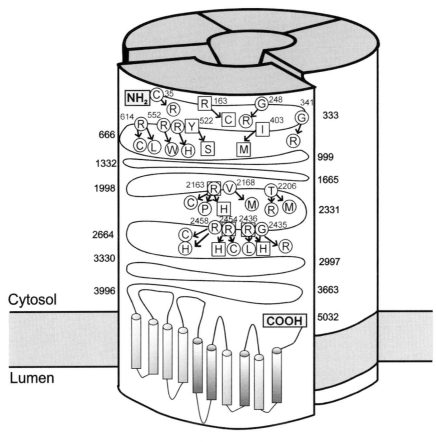

○ Malignant hyperthermia
□ Malignant hyperthermia/central core disease

Figure 6.2   Mutations predicted in the ryanodine receptor calcium channel in the membranes of the sarcoplasmic reticulum (SR). The functional channel is a homomeric tetramer. Ten transmembrane segments are indicated as cylinders at the carboxy-terminus. All published mutations are missense mutations situated in the foot protein bridging the gap between the t-tubular and the SR membrane. Central core disease patients carrying a RYR1 mutation are also susceptible to malignant hyperthermia. (Modified from W Melzer, A Herrmann-Frank, HC Lüttgau. The role of Ca^{2+} ions in excitation-contraction coupling of skeletal muscle fibers. Biochim Biophys Acta 1995;1241:59–116.)

Such diseases include central core disease, the King-Denborough syndrome, the nondystrophic myotonias, the periodic paralyses, myotonic dystrophy, and the dystrophin-deficient muscular dystrophies. Of these, only two disorders have an established predisposition to MH. It is certain that there is an increased susceptibility to MH in patients with central core disease, and this is likely also the case in King-Denborough syndrome.

Table 6.1   Mutations in proteins of the excitation-contraction coupling complex of skeletal muscle (ryanodine receptor [RYR1] and dihydropyridine receptor [DHPR]) causing malignant hyperthermia (MH), central core disease (CCD), or hypokalemic periodic paralysis (HypoPP)

RYR1: Malignant hyperthermia and/or central core disease

Nucleotide	Exon	Substitution	Disease state	Frequency	First report
T103C	2	Cys-35-Arg	MH	One family	181
C487T	6	Arg-163-Cys	MH, CCD	2%	182
G742A	9	Gly-248-Arg	MH	2%	183
G1021A	11	Gly-341-Arg	MH	6%	25
C1209G	12	Ile-403-Met	CCD	One family	182
A1565C	14	Tyr-522-Ser	MH, CCD	One family	184
C1654T	15	Arg-552-Trp	MH	One family	185
C1840T	17	Arg-614-Cys	MH	4%	24
G1841T	17	Arg-614-Leu	MH	2%	186
C6487T	39	Arg-2163-Cys	MH	4%	187
G6488A	39	Arg-2163-His	MH, CCD	One family	187
G6502A	39	Val-2168-Met	MH	7%	187
C6617T	40	Thr-2206-Met	MH	One family	187
G7300A	45	Gly-2435-Arg	MH	4%	188
G7304A	45	Arg-2436-His	MH, CCD	One family	189
C7372T	46	Arg-2458-Cys	MH	4%	190
G7373A	46	Arg-2458-His	MH	4%	190

DHPR: Hypokalemic periodic paralysis or malignant hyperthermia

Nucleotide	Exon	Substitution	Disease state	Frequency	First report
G1583A	11	R528H	HypoPP	40%	108
C3256T	26	R1086C	MH	One family	26
G3257A	26	R1086H	MH	One family	1
C3715G	30	R1239G	HypoPP	3%	109
G3716A	30	R1239H	HypoPP	40%	108
					109

Note: Numbering of RYR1 amino acids according to the revised version of Phillips et al. [207].

In the other disorders, although MH-like events have been described, no consistent triggering agent exists, and it seems likely that the molecular mechanisms responsible for these events differ from those of MH susceptibility. Of course, this does not obviate the need for caution when considering general anesthesia in those disorders in which MH-like events have been reported, as, for example, in cases of dystrophin-deficient dystrophies [35, 36]. Although MH susceptibility has been excluded by the in vitro contracture test in cases of dystrophin-deficient dystrophy, it is possible that the dystrophic process itself—which may increase the intramyoplasmic calcium concentration—may increase the sensitivity of skeletal muscle to inhalation narcotics and depolarizing narcotics. If

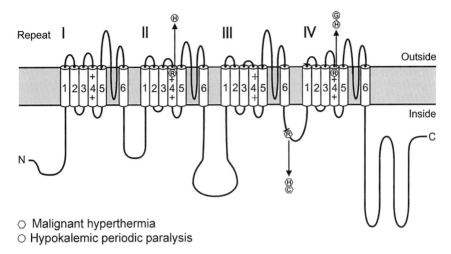

Figure 6.3 Mutations predicted in the α_1 subunit of the skeletal muscle L-type calcium (Ca^{2+}) channel (dihydropyridine receptor). Point mutations in the voltage-sensing S4 segments of this voltage-gated calcium channel cause hypokalemic periodic paralysis in more than 60% of the patients. Point mutations in the intracellular link connecting domains III and IV caused malignant hyperthermia in two families. (Modified from L Schleithoff, S Paul, T Deufel, et al. A novel DHP receptor mutation in a malignant hyperthermia family linked to another locus. Am J Hum Genet [submitted].)

doubt exists or previous events have occurred, the avoidance of possible triggering substances is appropriate.

THE PERIODIC PARALYSES

Hyperkalemic Periodic Paralysis

Hyperkalemic periodic paralysis was first described by Tyler [37] and Helweg-Larsen [38] and was extensively investigated by Gamstorp [39], who clearly differentiated it from paroxysmal familial paralysis and named it *adynamia episodica hereditaria.* Clinically, the most striking difference between the two diseases is that during the paralytic episodes, the serum potassium decreases in the former and increases in the latter. To stress this distinction, the names *hypokalemic periodic paralysis* and *hyperkalemic periodic paralysis,* respectively, are now preferred.

Hyperkalemic periodic paralysis is transmitted as an autosomal dominant trait with complete penetrance in both sexes, although incomplete penetrance has been reported for families with rare mutations [40, 41]. Sporadic cases have also been reported [42], and a de novo mutation was proven in a patient whose genetically confirmed father and mother did not carry the defective gene [43]. The disease has three clinically distinct variants. It can occur (1) without myotonia, (2) with clinical or electromyographic (EMG) myotonia, or (3) with paramyotonia. In some patients, a chronic progressive myopathy may develop that seems to be genetically determined [44–46].

Clinical Features

Attacks of hyperkalemic periodic paralysis usually begin in the first decade of life. Initially they are infrequent, but they increase in frequency. In severe cases, they may recur daily (Table 6.2). The attack commonly starts in the morning before breakfast, lasts from 15 minutes to 1 hour, and then spontaneously disappears. Rest often provokes the attack, particularly if preceded by strenuous exercise. Potassium loading usually precipitates an attack, and this is used in provocative testing. Cold environment, emotional stress, glucocorticoids, and pregnancy provoke or worsen the attacks. After strenuous exercise, weakness usually follows within a few minutes of rest. In some patients, paresthesia or the sensation of muscle tension heralds the attack. Sustained mild exercise after a period of strenuous exercise may postpone or prevent the weakness in the exercising muscle groups, while the resting muscles become weak.

The generalized weakness is usually accompanied by a significant increase of serum potassium (up to 5–6 mM). Sometimes, the serum potassium level remains within the upper normal range and rarely reaches cardiotoxic levels. When the serum potassium level begins to rise, the serum sodium level falls 3–9 mM. This fall is caused by sodium entry into muscle, which in turn causes movement of water into the muscle, resulting in hemoconcentration, which further increases the serum potassium level. During attacks, the urinary potassium excretion increases, and this may terminate the attack. Moderate exercise also hastens recovery. However, slight weakness may persist for days. Sometimes, transient hypokalemia occurs at the end of the attack [47]. Water diuresis, release of enzymes from muscle, creatinuria, and myalgia can also occur at the end of an attack. Between attacks, the serum potassium is normal. The frequency of attacks declines in the second half of life.

The course of the paralytic attacks is the same in all three forms of hyperkalemic periodic paralysis. Cooling can induce weakness but not stiffness, and reheating restores contractile force quickly (except in the paramyotonic form). EMG studies are required to determine the presence or absence of myotonia. In the nonmyotonic form, clinical and electrical myotonia are both absent. In families with the myotonic variant, the myotonic phenomena are present in all affected members. The clinical myotonia is usually very mild and never impedes voluntary movements. It is most readily observed in the facial, lingual, thenar, and finger extensor muscles. In the attack-free interval, the EMG shows typical myotonic discharges in almost every muscle. At the beginning of an attack, the EMG sometimes shows bursts of fibrillation potentials, which may explain the sensation of muscle tension. Cooling may provoke weakness but does not cause substantial myotonia. Paramyotonic hyperkalemic periodic paralysis is characterized by attacks of generalized muscle weakness associated with hyperkalemia and by paradoxical myotonia (for details, see the following section, Paramyotonia Congenita).

Table 6.2 Overview of the clinical, diagnostic, and therapeutic features for the muscle sodium channel diseases and familial hypokalemic periodic paralysis (a calcium channelopathy)

Disorder	Hyperkalemic periodic paralysis	Paramyotonia congenita	Potassium-aggravated myotonia	Familial hypokalemic periodic paralysis
Inheritance	Autosomal dominant. De novo mutations are known.	Autosomal dominant.	Autosomal dominant. De novo mutations are known.	Autosomal dominant. De novo mutations are known. Genetically heterogenous.
Gene and gene locus	SCN4A on 17q23.	SCN4A on 17q23.	SCN4A on 17q23.	CACNL1A3 on 1q32.
Symptoms	Generalized attacks of weakness. Weakness may become gradually permanent.	Muscular stiffness at the beginning of exposure to cold. Muscular weakness on prolonged exposure to cold.	Generalized muscle stiffness without weakness and without cold sensitivity.	Generalized attacks of weakness. Weakness may become gradually permanent.
First occurrence of symptoms	At the end of the first decade or beginning of the second decade.	At birth.	Early childhood.	Usually in the second decade.
Frequency of attacks	A few times per yr to daily.	On every exposure to a cold environment.	Depending on severity, occasionally or permanently.	Extremely variable: from one to two attacks in a lifetime to daily.
Severity of attacks	Occasionally, generalized paralysis. Frequently moderate weakness, often only in single muscle groups.	Stiffness and weakness that become more severe the heavier the work in the cold. The lower the temperature, the more severe the weakness.	Stiffness that becomes more severe the heavier the work. Low temperature has no influence on muscle stiffness.	Often, generalized paralysis. Less frequent moderate weakness (e.g., of the arms or legs).
Duration of attacks	Usually ½–1 hr, occasionally several hrs.	Stiffness only at the beginning of work in a cold environment. Weakness may last for hours after re-warming.	½–2 hrs	Several hrs to several days.
Time of day when symptoms appear	Early to late morning. Occasionally, at any time of day.	At any time when exposed to cold environment.	Any time during and after heavy exercise.	Second half of night. Early morning. Occasionally, late morning.

Table 6.2   (continued)

Disorder	Hyperkalemic periodic paralysis	Paramyotonia congenita	Potassium-aggravated myotonia	Familial hypokalemic periodic paralysis
Triggering factors	Muscular exercise with subsequent rest (attack 20–30 mins later). Cold. Hunger.	Cooling and heavy muscular work, particularly in combination.	Muscular exercise with subsequent rest. K$^+$ loading. Succinylcholine anesthesia.	Muscle exercise with subsequent rest (attack follows several hrs later). Carbohydrate-rich meals. Stress. Cold.
Diagnostic provocation	Muscular exercise (ergometer or running upstairs). Administration of K$^+$.	Cooling of lower arm for 30 mins in water of 12–15°C. Repeated forceful closure of the fist.	Muscle exercise and rest.	Administration of glucose and insulin (caution). Muscle exercise and carbohydrate-rich food the evening before the test.
Concomitant symptoms at the beginning of an attack	Myotonia, when present, increased. Cases without myotonia might present lid lag. Paresthesias common.	Sensations of tension in the muscles.	Sensations of tension in the muscles.	In rare cases, lid-lag phenomenon. No myotonia. No sensory disturbance.
K$^+$ in the serum during an attack	4.5–8.0 mM. After the attack, occasionally <3 mM.	3.5–4.5 mM.	3.5–4.5 mM.	2–3 mM.
Electromyogram	In cases with myotonia: bursts of fibrillationlike potentials in all muscles. During severe attacks, no spontaneous activity.	At the beginning of cooling, severe fibrillationlike spontaneous activity. During the weakness, no spontaneous activity.	Bursts of fibrillationlike potentials in all muscles. In severe cases, permanently present.	No spontaneous activity. In cases with permanent weakness, occasionally fibrillationlike potentials.
Therapy	*Preventive*: frequent meals, acetazolamide, dihydrochlorothiacide. *At the beginning of attack*: movement, salbutamol spray, injection of calcium gluconate.	*Preventive*: keeping the muscles warm, mexiletine. No therapeutic action known for relief of weakness.	Mexiletine depot or acetazolamide.	*Preventive*: acetazolamide, dichlorophenamide, spironolactone, low-sodium diet. *During an attack*: potassium tablets.

Diagnosis

The diagnosis of hyperkalemic periodic paralysis is based on the presence of typical attacks of weakness or paralysis, the positive family history, and the myotonic or paramyotonic phenomena if present. Except in some older patients with progressive myopathy, the muscles are well developed. Calf hypertrophy has been reported [48]. The serum CK is sometimes elevated to 200–300 U/liter. When the diagnosis is unclear, a provocative test can be performed, although the increased availability of DNA-based diagnosis may make such provocation unnecessary. This consists of the administration of 2–10 g of potassium chloride (26–130 mmol) in an unsweetened solution in the fasting state just after exercise, preferably in the morning. The test is contraindicated in subjects who are already hyperkalemic and in those who do not have adequate renal or adrenal reserve. An abnormally high serum potassium level between attacks suggests secondary rather than primary hyperkalemic periodic paralysis. The provocative test usually induces an attack within the next 1–2 hours.

An elegant alternative test consists of exercise on a bicycle ergometer for 30 minutes, so that the pulse increases to 120–160 beats per minute, followed by absolute rest in bed [47]. The serum potassium rises during exercise and then declines to almost the pre-exercise level, as in healthy individuals. Ten to 20 minutes after the onset of rest, a second hyperkalemic period occurs in the patients (in contrast to control subjects), and the patients become paralyzed. Recordings of the evoked compound muscle action potential during rest and exercise are also helpful in confirming the diagnosis of periodic paralysis [49] (Figure 6.4) and in differentiating between hyperkalemic periodic paralysis and paramyotonia congenita [50].

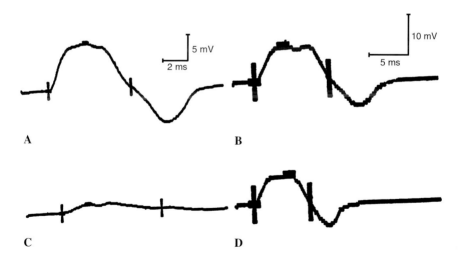

Figure 6.4   The exercise test in hyperkalemic periodic paralysis (after McManis et al. [49]). Pre-exercise status before (**A**) and after (**B**) treatment with 4 mg oral salbutamol in a patient having the Thr-704-Met point mutation in SCN4A. Postexercise decrement in M. abductor digiti minimi compound muscle action potential before (**C**) and after (**D**) treatment with 4 mg oral salbutamol in same patient. (Reprinted with permission from MG Hanna, J Stewart, AHV Schapira, et al. Salbutamol treatment in a patient with hyperkalemic periodic paralysis due to a mutation in the skeletal muscle sodium channel gene [SCN4A]. J Neurol Neurosurg Psychiatry 1998;68:248–250.)

Pathogenesis

In vitro electrophysiologic studies on muscle strips from patients with hyperkalemic periodic paralysis revealed abnormal inactivation of the sarcolemmal sodium channels [51–53]. As in the other sodium channelopathies, two types of sodium channels are expressed in the muscle fibers: one that inactivates (i.e., closes) normally, and another with impaired inactivation. The explanation of the paralysis in the disease is as follows [51–54]: Hyperkalemia induced by potassium intake or by activity causes slight membrane depolarization, even in normal muscle. In hyperkalemic periodic paralysis muscle, this small depolarization opens abnormally inactivating sodium channels. This allows sodium influx into the muscle fibers to be greater than normal, which prolongs and augments the depolarization. This in turn causes inactivation of the normally functioning sodium channels (i.e., those expressed by the normal gene) and renders the muscle fibers inexcitable. The sodium influx also causes a shift of water into the muscle fibers, which causes hemoconcentration and a further increase of serum potassium. This in turn causes additional muscle fibers to become depolarized and may result in paralysis of the entire muscle. The cycle is probably terminated when the hyperkalemia is relieved by kaliuresis. An increased activity of the sodium-potassium pump, stimulated by the increased concentration of intracellular sodium and extracellular potassium, may also help terminate the attack. When the serum potassium returns to normal, the defective sodium channels are likely to close, and a normal resting membrane potential is again attained.

Interestingly, patients never become weak during activity, despite an increase of the extracellular potassium level [55]. This seems to be connected to the work-related decrease in intracellular pH, because lowering the pH of the high-potassium bathing solution normalizes the contractile force exerted by muscle bundles obtained from hyperkalemic periodic paralysis patients [51]. In addition, physical activity is associated with enhanced adrenaline release. Adrenalin stimulates the sodium-potassium pump [56], which helps to compensate for the abnormal sodium influx into the muscle fibers.

The Sodium Channel of Adult Human Skeletal Muscle

After the cloning of SCN4A (the gene coding for the α subunit of the adult human skeletal muscle sodium channel, hSkm-1) in 1990, the demonstration of linkage of hyperkalemic periodic paralysis to its locus on chromosome 17q23 [57] provided the first proof for the existence of a human sodium channel disease. Soon after, three groups showed independently that paramyotonia congenita is also linked to the SCN4A locus [45, 58, 59].

SCN4A contains 24 exons distributed over approximately 30 kb. Intron-exon boundaries are known, and primer sets consisting of intron sequences allowing amplification of all 24 exons by polymerase chain reaction are available [60]. SCN4A is only expressed in skeletal muscle, and its product, the tetrodotoxin-sensitive hSkm1, is the only sodium channel detectable in the fully differentiated tissue.

The SCN4A gene product—a 260-kd glycoprotein containing approximately 2,000 amino acids—is distinguished by four domains of internal homology, each

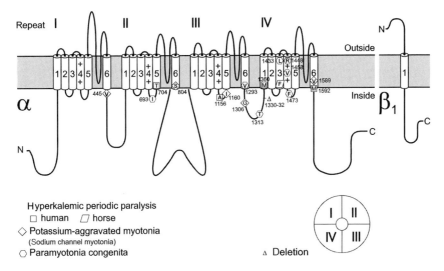

Figure 6.5 Mutations predicted in the sodium (Na⁺) channel α subunit of adult skeletal muscle, hSkm-1. When inserted in the membrane, the four repeats of the protein fold to generate a pore, as schematically indicated on the right-hand bottom of the figure. Conventional one-letter abbreviations are used for mutated amino acids (located at amino acid positions given by the respective numbers). In two positions (aa 1306, aa 1448), three different natural mutations have been detected. The different symbols used for the point mutations indicate the resulting diseases as explained at the bottom of the left-hand side. Included are the positions of mutations causing hyperkalemic periodic paralysis in the homologue horse gene. So far, no mutation has been found in the regulatory β subunit (far right). (Modified from F Lehmann-Horn, R Rüdel. Molecular pathophysiology of voltage-gated ion channels. Rev Physiol Biochem Pharmacol 1996;128:195–268.)

encompassing 225–325 amino acids (Figure 6.5). Each of these so-called repeats (I–IV) consists of six hydrophobic segments (S1–S6), putative transmembrane helices that are connected with each other by interlinkers. Between segments S5 and S6 of each repeat, the interlinkers consist of an extracellular part and a sequence that dips into the membrane. These four intramembrane loops are thought to form the lining of the channel pore as described in potassium channels. The S4 helices contain a repeating motif with a positively charged amino acid at every third position. The high-charge density suggests that it may function as a voltage sensor. The charges could shift in response to depolarization and may play an essential part in voltage-dependent activation or inactivation of the channel.

Another part of the protein to which a certain function has been assigned is the interlinker connecting repeat III-S6 with repeat IV-S1. It is likely that this part of the protein acts as the inactivation gate of the channel in a way that has been compared with a tethered ball [61]. The intracellular orifice of the pore or its surrounding protein parts may act as an acceptor of the ball. In the resting state, the ball is away from the pore; after activation, the ball is thought to swing into the mouth to block the ion pathway.

Table 6.3   Mutations of SCN4A, the gene encoding the α subunit of the human skeletal muscle sodium channel

Base exchange	Channel domain	Substitution	Exon	Phenotype	First report
Hyperkalemic periodic paralysis					
C2188T	IIS5$_i$	Thr-704-Met	13	Permanent weakness, nonmyotonic most frequent	45
G3466A	(IIIS4/5)$_i$	Ala-1156-Thr	19	Reduced penetrance	40
A4078G	IVS1	Met-1360-Val	23	Reduced penetrance	41
A4774G	IVS6$_i$	Met-1592-Val	24	Myotonic Frequent	43
Paramyotonia congenita					
T2078C	IIS4/5	Ile-693-Thr	13	No paralysis	191
G3877A	IIIS6$_i$	Val-1293-Ile	21	No paralysis	192
C3938T	(III/IV)$_i$	Thr-1313-Met	22	Frequent	129
T4298G	IVS3	Leu-1433-Arg	24	—	193
C4342T	IVS4	Arg-1448-Cys	24	Potential atrophy	127
G4343A	IVS4	Arg-1448-His	24	—	127
G4343C	IVS4	Arg-1448-Pro	24	Potential atrophy	70
T4364C	IVS4	Ile-1455-Thr	24	—	206
G4372T	IVS4	Val-1458-Phe	24	—	206
T4418C	IVS4/5$_i$	Phe-1473-Ser	24	—	69
Potassium-aggravated myotonias					
G1333A	IS6$_i$	Val-445-Met	9	Painful myotonia	194
C2411T	IIS6$_i$	Ser-804-Phe	14	Overlap Myotonia fluctuans	40, 176
A3478G	(III/IV)$_i$	Ile-1160-Val	19	Acetazolamide-responsive myotonia	171
G3917A	(III/IV)$_i$	Gly-1306-Glu	22	Myotonia permanens	64
G3917C	(III/IV)$_i$	Gly-1306-Ala	22	Myotonia fluctuans	64
G3917T	(III/IV)$_i$	Gly-1306-Val	22	Overlap Myotonia	129 64
G4765A	IVS6$_i$	Val-1589-Met	24	Myotonia	165

Molecular Genetics

To date, four mutations in SCN4A have been found to cause hyperkalemic periodic paralysis (see Figure 6.5; Table 6.3). Thr-704-Met is the most frequent SCN4A mutation, and in addition to hyperkalemic periodic paralysis with or without myotonia, it often causes a chronic progressive myopathy that can be significantly disabling in some patients [45]. The other three mutations cause myotonic hyperkalemic periodic paralysis without permanent weakness. Met-1592-Val, the first of all detected sodium channel mutations [43], always causes hyperkalemic periodic paralysis associated with myotonia. Two rare mutations (Ala-1156-Thr, Met-1360-Val) are of interest because they were discovered in families showing incomplete penetrance in females [40, 41, 46]. Finally, in one family with hyperkalemic periodic paralysis, no mutation was found when the cDNA coding for the α subunit of the sodium channel was sequenced, indicating that there is genetic heterogeneity [62].

Molecular Pathogenesis

The molecular pathogenesis of the sodium channel mutations that cause hyperkalemic periodic paralysis—as well as those responsible for the other two sodium channel diseases, described subsequently—has been studied by expressing the corresponding cDNAs in heterologous cell systems, such as the HEK-293 line (*h*uman *e*mbryonic *k*idney cell line). The findings in relation to the different mutations, which associate with the three recognized sodium channel diseases, are described here. The major observation from such expression studies is that all sodium channel mutations analyzed to date result in impairment of the fast-inactivation capability of the channel. Fast inactivation is responsible for the fast closing of the channel measured in milliseconds following its opening by a depolarizing stimulus. In all forms of sodium channel disease, fast inactivation has been shown to be incomplete (Figure 6.6A) or slowed (Figure 6.6B). Both these alterations are the result of pathologic channel reopenings (right-hand panel in Figure 6.6C). Incomplete inactivation causes a persistent steady-state, inward sodium current. It is much more pronounced in mutations causing hyperkalemic periodic paralysis [63] and is also seen in mutations causing potassium-aggravated myotonia [64–66]. On the other hand, a slowing of fast inactivation without much steady-state current is typically found with mutations causing paramyotonia congenita [67–70]. Mutations causing potassium-aggravated myotonia show such slowing only to a much lesser degree [64, 66].

The hypotheses derived from these results are that weakness or even paralysis in hyperkalemic periodic paralysis is due to the sustained depolarization caused by the persistent sodium current, whereas myotonia in paramyotonia congenita and potassium-aggravated myotonia is based on increased excitability caused by the delayed inactivation. The paradoxic increase of myotonia typical for paramyotonia congenita is explained by the cumulative increase of sodium influx during each action potential. In addition to fast inactivation, there is also the process of slow inactivation, which closes sodium channels on a time scale of seconds. This process would antagonize the building up of a steady-state current [71]. Slow inactivation was indeed found to be less pronounced in hyperkalemic periodic paralysis [72], but not in potassium-aggravated myotonia or paramyotonia congenita [73], in agreement with the earlier explanation for the paralysis in hyperkalemic periodic paralysis. Contrary to expectations, neither extracellular potassium nor reduced temperature had a direct effect on any of the mutant channels expressed in the heterologous system. It seems that these triggering factors exert their effects indirectly (e.g., they may increase a persistent sodium current by causing membrane depolarization according to physiologic mechanisms).

Therapy

Preventive therapy consists of frequent meals rich in carbohydrates; a low-potassium diet; and avoidance of fasting, strenuous work, and exposure to cold. Many patients

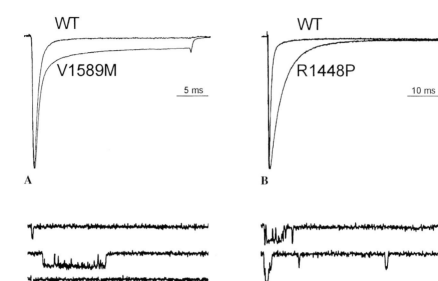

Figure 6.6 Impaired inactivation of sodium currents conducted by mutant channels expressed in a heterologous system (human embryonic kidney cells). The left-hand side of panel **C** shows six traces obtained in attached-patch technique with the wild-type (WT) for control. The membrane potential is clamped from a holding potential of 100 mV to 30 mV for 120 ms. Sodium current is activated and quickly inactivated on depolarization (downward deflections at the onset of traces). Only the second trace shows a 40-ms burst rather than the normal spike. With the mutant channel (right-hand side), almost every trace shows bursts and occasionally delayed openings. Averaging of 500 such traces results in smooth curves as illustrated in **A** for the Val-1589-Met mutation and in **B** for the Arg-1448-Pro mutation, in comparison with WT traces. (**A**) Shows persisting current as a typical finding for a mutation causing hyperkalemic periodic paralysis. (Modified from N Mitrovic, AL George Jr, R Heine, et al. Potassium-aggravated myotonia: the V1589M mutation destabilizes the inactivated state of the human muscle sodium channel. J Physiol 1994;478:395–402.) (**B**) Shows slowed inactivation as an example for paramyotonia congenita. (Modified from H Lerche, N Mitrovic, V Dubowitz, et al. Pathophysiology of paramyotonia congenita: the R1448P sodium channel mutation in adult human skeletal muscle. Ann Neurol 1996;39:599–608.)

are able to prevent or abort attacks by continuing slight exercise or ingesting carbohydrates at the onset of weakness (e.g., 2 g glucose per kg body weight). However, severe attacks may fail to respond to these measures [39]. Interestingly, attacks occur more frequently on holidays and weekends, when patients rest in bed longer than usual. Thus, patients are advised to rise early and have a full breakfast.

Some patients can abort or attenuate attacks by the prompt oral intake of a thiazide diuretic or acetazolamide, or by inhalation of a β-adrenergic agent. The beneficial effect of the diuretics is probably due to their capacity to lower the serum potassium level. The effect of the β-adrenergic agent is mediated via stimulation of the sodium-potassium pump [56, 74]. The inhalation of three puffs of 1.3 mg metaproterenol (repeatable after 15 minutes), two puffs of 0.18 mg albuterol [75], or two puffs of 0.1 mg salbutamol [47, 74, 76] (see Figure 6.4) has aborted acute attacks. Calcium gluconate, 0.5–2.0 g given intravenously, has also terminated attacks in some patients but not in others.

It is often advisable to prevent attacks by the continuous use of a thiazide diuretic [39] or acetazolamide [77, 78]. Diuretics that lower serum potassium are very effective in mild cases. The diuretics are used in modest dosages at intervals from twice daily to twice weekly [77]. Thiazide diuretics are preferable because of the possible complications of acetazolamide therapy [79]. The dosage should be kept as low as possible (e.g., 25 mg of hydrochlorothiazide daily or every other day). The drug should not lower the serum potassium below 3.3 mM or the serum sodium below 135 mM [77]. In severe cases, 50 or 75 mg of hydrochlorothiazide should be taken daily very early in the morning.

Normokalemic Periodic Paralysis

Normokalemic periodic paralysis, a rare disorder, is a variant of the hyperkalemic form. It resembles hyperkalemic periodic paralysis in many respects, but differs from it in that the serum potassium does not increase, even during serious attacks. The existence of normokalemic periodic paralysis as a nosologic entity has been questioned, because some patients with this condition are sensitive to oral potassium salts [80]. The disorder is transmitted as an autosomal dominant trait with high penetrance in both sexes. The attacks begin in the first decade of life and are provoked or worsened by rest after exercise, exposure to cold, and potassium loading. Large doses of sodium improve the weakness, but glucose loading has no effect. There are no consistent changes in the serum electrolytes, but increased sodium excretion and potassium retention occur during the attacks. The urinary potassium retention, lack of a beneficial effect of glucose, and failure of the serum potassium to increase in attacks distinguish this disease from primary hyperkalemic periodic paralysis. However, in at least one such family, the condition is caused by the common Val-704-Met mutation in SCN4A normally associated with hyperkalemic periodic paralysis (Lehmann-Horn F, Heine R, Pika U, et al., unpublished observation, 1994).

Hypokalemic Periodic Paralysis

The clinical symptoms of hypokalemic periodic paralysis were described in the eighteenth century. An early review summarizes what was known about the disease before 1941 [81]. Interestingly, it was not until 1934 that hypokalemia was recognized during the paralytic attacks [82]. The prevalence is estimated to be 1 in 100,000. Thus, the disease is the most common of the familial periodic paralyses. It is transmitted as an autosomal dominant trait with reduced penetrance in women (the male-to-female ratio is 3–4 to 1) [83].

Clinical Features

The disease is homogeneous, both clinically and electrophysiologically. Severe cases present in early childhood, mild cases present as late as the third decade of life, and approximately 60% present before age 16 years [81]. Initially, the attacks are infrequent, but after a few months or years, they increase in frequency and eventually may recur daily. An attack may range in severity from slight temporary weakness of an isolated muscle group to generalized paralysis. Paralytic attacks usually occur in the second half of the night or in the early morning hours. On awakening, the patient is unable to move his or her arms, legs, or trunk. In most cases, the cranial muscles are spared. The vital capacity is reduced in severe attacks, and death from ventilatory failure can occur [84]. Usually, strength increases gradually as the day passes. Occasionally, the weakness lasts 2–3 days.

The trigger for a nocturnal attack is often strenuous physical activity or a carbohydrate-rich meal on the preceding day. During the day, attacks can be provoked or worsened by high-carbohydrate and high-sodium intake and by excitement. Injection of a mixture of antiphlogistics and local anesthetics can trigger a severe attack after a few hours. Exposure to cold can induce local weakness. Slight physical activity can sometimes prevent or delay mild attacks. During major attacks, the serum potassium decreases, although not always below the normal range, and there is urinary retention of sodium, potassium, chloride, and water. The decrease in serum potassium is accompanied by a parallel decrease in serum phosphorus [85]. Oliguria, obstipation, and diaphoresis can occur during major attacks. Sinus bradycardia and electrocardiogram signs of hypokalemia (U waves in leads II, V-2, V-3, and V-4; progressive flattening of T waves; and depression of the ST segment) appear when the serum potassium falls below the normal range. Clinical or histopathologic signs of cardiomyopathy are absent [86].

Patients with mild forms of the disease may experience only a few attacks in their lifetime. Those with moderately severe disease experience fewer attacks after age 30 and may become attack-free in their 40s and 50s. Those with severe disease have attacks nearly daily, may not recover fully between the attacks, and show diurnal fluctuations of strength. These patients are usually weakest during the night and in the morning and become stronger later in the day.

Many patients develop a myopathy with permanent residual weakness independent of the severity and frequency of the paralytic attacks. In some families, all affected members develop a permanent myopathy. This myopathy is chronically progressive and affects especially pelvic-girdle and proximal and distal lower limb muscles. The computed tomography scan shows hypodense areas in the core of the muscles and replacement of muscle by fat [86].

Diagnosis

The diagnosis of familial hypokalemic periodic paralysis is suggested by a decrease of the serum potassium level during a major attack and by a positive family history. The serum CK is usually normal or slightly increased between the attacks and may increase transiently a few days after a major attack. Abnormally low serum potassium levels between attacks suggest secondary rather than primary periodic paralysis. In these cases, appropriate tests are needed to search for renal or gastrointestinal potassium wastage. Another secondary form is thyrotoxic periodic paralysis, which resembles the familial form with respect to changes in serum and urinary electrolytes during attacks and its response to glucose, insulin, potassium, and rest after exertion. The attacks cease when the euthyroid state is restored. Approximately 75% of the thyrotoxic cases occur in Asians. Because 95% of these cases are sporadic, this form is not discussed in this chapter (see reference 87 for further reading).

EMG evidence of myotonia usually excludes the diagnosis of hypokalemic periodic paralysis. In the absence of myotonia, one must still exclude the diagnosis of nonmyotonic hyperkalemic periodic paralysis. Lid lag without EMG evidence of myotonia has been noted in a few patients [88] but may also be observed in healthy subjects [89]. When there is no permanent weakness, the motor-unit potentials are normal between the attacks; patients presenting with permanent weakness show myopathic changes and fibrillation potentials or sometimes a peculiar pattern resembling neurogenic alterations. During a severe attack, no activity can be detected on insertion of the EMG needle; voluntary effort elicits few, if any, motor-unit potentials; and the evoked compound muscle action potential is either abnormally small or absent.

When the serum potassium of a patient cannot be investigated during a spontaneous attack, further tests may be required to establish the diagnosis of periodic paralysis and to determine its type. However, as with the hyperkalemic form, the increased availability of DNA testing may obviate the need for such provocation. The systemic provocative tests carry the risk of inducing a severe attack. Therefore, they must be performed by an experienced physician, and the serum potassium and glucose levels and the electrocardiogram must be closely monitored. Provocative tests with glucose, with or without the additional use of insulin, must never be done in patients who are already hypokalemic, and potassium chloride must not be given to patients unless they have adequate renal and adrenal function.

The simplest systemic provocative test exploits the physiologic potency of glucose—or of glucose plus insulin—to cause hypokalemia. The oral administration of glucose, 2 g per kg body weight, in the early morning, combined with 10–20 units of crystalline insulin given subcutaneously, may provoke a paralytic attack within 2–3 hours. Exercise and intake of carbohydrates the evening before increases the potency of the test. If the test is equivocal, intravenous administration of 1.5–3.0 g glucose per kg body weight over 60 minutes may provoke an attack. In cases difficult to diagnose, intravenous insulin in doses not exceeding 0.1 U/kg at 30 and 60 minutes during the glucose infusion may precipitate an attack [79]. Another form of the test uses prolonged glucose loading, 50 g glucose in 150 ml water administered hourly for up to 15 hours. Paresis normally appears within 7–15 hours and paralysis within 12–16 hours [90]. If these tests fail to induce an attack, they may be repeated after exercise and combined with salt loading (2 g of sodium chloride given orally every hour for a total of four doses). In general, a serum potassium level of 3.0 mM or less should be achieved. The test is positive when weakness ensues. A negative test does not exclude the diagnosis of primary hypokalemic periodic paralysis, because at times patients may be refractory.

Pathogenesis

The pathogenesis of the attacks is not understood. Forearm arteriovenous blood studies revealed that hypokalemia is generated by an insulin-dependent uptake of potassium from the extracellular space into the muscle fibers [91–94]. Increased insulin binding by muscle was found in one patient, but it was not clear whether the number or affinity of the insulin receptors was increased [95]. Another possibility tested was that the attacks are caused by episodic overactivity of the sarcolemmal sodium-potassium ATPase. Although the basal pumping activity of the enzyme was normal [96], insulin or epinephrine could abnormally enhance pumping activity in an intermittent manner.

In situ, muscle fiber inexcitability in hypokalemic periodic paralysis is caused by a depolarized sarcolemma [97, 98]. In vitro, a lowered extracellular potassium concentration causes membrane depolarization of hypokalemic periodic paralysis muscle but hyperpolarization of normal muscles [99]. The contractile apparatus is unaffected, because direct application of calcium to electrically inexcitable skinned muscle fibers produces a focal contraction [100]. The well-known enhancing effect of glucose and insulin on potassium uptake by muscle is likely to lower the serum potassium level. This induces an abnormal depolarization of the muscle fibers and initiates the attack. Cromakalim, a substance that activates sarcolemmal potassium channels, is able to depolarize hypokalemic periodic paralysis fibers in vitro so that they regain their contractile force [101, 102].

Molecular Genetics

A systematic genome-wide search in members of three families [103] demonstrated that the disease is linked to chromosome 1q31-32 and cosegregates with CACLN1A3, the gene encoding the L-type calcium channel (DHP receptor) α_1 subunit, which is mapped to this region [104, 105]. This subunit is part of the DHP receptor/calcium channel complex located in the transverse tubular system, which consists of the following subunits: α_1, α_2/δ, β, and γ [106]. The α_1 subunit (see Figure 6.3) contains the receptor for DHPs and other calcium channel antagonists and the pore. It is assumed to possess a dual function—as calcium channel and as voltage sensor for excitation-contraction coupling [107]—because it generates a voltage-dependent calcium release from the sarcoplasmic reticulum and thus mediates contraction.

Sequencing of cDNA derived from muscle biopsies of patients has revealed three mutations to date. Two of these are analogous, predicting arginine to histidine substitutions within the highly conserved S4 regions of repeats II and IV (Arg-528-His and Arg-1239-His, respectively); the third predicts an arginine to glycine substitution in IV-S4 (Arg-1239-Gly) [108–110]. The substitutions have corresponding counterparts in the α subunit of the sodium channel, and those cause paramyotonia congenita by uncoupling activation from inactivation [67]. The majority of families carry either the Arg-528-His or the Arg-1239-His substitution [111].

Molecular Pathogenesis

Expression of cDNA of CACLN1A3 results in functional channels only when (1) the cell system has a sarcoplasmic reticulum and triads necessary for excitation-contraction coupling and contraction, and (2) the other four subunits of the pentameric L-type calcium channel are coexpressed [112]. Thus, for the study of the dysfunction of mutant CACLN1A3, myotubes cultured from muscle specimens of patients are the preparation of choice, although they also contain normal channels. In such myotubes, the arginine-to-histidine exchanges reduced current amplitudes or enhanced inactivation of the channel [113, 114]. An L-type calcium current reduction was also found in a cell line derived from fibroblasts [115]. How L-type calcium current alterations are related to the hypokalemia-induced attacks of muscle weakness typical of this disease can only be speculated. The hypokalemia-induced membrane depolarization observed in excised muscle fibers [99] may reduce calcium release by inactivating sodium channels and by having a direct effect on its voltage control. Such potential effects of the mutation on the dual function of the L-type calcium channel need to be investigated further by studying the transmembrane calcium currents using patch-clamp techniques, as well as the transient changes of the intracellular calcium concentration using fluorescent indicators.

Therapy and Preventive Measures

Mild paralytic attacks need no treatment. Attacks of generalized paralysis should be treated with 2–10 g potassium chloride by mouth in an unsweetened 10–25% aqueous solution. In most cases, this causes muscle strength to recover considerably within 0.5–1.0 hour, especially when the patient uses every opportunity for physical activity as strength returns. If the patient shows no signs of recovery after 3–4 hours, the dose may be repeated [116]. Intravenous potassium administration is not recommended to terminate an acute attack, because it may produce life-threatening hyperkalemia. Some patients like to take potassium at the beginning of an attack. At first they take small doses, but with time they tend to increase the dose to relieve an attack more quickly or even to prevent one. This can lead to potassium dependency, and the disease becomes more difficult to control. In these patients, the daily paralytic attacks do not improve until the potassium is discontinued and other preventive measures are used. Nevertheless, occasional smaller doses of potassium are often unavoidable.

   In some families with mild disease, even simple therapy is effective. In other families, all forms of therapy fail. The basic recommendations are to avoid the ingestion of carbohydrate-rich meals and to avoid strenuous exertion. The medication of choice is acetazolamide [75]. The dosage should be as low as possible (e.g., 125 mg every other day). If the paralytic attacks continue, the dose can be increased up to a maximum of 250 mg twice daily. Adverse reactions to the drug include paresthesia, anorexia, transient myopia, and an increased incidence of nephrolithiasis. Few patients have developed renal failure during protracted acetazolamide therapy. In two families, one with the typical form and the other with a variant form of hypokalemic periodic paralysis, the drug precipitated muscle weakness [117, 118]. Like ammonium chloride, acetazolamide may act by inducing mild metabolic acidosis, which may prevent an intracellular shift of potassium [119]. Patients refractory to acetazolamide may respond favorably to dichlorphenamide, another carbonic anhydrase inhibitor, at doses of 25 mg three times daily [120]. Other medications have also been shown to be useful (see review in reference 87).

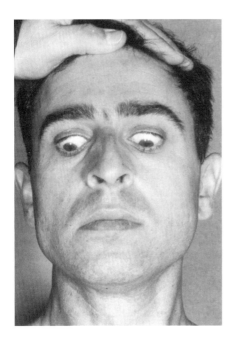

Figure 6.7   Lid-lag phenomenon in a patient with paramyotonia congenita. The patient is asked to gaze upward for 10 seconds, then suddenly downward. The lagging of the upper lids is obvious by the white rim over the iris.

PARAMYOTONIA CONGENITA

Clinical Features

The hallmarks of this disease, as first described by Eulenburg [121] and later confirmed in many families by Becker [122], are (1) paradoxical myotonia, defined as myotonia that appears during exercise and increases with continued exercise; (2) severe worsening of exercise-induced myotonia by cold; (3) a predilection of the myotonia for the face, neck, and distal upper extremity muscles; and (4) weakness after prolonged exercise and exposure to cold in most cases. In some families, patients have spontaneous attacks of weakness like those occurring in hyperkalemic periodic paralysis. The condition is transmitted as a dominant trait with complete penetrance.

Paramyotonic symptoms are present at birth and remain basically unchanged for the entire lifetime. If present, the attacks of weakness and hyperkalemia begin to appear in adolescence but not later. In warm conditions, the lid-lag phenomenon can usually easily be demonstrated (Figure 6.7). In cold conditions, the face may appear masklike, and the eyes cannot be opened for several seconds. Working in the cold makes the fingers so stiff that the patient becomes unable to move them within minutes. The stiffness then gives way to weakness. After warming, the hands may not regain strength for several hours. The legs are generally less affected. In warm conditions, many patients report no symptoms. Muscle pain, muscle atrophy, or hypertrophy are not typical for the disease.

In a number of families, the symptoms are clearly different from those found in most cases of paramyotonia. Some patients experience myotonic stiffness during work, even in warm conditions. Such patients require long-term medication. In some kinships, cold induces stiffness but no weakness. Still other patients are immediately paralyzed by cold. In some families, the patients have not only paramyotonic symptoms, but also temperature-independent paralytic attacks, resembling those in hyperkalemic periodic paralysis (see the previous section, Hyperkalemic Periodic Paralysis, under Clinical Features). The attacks usually begin early in the day and can last for several hours. Oral intake of potassium can induce such attacks.

Diagnosis

The diagnosis of paramyotonia congenita is suggested by work- and cold-induced muscle stiffness and by a positive family history. Permanent weakness and muscle atrophy are not signs of paramyotonia congenita. The EMG always shows myotonic discharges in all muscles, even at a normal muscle temperature. The serum CK is often elevated, sometimes to 5–10 times above normal.

The diagnosis can be verified by the following tests: (1) Cooling reduces the amplitude of the evoked compound muscle action potential [123–125]; and (2) cooled muscles are slow to relax and generate decreased force on maximal voluntary contraction [126]. The test is performed by determining the isometric force and relaxation time of the long finger flexor muscles before and after immersing the hand and forearm in a water bath at 15°C for 30 minutes. In some patients, the test reduces the force of contraction by more than 50% and prolongs the relaxation time from 0.5 seconds to 50 seconds. In other patients, the abnormalities appear after an additional maximal voluntary contraction lasting 1–2 minutes. The test is positive when the relaxation is markedly slowed. The isometric force exerted by the finger flexors often falls to 10% or less of the pretest value. The EMG shows dense fibrillationlike spontaneous activity in the cooled muscles that is different from the myotonic discharges present at normal muscle temperature. In some patients, the cooling increases the relaxation time but does not diminish the force. These patients have paramyotonia congenita without cold-induced weakness.

Pathogenesis

Electrophysiology on excised muscle specimens revealed that there was a non-inactivating component of the sodium current [51, 52]. Both stiffness and weakness are caused by the same mechanism (i.e., a long-lasting depolarization of the muscle fiber membranes). When the depolarization is mild (5–10 mV), this may fulfill exactly the condition for the voltage-dependent sodium channels to open again spontaneously after an action potential—in other words, for repetitive firing, which is the basis of the involuntary muscle activation that the patient experiences as muscle stiffness. When the depolarization is strong (20–30 mV), the normally functioning sodium channels adopt the state of inactivation—in other words, the muscle cells become inexcitable, which is the basis of the muscle weakness. When all fibers of a muscle are depolarized, the result is complete paralysis (fortunately, the heart muscle and the diaphragm are always spared).

Molecular Genetics

To date, 20 point mutations have been detected in different parts of SCN4A (see Table 6.3). The predicted amino acid substitutions are illustrated in Figure 6.5. Ten of them lead to paramyotonia congenita. Most of them involve the S4 transmembrane segment, which is thought to act as the voltage sensor for channel gating [70, 127, 128]. One mutation is situated in the III-IV interlinker, which is thought to form the inactivation gate of the channel (Thr-1313-Met) [129]. Expression studies of mutations causing paramyotonia congenita have been described earlier.

Therapy

Antiarrhythmic drugs, such as mexiletine, are effective in preventing muscle stiffness and weakness induced by physical activity or exposure to cold [130, 131]. However, the majority of paramyotonia congenita patients require no treatment and can cope with their symptoms.

In paramyotonic hyperkalemic periodic paralysis, the combined use of mexiletine and hydrochlorothiazide can prevent stiffness and weakness induced by cold, and the spontaneous attacks of hyperkalemic periodic paralysis, respectively [126].

THE MYOTONIAS

Molecular genetic advances have revealed that both forms of myotonia congenita are due to mutations in the skeletal muscle chloride channel gene. Furthermore, a number of previously imprecisely defined disorders are now known to be due to mutations in the muscle sodium channel gene and have been termed the *potassium-aggravated myotonias*. DNA studies can now be of considerable help in achieving a precise diagnosis in patients with myotonic disorders. This is reviewed at the end of this section.

Myotonia Congenita

The first description of a myotonic disorder was by Asmus Julius Thomsen in 1876, who in fact had myotonia congenita himself. In the 1950s, Becker [132] recognized that in many families diagnosed as having myotonia congenita, the inheritance was recessive. In these families, myotonia was more generalized than in Thomsen disease. Therefore, Becker named this type *recessive generalized myotonia*.

It is now clear that both the dominant and recessive forms are caused by mutations in the same gene, which codes for the major chloride channel of adult human skeletal muscle [133]. The intensive search for mutations that followed this discovery showed that the dominant form is very rare, as less than 10 different families have been identified at the molecular genetic level to date. The recessive form is much more common, and the estimation by Becker [134] of a frequency between 1 in 23,000 and 1 in 50,000 may still hold. Males seem to predominate at a ratio of 3 to 1 when the Becker-type propositi are counted. However, family studies disclose that women are affected at the same frequency, although to a much lesser degree.

Clinical Signs of Dominant Myotonia Congenita (Thomsen Disease)

Usually, Thomsen disease is recognized in early childhood, but the milder cases may go unrecognized until late childhood. The myotonia is generalized, with the

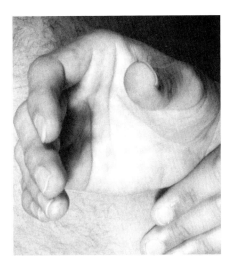

Figure 6.8 Myotonic stiffness of the hand of a patient with generalized myotonia (Becker). The patient was asked to rest his fingers for 5 minutes, then to make a tight fist as forcefully as possible for 3 seconds, and then to stretch his fingers. It took longer than 10 seconds for the patient to open his fist fully. This myotonic sign is more or less identical in the dominant and recessive forms.

legs being most affected, causing children to fall frequently. The cranial and upper limb musculature can be severely affected. Chewing is sometimes impaired. The myotonic stiffness is most pronounced when a forceful movement is abruptly initiated after the patient has rested for 5–10 minutes. For instance, after making a hard fist, the patient may not be able to extend the fingers fully for several seconds (Figure 6.8). The myotonia decreases or vanishes completely as the same movement is repeated several times (warm-up phenomenon), but it always recurs after a few minutes of rest. The patient may experience much difficulty while getting up from a chair or stepping into a bus in a hurry. Occasionally, a sudden noise may cause instantaneous generalized stiffness. The patient may then fall to the ground and remain rigid and helpless for some seconds or even minutes. Some patients have hypertrophied muscles and an athletic appearance (Figure 6.9). Their muscle strength is normal or even greater than normal, and they can be quite successful in sports in which strength is more important than speed. A slight contracture of the calves may limit dorsiflexion of the feet. Tapping a muscle produces an indentation that persists for a second or so (percussion myotonia, Figure 6.10). Lid lag is usually present (see Figure 6.7), and in some patients, myotonia of the lid muscles causes blepharospasm after forceful eye closure. The tendon reflexes are normal. In some families, the degree of myotonia fluctuates at a very slow and irregular periodicity of up to several months. In these families, afflicted members may sometimes suffer from muscle pain as a result of muscle spasms.

Clinical Signs of Becker-Type Myotonia

The clinical picture of recessive myotonia resembles that of the dominant form. A few special points are worth mentioning. In some patients, the myotonia does not manifest until age 10 years or even later, although in a few it is present by age 2–3 years. The severity of the myotonia may slowly increase for a number of years but usually not after age 25–30 years.

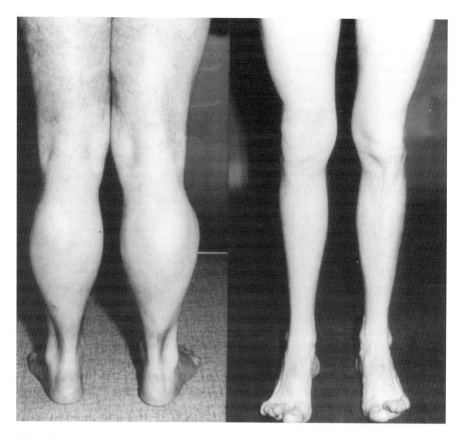

Figure 6.9   Left: hypertrophied calves of a patient with myotonia congenita (Thomsen). For comparison, the right panel shows the dystrophic calves of a patient with myotonic dystrophy.

In general, the myotonia is more severe in recessive than in dominant myotonia congenita. Patients with Becker myotonia are more handicapped in daily life. The disability stems mainly from myotonic stiffness affecting the leg muscles. In severely affected young patients, the stiffness may lead to toe-walking. Even more disabling in Becker patients is a peculiar transient weakness commonly encountered. This is best demonstrated when the patient makes a tight fist after a period of rest: The force exerted by the finger flexors vanishes almost completely within a few seconds. With repeated muscle contractions, the force returns within 20–60 seconds. This transient weakness is often generalized and troublesome, typically occurring when a patient attempts to rise from a recumbent position after rest or sleep. The leg and gluteal muscles are often markedly hypertrophied, and a lordotic appearance is common. By contrast, the neck, shoulder, and arm muscles appear poorly developed, resulting in a characteristic disproportionate figure. Patients with severe recessive myotonia congenita are limited in their choice of occupation, and they are unsuited for military service.

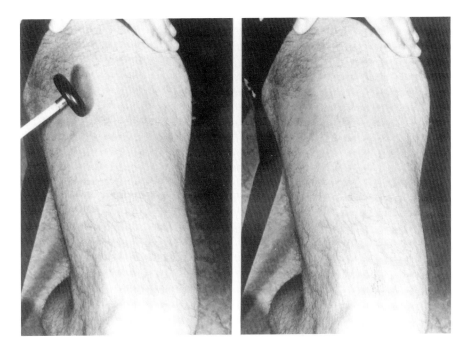

Figure 6.10   Percussion myotonia in the thigh of a patient with generalized myotonia (Becker).

Life expectancy is normal. In a few families, the heterozygotes can be identified by showing repetitive action potentials on EMG.

Pathogenesis

The muscle stiffness is due to the continued generation of runs of action potentials in the muscle fiber membrane for some seconds after a voluntary contraction. This continued activity prevents immediate muscle relaxation from occurring. Experiments with muscles of an animal model, the myotonic goat, showed that the overexcitability is caused by a permanent reduction of the resting chloride conductance of the muscle fiber membranes [135]. The high chloride conductance is necessary for a fast depolarization of the transverse tubular membrane, which becomes depolarized by potassium accumulation in the tubules during tetanic muscle excitation [136]. This pathologic mechanism was also demonstrated in human dominant and recessive myotonia congenita [137–139]. The skeletal muscle chloride channel was therefore an excellent candidate.

Molecular Genetics

The starting point for an understanding of myotonia congenita at the molecular level was expression cloning of the chloride channel in the electric organ of the

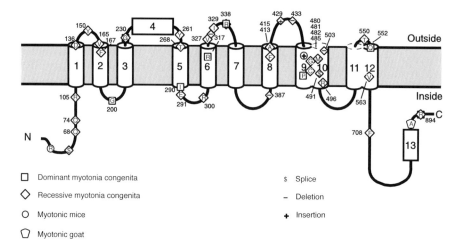

Figure 6.11 Mutations predicted in the skeletal muscle chloride channel monomer, ClC-1 (transmembrane segments indicated by cylinders). Conventional one-letter abbreviations are used for mutated amino acids (located at amino acid positions given by the respective numbers). The different symbols used for the mutations leading to Thomsen-type myotonia (dominant myotonia congenita) and Becker-type myotonia (recessive myotonia congenita), as well as to myotonia of the mouse and goat, are explained on the left-hand bottom. (Modified from F Lehmann-Horn, R Rüdel. Molecular pathophysiology of voltage-gated ion channels. Rev Physiol Biochem Pharmacol 1996;128:195–268.)

fish *Torpedo marmorata* [140]. Rat skeletal muscle chloride channel cDNA was then cloned by homology screening [141]. This was followed by demonstration of linkage of both dominant and recessive myotonia congenita to chromosome 7q35 [133]. A large number of mutations have subsequently been identified in this chloride channel gene in both forms of myotonia congenita.

CLCN1, the gene encoding the chloride channel responsible for the high resting membrane conductance of skeletal muscle cells, is a member of a newly identified multigene family encoding chloride channels that are structurally not related to any other known class of ion channels. It spans at least 40 kb and contains 23 exons with boundaries that have been located [142]. The complete coding sequence consists of 2,964 base pairs. ClC-1, the gene product, is a protein of 988 amino acids with a predicted molecular weight of 110 kd. Figure 6.11 is a revision [143–146] of the original membrane topology model that was based on hydropathy analysis [140].

Molecular Pathogenesis

Functional expression of CLCN1 has been accomplished in *Xenopus* oocytes [147–150], HEK-293 cells [151], and the insect cell line Sf-9 [152]. The resulting currents were similar to those found in native muscle fibers [153]. Electrophysiologic studies of wild-type and mutant channel proteins have provided the first insights into the pharmacology and structure-function relationships of ClC-

1 and led to the identification of regions involved in gating and permeation [151, 154–159]. Inferences from experiments with ClC-0 channel constructs [160, 161] and studies of ClC-1 constructs [162] strongly suggest that functional channels are formed as homodimers.

The 30 point mutations and three deletions that have been found in the channel gene may cause either dominant or recessive myotonia congenita (see Figure 6.11; Table 6.4) by producing change or loss of function of the gene product. Gene-dosage effects of loss-of-function mutations may lead to a recessive or dominant phenotype, depending on whether 50% of the gene product (supplied by the normal allele) is sufficient for normal function (i.e., haplosufficiency). Experiments with myotonia-generating drugs show that blockade of 50% of the physiologic chloride current is not sufficient to produce myotonic activity. This explains the existence of recessive transmission in the case of mutations that completely destroy the gene's coding functions. Dominant inheritance is explained by a mutant gene product that can bind to another protein and, in doing so, changes its function. The dominant trait of inheritance is therefore believed to be caused by mutations that result in a product able to form dimers with compromised channel function. The most common feature of the resulting chloride currents in dominant myotonia is a shift of the activation curve toward more positive membrane potentials. The chloride channel conductance is therefore markedly reduced in the physiologic range (Figure 6.12).

Therapy

Many myotonia congenita patients can manage their disease without medication. Should treatment be necessary, myotonic stiffness responds well to drugs that reduce the increased excitability of the cell membrane by interfering with the sodium channels (i.e., local anesthetics, antifibrillar and antiarrhythmic drugs, and related agents). These drugs suppress myotonic runs by decreasing the number of available sodium channels and have no known effect on chloride channels. Of the many drugs tested, mexiletine [163] is the drug of choice.

A simple method for scoring the severity of the myotonia before starting therapy and for evaluating the effect of the treatment is provided by the stair test [164]. The patient should rest for 10–15 minutes in a chair at the foot of the stairs, then get up and climb 10 steps as quickly as possible. A healthy person needs approximately 3 seconds; a patient with severe myotonia needs as many as 30 seconds. Immediate repetition of the test demonstrates the warm-up phenomenon.

Potassium-Aggravated Myotonia

Myotonia Fluctuans and Myotonia Permanens

These two diseases were newly defined when well-established clinical knowledge was combined with recent genetic and molecular biological information [64, 165]. Becker [134] had investigated more than 100 families with nondystrophic dominant myotonia and proposed several subtypes of what he thought was myotonia congenita. Molecular biology has revealed that these conditions are in fact caused by

Table 6.4   Disease-causing mutations of CLCN1, the gene encoding the chloride channel of human skeletal muscle

Genotype	Exon	Domain	Substitution	Inheritance	First report
+3/AT	Intron 1	N-term	Splice mutation	Recessive	195
C202T	2	N-term	Gln-68-Stop	Recessive	196
C220T	2	N-term	Gln-74-Stop	Recessive	197
C313T	3	N-term	Arg-105-Cys	Recessive	198
A407G	3	1	Asp-136-Gly	Recessive	199
A449G	4	1/2	Tyr-150-Cys	Recessive	197
T481G	4	1/2	Phe-161-Val	Recessive	208
T494G	4	2	Val-165-Gly	Recessive	198
C501G	4	2	Phe-167-Leu	Recessive	200
G598A	5	2/3	Gly-200-Arg	Dominant	197
G689A	5	3/4	Gly-230-Glu	Dominant or recessive	201
G706C	6	4	Val-236-Leu	Recessive	209
A782G	7	4/5	Tyr-261-Cys	Recessive	197
G854A	8	5	Splice mutation	Recessive	208
G854A	8	5	Gly-285-Glu	Recessive	209
T857C	8	5	Val-286-Ala	Dominant	209
C870G	8	5/6	Ile-290-Met	Dominant	114, 202
G871A	8	5/6	Glu-291-Lys	Recessive	198
C898T	8	5/6	Arg-300-Stop	Recessive	200
T920C	8	5/6	Phe-307-Ser	Dominant or recessive	208, 209
G937A	8	6	Ala-313-Thr	Dominant or recessive	208
G950A	8	6	Arg-317-Gln	Dominant	198
G979A	8	6/7	Splice mutation	Recessive	142
T986C	9	6/7	Ile-329-Thr	Recessive	198, 200
G1013A	9	6/7	Arg-338-Gln	Dominant or recessive	200
1095-96Δ	10	7	fs 387-Stop	Recessive	198
T1238G	11	8	Phe-413-Cys	Recessive	133
C1244T	11	8	Ala-415-Val	Recessive	197
1262insC	12	8/9	fs 429-Stop	Recessive	198
1278-81Δ	12	8/9	fs 433-Stop	Recessive	199
C1439T	13	9/10	Pro-480-Leu	Dominant	154
1437-50Δ	13	9/10	fs 503-Stop	Recessive	203
C1443A	13	9/10	Cys-481-Stop	Recessive	204
G1444A	13	9/10	Gly-482-Arg	Recessive	198
A1453G	13	9/10	Met-485-Val	Recessive	198
G1471A	13	10	Splice mutation	Recessive	198
G1488T	14	10/11	Arg-496-Ser	Recessive	142
C1649T	15	11/12	Thr-550-Met	Recessive	205
A1655G	15	12	Gln-552-Arg	Dominant, levior	114
T1667A	15	12	Ile-556-Asn	Dominant or recessive	208, 209
G1687A	15	12	Val-563-Ile	Recessive	204
C2124G	17	C-term	Phe-708-Leu	Recessive	204
G2149Δ	17	C-term	Glu-717-Stop	Recessive	208
C2680T	23	C-term	Arg-894-Stop	Dominant or recessive	198, 200

Δ = deletion; C-term = C-terminus; N-term = N-terminus.

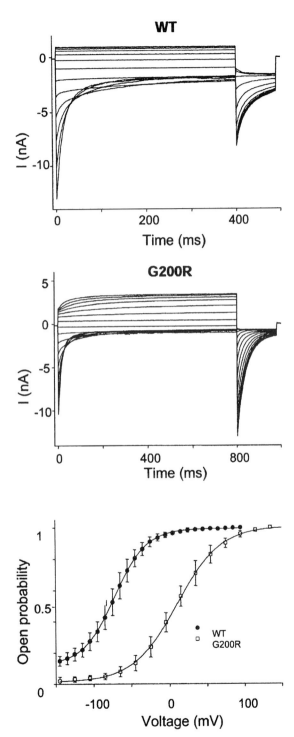

Figure 6.12 Functional expression of normal wild-type (WT) and Gly-200-Arg (G200R) mutant chloride channels in a mammalian cell line. The chloride currents shown in the upper and middle panel are responses to voltage steps going from a holding potential of 0 mV first to a variable prepotential (varied in 20-mV steps from –145 mV to 95 mV) and then to –105 mV. The instantaneous current amplitudes following the jump to –105 mV are used to determine the open probability (P_{open}). Its voltage dependence for normal channels (*full circles*, n = 5) and channels with the Gly-200-Arg mutation (*open squares*, n = 4) is given in the lower panel. P_{open} of the mutant channel is much reduced in the physiologic potential range.

mutations in the gene encoding the muscle sodium channel. Some of the forms could be classified as special types of paramyotonia, as they did show cold- and exercise-induced stiffness, albeit no cold-induced weakness. However, other forms could not be classified as paramyotonia congenita.

In one form, a characteristic finding is that affected individuals experience muscle stiffness that tends to fluctuate from day to day, hence the name myotonia *fluctuans* [166–168]. These patients never experience muscle weakness, and their muscle stiffness is not sensitive to cold. The muscle stiffness is, however, provoked by exercise, and often it occurs during rest after heavy exercise. The stiffness may then last for 0.5–2.0 hours. There may be periods lasting days or even weeks during which there is no muscle stiffness at all.

Another atypical but related disorder is acetazolamide-responsive myotonia [169], also known as *atypical* myotonia congenita [170, 171]. In this form, the muscle stiffness persists even in a warm environment, and in addition, muscle pain is induced by exercise. The stiffness and pain are alleviated by acetazolamide.

Another new disease is characterized by very severe and persisting myotonia and is therefore called myotonia *permanens* [64]. Continuous myotonic activity is noticeable on EMG, and molecular biology has revealed that this condition is caused by yet other mutations in SCN4A. The musculature of the neck and shoulders is markedly hypertrophied in these patients, and when the myotonia is aggravated—such as by intake of potassium-rich food—ventilation may be impaired because of stiffness of the thoracic muscles. Children are particularly at risk from suffering acute hypoventilation, leading to cyanosis and unconsciousness and sometimes causing confusion with epileptic seizures. In some cases, the misdiagnosis of epilepsy has resulted in treatment with anticonvulsants such as carbamazepine, which proved beneficial because of their antimyotonic property. Such patients would probably not survive without continuing treatment. One patient was misdiagnosed as having the myogenic type of Schwartz-Jampel syndrome [172], until electrophysiologic studies indicated that sodium channel inactivation was impaired [173]. Subsequent SCN4A analysis revealed that the patient had a typical myotonia permanens mutation [64]. A further indication of the severity of this disease is that all patients reported to date are sporadic cases harboring a de novo mutation.

In both myotonia fluctuans and myotonia permanens, depolarizing agents such as potassium or suxamethonium may aggravate the myotonia but do not induce weakness. It is well recognized that there is an increased incidence of adverse anesthesia-related events with the use of depolarizing relaxants in myotonic disorders. The incidence of such events seems to be highest in myotonia fluctuans families [167, 174]. There seems to be no biological reason for this, and it probably relates to the frequent absence of clinical myotonia in these patients, making the anesthesiologists unaware of the condition. Even during the spells of absence of clinical myotonia, EMG demonstrates subclinical myotonia.

Molecular Genetics

Six point mutations at four different positions are responsible for myotonia fluctuans and permanens. Four of the substitutions are located in the inactivation gate (see Figure 6.5). Three of them affect the same nucleotide, resulting in three different amino acid substitutions for one (Gly-1306) of a pair of glycines (1306/07) thought to be essential for proper inactivation. The more the substituted amino acid differs from glycine, by virtue of increasing complexity of its side-chain side, the greater the degree of membrane hyperexcitability and the more severe the clinical symptoms [40, 64]. Glutamic acid, which has a long side chain, causes myotonia permanens, the most severe form of sodium channel myotonia. Valine with a side chain of intermediate size causes moderate exercise-induced myotonia, and alanine, with the shortest side chain, results in the relatively benign myotonia fluctuans. Electrophysiologic experiments with some of these mutant genes expressed in human embryonic kidney cells to study the effect of these mutations on the channel properties [66] are discussed in the section Hyperkalemic Periodic Paralysis.

Differential Diagnosis in Patients Presenting with Myotonia

The discovery that sodium channel and chloride channel mutations can associate with different forms of myotonia has added to the increasing amount of molecular genetic data available on myotonic disorders. In addition to improving the classification of these disorders, molecular genetic testing can aid in achieving the correct diagnosis. A combined clinical and molecular genetic approach to patients with myotonia has been suggested at a workshop in 1997 [175].

Arguably, the most important myotonic disorder to identify is myotonic dystrophy, because of its potential systemic complications and genetic implications for female patients, who are much more likely than affected males to have offspring with the severe congenital form of the disease. The diagnosis is often clear clinically because of the associated features and should be confirmed by identifying the CTG expansion in the DM gene on chromosome 19. When there is clinical uncertainty, this test is very helpful.

A recently recognized disorder that may cause confusion in apparently CTG-repeat-negative cases of myotonic dystrophy is proximal myotonic myopathy (PROMM). This dominant disorder—although having some of the phenotypic features of myotonic dystrophy, such as frontal balding and a similar facies—is clinically distinct in that the muscle weakness and myotonia are proximal rather than distal. Genetic linkage in families with PROMM has not yet been established, but the myotonic dystrophy locus on 19q has been excluded [176–180].

CONCLUSION

Molecular genetic advances have revolutionized our understanding of the disorders caused by defective ion channels in skeletal muscle. It is now logical to classify them on the basis of the ion channel affected (Table 6.5). DNA-based diagnosis can be helpful, particularly in the periodic paralyses, and should be increasingly useful in identifying individuals at risk of developing malignant hyperthermia. In both situations, invasive diagnostic tests should be avoidable. Genetic heterogeneity is evident for hyperkalemic periodic paralysis and malig-

168   *Muscle Diseases*

Table 6.5   Diseases involving voltage-dependent channels of skeletal muscle: nondystrophic myotonias, periodic paralyses, and malignant hyperthermia

Chloride channelopathies (gene product: ClC-1)
  Dominant myotonia congenita (Thomsen type)
  Recessive myotonia congenita (Becker type)
Sodium channelopathies (gene product: Skm-1)
  Hyperkalemic periodic paralysis
  Paramyotonia congenita
  Potassium-aggravated myotonia
Calcium channelopathies (gene products: DHPR or RYR1)
  Hypokalemic periodic paralysis (L-type channel, DHPR)
  Malignant hyperthermia type 5 (L-type channel, DHPR)
  Malignant hyperthermia type 1 (calcium release channel, RYR1)

ClC-1 = muscle chloride channel; DHPR = dihydropyridine receptor; RYR1 = ryanodine receptor; Skm-1 = muscle sodium channel.

nant hyperthermia, and it is likely that more genes responsible for these disorders will be identified. A muscle potassium channel disorder has not yet been identified, although it seems likely that such a condition exists.

REFERENCES

1. Ackerman MJ, Clapham DE. Ion channels—basic science and clinical disease. N Engl J Med 1997;336:1575–1586.
2. Hoffman EP, Lehmann-Horn F, Rüdel R. Overexcited or inactive: ion channels in muscle disease. Cell 1995;80:681–686.
3. Lehmann-Horn F, Rüdel R. Molecular pathophysiology of voltage-gated ion channels. Rev Physiol Biochem Pharmacol 1996;128:195–268.
4. Hanna MG, Wood NW, Kullman DM. Ion channels and neurological disease: DNA based diagnosis is now possible, and ion channels may be important in common paroxysmal disorders. J Neurol Neurosurg Psychiatry 1998;65:427-431.
5. Denborough MA, Lovell RRH. Anaesthetic deaths in a family. Lancet 1960;ii:45.
6. Gronert GA. Malignant Hyperthermia. In AG Engel, C Franzini-Armstrong (eds), Myology. New York: McGraw-Hill, 1994;1661–1678.
7. Hogan K. To fire the train: a second malignant hyperthermia gene. Am J Hum Genet 1997;60:1303–1308.
8. Monnier N, Procaccio V, Stieglitz P, et al. Malignant-hyperthermia susceptibility is associated with a mutation of the alpha 1-subunit of the human dihydropyridine-sensitive L-type voltage-dependent calcium-channel receptor in skeletal muscle. Am J Hum Genet 1997;60:1316–1325.
9. Parness J, Palnitkar SS. Identification of dantrolene binding sites in porcine skeletal muscle sarcoplasmic reticulum. J Biol Chem 1996;270:18465-18472.
10. Kolb ME, Horne ML, Martz R. Dantrolene in human malignant hyperthermia: a multicenter study. Anesthesiology 1982;56:254–262.
11. European Malignant Hyperpyrexia Group. A protocol for the investigation of malignant hyperpyrexia (MH) susceptibility. Br J Anaesth 1984;56:1267–1269.
12. Ørding H. Diagnosis of susceptibility to malignant hyperthermia in man. Br J Anaesth 1988;60:287–302.
13. Mitchell G, Heffron JJA. Porcine stress syndromes. Adv Food Res 1982;8:167–230.
14. Archibald AL, Imlah P. The halothane sensitivity locus and its linkage relationships. Anim Blood Groups Biochem Genet 1985;16:253–263.
15. McCarthy TV, Healy JMS, Lehane M, et al. Localization of the malignant hyperthermia susceptibility locus to human chromosome 19q11.213.2. Nature 1990;343:562–563.

16. MacLennan DH, Duff C, Zorzato F, et al. Ryanodine receptor gene is a candidate for predisposition to malignant hyperthermia. Nature 1990;343:559–561.
17. Levitt RC, Nouri N, Jedlicka AE, et al. Evidence for genetic heterogeneity in malignant hyperthermia susceptibility. Genomics 1991;11:543–547.
18. Deufel T, Golla A, Iles D, et al. Evidence for genetic heterogeneity of malignant hyperthermia susceptibility. Am J Hum Genet 1992;50:1151–1161.
19. Fagerlund T, Islander G, Ranklev E, et al. Genetic recombination between malignant hyperthermia and calcium release channel in skeletal muscle. Clin Genet 1992;41:270-272.
20. Iles D, Lehmann-Horn F, Deufel T, et al. Localization of the gene encoding the α_2/δ-subunits of the L-type voltage-dependent calcium channel to chromosome 7q and segregation of flanking markers in malignant hyperthermia susceptible families. Hum Mol Genet 1994;3:969–975.
21. Robinson RL, Monnier N, Wolz W, et al. A genome-wide search for susceptibility loci in three European malignant hyperthermia pedigrees. Hum Mol Genet 1997;6:953–961.
22. Fujii J, Otsu K, Zorzato F, et al. Identification of a mutation in porcine ryanodine receptor associated with malignant hyperthermia. Science 1991;253:448–451.
23. Otsu K, Khanna VK, Archibald AL, et al. Co-segregation of porcine malignant hyperthermia and a probable causal mutation in the skeletal muscle ryanodine receptor gene in backcross families. Genomics 1991;11:744–750.
24. Gillard EF, Otsu K, Fujii J, et al. A substitution of cysteine for arginine 614 in the ryanodine receptor is potentially causative of human malignant hyperthermia. Genomics 1991;11:751–755.
25. Quane KA, Keating KE, Manning BM, et al. Detection of a novel mutation in the ryanodine receptor gene in malignant hyperthermia: implications for diagnosis and heterogeneity studies. Hum Mol Genet 1994;3:471–476.
26. Schleithoff L, Paul S, Deufel T, et al. A novel DHP receptor mutation in a malignant hyperthermia family linked to another locus. Am J Hum Genet (submitted).
27. Coronado R, Morrissette J, Sukhareva M, et al. Structure and function of ryanodine receptors. Am J Physiol 1994;266:C1485–C1504.
28. Meissner G. Ryanodine receptor/Ca^{2+} release channels and their regulation by endogenous effectors. Annu Rev Physiol 1994;56:485–508.
29. Melzer W, Herrmann-Frank A, Lüttgau HC. The role of Ca^{2+} ions in excitation-contraction coupling of skeletal muscle fibres. Biochim Biophys Acta 1995;1241:59–116.
30. Mickelson JR, Louis CF. Malignant hyperthermia: excitation-contraction coupling, Ca^{2+} release channel, and cell Ca^{2+} regulation defects. Physiol Rev 1996;76:537–592.
31. Tripathy A, Xu L, Mann G, Meissner G. Calmodulin activation and inhibition of skeletal muscle Ca^{2+} release channel (ryanodine receptor). Biophys J 1995;69:106–119.
32. O'Driscoll S, McCarthy TV, Eichinger HM, et al. Calmodulin sensitivity of the sarcoplasmic reticulum ryanodine receptor from normal and malignant hyperthermia susceptible muscle. Biochem J 1996;319:421–426.
33. Shomer NH, Mickelson JR, Louis CF. Caffeine stimulation of malignant hyperthermia-susceptible sarcoplasmic reticulum Ca^{2+} release channel. Am J Physiol 1994;36:C1253–C1261.
34. Herrmann-Frank A, Richter M, Lehmann-Horn F. 4-chloro-m-cresol: a specific tool to distinguish between malignant hyperthermia-susceptible and normal muscle. Biochem Pharmacol 1996;52:149–155.
35. Ohkoshi N, Yoshizawa T, Mizusawa H, et al. Malignant hyperthermia in a patient with Becker muscular dystrophy: dystrophin analysis and caffeine contracture study. Neuromuscul Disord 1995;5:53–58.
36. Gronert GA, Fowler W, Cardinet GH III, et al. Absence of malignant hyperthermia contractures in Becker-Duchenne dystrophy at age 2. Muscle Nerve 1992;15:52–56.
37. Tyler FH, Stephens FE, Gunn FD, Perkoff GT. Studies in disorders of muscle. VII. Clinical manifestations and inheritance of a type of periodic paralysis without hypopotassemia. J Clin Invest 1951;30:492–502.
38. Helweg-Larsen HF, Hauge M, Sagild U. Hereditary transient muscular paralysis in Denmark. Acta Genet Stat Med 1955;5:263–281.
39. Gamstorp I. Adynamia episodica hereditaria. Acta Paediatr 1956(suppl);108.
40. McClatchey AI, McKenna-Yasek D, Cros D, et al. Novel mutations in families with unusual and variable disorders of the skeletal muscle sodium channel. Nat Genet 1992;2:148–152.
41. Wagner S, Lerche H, Mitrovic N, et al. A novel sodium channel mutation causing a hyperkalemic paralytic and paramyotonic syndrome with reduced penetrance. Neurology 1997;49:1018–1025.
42. Dyken ML, Timmons GD. Hyperkalemic periodic paralysis with hypocalcemia episode. Arch Neurol 1963;9:508–517.

43. Rojas CV, Wang J, Schwartz L, et al. A Met-to-Val mutation in the skeletal muscle sodium channel alpha-subunit in hyperkalemic periodic paralysis. Nature 1991;354:387–389.
44. Bradley W, Taylor R, Rice D, et al. Progressive myopathy in hyperkalemic periodic paralysis. Arch Neurol 1989;47:1013–1017.
45. Ptáček LJ, George AL Jr, Griggs RC, et al. Identification of a mutation in the gene causing hyperkalemic periodic paralysis. Cell 1991;67:1021–1027.
46. Lehmann-Horn F, Rüdel R, Ricker K. Workshop report: non-dystrophic myotonias and periodic paralyses. Neuromuscul Disord 1993;3:161–168.
47. Ricker K, Camacho L, Grafe P, et al. Adynamia episodica hereditaria: what causes the weakness? Muscle Nerve 1989;10:883–891.
48. Venkateswarlu K, Taly A, Tharakan J, et al. Hyperkalemic periodic paralysis with calf hypertrophy: report of two cases from one family. J Assoc Physicians India 1986;34:381–383.
49. McManis PG, Lambert LH, Daube JR. The exercise test in periodic paralysis. Muscle Nerve 1986;9:704–710.
50. Subramony SH, Wee AS. Exercise and rest in hyperkalemic periodic paralysis. Neurology 1986;36:173–177.
51. Lehmann-Horn F, Küther G, Ricker K, et al. Adynamia episodica hereditaria with myotonia: a non-inactivating sodium current and the effect of extracellular pH. Muscle Nerve 1987;10:363–374.
52. Lehmann-Horn F, Rüdel R, Ricker K. Membrane defects in paramyotonia congenita (Eulenburg). Muscle Nerve 1987;10:633–641.
53. Lehmann-Horn F, Iaizzo PA, Hatt H, et al. Altered gating and reduced conductance of single sodium channels in hyperkalemic periodic paralysis. Pflügers Arch 1991;418:297–299.
54. Cannon SC, Brown RH Jr, Corey DP. A sodium channel defect in hyperkalemic periodic paralysis: potassium-induced failure of inactivation. Neuron 1991;6:619–626.
55. Gamstorp I. A study of transient muscular weakness. Acta Neurol Scand 1962;38:3–19.
56. Clausen T. Regulation of active Na⁺-K⁺ transport in skeletal muscle. Physiol Rev 1986;66:542–580.
57. Fontaine B, Khurana TS, Hoffman EP, et al. Hyperkalemic periodic paralysis and the adult muscle sodium channel alpha-subunit gene. Science 1990;250:1000–1003.
58. Ebers GC, George AL Jr, Barchi RL, et al. Paramyotonia congenita and hyperkalemic periodic paralysis are linked to the adult muscle sodium channel gene. Ann Neurol 1991;30:810–816.
59. Koch MC, Ricker K, Otto M, et al. Linkage data suggesting allelic heterogeneity for paramyotonia congenita and hyperkalemic periodic paralysis on chromosome 17. Hum Genet 1991;88:71–74.
60. George AL Jr, Iyer GS, Kleinfeld R, et al. Genomic organization of the human skeletal muscle sodium channel gene. Genomics 1993;15:598–606.
61. Armstrong CM, Bezanilla F, Rojas E. Destruction of sodium conductance in squid axons perfused with pronase. J Gen Physiol 1973;62:375–391.
62. Wang J, Zhou J, Todorovic SM, et al. Molecular genetics and genetic correlations in sodium channelopathies: lack of founder effect and evidence for a second gene. Am J Hum Genet 1993;52:1074–1084.
63. Cannon SC, Strittmatter SM. Functional expression of sodium channel mutations identified in families with periodic paralysis. Neuron 1993;10:317–326.
64. Lerche H, Heine R, Pika U, et al. Human sodium channel myotonia: slowed channel inactivation due to substitutions for glycine within the III/IV linker. J Physiol 1993;470:13–22.
65. Mitrovic N, George AL Jr, Heine R, et al. Potassium-aggravated myotonia: the V1589M mutation destabilizes the inactivated state of the human muscle sodium channel. J Physiol 1994;478:395–402.
66. Mitrovic N, George AL Jr, Lerche H, et al. Different effects on gating of three myotonia-causing mutations in the inactivation gate of the human muscle sodium channel. J Physiol 1995;487:107–114.
67. Chahine M, George AL Jr, Zhou M, et al. Sodium channel mutations in paramyotonia congenita uncouple inactivation from activation. Neuron 1994;12:281–294.
68. Yang N, Ji S, Zhou M, et al. Sodium channel mutations in paramyotonia congenita exhibit similar biophysical phenotypes in vitro. Proc Natl Acad Sci U S A 1994;91:12785–12789.
69. Mitrovic N, Lerche H, Heine R, et al. Role in fast inactivation of conserved amino acids in the IV/S4-S5 loop of the human muscle Na⁺ channel. Neurosci Lett 1996;214:9–12.
70. Lerche H, Mitrovic N, Dubowitz V, et al. Pathophysiology of paramyotonia congenita: the R1448P sodium channel mutation in adult human skeletal muscle. Ann Neurol 1996;39:599–608.
71. Ruff RL. Slow sodium channel inactivation must be disrupted to evoke prolonged depolarisation-induced paralysis. Biophys J 1994;66:542–545.
72. Cummins TR, Sigworth FJ. Impaired slow inactivation in mutant sodium channels. Biophys J 1996;71:227–236.
73. Hayward LJ, Brown RH, Cannon SC. Slow inactivation differs among mutant sodium channels associated with myotonia and periodic paralysis. Biophys J 1997;72:1204–1219.

74. Hanna MG, Stewart J, Schapira AHV, et al. Salbutamol treatment in a patient with hyperkalaemic periodic paralysis due to a mutation in the skeletal muscle sodium channel gene (SCN4A). J Neurol Neurosurg Psychiatry 1998;68:248–250.

75. Griggs RC, Engel WK, Resnick JS. Acetazolamide treatment of hypokalemic periodic paralysis. Ann Intern Med 1970;73:39–48.

76. Wang P, Clausen T. Treatment of attacks in hyperkalemic familial periodic paralysis by inhalation of salbutamol. Lancet 1976;ii:221–223.

77. McArdle B. Adynamia episodica hereditaria and its treatment. Brain 1962;85:121–148.

78. Riggs JE, Moxley RT, Griggs RC, Horner FA. Hyperkalemic periodic paralysis: an apparent sporadic case. Neurology 1981;31:1157–1159.

79. Riggs JE, Griggs RC. Diagnosis and Treatment of the Periodic Paralyses. In HL Klawans (ed), Clinical Neuropharmacology. New York: Raven Press, 1979;123–138.

80. Poskanzer DC, Kerr DNS. A third type of periodic paralysis with normokalemia and favorable response to sodium chloride. Am J Med 1961;31:328–342.

81. Talbott JH. Periodic paralysis. Medicine 1941;20:85–143.

82. Biemond A, Daniels AP. Familial periodic paralysis and its transition into spinal muscular atrophy. Brain 1934;57:91–108.

83. Cerny A, Katzenstein-Sutro E. Die paroxysmale Lähmung. Schweiz Arch Neurol Psych 1952;70:259–338.

84. Riggs JE. Periodic paralysis. A review. Clin Neuropharmacol 1989;12:249–257.

85. Delage R, Lebel M. Potential role of acute hypophosphatemia during hypokalemic periodic paralysis attack. Med Hypotheses 1990;32:273–275.

86. Links TP, Zwarts MJ, Wilmink JT, et al. Permanent muscle weakness in familial hypokalemic periodic paralysis. Brain 1990;113:1873–1889.

87. Lehmann-Horn F, Engel AG, Ricker K, et al. The Periodic Paralyses and Paramyotonia Congenita. In AG Engel, C Franzini-Armstrong (eds), Myology. New York: McGraw-Hill, 1994;1303–1334.

88. Odor DL, Patel AN, Pearce LA. Familial hypokalemic periodic paralysis with permanent myopathy. J Neuropathol Exp Neurol 1967;26:98–114.

89. Resnick JS, Engel WK. Myotonic lid lag in hypokalemic periodic paralysis. J Neurol Neurosurg Psychiatry 1967;30:47–51.

90. Johnsen T. A new standardized and effective method of inducing paralysis without administration of exogenous hormone in patients with familial periodic paralysis. Acta Neurol Scand 1976;54:167–172.

91. Zierler KL, Andres R. Movement of potassium into skeletal muscle during spontaneous attacks in familial periodic paralysis. J Clin Invest 1957;36:730–737.

92. Clausen T, Kohn PG. The effect of insulin on the transport of sodium and potassium in rat soleus muscle. J Physiol 1977;265:19–42.

93. Flatman JA, Clausen T. Combined effects of adrenaline and insulin on active electrogenic Na^+-K^+ transport in rat soleus muscle. Nature 1979;281:580–581.

94. Minaker KL, Meneilly GS, Flier JS, et al. Insulin-mediated hypokalemia and paralysis in familial hypokalemic paralysis. Am J Med 1988;84:1001–1006.

95. Hofmann WW, Adornator BT, Reich H. The relationship of insulin receptors to hypokalemic periodic paralysis. Muscle Nerve 1983;6:48–51.

96. Samaha FJ. Sodium-potassium adenosine triphosphate in diseased muscle: studied on periodic paralysis, myasthenia gravis, and Eaton-Lambert syndrome. Neurology 1969;19:551–552.

97. Grob D, Johns RJ, Liljestrand A. Potassium movement in patients with familial periodic paralysis. Am J Med 1957;23:356–375.

98. Riecker G, Bolte HD. Membranpotentiale einzelner Skelettmuskelzellen bei hypokaliämischer periodischer Muskelparalyse. Klin Wochenschr 1966;44:804–807.

99. Rüdel R, Lehmann-Horn F, Ricker K, Küther G. Hypokalemic periodic paralysis: in vitro investigation of muscle fiber membrane parameters. Muscle Nerve 1984;7:110–120.

100. Engel AG, Lambert EH. Calcium activation of electrically inexcitable muscle fibers in primary hypokalemic periodic paralysis. Neurology 1969;19:851–858.

101. Spuler A, Lehmann-Horn F, Grafe P. Cromakalim (BRL 34915) restores in vitro the membrane potential of depolarised human muscle fibres. Naunyn-Schmiedebergs Arch Pharmacol 1989;339:327–331.

102. Grafe P, Quasthoff S, Strupp M, et al. Enhancement of K^+ conductance improves in vitro the contraction force of skeletal muscle in hypokalemic periodic paralysis. Muscle Nerve 1990;13:451–457.

103. Fontaine B, Vale Santos JM, Jurkat-Rott K, et al. Mapping of hypokalemic periodic paralysis (HypoPP) to chromosome 1q31-q32 by a genome-wide search in three European families. Nat Genet 1994;6:267–272.

104. Gregg RG, Couch F, Hogan K, et al. Assignment of the human gene for the α_1-subunit of the skeletal muscle DHP-sensitive calcium channel (CACNL1A3) to chromosome 1q31-32. Genomics 1993;15:107–112.
105. Drouet B, Garcia L, Simon-Chazottes D, et al. The gene encoding for the α1 subunit of the skeletal dihydropyridine receptor (Cchl1a3=mdg) maps to mouse chromosome 1 and human 1q32. Mamm Genome 1993;4:499–503.
106. Catterall WA. Structure and function of voltage-sensitive ion channels. Science 1988;242:50-61.
107. Rios E, Pizarro G. Voltage sensor of excitation-contraction coupling in skeletal muscle. Physiol Rev 1991;71:849–908.
108. Jurkat-Rott K, Lehmann-Horn F, Elbaz A, et al. A calcium channel mutation causing hypokalemic periodic paralysis. Hum Mol Genet 1994;3:1415–1419.
109. Ptáček LJ, Tawil R, Griggs RC, et al. Dihydropyridine receptor mutations cause hypokalemic periodic paralysis. Cell 1994;77:863–868.
110. Grosson CLS, Esteban J, McKenna-Yasek D, et al. Hypokalemic periodic paralysis mutations: confirmation of mutation and analysis of founder effect. Neuromuscul Disord 1996;6:27–31.
111. Elbaz A, Vale-Santos J, Jurkat-Rott K, et al. Hypokalemic periodic paralysis (hypoPP) and the dihydropyridine receptor (CACNL1A3): genotype/phenotype correlations for two predominant mutations and evidence for the absence of a founder effect in 16 Caucasian families. Am J Hum Genet 1995;56:374–380.
112. Chaudhari N. A single nucleotide deletion in the skeletal muscle-specific calcium channel transcript of muscular dysgenesis (mdg) mice. J Biol Chem 1992;267:25636–25639.
113. Sipos I, Jurkat-Rott K, Harasztosi CS, et al. Skeletal muscle DHP receptor mutations alter calcium currents in human hypokalemic periodic paralysis myotubes. J Physiol 1995;483:299–306.
114. Lehmann-Horn F, Sipos I, Jurkat-Rott K, et al. Altered Calcium Currents in Human Hypokalemic Periodic Paralysis in Myotubes Expressing Mutant L-Type Calcium Channels. In DC Dawson, RA Frizzell (eds), Ion Channel and Genetic Diseases. New York: The Rockefeller University Press, 1995;101–113.
115. Lapie P, Goudet C, Nargeot J, et al. Electrophysiological properties of the hypokalemic periodic paralysis mutation (R528H) of the skeletal muscle alpha 1s subunit as expressed in mouse L cells. FEBS Lett 1996;382:244–248.
116. McArdle B. Metabolic myopathies. Am J Med 1963;35:661.
117. Torres CP, Griggs RC, Moxley RT, Bender AN. Hypokalemic periodic paralysis exacerbated by acetazolamide. Neurology 1981;31:1423–1528.
118. Vern B, Danon M, Hanlon K. Hypokalemic periodic paralysis with unusual responses to acetazolamide and sympathomimetics. J Neurol Sci 1987;81:159–172.
119. Resnick JS, Engel WK, Griggs RC, Stam AC. Acetazolamide prophylaxis in hypokalemic periodic paralysis. N Engl J Med 1968;278:582–586.
120. Dalakas MC, Engel WK. Treatment of "permanent" muscle weakness in familial hypokalemic periodic paralysis. Muscle Nerve 1983;6:182–186.
121. Eulenburg A. Über eine familiäre durch 6 Generationen verfolgbare Form congenitaler Paramyotonie. Neurologisches Zentralblatt 1886;5:265–272.
122. Becker PE. Paramyotonia Congenita (Eulenburg). Fortschritte der Allgemeinen und Klinischen Humangenetik. Stuttgart, Germany: Georg Thieme, 1970.
123. Subramony SH, Malhotra CP, Mishra SK. Distinguishing paramyotonia congenita and myotonia congenita by electromyography. Muscle Nerve 1983;6:374–379.
124. Gutmann L, Riggs J, Brick J. Exercise-induced membrane failure in paramyotonia congenita. Neurology 1986;36:130–132.
125. Jackson CE, Barohn RJ, Ptáček L. Paramyotonia congenita: abnormal short exercise test, and improvement after mexiletine therapy. Muscle Nerve 1994;17:763–768.
126. Ricker K, Rohkamm R, Böhlen R. Adynamia episodica and paralysis periodica paramyotonica. Neurology 1986;36:682–686.
127. Ptáček LJ, George AL Jr, Barchi RL, et al. Mutations in an S4 segment of the adult skeletal muscle sodium channel cause paramyotonia congenita. Neuron 1992;8:891–897.
128. Wang J, Dubowitz V, Lehmann-Horn F, et al. In Vivo Structure/Function Studies: Consecutive Arg1448 Changes to Cys, His and Pro at the Extracellular Surface of IVS4. In DC Dawson, RA Frizzell (eds), Ion Channel and Genetic Diseases. New York: The Rockefeller University Press, 1995;77–88.
129. McClatchey AI, van den Bergh P, Pericak-Vance MA, et al. Temperature-sensitive mutations in the III-IV cytoplasmic loop region of the skeletal muscle sodium channel gene in paramyotonia congenita. Cell 1992;8:769–774.
130. Ricker K, Haass A, Rüdel R, et al. Successful treatment of paramyotonia congenita (Eulenburg). Muscle stiffness and weakness prevented by tocainide. J Neurol Neurosurg Psychiatry 1980;43:268–271.

131. Streib EW. Paramyotonia congenita: successful treatment with tocainide. Clinical and electrophysiologic findings in seven patients. Muscle Nerve 1987;10:155–162.

132. Becker P. Zur Frage der Heterogenie der erblichen Myotonien. Nervenarzt 1957;28:455–460.

133. Koch MC, Steinmeyer K, Lorenz C, et al. The skeletal muscle chloride channel in dominant and recessive human myotonia. Science 1992;257:797–800.

134. Becker PE. Myotonia Congenita and Syndromes Associated with Myotonia. Stuttgart, Germany: Georg Thieme, 1977.

135. Bryant SH. Cable properties of external intercostal muscle fibres from myotonic and non-myotonic goats. J Physiol 1969;204:539–550.

136. Adrian RH, Bryant SH. On the repetitive discharge in myotonic muscle fibres. J Physiol 1974;240:505–515.

137. Lipicky RJ. Myotonic Syndromes Other Than Myotonic Dystrophy. In PJ Vinken, GW Bruyn (eds), Handbook of Clinical Neurology (Vol 40). Amsterdam, the Netherlands: Elsevier, 1979;533–571.

138. Rüdel R, Ricker K, Lehmann-Horn F. Transient weakness and altered membrane characteristic in recessive generalized myotonia (Becker). Muscle Nerve 1988;11:202–211.

139. Franke C, Iaizzo PA, Hatt H, et al. Altered Na channel activity and reduced Cl conductance cause hyperexcitability in recessive generalized myotonia (Becker). Muscle Nerve 1991;14:762–770.

140. Jentsch TJ, Steinmeyer K, Schwarz G. Primary structure of *Torpedo marmorata* chloride channel isolated by expression cloning in *Xenopus* oocytes. Nature 1990;348:510–514.

141. Steinmeyer K, Klocke R, Ortland C, et al. Inactivation of muscle chloride channel by transposon insertion in myotonic mice. Nature 1991;354:304–308.

142. Lorenz C, Meyer-Kleine CH, Steinmeyer K, et al. Genomic organization of the human muscle chloride channel ClC-1 and analysis of novel mutations leading to Becker-type myotonia. Hum Mol Genet 1994;3:941–946.

143. Kieferle S, Fong P, Bens M, et al. Two highly homologous members of the ClC chloride channel family in both rat and human kidney. Proc Natl Acad Sci U S A 1994;91:6943–6947.

144. Middleton RE, Pheasant DJ, Miller C. Purification, reconstitution, and subunit composition of a voltage-gated chloride channel from *Torpedo electroplax*. Biochemistry 1994;33:1389–1398.

145. Schmidt-Rose T, Jentsch TJ. Reconstitution of functional voltage-gated chloride channels from complementary fragments of ClC-1. J Biol Chem 1997;272:20515–20521.

146. Schmidt-Rose T, Jentsch TJ. Transmembrane topology of a ClC chloride channel. Proc Natl Acad Sci U S A 1997;94:7633–7638.

147. Steinmeyer K, Ortland C, Jentsch TJ. Primary structure and functional expression of a developmentally regulated skeletal muscle chloride channel. Nature 1991;354:301–304.

148. Pusch M, Steinmeyer K, Jentsch TJ. Low single channel conductance of the major skeletal muscle chloride channel, ClC-1. Biophys J 1994;66:149–152.

149. Pusch M, Jentsch TJ. Molecular physiology of voltage-gated chloride channels. Physiol Rev 1994;74:813–827.

150. Jentsch TJ, Günther W, Pusch M, et al. Properties of voltage-gated chloride channels of the ClC gene family. J Physiol 1995;482:19S–25S.

151. Fahlke C, Rüdel R, Mitrovic N, et al. An aspartic acid residue important for voltage-dependent gating of human muscle chloride channels. Neuron 1995;15:463–472.

152. Astill DSJ, Rychkov G, Clarke JD, et al. Characteristics of skeletal muscle chloride channel ClC-1 and point mutant R304E expressed in Sf-9 insect cells. Biochim Biophys Acta 1996;1280:178–186.

153. Fahlke C, Rüdel R. Chloride currents across the membrane of mammalian skeletal muscle fibres. J Physiol 1995;484:355–368.

154. Steinmeyer K, Lorenz C, Pusch M, et al. Multimeric structure of ClC-1 chloride channel revealed by mutations in dominant myotonia congenita (Thomsen). EMBO J 1994;13:737–743.

155. Fahlke C, Rosenbohm A, Mitrovic N, et al. Mechanism of voltage-dependent gating in skeletal muscle chloride channels. Biophys J 1996;71:695–706.

156. Fahlke C, Beck CL, George AL Jr. A mutation in autosomal dominant myotonia congenita affects pore properties of the muscle chloride channel. Proc Natl Acad Sci U S A 1997;94:2729–2734.

157. Pusch M, Steinmeyer K, Koch MC, Jentsch TJ. Mutations in dominant human myotonia congenita drastically alter the voltage dependence of the ClC-1 chloride channel. Neuron 1995;15:1455–1463.

158. Kürz L, Wagner S, George AL Jr, et al. Probing the major skeletal muscle chloride channel with Zn^{2+} and other sulfhydryl-reactive compounds. Pflügers Arch 1997;433:357–363.

159. Rychkov GY, Astill D, Bennetts B, et al. pH-dependent interactions of Cd^{2+} and a carboxylate blocker with the rat ClC-1 chloride channel and its R304E mutant in the Sf-9 insect cell line. J Physiol 1997;501:355–362.

160. Middleton RE, Pheasant DJ, Miller C. Homodimeric architecture of a ClC-type chloride ion channel. Nature 1996;383:337–340.

161. Ludewig U, Pusch M, Jentsch T. Two physically distinct pores in the dimeric ClC-0 chloride channel. Nature 1996;383:340–343.
162. Fahlke C, Knittle T, Gurnett CA, et al. Subunit stoichiometry of human muscle chloride channels. J Gen Physiol 1997;109:93–104.
163. Leheup B, Himon F, Morali A, et al. Value of mexiletine in the treatment of Thomsen-Becker myotonia. Arch Fr Pédiatr 1986;43:49–50.
164. Birnberger KL, Rüdel R, Struppler A. Clinical and electrophysiological observations in patients with myotonic muscle disease and the therapeutic effect of N-propyl-ajmaline. J Neurol 1975;210:99–110.
165. Heine R, Pika U, Lehmann-Horn F. A novel SCN4A mutation causing myotonia aggravated by cold and potassium. Hum Mol Genet 1993;2:1349–1353.
166. Ricker K, Lehmann-Horn F, Moxley RT. Myotonia fluctuans. Arch Neurol 1990;47:268–272.
167. Ricker K, Koch M, Lehmann-Horn F, et al. Proximal myotonic myopathy (PROMM), a disorder resembling atypical myotonic dystrophy without CTG repeat expansion. Neurology 1994;44:1448–1452.
168. Lennox G, Purves A, Marsden D. Myotonia fluctuans. Arch Neurol 1992;49:1010–1011.
169. Trudell RG, Kaiser KK, Griggs RC. Acetazolamide responsive myotonia congenita. Neurology 1987;37:488–491.
170. Ptáček LJ, Tawil R, Griggs RC, et al. Linkage of atypical myotonia congenita to sodium channel locus. Neurology 1992;42:431–433.
171. Ptáček LJ, Tawil R, Griggs RC, et al. Sodium channel mutations in acetazolamide-responsive myotonia congenita, paramyotonia congenita and hyperkalemic periodic paralysis. Neurology 1994;44:1500–1503.
172. Spaans F, Theunissen P, Reekers A, et al. Schwartz-Jampel syndrome: part I. Clinical, electromyographic, and histologic studies. Muscle Nerve 1990;13:516–527.
173. Lehmann-Horn F, Iaizzo PA. Are myotonias and periodic paralyses associated with susceptibility to malignant hyperthermia? Br J Anaesth 1990;65:692–697.
174. Vita GM, Olckers A, Jedlicka AE, et al. Masseter muscle rigidity associated with glycine[1306]-to-alanine mutation in adult muscle sodium channel-subunit gene. Anesthesiology 1995;82:1097–1103.
175. Rüdel R, Lehmann-Horn F. Paramyotonia, potassium-aggravated myotonias and periodic paralyses. Neuromuscul Disord 1997;7:127–132.
176. Ricker K, Moxley RT, Heine R, Lehmann-Horn F. Myotonia fluctuans, a third type of muscle sodium channel disease. Arch Neurol 1994;51:1095–1102.
177. Ricker K, Koch MC, Lehmann-Horn F, et al. Proximal myotonic myopathy. Clinical features of a multisystem disorder similar to myotonic dystrophy. Arch Neurol 1995;52:25–31.
178. Meola G, Sansone V, Radice S, et al. A family with an unusual myotonic and myopathic phenotype and no CTG expansion (proximal myotonic myopathy syndrome): a challenge for future molecular studies. Neuromuscul Disord 1996;6:143–150.
179. Sander HW, Tavoulareas GP, Chokroverty S. Heat-sensitive myotonia in proximal myotonic myopathy. Neurology 1996;47:956–962.
180. Sander HW, Tavoulareas GP, Quinto CM, et al. The exercise test distinguishes proximal myotonic myopathy from myotonic dystrophy. Muscle Nerve 1997;20:235–237.
181. Lynch PJ, Krivosic-Horber R, Reyford H, et al. Identification of heterozygous and homozygous individuals with a novel RYR1 mutation in a large kindred. Anesthesiology 1997;86:620–626.
182. Quane KA, Healy JMS, Keating KE, et al. Mutations in the ryanodine receptor gene in central core disease and malignant hyperthermia. Nat Genet 1993;5:51–55.
183. Gillard EF, Otsu K, Fujii J, et al. Polymorphisms and deduced amino acid substitutions in the coding sequence of the ryanodine receptor (RYR1) gene in individuals with malignant hyperthermia. Genomics 1992;13:1247–1254.
184. Quane KA, Keating KE, Healy JMS, et al. Mutation screening of the RYR1 gene in malignant hyperthermia: detection of a novel Tyr to Ser mutation in a pedigree with associated central cores. Genomics 1994;23:236–239.
185. Keating KE, Giblin L, Lynch PJ, et al. Detection of a novel mutation in the ryanodine receptor gene in an Irish malignant hyperthermia pedigree: correlation of the IVCT response with the affected and unaffected haplotypes. J Med Genet 1997;34:291–296.
186. Quane KA, Ørding H, Keating KE, et al. Detection of a novel mutation at amino acid position 614 in the ryanodine receptor in malignant hyperthermia. Br J Anaesth 1997;79:332–337.
187. Manning BM, Quane KA, Ørding H, et al. Identification of novel mutations in the ryanodine-receptor gene (RYR1) in malignant hyperthermia: genotype-phenotype correlation. Am J Hum Genet 1998;62:599–609.

188. Keating KE, Quane KA, Manning BM, et al. Detection of a novel RYR1 mutation in four malignant hyperthermia pedigrees. Hum Mol Genet 1994;10:1855–1858.
189. Zhang Y, Chen HS, Khanna VK, et al. A mutation in the human ryanodine receptor gene associated with central core disease. Nat Genet 1993;5:46–49.
190. Manning BM, Quane KA, Lynch PJ, et al. Novel mutations at a CpG dinucleotide in the ryanodine receptor in malignant hyperthermia. Hum Mutat 1998;11:45–50.
191. Plassart E, Eymard B, Maurs L, et al. Paramyotonia congenita: genotype to phenotype correlations in two families and report of a new mutation in the sodium channel gene. J Neurol Sci 1996;142:126–133.
192. Koch MC, Baumbach K, George AL Jr, et al. Paramyotonia congenita without paralysis on exposure to cold: a novel mutation in the SCN4A gene (Val1293Ile). Neuroreport 1995;6:2001–2004.
193. Ptáček LJ, Gouw L, Kwiecinski H, et al. Sodium channel mutations in paramyotonia congenita and hyperkalemic periodic paralysis. Ann Neurol 1993;33:300–307.
194. Rosenfeld J, Sloan-Brown K, George AL Jr. A novel muscle sodium channel mutation causes painful congenital myotonia. Ann Neurol 1997;42:811–814.
195. Sloan-Brown K, George AL Jr. Inheritance of three distinct muscle chloride channel gene (CLCN1) mutations in a single recessive myotonia congenita family. Neurology 1997;48:542–543.
196. Zhang J, George AL Jr, Griggs RC, et al. Mutations in the human skeletal muscle chloride channel gene (CLCN1) associated with dominant and recessive myotonia congenita. Neurology 1996;47:993–998.
197. Mailänder V, Heine R, Deymeer F, et al. Novel muscle chloride channel mutations and their effects on heterozygous carriers. Am J Hum Genet 1996;58:317–324.
198. Meyer-Kleine C, Steinmeyer K, Ricker K, et al. Spectrum of mutations in the major human skeletal muscle chloride channel gene (CLCNl) leading to myotonia. Am J Hum Genet 1995;57: 1325–1334.
199. Heine R, George AL Jr, Pika U, et al. Proof of a non-functional muscle chloride channel in recessive myotonia congenita (Becker) by detection of a 4 base pair deletion. Hum Mol Genet 1994;3:1123–1128.
200. George AL Jr, Sloan-Brown K, Fenichel GM, et al. Nonsense and missense mutations of the muscle chloride channel gene in patients with myotonia congenita. Hum Mol Genet 1994;3:2071–2072.
201. George AL Jr, Crackover MA, Abdalla JA, et al. Molecular basis of Thomsen's disease (autosomal dominant myotonia congenita). Nat Genet 1993;3:305–310.
202. Koty PP, Pegoraro E, Hobson G, et al. Myotonia and the muscle chloride channel: dominant mutations show variable penetrance and founder effect. Neurology 1996;47:963–968.
203. Meyer-Kleine C, Ricker K, Otto M, et al. A recurrent 14 bp deletion in the CLCN1 gene associated with generalized myotonia (Becker). Hum Mol Genet 1994;3:1015–1016.
204. Sangiuolo F, Botta A, Mesoraca A, et al. Identification of five new mutations and three novel polymorphisms in the muscle chloride channel gene (CLCN1) in 20 Italian patients with dominant and recessive myotonia congenita. Hum Mutat 1997;11:331.
205. Sejersen T, Anvret M, George AL Jr. Autosomal recessive myotonia congenita with missense mutation (T550M) in chloride channel gene (CLCN1). Neuromuscul Disord 1996(suppl);S47.
206. Jurkat-Rott K, Herzog J, Deymeer F, et al. Genotype-phenotype relations in paramyotonia congenita. (submitted).
207. Phillips MS, Fujii J, Khanna VK, et al. The structural organization of the human skeletal muscle ryanodine receptor (RYRl) gene. Genomics 1996;34:24–41.
208. Plassart-Schiess E, Gervais A, Eymard B, et al. Novel muscle chloride channel (CLCN1) mutations in myotonia congenita with various modes of inheritance including incomplete dominance and penetrance. Neurology 1998;50:1176–1179.
209. Kubisch C, Schmidt-Rose T, Fontaine B, et al. ClC-1 chloride channel mutations in myotonia congenita: variable penetrance of mutations shifting the voltage dependence. Hum Mol Genet 1998;11: 1753–1760.

7
Mitochondrial Myopathies: Clinical Features, Molecular Genetics, Investigation, and Management

Shamima Rahman and Anthony H. V. Schapira

The mitochondrion is an intracellular organelle and the site of the cell's major energy-producing pathways. The mitochondrial outer membrane encompasses the multiple folded inner membrane, the intermembranous space, and the matrix. Although traditionally depicted as sausage- or rod-shaped structures, mitochondria may derive from a network of tubular forms that constitute a single interconnecting mitochondrion. The matrix space is the site of fatty acid β-oxidation and the Krebs citric acid (tricarboxylic acid) cycle. Diseases caused by defects of these and other pathways of intermediary metabolism are briefly covered in this chapter and are covered in greater detail in Chapter 8. This chapter focuses on muscle disorders that are due to defects of oxidative phosphorylation.

OXIDATIVE PHOSPHORYLATION

The mitochondrial respiratory chain (complexes I–IV) and oxidative phosphorylation (OXPHOS) system (complexes I–V) are responsible for adenosine triphosphate (ATP) production by aerobic metabolism. The OXPHOS complexes are located in the inner mitochondrial membrane (Figure 7.1), with a stoichiometry of 1:2:3:6:6 for complexes I–V.

Mammalian complex I comprises approximately 41 polypeptide subunits, seven of which are encoded by mtDNA (Figure 7.2; Table 7.1). Chaotropic agents resolve complex I into two water soluble fractions: the flavoprotein (FP) and iron protein (IP) fragments. The FP fractions contain the 51-kd reduced form of nicotinamide-adenine dinucleotide (NADH) binding site; the IP fraction contains at least nine subunits and the major iron-sulfur (FeS) proteins of the complex. The hydrophobic fraction of complex I comprises the majority of subunits, including the mtDNA-encoded subunits, which form the membrane-bound core of the complex. The structure, function, and pathology of complex I were the subjects of an extensive review in 1998 [1].

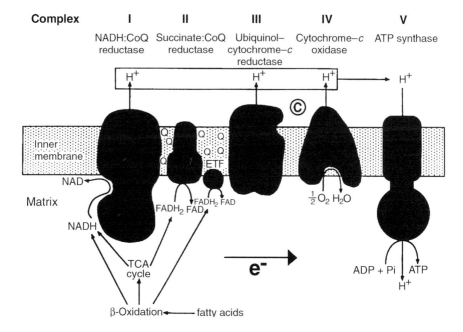

Figure 7.1   The mitochondrial respiratory chain and oxidative phosphorylation system. (NADH = the reduced form of nicotinamide-adenine dinucleotide; CoQ = ubiquinone; ATP = adenosine triphosphate; NAD = nicotinamide adenine dinucleotide; TCA = tricarboxylic acid cycle; $FADH_2$ = the reduced form of flavin adenine dinucleotide; FAD = flavin adenine dinucleotide; ETF = electron transfer flavoprotein; e^- = electron; ADP = adenosine diphosphate; Pi = inorganic phosphate.) (Reprinted with permission from JM Cooper, J Clark. The Structural Organisation of the Mitochondrial Respiratory Chain. In AHV Schapira, S Di-Mauro [eds], Mitochondrial Disorders in Neurology. Oxford, UK: Butterworth–Heinemann Oxford International Medical Reviews, Neurology 14, 1994;1–30.)

Complex II has only four subunits, all encoded by nuclear genes. These include the 70-kd flavin adenine dinucleotide–containing protein, the 27-kd FeS protein, and two cytochrome *b*–type subunits. Complex II can be resolved into the succinate dehydrogenase (SDH) fraction containing the FP and FeS components, and the hydrophobic fraction associated with the hydrophobic cytochrome *b* peptides. SDH catalyzes the oxidation of succinate to fumarate and serves in the tricarboxylic acid cycle. Complex III is composed of 11 subunits, only one of which (cytochrome *b*) is encoded by mtDNA. The FeS clusters are contained within the Rieske protein.

Complex IV (cytochrome oxidase, COX) comprises 13 polypeptides, three of which (COI, COII, and COIII) are encoded by mtDNA. The crystal structure of bovine heart complex IV was described in 1996 [2]. Isoforms of some of the nuclear-encoded subunits have been described, but their functional relevance is uncertain [3]. COI contains heme a and the heme a_3–Cu_B center, where oxygen is reduced. COII also contains a Cu_B center and accepts electrons from cytochrome *c*. COIII does not contain any prosthetic groups, and its removal in some systems does not appear to affect complex IV activity [4]. The structure and

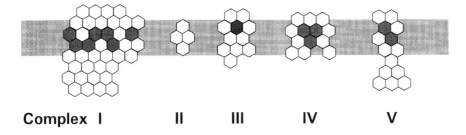

Figure 7.2 The mitochondrial (mt) respiratory chain and the oxidative phosphorylation system. Each hexagon represents a polypeptide subunit. White subunits are encoded by nuclear genes; shaded subunits are encoded by mtDNA. (Reprinted with permission from AHV Schapira. Inborn and induced defects of mitochondria. Arch Neurol 1998;55:1293–1296.)

function of mammalian complex IV was reviewed in detail in 1997 [5]. Complex V (ATPase) comprises the F_0 and F_1 fractions; F_0 is the membrane anchor, and F_1 is the coupling factor. Approximately 13–14 subunits constitute mammalian complex V, of which two (ATPase 6 and 8) are encoded by mtDNA.

The functional arrangement of the OXPHOS system is shown in Figure 7.3. In essence, electrons are passed down the respiratory chain from low-redox-potential centers—such as NADH—to those of higher-redox potential, and ultimately to molecular oxygen. The transfer of electrons is used to build up an electrochemical gradient of protons. Ubiquinone (coenzyme Q_{10}, CoQ) may serve as an electron acceptor to both complex I and complex II and, in turn, transfer electrons to cytochrome *c*. Protons are pumped at three coupling sites: complexes I, III, and IV. The proton motive force (~150 mV) generated is used by complex V to drive ATP synthesis by free energy transduction.

MITOCHONDRIAL GENETICS

Mitochondria are the only subcellular organelles to contain their own genetic material. The mitochondrial genome is a 16.5-kb, circular, double-stranded DNA mol-

Table 7.1 Oxidative phosphorylation polypeptides

Enzyme complex		mtDNA-encoded subunits	Nuclear-encoded subunits
I	NADH ubiquinone oxidoreductase	7 (ND1,2,3,4,4L,5,6)	~34
II	Succinate ubiquinone oxidoreductase	0	4
III	Ubiquinol cytochrome *c* oxidoreductase	1 (cytochrome *b*)	10
IV	Cytochrome *c* oxidase	3 (CO I, II, III)	10
V	Adenosine triphosphate synthase	2 (ATPase 6, 8)	11 or 12

NADH = the reduced form of nicotinamide-adenine dinucleotide; CO = cytochrome oxidase.

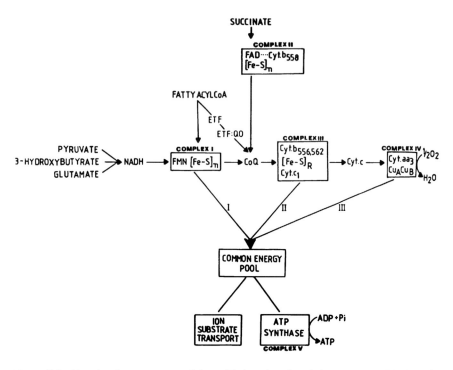

Figure 7.3   Functional arrangement of the oxidative phosphorylation system. (NADH = the reduced form of nicotinamide adenine dinucleotide; ACYL CoA = acyl coenzyme A; FMN = flavin mononucleotide; FAD = flavin adenine dinucleotide; ETF = electron transfer flavoprotein; ETF:QO = electron transfer flavoprotein–ubiquinone oxidoreductase; CoQ = ubiquinone; ATP = adenosine triphosphate; ADP = adenosine diphosphate; Pi = inorganic phosphate.)

ecule with unique genetic characteristics (Figure 7.4). It is exclusively maternally inherited, has its own genetic code, and has virtually no introns. The nucleotide sequence was fully elucidated in 1981 and encodes 13 structural components of the respiratory chain/OXPHOS system, 22 transfer RNAs (tRNAs), and 2 ribosomal RNAs (rRNAs) [6]. The presence of multiple copies of the mitochondrial genome leads to the phenomenon of heteroplasty, in which differing proportions of mutant and wild-type mtDNA coexist in the mitochondria of a cell. This in turn means that mitochondrial genetics bears greater similarities to population genetics than to traditional Mendelian genetics. The remaining 69 polypeptides of the OXPHOS system, all components of other mitochondrial biochemical pathways (numbering several hundred) and all proteins required for their import and assembly, are encoded on the nuclear genome. These are synthesized on cytosolic ribosomes, usually with a cleavable N-terminal presequence for mitochondrial targeting, and are

Figure 7.4 ➤   Human mitochondrial DNA (mtDNA). O_H and O_L are the origins of heavy- and light-strand replication, respectively. The more common mtDNA mutations associated with mitochondrial encephalomyopathies are shown. (NADH = the reduced form of nicotinamide-adenine dinucleotide; ATP = adenosine triphosphate.)

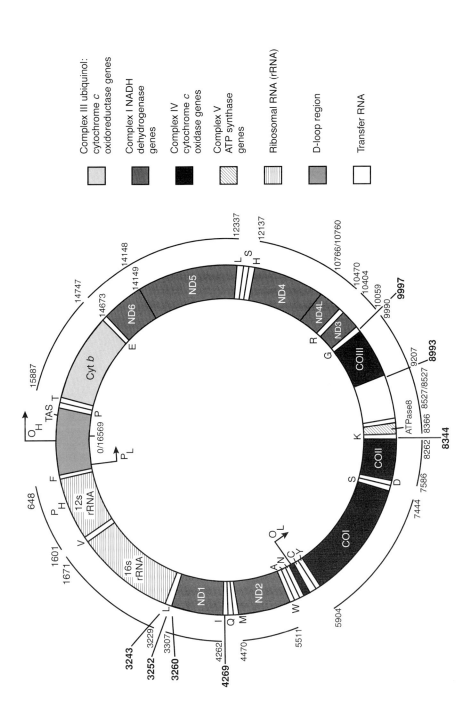

subsequently imported into the mitochondrion and sorted to the appropriate compartment (intermembrane or matrix spaces, or inner membrane) [7].

The mechanisms of mtDNA replication, transcription, and translation are fairly well characterized, and several of the *trans*-acting nuclear factors involved have been isolated, the corresponding cDNAs sequenced, and their genes localized to chromosomes. This was reviewed by Taanman in 1999 [8]. Rapid segregation of different mitochondrial genomes to homoplasmy, sometimes even completely switching between homoplasmy for one base to another within a single generation, has been observed both for neutral polymorphisms in Holstein cows [9] and for mutant mtDNA molecules in human disease [10, 11]. A genetic bottleneck occurring during oogenesis has been proposed to explain this rapid and preferential expansion of one genome over another and is the subject of a 1997 review [12].

There has been renewed interest in mitochondria since the recognition that mutations of mtDNA cause human disease. These mutations include large- and small-scale rearrangements and approximately 70 different point mutations [13]. This large number of mutations is related to the high mutation rate of mtDNA, 10–20 times greater than nuclear DNA. mtDNA lacks protective histones, the repair mechanisms for mtDNA are comparatively inefficient, and mtDNA incurs a higher rate of damage because of exposure to OXPHOS-generated free radicals. All these factors may contribute to mtDNA mutations. Large-scale rearrangements of mtDNA are usually sporadic, whereas most point mutations are maternally inherited. Inhibition of mitochondrial protein synthesis by deletions or point mutations involving tRNA genes commonly leads to mitochondrial proliferation, which appears as ragged red fibers (RRF) in biopsied muscle. Mutations are found in the mitochondrial genome in approximately one-third of adults but in only 4% of children with OXPHOS disorders [14]. The mechanism by which mtDNA mutations cause disease is still incompletely understood [15]. This is discussed in detail in the section Molecular Genetics.

CLINICAL PRESENTATIONS OF MITOCHONDRIAL DISEASE

In 1962, Luft reported the first case of a mitochondrial disorder: a Swedish woman with hypermetabolism but without any evidence of thyroid dysfunction [16]. Further studies demonstrated abnormal mitochondrial structure and loose coupling of oxidation and phosphorylation. The following year, Engel and Cunningham, using a modification of the Gomori trichrome stain, described the morphologic hallmark of the mitochondrial myopathies, the RRF, in which intense subsarcolemmal red staining represents mitochondrial proliferation [17]. Ultrastructural abnormalities of mitochondrial size, number, and morphology are also often observed in patients with mitochondrial myopathies. The first mutations of mtDNA associated with human disease were described in 1988 [18].

Mitochondrial Myopathies

Progressive External Ophthalmoplegia

Progressive external ophthalmoplegia (PEO) is one of the most common manifestations of mitochondrial myopathy. Patients may present with an isolated ocu-

Table 7.2 Point mutations of mitochondrial DNA associated with progressive external opthalmoplegia (PEO)

Mutation	Gene	Phenotype	Reference
A3243G	tRNA leucine[UUR]	PEO	50
A3251G	tRNA leucine[UUR]	PEO, myopathy, sudden death	306
C3256T	tRNA leucine[UUR]	Multisystem/PEO	263
T4274C	tRNA isoleucine	PEO	307
T4285C	tRNA isoleucine	PEO	308
G4298A	tRNA isoleucine	PEO/MS	309
A5692G	tRNA asparagine	PEO	310
G5703A	tRNA asparagine	PEO	263
T12311C	tRNA leucine[CUN]	PEO	311
G12315A	tRNA leucine[CUN]	PEO	312

MS = multiple sclerosis; tRNA = transfer RNA.

lar myopathy with bilateral ptosis and weakness of extraocular muscles, but frequently there is also associated proximal muscle weakness with exercise intolerance. Less commonly, there may be encephalopathic features or retinopathy [19]. Onset of the ocular myopathy is usually insidious in adolescence or early adulthood, with usually symmetric ptosis and limitation of eye movements in all directions, but particularly upgaze. The clinical course is usually only slowly progressive. Muscle histology characteristically reveals RRF and a mosaic distribution of fibers staining negatively for COX activity (COX-negative fibers).

More than one-half of patients with PEO have a single large deletion or duplication (or both) of their mtDNA [20]. In other patients, PEO is maternally inherited and is due to mtDNA point mutations—most commonly, the A3243G mutation in the tRNA leucine[UUR] gene associated with the mitochondrial encephalomyopathy with lactic acidosis and strokelike episodes (MELAS) syndrome (see the section Mitochondrial Encephalomyelopathy with Lactic Acidosis and Strokelike Episodes) [21]. Several other point mutations associated with PEO are listed in Table 7.2. In other pedigrees, autosomally inherited (dominant, adPEO, or recessive, arPEO) PEO is associated with multiple mtDNA deletions that are secondary to nuclear gene defects [22, 23]. Genetic loci predisposing to multiple deletions have been mapped to chromosome 10q23.3-24.3 in a Finnish family [24] and to chromosome 3p14.1-21.2 in three Italian families [25], all with adPEO, but the responsible nuclear genes have not yet been isolated. Multiple deletions have also been found in patients with recurrent myoglobinuria [26], with mitochondrial neurogastrointestinal encephalopathy (MNGIE—see the section titled Mitochondrial Neurogastrointestinal Encephalopathy), with the myoclonic epilepsy with RRF (MERRF) syndrome [27], and at low levels in inclusion body myositis [28].

Isolated Skeletal Myopathy

Exercise intolerance may be the sole clinical feature of mitochondrial disease. Weakness is mainly proximal, mild, and most easily detected in the upper limbs [19]. Fatigue characteristically occurs after sustained or repeated contraction. Weakness and exercise intolerance may occasionally be accompanied by recurrent exertional myoglobinuria. As with PEO, the clinical course is usually relatively benign. MtDNA defects associated with isolated skeletal myopathy include multiple deletions [26]; point mutations in tRNA genes, including the A3243G MELAS mutation [29] and other mutations (e.g., T3250C [30] and A3302G [31] in tRNA leucine[UUR], C15990T in tRNA proline [32], A12320G in tRNA leucine[CUN] [33], and A606G in tRNA phenylalanine [34]); a point mutation G15615A in the cytochrome *b* gene [35]; and a 15-bp microdeletion in the CO III gene [36].

Kearns-Sayre Syndrome

In Kearns-Sayre syndrome, PEO presents as part of a clinical triad—with retinal degeneration and onset before age 20 years—and is variably associated with cerebellar ataxia, growth failure, sensorineural deafness, heart block, and raised cerebrospinal fluid (CSF) protein [37]. Cardiac conduction defects in Kearns-Sayre syndrome include left anterior hemiblock, right bundle branch block, Mobitz type II atrioventricular block, and complete heart block [38]. Diabetes mellitus, hypoparathyroidism, growth hormone deficiency, and other endocrine disturbances may also occur [37, 39, 40]. Both RRF and COX-negative fibers are present in biopsied muscle. As might be expected from the multisystem nature of the disease, the prognosis is much worse than in patients with isolated PEO or skeletal myopathy. The course is usually progressively downhill, leading to death during the second or third decade.

Ninety percent of patients with Kearns-Sayre syndrome have a large-scale rearrangement (deletion, duplication, or both) of their muscle mtDNA [20, 41–43]. The syndrome is nearly always sporadic [41].

Mitochondrial Encephalomyopathies

A number of maternally inherited encephalomyopathy syndromes are recognized, and these are described in detail in the following sections. However, clinical presentations that do not fit discretely into one of these syndromes are well recognized, as is overlap between the different syndromes, resulting in continued debate about the validity of clinical classification of mitochondrial disorders. Although a rapidly increasing number of molecular defects has been identified, a rational molecular classification of mitochondrial disorders is still far from complete, so a clinical classification is presented in the following section.

Mitochondrial Encephalomyopathy with Lactic Acidosis and Strokelike Episodes

The MELAS syndrome was first defined by Pavlakis in 1984 and is characterized by strokelike episodes consisting of episodic headache with vomiting, seizures, and transient hemiplegia or hemianopia, together with lactic acidosis and biochemical (reduced OXPHOS enzyme activities) or morphologic (RRF) evidence of mitochondrial dysfunction [44]. Duration of the strokes usually varies from a

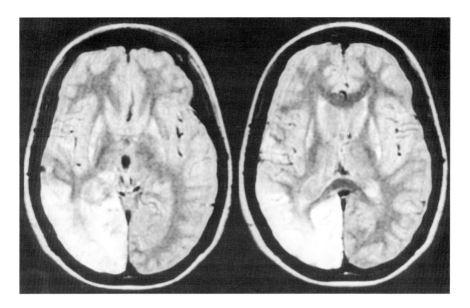

Figure 7.5 T$_2$-weighted brain magnetic resonance images of a mitochondrial encephalomyopathy with lactic acidosis and strokelike episodes patient with typical parieto-occipital changes in an acute strokelike episode.

few hours to several days, but hemiplegia or hemianopia may persist for several weeks. The encephalopathy may manifest as seizures, dementia, or both. Myopathy is usually proximal, presenting with exercise intolerance or weakness, and musculature is generally thin. The facies may be myopathic. The first strokelike episode usually occurs between ages 5 and 15 years, but onset may occasionally be in infancy (with developmental delay) or in adult life, usually before age 40 years. Short stature may be the presenting feature.

The cause of the strokes is not known, but they may be due to small vessel angiopathy or to a direct effect of OXPHOS disturbance on the brain parenchyma [45]. The finding of strongly SDH-positive blood vessels in MELAS patients, indicating mitochondrial proliferation in the vessel walls, provides evidence to support this view [46]. The most frequent abnormality on neuroimaging in MELAS is bilateral symmetric basal ganglia calcification [47]. There may also be focal lucencies on computed tomography (CT), or increased signal on T$_2$-weighted magnetic resonance imaging (MRI), usually located in the occipital or parietal lobes (Figure 7.5). These represent infarcts but do not always correspond to vascular territories [44].

Lactate may be 10–20 mmol/liter during episodes of acute encephalopathy but can be normal between episodes of metabolic decompensation. In contrast, the CSF lactate is usually persistently elevated to two to three times greater than normal. Biochemical studies of muscle may demonstrate an isolated defect of complex I [48] or combined defects of complexes I, III, and IV [49]. Unlike other mitochondrial myopathies, the RRFs in MELAS stain positively for COX, as do

Table 7.3   Point mutations of mitochondrial DNA associated with mitochondrial encephalomyopathy with lactic acidosis and strokelike episodes

Mutation	Gene	Reference
G1642A	tRNA valine	313
A3243G	tRNA leucine[UUR]	52
A3252G	tRNA leucine[UUR]	314
A3260G	tRNA leucine[UUR]	315
T3271C	tRNA leucine[UUR]	316
T3291C	tRNA leucine[UUR]	317
A5814G	tRNA cysteine	318
T9957C	CO III	266
G13513A	ND5	264

CO = cytochrome oxidase; tRNA = transfer RNA.

the SDH-positive blood vessels, and it is rare to find more than a few COX-negative fibers in biopsied muscle from MELAS patients [50, 51].

MELAS is the most common maternally inherited mitochondrial disease and is associated with at least nine different mtDNA point mutations, five of which are located in the tRNA leucine[UUR] gene (Table 7.3). The most common mutation, A3243G, is found in approximately 80% of patients with MELAS [52, 53]. Phenotypes associated with this mutation are very heterogeneous, however, and include PEO, diabetes mellitus, sensorineural hearing loss, pigmentary retinopathy, and cardiomyopathy, usually hypertrophic [50, 51]. Furthermore, pedigree analysis in MELAS cases often reveals the presence of oligo- and asymptomatic maternal relatives with the A3243G mutation [49]. Other mtDNA point mutations associated with MELAS are listed in Table 7.3. MELAS syndrome caused by a single large mtDNA deletion has also been reported [54].

Myoclonic Epilepsy with Ragged Red Fibers

MERRF was first recognized as a distinct clinical entity by Fukuhara in 1980 [55] and was subsequently noted to be associated with a mtDNA mutation [56]. The core clinical features of this syndrome are myoclonus, seizures, and ataxia with an RRF myopathy, but presentation is very heterogeneous, even within a single pedigree, and includes dementia, peripheral neuropathy, hearing loss, optic atrophy, short stature, multiple lipomata, and spastic paraparesis [57, 58]. Onset is usually in late childhood or in adulthood, and the clinical course is variable, slowly progressing in some cases and moving rapidly downhill in others. Incomplete presentations are common, and not all patients have RRF. As with MELAS, pedigree analysis frequently reveals oligo- and asymptomatic maternal relatives carrying the responsible mtDNA mutation. Plasma and CSF lactate may be elevated, but this is not a universal feature. In addition to RRF, there are frequently COX-negative fibers in biopsied muscle. Neuropathology has been performed in some patients and revealed neuronal loss and gliosis, particularly in the dentate nucleus and inferior olivary complex [55].

The majority (80%) of patients with MERRF have a point mutation A8344G in the tRNA lysine gene [56], but some have point mutations at other nucleotides—T8356C [59] and G8363A [60]—in the same gene. A single C-base insertion at nucleotide 7472 in the tRNA serine^{UCN} gene was associated with a syndrome of hearing loss, ataxia, and myoclonus similar to MERRF [61]. In 1995, MERRF was reported in a patient with multiple mtDNA deletions [27]. In addition, patients with clinical features overlapping those of both the MELAS and MERRF syndromes are well recognized, and mutations associated with this phenotype are T7512C in the tRNA serine^{UCN} gene [62] and T8356C [63].

Leber Hereditary Optic Neuropathy

Leber hereditary optic neuropathy (LHON) is a maternally inherited bilateral acute or subacute painless loss of central vision that is due to optic atrophy. The mean age at onset is 23 years, with 90% of patients presenting by age 45. Almost 85% of affected individuals are male. Patients have centrocecal scotomas and abnormal color vision. Vision loss is severe and permanent in most cases, with acuities falling to 6/60 or less over a period of a few weeks [64].

Three primary mtDNA point mutations are recognized in LHON, all involving complex I genes: G11778A in ND4 (in 50–70% of cases), G3460A in ND1 (in 15–25% of cases), and T14484C in ND6 [65–67]. The T14484C mutation is associated with a better prognosis [68], with some visual recovery in as many as 70% of patients. These three mutations are responsible for more than 90% of cases of LHON [69] and have never been reported in controls. They are often homoplasmic and can be detected in blood. A large number of other point mutations affecting mtDNA complex I, III, and IV genes have been reported in LHON pedigrees, but all these mutations have also been found in healthy controls and are therefore unlikely to be primary pathogenic mutations [70]. However, they may act synergistically with the primary mutations.

The pathogenesis of LHON is not clear. All the primary mtDNA mutations are in complex I genes, and complex I deficiency has been documented biochemically in platelets and muscle in some patients [71, 72]. However, it seems unlikely that mtDNA mutations are solely responsible for the LHON phenotype, as only 15% of females carrying a primary mtDNA mutation are clinically affected. An X-linked vision loss susceptibility locus has been postulated to explain the male preponderance of clinically affected individuals [73], but evidence for this from linkage studies is not supportive [74]. Another possibility is that novel antigens may arise secondary to the mtDNA complex I gene mutations and that autoimmune mechanisms may play a role in disease pathogenesis [75]. The coexistence of LHON and multiple sclerosis in some patients lends support to this hypothesis [76].

Myopathy is not a feature of LHON, but dystonia and striatal degeneration have been noted in some families, particularly in association with point mutations G14459A, A11696G, and T14596A in mitochondrial complex I subunit genes [77, 78]. Other clinical features seen in LHON pedigrees include various neurologic abnormalities [70] and cardiac conduction defects (pre-excitation syndrome) [79]. LHON is not discussed in detail in this chapter but was the subject of reviews in 1997 [70] and 1999 [80].

Neuropathy, Ataxia, and Retinitis Pigmentosa

Neuropathy, ataxia, and retinitis pigmentosa (NARP) is a maternally inherited syndrome that is characterized by proximal neurogenic muscle weakness with sensory neuropathy, pigmentary retinopathy, seizures, ataxia, learning difficulties, and dementia [81]. RRF are not a feature of this syndrome. The syndrome is associated with a T→G transversion and a T→C transition, both at nucleotide 8993 of the mitochondrial genome [81, 82]. A notable feature of these mutations is the apparently good correlation between mutant load and disease severity. Family members with moderate levels of these mutations present with the NARP syndrome, whereas individuals with a mutant load higher than 90% have maternally inherited Leigh syndrome [83].

Leigh Syndrome

Leigh syndrome (LS), or subacute necrotizing encephalomyelopathy, is a progressive neurodegenerative disorder with characteristic neuropathologic features. In 1951, Denis Leigh reported the neuropathology of a 7-month-old infant who died following a progressive neurologic illness of 6 weeks' duration, with somnolence, blindness, deafness, and generalized limb spasticity [84]. Leigh's findings were focal, bilaterally symmetric, subacute necrotic lesions in the thalamus extending to the pons, and in the inferior olives and spinal cord. Histologic characteristics of these lesions were intense capillary proliferation, gliosis, demyelination, and vacuolation, with relative preservation of neurons.

Clinical features associated with LS neuropathology include psychomotor retardation, hypotonia, failure to thrive, breathing abnormalities, oculomotor disturbances, optic atrophy, seizures, and lactic acidosis. Biochemical defects reported in patients with LS include OXPHOS defects, particularly of complex I [85] or complex IV [86]; deficiency of the pyruvate dehydrogenase complex (PDHC) [87]; and biotinidase deficiency [88]. Thus, the syndrome appears to represent the neuropathologic endpoint of disordered cerebral mitochondrial energy production.

Mitochondrial DNA point mutations—particularly at nucleotide 8993 (base change T to G or C) in the mitochondrial ATPase 6 gene, which encodes a component of complex V—are found in as many as 20% of LS cases [82, 83, 89, 90]. These mutations are present at very high loads (>90%) in patients with LS, but at lower levels may produce the milder NARP syndrome, as discussed in the Neuropathy, Ataxia, and Retinitis Pigmentosa section. The tRNA point mutations A8344G and A3243G, associated with MERRF and MELAS syndromes respectively, may also cause LS if present at very high mutant loads [29, 90, 91], and an adult with LS had a point mutation G1644T in the tRNA valine gene [92]. Occasional LS patients with mtDNA deletions [90, 93, 94] or depletion [95] have been reported. Other point mutations in the ATPase 6 gene, T8851C and T9176C, are also associated with bilateral striatal necrosis and with maternally inherited LS [96–98]. The reason for the frequency of ATPase 6 mutations in LS is not clear.

Most cases of LS, however, are thought to be caused by nuclear gene defects [90]. These have been proved for LS with PDHC deficiency [99], complex I deficiency [100], complex II deficiency [101], and complex IV deficiency [102, 103]; are presumed in biotinidase deficiency; and are postulated for LS patients with defects of complex I of the respiratory chain.

Mitochondrial DNA Depletion

A quantitative defect of mtDNA, with severe tissue-specific reduction in mtDNA copy number, was first described in 1991 [104]. mtDNA is depleted by as much as 99% in affected tissues compared with age-matched control subjects. More than 30 cases have now been reported [105], making this a relatively common cause of lactic acidosis in infancy. As with other mitochondrial disorders, clinical features are heterogeneous, but typically, neonatal or infantile onset fatal lactic acidosis is associated with severe hypotonia and progressive liver failure. Variable features include seizures, ophthalmoplegia, Fanconi syndrome, and congestive heart failure. This multisystem disorder is often fatal in infancy, but cases with less severe depletion of mtDNA, associated with onset of myopathy later in childhood and slower progression of disease, have been reported [106].

Family studies have suggested autosomal recessive inheritance, but some cases are sporadic. There is no evidence of maternal inheritance, and cell fusion studies have demonstrated complementation of the defect by a donor nucleus [107]. The precise molecular mechanisms are still sought. Although it has been suggested that depletion may be due to the absence of mitochondrial transcription factor A (mtTFA) [108, 109], reduction in mtTFA protein levels are likely to be a secondary effect. Mouse embryos in which both copies of the gene encoding mtTFA have been disrupted exhibit severe mtDNA depletion, but die in utero [110].

Mitochondrial Neurogastrointestinal Encephalopathy

MNGIE syndrome was first described in 1987 as myoneurogastrointestinal encephalopathy [111], and subsequently described again under several different acronyms: POLIP (*p*olyneuropathy, *o*phthalmoplegia, *l*eukoencephalopathy, and *i*ntestinal *p*seudo-obstruction), OGIMD (*o*culo*g*astro*i*ntestinal *m*uscular *d*ystrophy), MEPOP (*m*itochondrial *e*ncephalomyopathy with sensorimotor *p*olyneuropathy, *o*phthalmoplegia, and *p*seudo-obstruction), and CIPO (*c*hronic *i*ntestinal *p*seudo-obstruction with myopathy and *o*phthalmoplegia) [112]. In 1994, Hirano proposed the name *mitochondrial* neurogastrointestinal encephalopathy and suggested diagnostic criteria comprising peripheral neuropathy, PEO, and gastrointestinal dysmotility, together with histologic features of mitochondrial myopathy (RRF, increased SDH staining, or ultrastructurally abnormal mitochondria) [112]. The most frequent gastrointestinal symptoms in these patients are recurrent nausea, vomiting, and diarrhea. Neuroimaging may demonstrate leukodystrophy, and neurophysiologic studies may demonstrate a sensorimotor polyneuropathy. Various OXPHOS enzyme defects have been reported in these patients. The molecular defect is usually multiple mtDNA deletions, which are thought to be recessively inherited, and a locus was mapped to chromosome 22q13.32-qter in 1998 [113]; mutations in the thymidine phosphorylase gene have now been identified [114].

Alpers Disease

Alpers disease, or progressive neuronal degeneration of childhood with liver disease, is a rare familial disorder of unknown etiology [115]. There is continuing debate as to whether this may be a mitochondrial disorder. Typically, onset of symptoms follows normal delivery and early development. Infants most often present with intractable generalized convulsions associated with developmental delay, marked hypotonia, episodes of vomiting, and failure to thrive. There may be signs of liver disease at presentation, although these may not occur until later. Investigations reveal occipital and posterior temporal hypodensities and atrophy on CT scan, characteristic electroencephalogram (EEG) features (very slow activity of very high amplitude interspersed by lower amplitude polyspikes [116]), absent visual evoked responses, and abnormal liver histology [115]. The latter may involve fatty change, hepatocyte loss, bile duct proliferation, fibrosis, or frank cirrhosis. The clinical course is progressively downhill, and death usually occurs before age 3 years, although presentation in adulthood has been reported [117]. Neuropathology reveals patchy cortical thinning and discoloration, particularly of the striate cortex, with spongiosis, neuronal loss, and astrocytosis on histologic examination [115].

The underlying metabolic defect remains unknown. Evidence for a mitochondrial disorder includes reports of disordered pyruvate oxidation or OXPHOS function in occasional families [118–121]. Inheritance has been suggested to be autosomal recessive [122].

Nonneuromuscular Involvement in Oxidative Phosphorylation Disorders

The number of recognized clinical phenotypes associated with OXPHOS disorders is continually increasing, and in children, at least, isolated neuromuscular disease seems to be the exception rather than the rule. In a 1996 French series of 100 children with OXPHOS disease, 56% presented with nonneuromuscular symptoms [123]. OXPHOS disturbance can affect virtually any tissue, and reported clinical features include cardiomyopathy, pancytopenia, renal tubulopathy, chronic diarrhea, liver failure, and various endocrinopathies.

Cardiomyopathy

Cardiac manifestations of mitochondrial disorders are increasingly recognized and may either occur in association with neuromuscular symptoms or, more rarely, as the main or even sole clinical feature. Conduction defects are a frequent feature of the Kearns-Sayre syndrome and were described in the section covering it. They may also be seen in patients with other mitochondrial disorders—for example, both heart block and Wolff-Parkinson-White syndrome have been reported in patients with the A3243G MELAS mutation [50, 51].

The other main cardiac manifestation of OXPHOS defects is cardiomyopathy, which is usually hypertrophic but may occasionally be dilated. Hypertrophic cardiomyopathy has been reported in pedigrees bearing the MELAS A3243G mutation [51] and the MERRF A8344G mutation [56], and in an infant with maternally inherited LS caused by the T8993G mutation in the ATPase 6 gene [124]. In other cases, cardiomyopathy may be associated with multiple mtDNA deletions, either as the main clinical feature [125] or associated with adPEO [126] or arPEO [127]. A number of mtDNA point mutations, mainly clustered in the

Table 7.4 Point mutations of mitochondrial DNA associated with cardiomyopathy

Mutation	Gene	Phenotype	Reference
A3243G	tRNA leucine^{UUR}	MELAS	51
C3254G	tRNA leucine^{UUR}	MiMyCa	320
A3260G	tRNA leucine^{UUR}	MiMyCa	321
C3303T	tRNA leucine^{UUR}	MiMyCa	322
A4269G	tRNA isoleucine	Multisystem disease	323
A4295G	tRNA isoleucine	HCM	324
A4300G	tRNA isoleucine	HCM	325
A4317G	tRNA isoleucine	HCM	326
C4320T	tRNA isoleucine	Multisystem disease	327
A8344G	tRNA lysine	MERRF	56
G8363A	tRNA lysine	Multisystem disease	328
T8993G	ATPase 6	NARP, LS	124
T9997C	tRNA glycine	HCM	329

tRNA = transfer RNA; MELAS = mitochondrial encephalomyopathy with lactic acidosis and strokelike episodes; MiMyCa = mitochondrial myopathy and cardiomyopathy; HCM = hypertrophic cardiomyopathy; MERRF = myoclonic epilepsy with ragged red fibers; NARP = neuropathy, ataxia, and retinitis pigmentosa; LS = Leigh syndrome.

tRNA leucine and isoleucine genes, are associated with maternally inherited cardiomyopathy syndromes (Table 7.4). In other patients with cardiomyopathy secondary to defects of complex I or IV, mtDNA mutations have not been identified, and nuclear gene defects may be responsible. Overall, the frequency of mtDNA mutations in cardiomyopathy appears low [128].

The association of cardiomyopathy with cataracts in patients with OXPHOS defects was first noted in 1975 [129], and the underlying biochemical basis of this syndrome has been elucidated. The adenine nucleotide translocase exchanges mitochondrial ATP with cytosolic adenosine diphosphate. Defects in this translocator were described in 1997 in several patients with the Sengers syndrome of congenital cataract, hypertrophic cardiomyopathy, mitochondrial myopathy, and lactic acidosis after minimal exercise [130]. A mouse model with an ANT1 null mutation has a similar phenotype to the human disorder, with cardiomyopathy, proliferation of muscle mitochondria, RRFs, lactic acidosis, and exercise intolerance [131].

Hematologic Manifestations

In 1979, Pearson et al. reported four unrelated children with refractory sideroblastic anemia of infantile onset associated with striking vacuolation of erythroid and myeloid marrow precursors and exocrine pancreatic dysfunction [132]. In the subsequent two decades, further cases have been reported, and it is now clear that the Pearson marrow pancreas syndrome is a mitochondrial disorder. In 1989, large-scale mtDNA rearrangements (deletions, duplications, or both) were described in patients with Pearson syndrome and have been found in all cases reported in the literature [133]. These are usually sporadic, but maternal inheritance has been reported in a boy with Pearson syndrome. He had an identical mtDNA deletion to his mother, who had PEO [134].

Other clinical features frequently encountered in Pearson syndrome include variable neutropenia or thrombocytopenia, diabetes mellitus, lactic acidosis, liver disease, growth failure, renal tubulopathy, and partial villous atrophy. Mortality is high, particularly because of liver failure. Two of Pearson's original cases died in the third year of life, one with metabolic acidosis and sepsis and the other because of acidosis and hepatic failure. In a 1995 French series, 12 of 21 patients died, all before age 4 years [135]. Spontaneous improvement of the anemia is characteristically seen in the few survivors, and transfusion requirements may cease, as was the case for Pearson's remaining two patients. This clinical improvement reflects clearance of mutant mtDNA from rapidly dividing hematopoietic tissues. However, mutant mtDNA accumulates in slowly dividing tissues [136], and multisystem features gradually become apparent. In particular, survivors of Pearson syndrome may later develop symptoms of Kearns-Sayre syndrome (see earlier section, Kearns-Sayre Syndrome) [137]. The spectrum of mtDNA rearrangements is similar in the two syndromes, so they may be considered to be diverse presentations of the same disease entity. There is no obvious correlation between the type, size, or location of the rearrangements and the clinical course.

Marrow involvement by OXPHOS defects is most often seen in infants with Pearson syndrome, but adults with acquired sideroblastic anemia associated with point mutations in mtDNA tRNA (G12301A in tRNA leucine^{CUN}) and protein-coding (T6721C and T6742C in COX I) genes have been reported [138, 139]. A pedigree with maternally inherited sideroblastic anemia has been described [140]. In another family, two brothers with sideroblastic anemia had multiple mtDNA deletions, as did their asymptomatic mother [141]. Autosomal dominant inheritance was postulated in this family. In another pedigree, a syndrome of myopathy, lactic acidosis, and sideroblastic anemia, associated with mental retardation and dysmorphic features, appeared to be inherited as an autosomal recessive trait in two siblings born to first cousin parents [142]. No mtDNA rearrangements were identified in these siblings.

Renal Disease

Renal involvement is rare in adults with mitochondrial disease (only one of Petty's 66 patients with mitochondrial myopathy had associated renal disease [19]), but it is a frequent finding in the pediatric population. Extrarenal symptoms are always present in these patients. Proximal tubular defects of the Fanconi type are the most common renal manifestation of OXPHOS defects, especially in association with COX deficiency (in 16 of 31 cases in a literature review [143]), and in the Pearson, Kearns-Sayre, Leigh, and mtDNA depletion syndromes. More rarely, patients may have renal tubular acidosis, and one patient with Kearns-Sayre and an 8.8-kb mtDNA deletion had features of Bartter syndrome [144]. Occasional patients with glomerular disease (focal segmental glomerular sclerosis presenting as nephrotic syndrome) have been reported, as have patients with chronic renal insufficiency secondary to tubulointerstitial nephritis [143].

Endocrine Disease

Endocrine disease is also more common in childhood mitochondrial disorders, although insulin-dependent diabetes mellitus is frequently seen in pedigrees with the MELAS A3243G mutation, often in association with deafness [145]. Diabetes mellitus may also be caused by mtDNA deletions/duplications [146], often in patients with other features of the Kearns-Sayre or Pearson syndromes (see previous sections: Kearns-Sayre Syndrome and Hematologic Manifestations). Single mtDNA deletions are also responsible for some cases of Wolfram syndrome (diabetes insipidus, diabetes mellitus, optic atrophy, and deafness) [147]. Autosomal recessively inherited Wolfram syndrome that is due to multiple mtDNA deletions has been described, and linkage to a nuclear locus 4p16 has been reported in these families [148]. Other endocrine manifestations of OXPHOS disease include hypoparathyroidism, hypothyroidism, adrenal insufficiency, hypogonadism, and short stature that is due to growth hormone deficiency [123].

Gastrointestinal and Liver Disease

In adults, gastrointestinal symptoms are most frequently seen in patients with the MNGIE syndrome (see section Mitochondrial Neurogastrointestinal Encephalopathy) and include recurrent vomiting, diarrhea, and intestinal pseudo-obstruction. These symptoms may also occur in other mitochondrial syndromes. A point mutation G8313A in the tRNA lysine gene has been reported in association with gastrointestinal symptoms and encephalopathy [149], and mtDNA rearrangements were found in two children with chronic diarrhea and villous atrophy [150].

In children, liver disease is common, particularly complicating the Pearson and mtDNA depletion syndromes, and is often the cause of death in these patients. In a 1997 French series, 10% of children found to have OXPHOS defects had been referred because of liver dysfunction [151]. Clinical features of these patients included hypoglycemia, jaundice, hepatomegaly, and liver failure. Liver histology was performed in 15 cases and revealed steatosis in seven cases, cirrhosis (usually micronodular) in seven cases, and both steatosis and micronodular cirrhosis in one case. OXPHOS defects in the liver of these patients were isolated defects of complex I or IV or a generalized defect. There was no correlation between enzyme defect and clinical course.

Biochemically Defined Defects of Oxidative Phosphorylation

Another method of classifying mitochondrial disorders is according to the site of biochemical defect. Patients may have either an isolated defect of one of the OXPHOS complexes, or a combined defect involving two or more complexes. As with clinical classification, the biochemical classification is only of limited use, as the same clinical picture (e.g., LS) may be produced by a number of different biochemical defects and—with the exception of complex II, which has only nuclear-encoded subunits—the nature of the biochemical defect does not provide any information about the likely mode of inheritance.

Complex I Deficiency

Complex I deficiency is probably one of the most common OXPHOS defects, with more than 100 patients reported in the literature. Technical difficulties with assays of this enzyme complex mean that ascertainment of cases may be incomplete [90]. Patients present with either an isolated myopathy or a multisystem disorder [152]. The latter may be subclassified into fatal infantile lactic acidosis, LS, or a recognized syndrome associated with mitochondrial mutations, such as MELAS or MERRF. There has been a single case report of a benign, spontaneously reversible, infantile complex I deficient myopathy [153]. Some forms of complex I deficiency may not be associated with lactic acidosis—for example, in LHON. Mutations in mtDNA-encoded complex I subunits have been described in LHON (see earlier section, Leber Hereditary Optic Neuropathy), and in 1998 a mutation was identified in a nuclear-encoded subunit in a child with fatal complex I deficiency [154].

Complex II Deficiency

Isolated complex II deficiency is rare. This is the only OXPHOS complex with no mitochondrially encoded subunits, and the first complex in which a nuclear gene mutation was identified: a homozygous point mutation in the gene encoding the FP subunit of SDH in two French sisters with LS [101]. So far, this mutation has not been identified in any other patient with SDH deficiency.

Complex III Deficiency

Isolated complex III deficiency is also rare, with fewer than 25 cases reported in the literature. As with other OXPHOS disorders, presentation may be at any age, and clinical features are heterogeneous, ranging from a severe neonatal multiorgan disorder including lactic acidosis and renal Fanconi syndrome to isolated myopathy [155]. A point mutation in cytochrome *b* has been reported in a patient with isolated complex III deficiency and exercise intolerance [35].

Complex IV Deficiency

Complex IV deficiency is the most commonly identified OXPHOS defect. In an Italian series of 60 patients with OXPHOS defects, 70% had COX deficiency [156]. Onset is usually between the neonatal period and 3 years of age, but it may be later. Cases of isolated COX deficiency with adult onset have been described [157]. Clinical presentation is heterogeneous [158]. The most frequent presentation is a fatal infantile myopathy [159]. Initial features include failure to thrive, weakness, hypotonia, and severe lactic acidosis. There may be associated multisystem features, including hepatic involvement, renal tubulopathy of a Fanconi type, and cardiomyopathy. Most of these infants succumb to overwhelming lactic acidosis in the first year of life.

A few children have been described in whom a severe COX-deficient myopathy resolved spontaneously by age 3 years [160]. These children presented at birth with profound hypotonia and weakness leading to feeding and breathing difficulties, with associated lactic acidosis. Clinical improvement began between 6 and 9 months of age. This benign, reversible infantile myopathy may be due to a defect in a developmentally regulated COX subunit, with resolution of the COX deficiency being secondary to isoform switching [161].

In other cases, cardiomyopathy may be the only clinical feature [162]. Isolated COX deficiency is also a common biochemical defect in LS [90]. Focal COX deficiency is observed in muscle biopsies from many patients with mtDNA deletions or point mutations, but may not involve sufficient fibers to produce a demonstrable defect on enzyme assay. Several mutations have been identified in mitochondrial COX genes. These are discussed in the Molecular Genetics section under Protein Coding Mutations.

Complex V Deficiency

Complex V deficiency is rarely described, and activity of this complex is only partially reduced, even in patients with known mutations in the mitochondrial gene for ATP synthase subunit 6, such as the NARP T8993G/C mutations (see earlier section, Neuropathy, Ataxia, and Retinitis Pigmentosa) [163]. Complex V deficiency may be associated with 3-methylglutaconic aciduria [164].

Combined Deficiencies of Oxidative Phosphorylation Complexes

Combined deficiencies of complexes I and IV are most commonly seen in mtDNA mutations involving tRNAs, such as those associated with the MERRF and MELAS syndromes. Complex III may also be involved, because it has a single mtDNA-encoded subunit cytochrome *b*, but complex II is typically unaffected, because it is entirely nuclear encoded. Other combinations of OXPHOS defects also occur and may be due to mutations in nuclear regulatory genes [165]. In some cases, OXPHOS defects are associated with deficiency of the PDHC [166, 167].

Coenzyme Q_{10} Deficiency

Deficiency of CoQ, which shuttles electrons between complexes I and II and complex III, has been described in two families with mitochondrial encephalomyopathy and lactic acidosis. In the first family, two sisters had progressive muscle weakness of childhood onset, recurrent myoglobinuria, and central nervous system dysfunction (seizures, cerebellar symptoms, and learning difficulties) [168]. Activities of individual OXPHOS enzyme complexes I, II, III, and IV were normal, but activities of complex I–III and complex II–III, which both need CoQ, were abnormally low. The other case had a similar phenotype [169]. Muscle biopsy revealed RRF, COX-negative fibers, and excess lipid. CoQ levels were less than 4% of controls in the two sisters and less than 25% in the third patient. Clinical improvement followed treatment with oral CoQ (150 mg daily). These patients are thought to have a defect in one of the steps of CoQ biosynthesis.

Mitochondrial Myopathies not Due to Oxidative Phosphorylation Defects

Disorders of Fatty Acid Oxidation

The disorders of fatty acid oxidation encompass defects of enzymes involved in transport of fatty acids across the inner mitochondrial membrane and defects of the fatty acid β-oxidation spiral. All the defects described so far are inherited as autosomal recessive traits. Transport of long-chain fatty acyl-coenzyme As (CoAs) across the inner mitochondrial membrane involves esterification with carnitine and the activities of three enzymes: carnitine palmitoyl transferase (CPT) I, carnitine-acylcarnitine translocase, and CPT II. CPT I is located on the inner side of the outer mitochondrial membrane and CPT II on the inner side of the inner mitochondrial membrane, whereas the translocase is embedded in the inner mitochondrial membrane. Inherited defects have been described for each of these three enzymes. In addition, impaired carnitine transport across the plasma membrane may also cause human disease (primary systemic carnitine deficiency).

Defects have been described for the following enzymes involved in β-oxidation: short-chain acyl coenzyme A (acyl-CoA) dehydrogenase (SCAD), short-chain 3-hydroxyacyl-CoA dehydrogenase (SCHAD), medium-chain acyl-CoA dehydrogenase (MCAD), long-chain acyl-CoA dehydrogenase (LCAD), the mitochondrial trifunctional protein (encompassing activities of long-chain 3-hydroxy acyl-CoA dehydrogenase [LCHAD], 2-enoyl CoA hydratase, and 3-oxo acyl-CoA hydratase), and very-long-chain acyl-CoA dehydrogenase (VLCAD). All are rare, with the exception of MCAD and trifunctional protein deficiencies. MCAD deficiency is one of the most commonly recognized inborn errors of metabolism, with an estimated incidence of 1 in 6,000–10,000 births in white populations [170]. The genes encoding many of these enzymes have been cloned, sequenced, and localized to chromosomes and mutations identified in affected patients. MCAD and LCHAD deficiencies are unusual in that a single common mutation is responsible for the majority of cases.

Disorders of fatty acid oxidation typically present with recurrent episodes of hypoketotic hypoglycemia, triggered by fasting or intercurrent illness, which may be associated with Reye syndrome–like features of encephalopathy, hepatomegaly, and hepatocellular dysfunction. There may also be skeletal myopathy, with lipid storage, and cardiomyopathy, which may be dilated or hypertrophic. Onset of symptoms is frequently during infancy but may be delayed until adolescence or adulthood with recurrent episodes of myoglobinuria. Age at presentation may be related to residual enzyme activity. Long-chain fatty acid oxidation defects characteristically have a moderate lactic acidosis that is postulated to be secondary to the disturbed mitochondrial function.

Primary Systemic Carnitine Deficiency

Childhood onset of progressive dilated cardiomyopathy is associated with lipid storage skeletal myopathy, hypoketotic hypoglycemic episodes, and hyperammonemia [171, 172]. The phenotype is variable, even within a family, and presentation may be as sudden infant death [173]. Plasma carnitine levels are extremely low, typically less than 10 mmol/liter. There is a dramatic clinical response to large doses of oral carnitine. In 1998, linkage analysis in a large

Japanese family localized the gene to chromosome 5q31.1-32 [174], and a number of mutations have subsequently been reported [175–178].

Carnitine Palmitoyl Transferase Type I Deficiency

CPT I deficiency is also rare. Episodes of hypoketotic hypoglycemia, triggered by fasting or intercurrent illness and associated with hepatomegaly, typically start in infancy [179]. Myopathy and cardiomyopathy have not been reported in this disorder. The gene for CPT I has been localized to chromosome 11q [180].

Carnitine Palmitoyl Transferase Type II Deficiency

CPT II deficiency was the first disorder of fatty acid metabolism to be described [181] and is more common than CPT I deficiency. Onset is most often in late adolescence or early adulthood with exercise-induced muscle pain, frequently with myoglobinuria, but infantile and fatal neonatal variants are recognized. The latter may be associated with congenital malformations. Rhabdomyolysis may precipitate acute renal failure. Point mutations have been characterized in the CPT II gene on chromosome 1p32 in affected patients, including a common missense mutation S113L in adults with recurrent myoglobinuria [182].

Carnitine-Acylcarnitine Translocase Deficiency

The first report of this rare defect was of a severe neonatal presentation with hypoglycemic coma associated with seizures, muscle weakness, cardiomyopathy, and liver dysfunction [183]. A second case had heart block [184], and a third presented as sudden neonatal death [185]. A milder phenotype was described in 1998 [186]. The translocase gene has been cloned [187] and a frameshift mutation identified in an affected patient [188].

Short-Chain Acyl-CoA Dehydrogenase Deficiency

Few cases of SCAD deficiency have been reported, and clinical presentation is extremely variable. Neonates may present with failure to thrive, hypotonia, muscle weakness, and metabolic acidosis [189]. Unlike other β-oxidation defects, hypoketotic hypoglycemia does not seem to occur. This may be because longer-chain fatty acyl-CoAs can be metabolized to maintain normoglycemia [190]. The gene has been localized to 12q22-ter and a number of mutations reported [191].

Short-Chain 3-Hydroxy Acyl-CoA Dehydrogenase Deficiency

SCHAD deficiency was first described by Tein et al. in 1991 [192] in a teenage girl with recurrent myoglobinuria and hypoketotic hypoglycemia. Two other children presenting with hypoglycemic episodes also had this defect [193]. The gene has been mapped to chromosome 4q22-26 [194].

Medium-Chain Acyl-CoA Dehydrogenase Deficiency

MCAD deficiency is the most frequent disorder of fatty acid oxidation and typically presents with hypoketotic hypoglycemia in the first or second year of life, after an episode of metabolic stress such as fasting or intercurrent illness. There is often associated encephalopathy and hepatomegaly. Patients are usually well between acute episodes of hypoglycemia, but the range of clinical features associated with MCAD deficiency includes lipid storage myopathy, cardiomyopathy, and sudden unexpected death in infancy [195]. A common point mutation G985A has been identified in 90% of mutant alleles [196].

Long-Chain Acyl-CoA Dehydrogenase Deficiency

Clinical features of LCAD deficiency are similar to MCAD deficiency, with hypoketotic hypoglycemia, myopathy, cardiomyopathy, and hepatomegaly [197], but older children may present with muscle pain and myoglobinuria, as in CPT II deficiency. Some cases previously thought to have LCAD deficiency have subsequently been shown to have VLCAD deficiency [198]. The LCAD gene has been cloned, sequenced, and localized to chromosome 2q34-35 [199].

Trifunctional Protein Deficiency

As in MCAD deficiency, presentation of LCHAD deficiency is usually in late infancy with recurrent attacks of hypoketotic hypoglycemia, hypotonia, cardiomyopathy, and hepatomegaly [200]. Liver disease tends to be more marked than in other β-oxidation defects. Presentation with isolated myopathy, rapidly progressive fatal cardiomyopathy, or sudden infant death is recognized [201, 202]. Long-term complications of pigmentary retinopathy and peripheral neuropathy may be due to the accumulation of toxic metabolites [190]. The gene has been cloned and localized to 2p23.3-24.1, and a common mutation G1528C has been identified [203]. Heterozygote mothers may develop acute fatty liver of pregnancy [204].

Very-Long-Chain Acyl-CoA Dehydrogenase Deficiency

VLCAD deficiency usually presents in infancy with hypoketotic hypoglycemia, hepatic dysfunction, or hypertrophic cardiomyopathy [205, 206] but can cause sudden death. The defect may also present in adulthood with episodes of painful rhabdomyolysis induced by fasting or exercise [207, 208]. The gene has been cloned, sequenced, and localized to chromosome 17p11, and mutations have been identified in both infantile-onset and adult cases [209].

Glutaric Aciduria Type II

Multiple acyl-CoA dehydrogenase deficiency or glutaric aciduria type II is due to deficiency of electron transfer flavoprotein (ETF) or its dehydrogenase (ETF-QO). Presentation is usually in the neonatal period with severe metabolic acidosis, hypoketotic hypoglycemia, hyperammonemia, and congenital abnormalities (polycystic kidneys), but may be later with episodic hypoglycemia and lipid storage myopathy [210].

Disorders of Pyruvate Metabolism

Pyruvate Dehydrogenase Deficiency

The PDHC contains three catalytic (pyruvate decarboxylase E1, dihydrolipoyl transacetylase E2, and lipoamide dehydrogenase E3) and two regulatory (PDH kinase and phosphatase) components. A sixth component—protein X—is thought to have a structural role. Most patients have E1 deficiency, and mutations have been described in the E1α gene, which is located on the X chromosome [211].

PDHC deficiency is one of the most commonly defined disorders of mitochondrial energy production and represents 10–15% of congenital lactic acidosis [212]. Several hundred patients have been reported [211]. Clinical presentation of PDHC deficiency is extremely heterogeneous. In the severe form, presentation is in the newborn period with severe, persistent lactic acidosis, sometimes associated with agenesis of the corpus callosum, and invariably resulting in death within a few weeks or months. Presentation later in infancy is associated with global developmental delay, hypotonia, seizures, failure to thrive, and sometimes with dysmorphic features. Characteristically, there are intermittent episodes of severe lactic acidosis, usually precipitated by intercurrent infection. The clinical spectrum overlaps with classical LS, including typical neuropathology [87]. Although there is an equal sex incidence in PDHC deficiency, clinical presentation differs markedly between the sexes. Severe neonatal lactic acidosis is more common in males, whereas chronic neurodegenerative disease is seen more often in females. A third group of patients, all boys, have a benign course with ataxia precipitated by carbohydrate loads. These patients may respond to a high-fat, low-carbohydrate (ketogenic) diet [213].

Lipoamide dehydrogenase (E3) is an FP common to the pyruvate, α-ketoglutarate and branched chain α-ketoacid dehydrogenase complexes. Seven infants with E3 deficiency have been reported [214–220]. All presented in early infancy with failure to thrive and hypotonia and subsequently suffered progressive neurologic deterioration after episodes of acute metabolic decompensation. Basal ganglia lesions were observed in three cases. Biochemical features were elevated levels of plasma lactate, pyruvate, and branched chain amino acids, together with α-ketoglutaric aciduria. The E3 gene has been localized to chromosome 7q31-32, and mutations have been identified in two affected infants [221]. Prognosis is generally poor. Dietary and pharmacologic interventions have largely been unsuccessful, except for response to oral lipoic acid in a single case and to dichloroacetate in an Israeli boy who had normal cognitive function at the age of 5 years [219]. E3 deficiency may also present as recurrent myoglobinuria with lactic acidosis in adulthood [222].

Pyruvate Carboxylase Deficiency

Pyruvate carboxylase deficiency is a rare autosomal recessive disorder that has two major modes of presentation. Type A presents with global developmental delay and intermittent acute lactic acidosis in the first few months of life. Hypoglycemia is unusual, whereas plasma alanine and proline are high, with raised urinary lactate and 2-ketoglutarate. This presentation is most commonly seen in certain North American native tribes and is associated with a common founder mutation. Type B, the severe neonatal form of the disease, has a more fulminant lactic acidosis with rapid progression to death. Associated biochemical abnormalities are hyperammonemia and raised plasma citrulline, lysine, and proline. The lactate/pyruvate (L/P) ratio is high in type B but usually normal in type A disease. Type B disease is more frequent in patients of Arab descent. The difference in clinical features between the two groups is probably related to the residual enzyme activity, which is higher in type A [223].

Krebs Cycle Defects

Defects of the Krebs cycle have been identified only rarely, suggesting that some defects in this pathway may be incompatible with survival beyond the intrauterine period. Two autosomal recessively inherited defects specific to the Krebs cycle have been reported: α-ketoglutarate dehydrogenase (α-KGD) deficiency and fumarase deficiency [224, 225]. SDH is also part of complex II of the OXPHOS, and defects of this enzyme have been discussed previously. One patient with combined SDH and aconitase deficiency in skeletal muscle had limb weakness and exercise intolerance [226].

Deficiency of the multienzyme complex α-KGD has been described in 7 patients from three consanguineous families [224, 227, 228]. Lactic acidosis was associated with progressive encephalomyopathy with hypotonia, muscle weakness, pyramidal and extrapyramidal signs, failure to thrive, and developmental delay. The L/P ratio was high, particularly in the fed state, whereas the ketone body molar ratio was low normal. Residual α-KGD activity was 5% in muscle and up to 25% in fibroblasts. Prognosis was poor in nearly all cases, although the lactic acidosis seems to have responded to a low carbohydrate diet in one child [228]. Deficiency of lipoamide dehydrogenase (E3), which is common to α-KGD, PDHC, and branched-chain ketoacid decarboxylase, has been discussed earlier.

Ten children with fumarase deficiency had progressive encephalomyopathy with hypotonia, hyporeflexia, and cerebral atrophy [229–235]. Lactate was raised, particularly in the CSF, and variable other features included neutropenia, dystonia, choreoathetoid movements, microcephaly, and congenital hydrocephalus. The diagnosis was suspected by finding fumaric aciduria and confirmed by enzyme assay. Residual enzyme activity varied between 0% and 10%. Both mitochondrial and cytosolic enzymes were equally affected. Both isoforms are encoded by a single gene located on chromosome 1q42.1, and a homozygous missense mutation was identified in a conserved part of the cDNA in a Moroccan sibling pair [234]. Other mutations have subsequently been reported [236].

MOLECULAR GENETICS

More than 70 pathogenic mtDNA point mutations have now been described, in addition to a large number of deletion species [13]. Much is still unknown regarding the molecular pathogenesis of these mutations, but some patterns are beginning to emerge, and these are discussed in the following sections. Cell culture systems using transmitochondrial cybrids have been particularly helpful in beginning to unravel the molecular mechanisms involved. In these model systems, cells lacking mtDNA (ρ^0 cells) are fused with enucleated cells containing the mutation of interest to produce transmitochondrial cybrids in which the mtDNA mutation may be studied in the context of a different nuclear background [237].

However, despite many detailed studies, it is still difficult to explain the lack of correlation between genotype and phenotype for many mtDNA mutations. Although some variation in phenotype may be explained by differing tissue distributions of heteroplasmic mutations, other factors are likely to be involved. These include other modifying mutations or polymorphisms (either mitochondrial [238] or nuclear [239]), immunologic mechanisms [76], and environmental factors [240].

Mitochondrial DNA Mutations

Deletions and Duplications

Large-scale rearrangements of the mitochondrial genome are always heteroplasmic and may involve single or multiple deletions or partial duplications. The clinical phenotypes most commonly associated with these mutations are PEO and the Kearns-Sayre and Pearson syndromes [20, 43, 133]. There is no obvious relationship between the clinical phenotype and size, location, or percentage of the mtDNA deletion(s) in muscle. However, the proportion of deleted mtDNA molecules varies widely between tissues, and tissue distribution and segregation is likely to be important in determining the phenotype. Evolution of a phenotype (e.g., in patients with Pearson syndrome who later develop Kearns-Sayre syndrome) may be explained by selection against deleted mtDNA molecules in rapidly dividing tissues, such as bone marrow, paralleled by accumulation of deleted molecules in nondividing tissues, such as muscle and the central nervous system [136].

Although many different mtDNA deletion molecules have been described, ranging in size from 1 to 10 kb, 30–40% of all deletions are identical, spanning 4,977 bp from ATPase 8 to ND5 and flanked by a perfect 13-bp direct repeat [241]. This has led to speculation that the deletion may be produced by homologous recombination, or else slippage during replication [242, 243]. The mechanism of production is not clear in other cases, in which the deletions are not flanked by repeats, but may involve breakage and ligation of replication intermediates. Single deletions are usually sporadic, although they may occasionally be maternally inherited [134]. They are present at low levels in human oocytes [244], but transmission is thought to be prevented in most cases by the bottleneck effect [12]. Multiple deletions, however, are inherited as Mendelian traits, either recessive or dominant, and are discussed in the section Nuclear Gene Defects.

The mechanism of pathogenesis of deletions is thought to be via impaired mitochondrial translation, and this has been supported by cybrid studies. Impaired mitochondrial translation has been observed in transmitochondrial cybrids containing 60% or more deleted mtDNA [245]. Single-fiber analysis of muscle from patients with mtDNA deletions, demonstrating a higher percentage of deleted mtDNA in COX-negative fibers compared with COX-positive fibers, also provides evidence for impaired mitochondrial translation secondary to the deletion [246]. Impairment of mitochondrial translation most probably follows insufficiency of tRNAs that is due to deletion of tRNA genes.

Duplications are seen in the Kearns-Sayre and Pearson syndromes and in patients with diabetes and deafness [247–249]. It has been proposed that duplications may be an intermediate in forming all deletions [250, 251]. Maternal inheritance of duplications has been reported [146, 249, 252]. The pathogenic mechanism of duplications is uncertain, but those involving the D-loop may interfere with the binding and function of *trans*-acting nuclear factors. However, there is much controversy regarding whether duplications are intrinsically pathogenic [253].

Transfer RNA Point Mutations

Point mutations in mitochondrial tRNA genes are usually heteroplasmic and often display marked phenotypic heterogeneity. This has been discussed earlier in relation to the A3243G and A8344G mutations most commonly associated with MELAS and MERRF syndromes, respectively. A8344G is found in 80–90% of cases of MERRF [56], and two other mutations in the tRNA lysine gene, T8356C and G8363A, have also been reported in families with this phenotype [59, 60]. Studies of cultured myotubes bearing the A8344G mutation revealed a threshold of 85% mutant load for pathogenicity [254]. Cybrids containing the A8344G and T8356C point mutations had decreased mitochondrial protein synthesis, with concomitant reduction in the activities of complexes I and IV [255, 256]. Further cybrid studies demonstrated defective aminoacylation of the mutant tRNA lysine in cell lines containing the A8344G mutation, leading to premature termination of translation at lysine codons [257].

Pathogenic mechanisms are less clear for the MELAS mutations. Reductions in both protein synthesis and complex I activity were observed in cybrids containing greater than 95% A3243G and T3271C mutations [258, 259]. In addition, a partially processed polycistronic RNA—RNA 19—has been observed in A3243G mutant cell lines, but its pathogenic significance is unclear, because it is also found at low levels in normal tissues [258, 260]. The large number of tRNA leucine[UUR] mutations documented may be due to the critical role of this gene in controlling mtDNA transcription rates. Transcription of mitochondrial ribosomal RNA genes is modulated by a termination factor, mTERF, which binds to a 13-bp sequence within the tRNA leucine[UUR] gene to promote transcription termination. In vitro studies have demonstrated impaired mTERF binding and decreased efficiency of transcription termination in cell lines containing the A3243G mutation [261], but there is no evidence for this occurring in vivo [262, 263].

Ribosomal RNA Point Mutations

A single homoplasmic point mutation, A1555G, has been described in the 12S rRNA gene in families with nonsyndromic congenital hearing loss and in aminoglycoside-induced deafness [240].

Protein-Coding Mutations

Although most reported mtDNA point mutations involve tRNA genes, an increasing number of protein-coding mutations is being described. The reason for this is (at least partly) that tRNA genes were initially regarded as hot spots for mtDNA mutations and were therefore targeted in initial sequencing studies [264], which have only more recently been extended to include protein-coding genes. However, it is also possible that tRNA mutations are indeed more common than mutations in protein-coding genes, for reasons that are not clear at present. A general characteristic of protein-coding mutations is that the phenotype associated with each mutation has tended to be more homogeneous than for tRNA point mutations.

The first point mutations in mtDNA protein-coding genes were described in association with LHON, in subunits ND1, ND4, and ND6 of complex I [65–67]. These are often homoplasmic. Other mtDNA complex I gene mutations are associated with LHON plus dystonia [77, 78] and with MELAS [265]. Base changes in cytochrome *b* and in COX subunit genes have also been reported in LHON pedigrees, but these do not appear to be primary pathogenic mutations [70].

Point mutations causing LS, NARP, and familial bilateral striatal necrosis appear to be clustered in the gene-encoding subunit 6 of the ATP synthase [81, 82, 96, 97]. Cell culture studies of the T8993G mutation have revealed reduced respiratory rates and decreased synthesis of ATP [163, 266].

Since 1995, mutations have been reported in the mitochondrial COX subunit genes in association with a range of different phenotypes. A 15-bp in-frame microdeletion in CO III was associated with severe isolated COX deficiency in a girl with recurrent myoglobinuria and muscle cramps [36]. Two other mutations in CO III have been described—both point mutations—and associated with different phenotypes. These are T9957C in a patient with MELAS [267] and a stop mutation G9952A leading to the production of a truncated protein in a 36-year-old woman with recurrent episodes of encephalopathy [268]. A heteroplasmic 5-bp out-of-frame deletion in CO I was reported in a man with a motor neuron disease–like syndrome with progressive spastic quadriparesis, and speech and swallowing difficulties [269]. We have identified a missense mutation T7671A in the CO II gene in a boy with isolated skeletal myopathy [270].

Nuclear Gene Defects

In contrast to the exponentially expanding number of reported mtDNA mutations, very few nuclear gene defects have been described in OXPHOS proteins. The first nuclear mutation reported in an OXPHOS subunit was a homozygous point mutation in the FP subunit of SDH in two French sisters with LS [101]. In 1998, the first mutations were identified in nuclear-encoded subunits of complex I: in the 18-kd subunit in an Israeli child with fatal infantile complex I deficiency [154] and in the NDUFS8 subunit in an infant with LS [100].

COX-deficient LS appears to be inherited as an autosomal recessive trait [90]. Cell fusion studies suggest that most patients belong to a single complementation group [271, 272]. Sequence analysis failed to identify pathogenic mutations in either mitochondrial [273] or nuclear [274] COX structural subunits in COX-deficient LS. In 1998, mutations were found in SURF1, a nuclear gene located on chromosome 9q34, which encodes a putative assembly or maintenance factor specific for the COX complex [102, 103].

Mutations in nuclear genes responsible for regulating mtDNA transcription, replication, and repair may also produce human disease. Such mutations are postulated to be responsible for autosomally inherited multiple mtDNA deletion syndromes and the mtDNA depletion syndrome of infancy and childhood. Linkage studies have identified some loci for these disorders of intergenomic communication [24, 25], but no candidate gene has been isolated to date.

Many of the nuclear genes responsible for non-OXPHOS mitochondrial disorders have been isolated and mutations reported. These are discussed in the relevant previous sections.

INVESTIGATION OF MITOCHONDRIAL DISEASE

As there is no single diagnostic investigation for OXPHOS disorders, a multidisciplinary approach to diagnosis is required, incorporating clinical assessment, biochemical investigations, histochemistry, and molecular genetic techniques. Although a specific molecular diagnosis is still achieved only in a minority of cases, the chances of doing this may be optimized by coordinated investigation in a specialized center.

Clinical Assessment

There are no individually diagnostic clinical features of mitochondrial disease, but the constellation of signs and symptoms may be suggestive of OXPHOS disease, particularly if there is involvement of a number of apparently unrelated systems. Furthermore, certain clinical features should in themselves arouse suspicion of OXPHOS disease—for example, recurrent strokelike episodes and myoclonus. Family history is also useful, particularly if there is maternal inheritance, as subsequent investigations can then be directed at the mitochondrial genome.

Ophthalmologic assessment for retinopathy and optic atrophy, echocardiography, and electrocardiography are useful to determine the extent of organ involvement, particularly in children, as isolated myopathy is an unusual presentation of mitochondrial disease in this age group. It is important to identify multisystem features early to provide adequate supportive therapy and as an approximate prognostic guide.

Metabolites

Persistent unexplained lactic acidosis may be the only clue to an underlying OXPHOS disorder. However, the lactate is often normal or only marginally elevated in patients with OXPHOS disease, or may only be abnormal on provocation—for example, after exercise. In adults, some centers measure blood lactate after a formal exercise test (e.g., the subanaerobic threshold exercise test [275]), but this is rarely practical in young children. Great care should be taken when measuring and interpreting blood lactates, particularly in children. Artifactual elevation may follow venous stasis or screaming and struggling during venepuncture. This may be avoided by sampling from a previously inserted cannula. Ideally, the sample should be deproteinized immediately by collecting it into a tube containing perchloric acid. CSF lactate is thought to be less prone to artifactual elevation. However, CSF lactate may be raised after seizure or stroke in the absence of mitochondrial disease, and results should therefore be interpreted with caution. CSF protein is characteristically raised in Kearns-Sayre syndrome and may be elevated in MERRF, but it is usually normal in most OXPHOS disorders.

The L/P ratio is a useful measure of cytoplasmic redox status, although it may sometimes be misleading. The ketone body molar ratio (β-hydroxybutyrate/acetoacetate) may also be helpful as a measure of mitochondrial redox status [123]. In children with lactic acidosis, other metabolic causes should be sought. Blood glucose, pH, and electrolytes should be measured, along with ammonia and quantitative assessment of plasma amino acids. Hyperammonemia often accompanies lactic acidosis in pyruvate carboxylase deficiency, fatty acid oxidation defects, and organic acidemias. Activities of PDHC and pyruvate carboxylase may be determined in cultured skin fibroblasts and biotinidase in blood. Plasma free and acyl carnitines may be diagnostic in fatty acid oxidation defects, and urinary organic acids (measured by gas chromatography and mass spectrometry) may be diagnostic in organic acidemias. There are no diagnostic urinary metabolites in OXPHOS disorders.

The blood creatine kinase is usually normal in OXPHOS disorders, except in those cases presenting with acute rhabdomyolysis, and was raised in only four of a series of 51 affected patients [276]. Three of these four patients had isolated myopathy, whereas the fourth had PEO with proximal weakness. Renal tubular and hepatic function should also be evaluated as part of the screen for multisystem involvement.

Neuroimaging

No diagnostic imaging features of mitochondrial disease exist, but characteristic distributions of abnormalities are recognized in MELAS and LS. In the former, parieto-occipital lesions and symmetric basal ganglia calcification are the most frequent findings [47]. After an acute strokelike episode, CT may reveal hypodensity, and MRI may reveal high signal on T2-weighted scans consistent with infarction (see Figure 7.5). These changes may resolve over the subsequent hours or days, but in some cases, cerebral atrophy and calcification may develop. In LS, bilateral symmetric basal ganglia lesions are typical. These appear as hypodensities on CT [277] and as areas of high-signal intensity on T2-weighted MRI scans (Figure 7.6) [278]. MRI findings in other mitochondrial syndromes, including PEO and Kearns-Sayre, are nonspecific and include cerebral and cerebellar atrophy; white-matter hyperintense signal abnormalities on T2 scans; and basal ganglia, thalamic, or brain stem lesions [279]. There is poor correlation between individual neurologic features and the MRI abnormalities. Scans may be normal, particularly if the clinical presentation is of isolated skeletal myopathy [19, 279]. In a 1998 review of 25 children with mitochondrial disorders, no patient with clinical encephalopathy had a normal scan, but findings were nonspecific in many cases [280]. Magnetic resonance spectroscopy (MRS) of brain or muscle may demonstrate impaired mitochondrial energy metabolism, with increased inorganic phosphate to phosphocreatine ratio on ^{31}P-MRS of

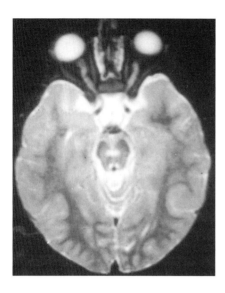

Figure 7.6   T2-weighted brain MRI of a patient with Leigh syndrome demonstrating bilateral, symmetric, high-density lesions in the midbrain.

muscle [281] and increased regional brain lactates on proton MRS of brain [282].

Neurophysiologic Studies

Neurophysiologic findings are variable in mitochondrial encephalomyopathies. A number of EEG abnormalities were observed in a series of 25 patients [283]. The most frequent findings were epileptiform discharges and generalized slow waves consistent with a subacute encephalopathy. The electromyogram may be mildly myopathic in mitochondrial disorders, but it is frequently normal, even in patients with clinically apparent myopathy [276]. Peripheral neuropathy is common [284], and nerve conduction studies may reveal axonal or mixed axonal–demyelinating peripheral sensorimotor neuropathy. Visual evoked responses were altered in one study of MERRF [285], and the electroretino-gram was abnormal in all 11 patients with pigmentary retinopathy in Petty's series of 66 patients with mitochondrial myopathy [19] and in a patient with NARP syndrome [81].

Muscle Biopsy

Muscle biopsy is often regarded as the best and most definitive means to diag-nose mitochondrial respiratory chain disease. The muscle obtained may be used for histochemical, biochemical, and molecular genetic analysis. The morphologic hallmark of OXPHOS diseases is the RRF, as seen on the modified Gomori

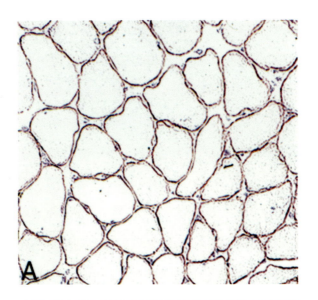

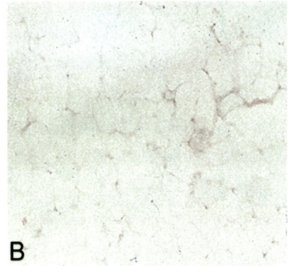

Color Plate 1 These transverse cryostat sections of muscle biopsies show immunoreactive dystrophin using a monoclonal antibody that recognizes rod-domain epitopes. The bound antibodies are displayed by peroxidase reaction. (**A**) The normal pattern. (**B**) Complete deficiency in Duchenne dystrophy.

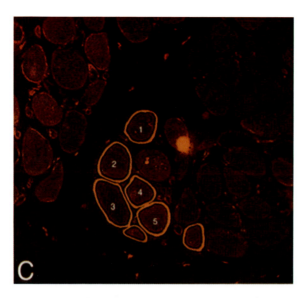

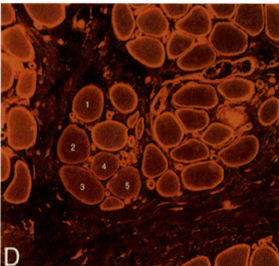

Color Plate 1 (continued) (**C, D**) Serial sections from a Duchenne muscle biopsy. Using the monoclonal antibody that recognizes rod-domain epitopes, (**C**) is stained for dystrophin. Using a monoclonal antibody for the NH$_2$-terminus, (**D**) is stained for utrophin. (**C**) Several "revertant" fibers are shown with dystrophin immunostaining, and most fibers are devoid of dystrophin. (**D**) By contrast, utrophin is strongly expressed in all dystrophin-negative muscle fibers but weakly expressed in the revertants.

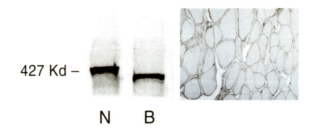

427 Kd –

N   B

Color Plate 2   On the left, an immunoblot shows abundant normal-sized, 427-kd dystrophin from a normal muscle biopsy (N). The band from a patient with Becker muscular dystrophy shows a smaller amount of low-molecular-weight dystrophin (B). On the right, muscle biopsy of the same patient shows weak and interrupted dystrophin immunoperoxidase staining.

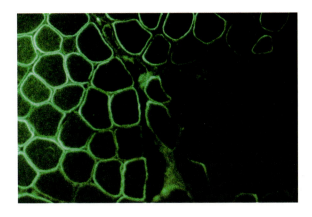

Color Plate 3 Dystrophin immunofluorescence from a definite carrier shows a cluster of dystrophin-negative muscle fibers that had normal spectrin and laminin immunostaining (not shown).

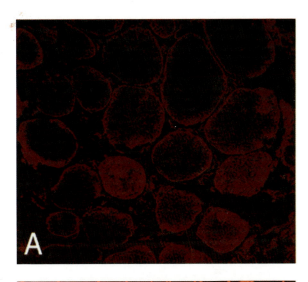

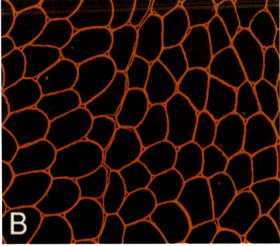

Color Plate 4 (**A**) Complete lack of immuno-reactive α-sarcoglycan in a 13-year-old boy who presented with a Duchenne-type muscular dystrophy. He had a missense mutation in the α-sarcoglycan gene. (**B**) Normal α-sarcoglycan immunostaining.

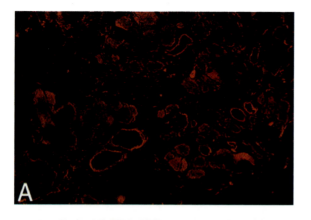

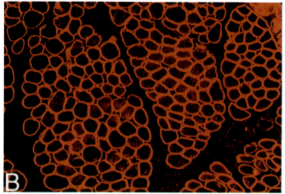

Color Plate 5 (**A**) Near-complete deficiency of merosin in a patient with congenital muscular dystrophy. A few fibers retained some immunoreactive merosin. (**B**) Normal merosin immunostaining.

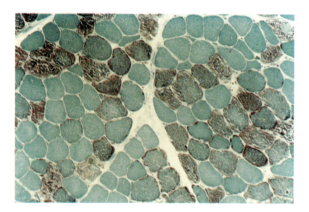

Color Plate 6 Modified Gomori trichrome stain demonstrating ragged red fibers. Lipid droplets are also visible in some fibers.

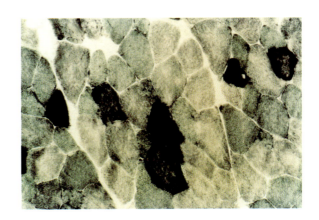

Color Plate 7   Succinate dehydrogenase stain demonstrates intense activity in some fibers.

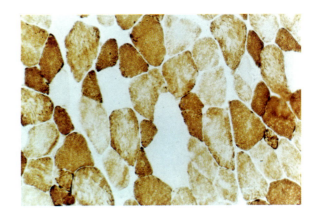

Color Plate 8   Cytochrome oxidase stain in serial section to Color Plate 7. The succinate dehydrogenase-positive fibers are negative for cytochrome oxidase.

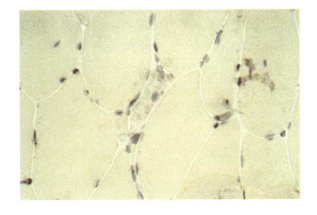

Color Plate 9   In this patient with inclusion body myositis, amyloid deposition in a muscle fiber is seen. Congo red–stained and viewed with polarized light.

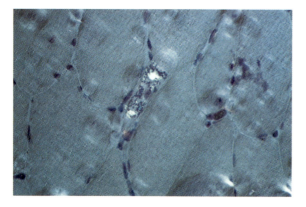

Color Plate 10　In this patient with inclusion body myositis, amyloid deposition in a muscle fiber is seen. Congo red staining used with polarized light shows birefringent amyloid.

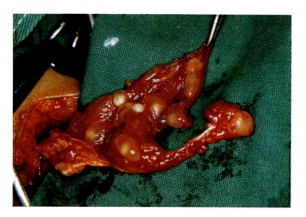

Color Plate 11　In this muscle biopsy, live cysticerci are seen pouring out of the muscle.

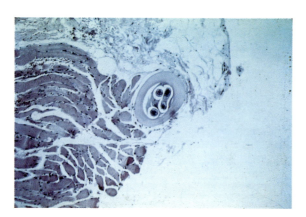

Color Plate 12　In this muscle biopsy, the larva of *Trichinella spiralis* is seen.

trichrome stain (see Color Plate 6). This demonstrates subsarcolemmal accumulations of mitochondrial material, often in association with excess glycogen or lipid. The proportion of fibers affected in a transverse section varies considerably between patients, but the ragged red appearances are segmental, so more fibers may be affected along their length. The RRF stain strongly for SDH, and indeed, this stain is more sensitive in detecting abnormal fibers (see Color Plate 7). The COX stain may demonstrate the abnormal fibers to be COX positive or COX negative. In chronic progressive external ophthalmoplegia (CPEO), Kearns-Sayre syndrome, and MERRF, a high proportion of RRF are COX negative (see Color Plate 8), whereas in MELAS, the abnormal fibers are more frequently COX positive. In some patients, particularly those with CPEO, COX-negative fibers may be the only morphologic abnormality with the oxidative stains.

Ragged red, SDH-positive, COX-negative fibers are not specific to mitochondrial respiratory chain diseases and have been observed in the inflammatory myopathies and in inclusion body myositis. COX-negative fibers are seen as a normal consequence of aging, although they should not exceed 5% of the fibers [286].

Some patients have been classified as having mitochondrial myopathy on the basis of defective biochemistry or molecular genetic analysis, even in the absence of the morphologic changes described in the preceding paragraphs [29, 287].

The presence or absence of RRF does not appear to relate directly to the mtDNA mutation when present. For some time, it was believed that mutations involving tRNA genes (deletions, point mutations) were associated with RRF, and those involving coding genes (LHON, NARP) were not. However, there are now several examples of patients with mitochondrial myopathy or encephalomyopathy phenotypes, ND gene mutations, and RRF on biopsy [265].

Isolated SDH or COX deficiency may be seen in some patients. In SDH deficiency, the extrafusal fibers may show severe depletion of activity, whereas staining may appear normal in the intrafusal fibers of the muscle spindles and the smooth muscle of arterioles. A similar pattern may be seen in primary COX deficiency because of a mutation in one of the mtDNA COX genes.

Ultrastructural analysis by electron microscopy may identify paracrystalline inclusions within the mitochondria of a proportion of patients (Figure 7.7). These may be located within the matrix or intermembranous space and appear as "parking lot" (type I) or large rectangular (type II) arrangements. The crystals are immunoreactive for creatine kinase [288]. Other changes may include a proliferation of enlarged mitochondria, many of which may contain abnormal cristae. There is often an excess of glycogen.

In situ hybridization studies have demonstrated that in the case of mtDNA deletions, the abnormal molecules are present in highest proportion in the RRF and COX-negative fibers [262, 289–291]. The deleted mtDNAs are transcribed but not translated, presumably because of the lack of appropriate tRNAs.

Mitochondrial DNA Analysis

Skeletal muscle is the tissue of choice for mtDNA studies, because mutations may not always be detected in blood. Most centers screen for the relatively com-

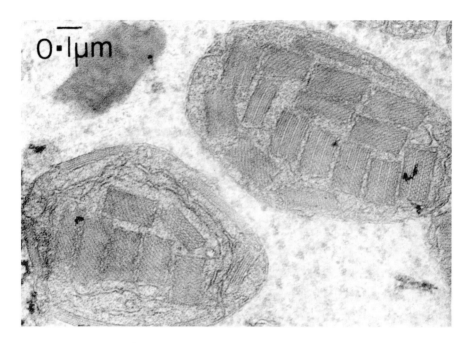

Figure 7.7 Electron micrograph of mitochondrion with paracrystalline inclusions.

mon mtDNA mutations at nucleotides 3243, 8344, and 8993 by using polymerase chain reaction amplification and restriction analysis and—for large-scale rearrangements—by using Southern blot analysis. Some centers are now using long-range polymerase chain reaction to detect mtDNA rearrangements. In childhood, the yield is low, because these mutations are all rare in this age group [14]. To diagnose mtDNA depletion, it is important to quantitate the Southern blot of mtDNA from an affected tissue carefully, using age-matched controls.

Sequencing of the entire mitochondrial genome may be indicated in selected cases, particularly in which there is maternal inheritance, but this is currently only available as a research investigation; because it is costly and time-consuming. Once a mutation has been identified, studies of single muscle fibers and transmitochondrial cell lines may be used to establish pathogenicity of the mutation. It is often difficult to differentiate a pathogenic mtDNA mutation from a neutral polymorphism, but some criteria for pathogenicity that have been suggested include absence of the mutation in controls, mutation of a nucleotide that is highly conserved through evolution, a mutation resulting in a significant amino acid change (for protein-coding genes), segregation of the mutation with the phenotype, correlation between degree of heteroplasmy and the phenotype, and identification of the mutation in affected patients from ethnically distinct populations.

GENETIC COUNSELING AND TREATMENT

Genetic Counseling

Genetic counseling of OXPHOS disorders is difficult because of the number of different modes of inheritance involved. Few studies have examined recurrence risks in families with mitochondrial myopathies. One report suggested that transmission of MERRF to offspring does not occur until the mother's mutant load is more than 35–40%, but the number of families studied was small [292]. A detailed study of LHON pedigrees with the three primary mutations indicated risks of 30% for brothers, 8% for sisters, 46% for nephews, 10% for nieces, and 31% for male and 6% for female matrilineal first cousins of affected individuals [293]. The usual recurrence risk quoted for other OXPHOS defects is higher than 25% because of the possibility of maternal inheritance. Recurrence in maternally inherited defects may be as much as 100% and can only be reliably avoided by in vitro fertilization of a donor ovum.

Attempts at prenatal diagnosis of mtDNA defects are not recommended, because little is known about drift of mtDNA point mutations in intrauterine life and because of a risk of maternal contamination of the sample [294]. Prenatal diagnosis may be possible for some families with isolated defects of complex I or IV, providing the defect is expressed in cultured cells.

Supportive Management

No specific treatments exist for OXPHOS disorders. Supportive measures are therefore the mainstay of management. These include sodium bicarbonate to correct the acidosis, anticonvulsants for seizures, and pacing for cardiac conduction defects. Valproate should be avoided, because this may precipitate liver failure [120] or seizures [295], and care should be taken with general anesthesia [296]. A multidisciplinary approach is essential if potential systemic features are to be recognized and treated early. Psychological support for patients and their families is vital.

Drugs

Pharmacologic interventions that have been tried in OXPHOS disorders include dichloroacetate; cofactors, such as riboflavin, thiamine, CoQ, and carnitine; and artificial electron acceptors, including ascorbate and menadione. Ascorbate, menadione, and CoQ may also have an antioxidant function. Reports of benefit are anecdotal only (see, for example, references 297–299) and have not been substantiated by the few clinical trials performed. CoQ is probably only beneficial in cases of isolated CoQ deficiency [168, 169]. One multicenter trial of CoQ in mitochondrial patients with OXPHOS deficiency suggested partial response in a few patients [300], but this was not maintained. Another study documented increased serum levels of CoQ after treatment, but this was not accompanied by any improvement in oxidative metabolism or any objective clinical improvement [301]. Similarly, trials of dichloroacetate demonstrated reduction in arterial [302] and cerebral [303] lactate levels but no clinical improvement. Further clinical trials are needed but are hampered by the small numbers of patients in each group of disorders; by the lack of clinical, biochemical, or genetic homogeneity; and by the unpredictable natural history of these diseases.

Treatment of Nonoxidative Phosphorylation Defects

Treatments that may be of benefit in PDHC deficiency include a ketogenic diet and dichloroacetate. The latter inhibits the PDH kinase, which normally inactivates PDHC by phosphorylation. Appropriate dietary intervention should be instituted for disorders of fatty acid oxidation, together with medium-chain triglyceride and carnitine supplements when indicated.

Novel Therapeutic Strategies

Some centers consider gene therapy to be the only possible long-term approach to treating OXPHOS disorders. However, this is complicated by the dual genetic input involved and by the inaccessibility of the mitochondrion, which means that special gene targeting methods need to be devised. Methods that have been tried in vitro include sequence-specific inhibition of mutant mtDNA replication by antisense oligonucleotides and peptide nucleic acids, cytosolic synthesis of mitochondrially encoded proteins, and intramitochondrial import of wild-type mtDNA by specialized vector systems [304].

In one patient with an mtDNA point mutation, bupivacaine-induced muscle necrosis led to regeneration by normal muscle lacking the mutant mtDNA [305]. However, only a 2-cm block of muscle was treated, and it is difficult to envisage how this method might be used on a large scale to treat generalized myopathy. Eccentric exercise has been suggested as a therapeutic rationale to attempt to induce widespread muscle necrosis [306], but so far there have not been any clinical trials of this.

REFERENCES

1. Brandt U (ed). Structure and function of complex I. Biochim Biophys Acta 1998;1364:1–296.
2. Tsukihara T, Aoyama H, Yamashita E, et al. The whole structure of the 13-subunit oxidized cytochrome c oxidase at 2.8 A. Science 1996;272:1136–1144.
3. Linder D, Freund R, Kadenbach B. Species-specific expression of cytochrome c oxidase isozymes. Comp Biochem Physiol B Biochem Mol Biol 1995;112:461–469.
4. Hendler RW, Pardhasaradhi K, Reynafarje B, et al. Comparison of energy-transducing capabilities of the two- and three-subunit cytochromes aa$_3$ from Paracoccus denitrificans and the 13-subunit beef heart enzyme. Biophys J 1991;60:415–423.
5. Taanman JW. Human cytochrome c oxidase: structure, function, and deficiency. J Bioenerg Biomembr 1997;29:151–163.
6. Anderson S, Bankier AT, Barrell BG, et al. Sequence and organization of the human mitochondrial genome. Nature 1981;290:457–465.
7. Schatz G. The protein import system of mitochondria. J Biol Chem 1996;271:31763–31766.
8. Taanman JW. The human genome: structure, transcription, translation and replication. Biochim Biophys Acta 1999;1410:103–123.

9. Hauswirth WW, Laipis PJ. Mitochondrial DNA polymorphism in a maternal lineage of Holstein cows. Proc Natl Acad Sci U S A 1982;79:4686–4690.
10. Degoul F, Francois D, Diry M, et al. A near homoplasmic T8993G mtDNA mutation in a patient with atypic Leigh syndrome not present in the mother's tissues. J Inherit Metab Dis 1997;20:49–53.
11. Seller A, Kennedy CR, Temple IK, et al. Leigh syndrome resulting from de novo mutation at position 8993 of mitochondrial DNA. J Inherit Metab Dis 1997;20:102–103.
12. Brown GK. Bottlenecks and beyond: mitochondrial DNA segregation in health and disease. J Inherit Metab Dis 1997;20:2–8.
13. Servidei S. Mitochondrial encephalomyopathies: gene mutation. Neuromuscul Disord 1998;8:8–11.
14. Shoffner JM. Maternal inheritance and the evaluation of oxidative phosphorylation diseases. Lancet 1996;348:1283–1288.
15. Schon EA, Bonilla E, DiMauro S. Mitochondrial DNA mutations and pathogenesis. J Bioenerg Biomembr 1997;29:131–149.
16. Luft R, Ikkos D, Palmieri G, et al. A case of severe hypermetabolism of nonthyroid origin with a defect in the maintenance of mitochondrial respiratory control: a correlated clinical, biochemical, and morphological study. J Clin Invest 1962;41:1776–1804.
17. Engel WK, Cunningham GG. Rapid examination of muscle tissue; an improved trichrome stain method for fresh-frozen biopsy sections. Neurology 1963;13:919–923.
18. Holt IJ, Harding AE, Morgan Hughes JA. Deletions of muscle mitochondrial DNA in patients with mitochondrial myopathies. Nature 1988;331:717–719.
19. Petty RK, Harding AE, Morgan Hughes JA. The clinical features of mitochondrial myopathy. Brain 1986;109:915–938.
20. Moraes CT, DiMauro S, Zeviani M, et al. Mitochondrial DNA deletions in progressive external ophthalmoplegia and Kearns-Sayre syndrome. N Engl J Med 1989;320:1293–1299.
21. Mariotti C, Savarese N, Suomalainen A, et al. Genotype to phenotype correlations in mitochondrial encephalomyopathies associated with the A3243G mutation of mitochondrial DNA. J Neurol 1995;242:304–312.
22. Zeviani M, Servidei S, Gellera C, et al. An autosomal dominant disorder with multiple deletions of mitochondrial DNA starting at the D-loop region. Nature 1989;339:309–311.
23. Servidei S, Zeviani M, Manfredi G, et al. Dominantly inherited mitochondrial myopathy with multiple deletions of mitochondrial DNA: clinical, morphologic, and biochemical studies. Neurology 1991;41:1053–1059.
24. Suomalainen A, Kaukonen J, Amati P, et al. An autosomal locus predisposing to deletions of mitochondrial DNA. Nat Genet 1995;9:146–151.
25. Kaukonen JA, Amati P, Suomalainen A, et al. An autosomal locus predisposing to multiple deletions of mtDNA on chromosome 3p. Am J Hum Genet 1996;58:763–769.
26. Ohno K, Tanaka M, Sahashi K, et al. Mitochondrial DNA deletions in inherited recurrent myoglobinuria. Ann Neurol 1991;29:364–369.
27. Blumenthal DT, Shanske S, Schochet SS, et al. Myoclonus epilepsy with ragged red fibers and multiple mtDNA deletions. Neurology 1998;50:524–525.
28. Oldfors A, Larsson NG, Lindberg C, et al. Mitochondrial DNA deletions in inclusion body myositis. Brain 1993;116:325–336.
29. Hammans SR, Sweeney MG, Brockington M, et al. Mitochondrial encephalopathies: molecular genetic diagnosis from blood samples. Lancet 1991;337:1311–1313.
30. Goto Y, Tojo M, Tohyama J, et al. A novel point mutation in the mitochondrial tRNA(Leu)(UUR) gene in a family with mitochondrial myopathy. Ann Neurol 1992;31:672–675.
31. Bindoff LA, Howell N, Poulton J, et al. Abnormal RNA processing associated with a novel tRNA mutation in mitochondrial DNA. A potential disease mechanism. J Biol Chem 1993;268:19559–19564.
32. Moraes CT, Ciacci F, Bonilla E, et al. A mitochondrial tRNA anticodon swap associated with a muscle disease. Nat Genet 1993;4:284–288.
33. Weber K, Wilson JN, Taylor L, et al. A new mtDNA mutation showing accumulation with time and restriction to skeletal muscle. Am J Hum Genet 1997;60:373–380.
34. Chinnery PF, Johnson MA, Taylor RW, et al. A novel mitochondrial tRNA phenylalanine mutation presenting with acute rhabdomyolysis. Ann Neurol 1997;41:408–410.
35. Dumoulin R, Sagnol I, Ferlin T, et al. A novel gly290asp mitochondrial cytochrome b mutation linked to a complex III deficiency in progressive exercise intolerance. Mol Cell Probes 1996;10:389–391.
36. Keightley JA, Hoffbuhr KC, Burton MD, et al. A microdeletion in cytochrome c oxidase (COX) subunit III associated with COX deficiency and recurrent myoglobinuria. Nat Genet 1996;12:410–416.

37. Berenberg RA, Pellock JM, DiMauro S, et al. Lumping or splitting? "Ophthalmoplegia-plus" or Kearns-Sayre syndrome? Ann Neurol 1977;1:37–54.
38. Roberts NK, Perloff JK, Kark RA. Cardiac conduction in the Kearns-Sayre syndrome (a neuromuscular disorder associated with progressive external ophthalmoplegia and pigmentary retinopathy). Report of 2 cases and review of 17 published cases. Am J Cardiol 1979;44:1396–1400.
39. Quade A, Zierz S, Klingmuller D. Endocrine abnormalities in mitochondrial myopathy with external ophthalmoplegia. Clin Invest 1992;70:396–402.
40. Harvey JN, Barnett D. Endocrine dysfunction in Kearns-Sayre syndrome. Clin Endocrinol (Oxf) 1992;37:97–103.
41. Zeviani M, Moraes CT, DiMauro S, et al. Deletions of mitochondrial DNA in Kearns-Sayre syndrome. Neurology 1988;38:1339–1346.
42. Lestienne P, Ponsot G. Kearns-Sayre syndrome with muscle mitochondrial DNA deletion. Lancet 1988;1:885.
43. Holt IJ, Harding AE, Cooper JM, et al. Mitochondrial myopathies: clinical and biochemical features of 30 patients with major deletions of muscle mitochondrial DNA. Ann Neurol 1989;26:699–708.
44. Pavlakis SG, Phillips PC, DiMauro S, et al. Mitochondrial myopathy, encephalopathy, lactic acidosis, and strokelike episodes: a distinctive clinical syndrome. Ann Neurol 1984;16:481–488.
45. Sakuta R, Nonaka I. Vascular involvement in mitochondrial myopathy. Ann Neurol 1989;25:594–601.
46. Hasegawa H, Matsuoka T, Goto Y, et al. Strongly succinate dehydrogenase-reactive blood vessels in muscles from patients with mitochondrial myopathy, encephalopathy, lactic acidosis, and stroke-like episodes. Ann Neurol 1991;29:601–605.
47. Sue CM, Crimmins DS, Soo YS, et al. Neuroradiological features of six kindreds with MELAS tRNA(Leu) A2343G point mutation: implications for pathogenesis. J Neurol Neurosurg Psychiatry 1998;65:233–240.
48. Koga Y, Nonaka I, Kobayashi M, et al. Findings in muscle in complex I (NADH coenzyme Q reductase) deficiency. Ann Neurol 1988;24:749–756.
49. Ciafaloni E, Ricci E, Shanske S, et al. MELAS: clinical features, biochemistry, and molecular genetics. Ann Neurol 1992;31:391–398.
50. Moraes CT, Ciacci F, Silvestri G, et al. Atypical clinical presentations associated with the MELAS mutation at position 3243 of human mitochondrial DNA. Neuromuscul Disord 1993;3:43–50.
51. Hammans SR, Sweeney MG, Hanna MG, et al. The mitochondrial DNA transfer RNALeu(UUR) A→G(3243) mutation. A clinical and genetic study. Brain 1995;118:721–734.
52. Goto Y, Nonaka I, Horai S. A mutation in the tRNA(Leu)(UUR) gene associated with the MELAS subgroup of mitochondrial encephalomyopathies. Nature 1990;348:651–653.
53. Kobayashi Y, Momoi MY, Tominaga K, et al. A point mutation in the mitochondrial tRNA(Leu)(UUR) gene in MELAS (mitochondrial myopathy, encephalopathy, lactic acidosis and stroke-like episodes). Biochem Biophys Res Commun 1990;173:816–822.
54. Campos Y, Garcia-Silva T, Barrionuevo CR, et al. Mitochondrial DNA deletion in a patient with mitochondrial myopathy, lactic acidosis, and stroke-like episodes (MELAS) and Fanconi syndrome. Pediatr Neurol 1995;13:69–72.
55. Fukuhara N, Tokiguchi S, Shirakawa K, et al. Myoclonus epilepsy associated with ragged-red fibres (mitochondrial abnormalities): disease entity or a syndrome? Light- and electron-microscopic studies of two cases and review of literature. J Neurol Sci 1980;47:117–133.
56. Shoffner JM, Lott MT, Lezza AM, et al. Myoclonic epilepsy and ragged-red fiber disease (MERRF) is associated with a mitochondrial DNA tRNA(Lys) mutation. Cell 1990;61:931–937.
57. Silvestri G, Ciafaloni E, Santorelli FM, et al. Clinical features associated with the A→G transition at nucleotide 8344 of mtDNA ("MERRF mutation"). Neurology 1993;43:1200–1206.
58. Hammans SR, Sweeney MG, Brockington M, et al. The mitochondrial DNA transfer RNA(Lys)A→G(8344) mutation and the syndrome of myoclonic epilepsy with ragged red fibres (MERRF). Relationship of clinical phenotype to proportion of mutant mitochondrial DNA. Brain 1993;116:617–632.
59. Silvestri G, Moraes CT, Shanske S, et al. A new mtDNA mutation in the tRNA(Lys) gene associated with myoclonic epilepsy and ragged-red fibers (MERRF). Am J Hum Genet 1992;51:1213–1217.
60. Ozawa M, Nishino I, Horai S, et al. Myoclonus epilepsy associated with ragged-red fibers: a G-to-A mutation at nucleotide pair 8363 in mitochondrial tRNA(Lys) in two families. Muscle Nerve 1997;20:271–278.
61. Tiranti V, Chariot P, Carella F, et al. Maternally inherited hearing loss, ataxia and myoclonus associated with a novel point mutation in mitochondrial tRNASer(UCN) gene. Hum Mol Genet 1995;4:1421–1427.
62. Nakamura M, Nakano S, Goto Y, et al. A novel point mutation in the mitochondrial tRNA(Ser(UCN)) gene detected in a family with MERRF/MELAS overlap syndrome. Biochem Biophys Res Commun 1995;214:86–93.

63. Zeviani M, Muntoni F, Savarese N, et al. A MERRF/MELAS overlap syndrome associated with a new point mutation in the mitochondrial DNA tRNA(Lys) gene. Eur J Hum Genet 1993;1:80–87. [Published erratum appears in Eur J Hum Genet 1993;1:124.]
64. Harding AE, Sweeney MG. Leber's Hereditary Optic Neuropathy. In AHV Schapira, S DiMauro (eds), Mitochondrial Disorders in Neurology. Oxford, UK: Butterworth–Heinemann, 1994;181–198.
65. Wallace DC, Singh G, Lott MT, et al. Mitochondrial DNA mutation associated with Leber's hereditary optic neuropathy. Science 1988;242:1427–1430.
66. Huoponen K, Vilkki J, Aula P, et al. A new mtDNA mutation associated with Leber hereditary optic neuroretinopathy. Am J Hum Genet 1991;48:1147–1153.
67. Johns DR, Neufeld MJ, Park RD. An ND-6 mitochondrial DNA mutation associated with Leber hereditary optic neuropathy. Biochem Biophys Res Commun 1992;187:1551–1557.
68. Mackey D, Howell N. A variant of Leber hereditary optic neuropathy characterized by recovery of vision and by an unusual mitochondrial genetic etiology. Am J Hum Genet 1992;51:1218–1228.
69. Mackey DA, Oostra RJ, Rosenberg T, et al. Primary pathogenic mtDNA mutations in multigeneration pedigrees with Leber hereditary optic neuropathy. Am J Hum Genet 1996;59:481–485.
70. Howell N. Leber hereditary optic neuropathy: how do mitochondrial DNA mutations cause degeneration of the optic nerve? J Bioenerg Biomembr 1997;29:165–173.
71. Smith PR, Cooper JM, Govan GG, et al. Platelet mitochondrial function in Leber's hereditary optic neuropathy. J Neurol Sci 1994;122:80–83.
72. Larsson NG, Andersen O, Holme E, et al. Leber's hereditary optic neuropathy and complex I deficiency in muscle. Ann Neurol 1991;30:701–708.
73. Bu XD, Rotter JI. X chromosome-linked and mitochondrial gene control of Leber hereditary optic neuropathy: evidence from segregation analysis for dependence on X chromosome inactivation. Proc Natl Acad Sci U S A 1991;88:8198–8202.
74. Chalmers RM, Davis MB, Sweeney MG, et al. Evidence against an X-linked visual loss susceptibility locus in Leber hereditary optic neuropathy. Am J Hum Genet 1996;59:103–108.
75. Smith PR, Cooper JM, Govan GG, et al. Antibodies to human optic nerve in Leber's hereditary optic neuropathy. J Neurol Sci 1995;130:134–138.
76. Harding AE, Sweeney MG, Miller DH, et al. Occurrence of a multiple sclerosis-like illness in women who have a Leber's hereditary optic neuropathy mitochondrial DNA mutation. Brain 1992;115:979–989.
77. Jun AS, Brown MD, Wallace DC. A mitochondrial DNA mutation at nucleotide pair 14459 of the NADH dehydrogenase subunit 6 gene associated with maternally inherited Leber hereditary optic neuropathy and dystonia. Proc Natl Acad Sci U S A 1994;91:6206–6210.
78. De Vries DD, Went LN, Bruyn GW, et al. Genetic and biochemical impairment of mitochondrial complex I activity in a family with Leber hereditary optic neuropathy and hereditary spastic dystonia. Am J Hum Genet 1996;58:703–711.
79. Nikoskelainen E, Wanne O, Dahl M. Pre-excitation syndrome and Leber's hereditary optic neuroretinopathy. Lancet 1985;1:696.
80. Chalmers RM, Schapira AHV. Clinical, biochemical and molecular genetic features of Lebers hereditary optic neuropathy. Biochim Biophys Acta 1999;1410:147–158.
81. Holt IJ, Harding AE, Petty RK, et al. A new mitochondrial disease associated with mitochondrial DNA heteroplasmy. Am J Hum Genet 1990;46:428–433.
82. De Vries DD, van Engelen BG, Gabreels FJ, et al. A second missense mutation in the mitochondrial ATPase 6 gene in Leigh's syndrome. Ann Neurol 1993;34:410–412.
83. Tatuch Y, Christodoulou J, Feigenbaum A, et al. Heteroplasmic mtDNA mutation (T→G) at 8993 can cause Leigh disease when the percentage of abnormal mtDNA is high. Am J Hum Genet 1992;50: 852–858.
84. Leigh D. Subacute necrotizing encephalomyelopathy in an infant. J Neurol Neurosurg Psychiatry 1951;14216–14221.
85. van Erven PM, Gabreels FJ, Ruitenbeek W, et al. Mitochondrial encephalomyopathy. Association with an NADH dehydrogenase deficiency. Arch Neurol 1987;44:775–778.
86. Willems JL, Monnens LA, Trijbels JM, et al. Leigh's encephalomyelopathy in a patient with cytochrome c oxidase deficiency in muscle tissue. Pediatrics 1977;60:850–857.
87. Kretzschmar HA, DeArmond SJ, Koch TK, et al. Pyruvate dehydrogenase complex deficiency as a cause of subacute necrotizing encephalopathy (Leigh disease). Pediatrics 1987;79:370–373.
88. Baumgartner ER, Suormala TM, Wick H, et al. Biotinidase deficiency: a cause of subacute necrotizing encephalomyelopathy (Leigh syndrome). Report of a case with lethal outcome. Pediatr Res 1989;26:260–266.
89. Santorelli FM, Shanske S, Macaya A, et al. The mutation at nt 8993 of mitochondrial DNA is a common cause of Leigh's syndrome. Ann Neurol 1993;34:827–834.

90. Rahman S, Blok RB, Dahl HH, et al. Leigh syndrome: clinical features and biochemical and DNA abnormalities. Ann Neurol 1996;39:343–351.

91. Koga Y, Yoshino M, Kato H. MELAS exhibits dominant negative effects on mitochondrial RNA processing. Ann Neurol 1998;43:835.

92. Chalmers RM, Lamont PJ, Nelson I, et al. A mitochondrial DNA tRNA(Val) point mutation associated with adult-onset Leigh syndrome. Neurology 1997;49:589–592.

93. Yamamoto M, Clemens PR, Engel AG. Mitochondrial DNA deletions in mitochondrial cytopathies: observations in 19 patients. Neurology 1991;41:1822–1828.

94. Yamadori I, Kurose A, Kobayashi S, et al. Brain lesions of the Leigh-type distribution associated with a mitochondriopathy of Pearson's syndrome: light and electron microscopic study. Acta Neuropathol 1992;84:337–341.

95. Morris AA, Taanman JW, Blake J, et al. Liver failure associated with mitochondrial DNA depletion. J Hepatol 1998;28:556–563.

96. De Meirleir L, Seneca S, Lissens W, et al. Bilateral striatal necrosis with a novel point mutation in the mitochondrial ATPase 6 gene. Pediatr Neurol 1995;13:242–246.

97. Thyagarajan D, Shanske S, Vazquez Memije M, et al. A novel mitochondrial ATPase 6 point mutation in familial bilateral striatal necrosis. Ann Neurol 1995;38:468–472.

98. Campos Y, Martin MA, Rubio JC, et al. Leigh syndrome associated with the T9176C mutation in the ATPase 6 gene of mitochondrial DNA. Neurology 1997;49:595–597.

99. Matthews PM, Marchington DR, Squier M, et al. Molecular genetic characterization of an X-linked form of Leigh's syndrome. Ann Neurol 1993;33:652–655.

100. Loeffen J, Smeitink J, Triepels R, et al. The first nuclear-encoded complex I mutation in a patient with Leigh syndrome. Am J Hum Genet 1998;6:1598–1608.

101. Bourgeron T, Rustin P, Chretien D, et al. Mutation of a nuclear succinate dehydrogenase gene results in mitochondrial respiratory chain deficiency. Nat Genet 1995;11:144–149.

102. Zhu Z, Yao J, Johns T, et al. *SURF1*, encoding a factor involved in the biogenesis of cytochrome *c* oxidase, is mutated in Leigh syndrome. Nat Genet 1998;20:328–343.

103. Tiranti V, Hoertnagel K, Carrozzo R, et al. Mutations of SURF-1 in Leigh disease associated with cytochrome c oxidase deficiency. Am J Hum Genet 1998;63:1609–1621.

104. Moraes CT, Shanske S, Tritschler HJ, et al. mtDNA depletion with variable tissue expression: a novel genetic abnormality in mitochondrial diseases. Am J Hum Genet 1991;48:492–501.

105. Taanman JW, Bodnar AG, Cooper JM, et al. Molecular mechanisms in mitochondrial DNA depletion syndrome. Hum Mol Genet 1997;6:935–942.

106. Vu TH, Sciacco M, Tanji K, et al. Clinical manifestations of mitochondrial DNA depletion. Neurology 1998;50:1783–1790.

107. Bodnar AG, Cooper JM, Holt IJ, et al. Nuclear complementation restores mtDNA levels in cultured cells from a patient with mtDNA depletion. Am J Hum Genet 1993;53:663–669.

108. Larsson NG, Oldfors A, Holme E, et al. Low levels of mitochondrial transcription factor A in mitochondrial DNA depletion. Biochem Biophys Res Commun 1994;200:1374–1381.

109. Poulton J, Morten K, Freeman Emmerson C, et al. Deficiency of the human mitochondrial transcription factor h-mtTFA in infantile mitochondrial myopathy is associated with mtDNA depletion. Hum Mol Genet 1994;3:1763–1769.

110. Larsson NG, Wang J, Wilhelmsson H, et al. Mitochondrial transcription factor A is necessary for mtDNA maintenance and embryogenesis in mice. Nat Genet 1998;18:231–236.

111. Bardosi A, Creutzfeldt W, DiMauro S, et al. Myo-, neuro-, gastrointestinal encephalopathy (MNGIE syndrome) due to partial deficiency of cytochrome-c-oxidase. A new mitochondrial multisystem disorder. Acta Neuropathol 1987;74:248–258.

112. Hirano M, Silvestri G, Blake DM, et al. Mitochondrial neurogastrointestinal encephalomyopathy (MNGIE): clinical, biochemical, and genetic features of an autosomal recessive mitochondrial disorder. Neurology 1994;44:721–727.

113. Hirano M, Garcia-de-Yebenes J, Jones AC, et al. Mitochondrial neurogastrointestinal encephalomyopathy syndrome maps to chromosome 22q13.32-qter. Am J Hum Genet 1998;63:526–533.

114. Nishino I, Spinazzola A, Hirano M. Thymidine phosphorylase gene mutations in MNGIE: a human mitochondrial disorder. Science 1999;283:689–692.

115. Harding BN. Progressive neuronal degeneration of childhood with liver disease (Alpers-Huttenlocher syndrome): a personal review. J Child Neurol 1990;5:273–287.

116. Boyd SG, Harden A, Egger J, et al. Progressive neuronal degeneration of childhood with liver disease ("Alpers' disease"): characteristic neurophysiological features. Neuropediatrics 1986;17:75–80.

117. Harding BN, Alsanjari N, Smith SJ, et al. Progressive neuronal degeneration of childhood with liver disease (Alpers' disease) presenting in young adults. J Neurol Neurosurg Psychiatry 1995;58:320–325.

118. Prick MJ, Gabreels FJ, Renier WO, et al. Progressive infantile poliodystrophy. Association with disturbed pyruvate oxidation in muscle and liver. Arch Neurol 1981;38:767–772.
119. Prick MJ, Gabreels FJ, Trijbels JM, et al. Progressive poliodystrophy (Alpers' disease) with a defect in cytochrome aa3 in muscle: a report of two unrelated patients. Clin Neurol Neurosurg 1983;85:57–70.
120. Chabrol B, Mancini J, Chretien D, et al. Valproate-induced hepatic failure in a case of cytochrome c oxidase deficiency. Eur J Pediatr 1994;153:133–135.
121. Morris AA, Singh Kler R, Perry RH, et al. Respiratory chain dysfunction in progressive neuronal degeneration of childhood with liver disease. J Child Neurol 1996;11:417–419.
122. Huttenlocher PR, Solitare GB, Adams G. Infantile diffuse cerebral degeneration with hepatic cirrhosis. Arch Neurol 1976;33:186–192.
123. Munnich A, Rotig A, Chretien D, et al. Clinical presentations and laboratory investigations in respiratory chain deficiency. Eur J Pediatr 1996;155:262–274.
124. Pastores GM, Santorelli FM, Shanske S, et al. Leigh syndrome and hypertrophic cardiomyopathy in an infant with a mitochondrial DNA point mutation (T8993G). Am J Med Genet 1994;50:265–271.
125. Takei Y, Ikeda S, Yanagisawa N, et al. Multiple mitochondrial DNA deletions in a patient with mitochondrial myopathy and cardiomyopathy but no ophthalmoplegia. Muscle Nerve 1995;18: 1321–1325.
126. Suomalainen A, Paetau A, Leinonen H, et al. Inherited idiopathic dilated cardiomyopathy with multiple deletions of mitochondrial DNA. Lancet 1992;340:1319–1320.
127. Bohlega S, Tanji K, Santorelli FM, et al. Multiple mitochondrial DNA deletions associated with autosomal recessive ophthalmoplegia and severe cardiomyopathy. Neurology 1996;46:1329–1334.
128. Turner LF, Kaddoura S, Harrington D, et al. Mitochondrial DNA in idiopathic cardiomyopathy. Eur Heart J 1998;191725–191729.
129. Sengers RC, Trijbels JM, Willems JL, et al. Congenital cataract and mitochondrial myopathy of skeletal and heart muscle associated with lactic acidosis after exercise. J Pediatr 1975;86:873–880.
130. Smeitink J, Huizing M, Ruitenbeek W, et al. Adenine nucleotide translocator deficiency in a patient with fatal congenital cardiomyopathy, cataract and mitochondrial myopathy. J Inherit Metab Dis 1997;20:7.
131. Graham BH, Waymire KG, Cottrell B, et al. A mouse model for mitochondrial myopathy and cardiomyopathy resulting from a deficiency in the heart/muscle isoform of the adenine nucleotide translocator. Nat Genet 1997;16:226–234.
132. Pearson HA, Lobel JS, Kocoshis SA, et al. A new syndrome of refractory sideroblastic anemia with vacuolization of marrow precursors and exocrine pancreatic dysfunction. J Pediatr 1979;95:976–984.
133. Rotig A, Colonna M, Bonnefont JP, et al. Mitochondrial DNA deletion in Pearson's marrow/pancreas syndrome. Lancet 1989;1:902–903.
134. Bernes SM, Bacino C, Prezant TR, et al. Identical mitochondrial DNA deletion in mother with progressive external ophthalmoplegia and son with Pearson marrow-pancreas syndrome. J Pediatr 1993;123:598–602.
135. Rotig A, Bourgeron T, Chretien D, et al. Spectrum of mitochondrial DNA rearrangements in the Pearson marrow-pancreas syndrome. Hum Mol Genet 1995;4:1327–1330.
136. Larsson NG, Holme E, Kristiansson B, et al. Progressive increase of the mutated mitochondrial DNA fraction in Kearns-Sayre syndrome. Pediatr Res 1990;28:131–136.
137. McShane MA, Hammans SR, Sweeney M, et al. Pearson syndrome and mitochondrial encephalomyopathy in a patient with a deletion of mtDNA. Am J Hum Genet 1991;48:39–42.
138. Gattermann N, Retzlaff S, Wang YL, et al. A heteroplasmic point mutation of mitochondrial tRNALeu(CUN) in non-lymphoid haemopoietic cell lineages from a patient with acquired idiopathic sideroblastic anaemia. Br J Haematol 1996;93:845–855.
139. Gattermann N, Retzlaff S, Wang YL, et al. Heteroplasmic point mutations of mitochondrial DNA affecting subunit I of cytochrome c oxidase in two patients with acquired idiopathic sideroblastic anemia. Blood 1997;90:4961–4972.
140. Tuckfield A, Ratnaike S, Hussein S, et al. A novel form of hereditary sideroblastic anaemia with macrocytosis. Br J Haematol 1997;97:279–285.
141. Casademont J, Barrientos A, Cardellach F, et al. Multiple deletions of mtDNA in two brothers with sideroblastic anemia and mitochondrial myopathy and in their asymptomatic mother. Hum Mol Genet 1994;3:1945–1949.
142. Inbal A, Avissar N, Shaklai M, et al. Myopathy, lactic acidosis, and sideroblastic anemia: a new syndrome. Am J Med Genet 1995;55:372–378.
143. Niaudet P, Rotig A. Renal involvement in mitochondrial cytopathies. Pediatr Nephrol 1996;10: 368–373.
144. Goto Y, Itami N, Kajii N, et al. Renal tubular involvement mimicking Bartter syndrome in a patient with Kearns-Sayre syndrome. J Pediatr 1990;116:904–910.

145. van den Ouweland JM, Lemkes HH, Ruitenbeek W, et al. Mutation in mitochondrial tRNA(Leu)(UUR) gene in a large pedigree with maternally transmitted type II diabetes mellitus and deafness. Nat Genet 1992;1:368–371.
146. Ballinger SW, Shoffner JM, Hedaya EV, et al. Maternally transmitted diabetes and deafness associated with a 10.4 kb mitochondrial DNA deletion. Nat Genet 1992;1:11–15.
147. Rotig A, Cormier V, Chatelain P, et al. Deletion of mitochondrial DNA in a case of early-onset diabetes mellitus, optic atrophy, and deafness (Wolfram syndrome, MIM 222300). J Clin Invest 1993;91:1095–1098.
148. Barrientos A, Volpini V, Casademont J, et al. A nuclear defect in the 4p16 region predisposes to multiple mitochondrial DNA deletions in families with Wolfram syndrome. J Clin Invest 1996;97:1570–1576.
149. Verma A, Piccoli DA, Bonilla E, et al. A novel mitochondrial G8313A mutation associated with prominent initial gastrointestinal symptoms and progressive encephaloneuropathy. Pediatr Res 1997;42:448–454.
150. Cormier Daire V, Bonnefont JP, Rustin P, et al. Mitochondrial DNA rearrangements with onset as chronic diarrhea with villous atrophy. J Pediatr 1994;124:63–70.
151. Cormier Daire V, Chretien D, Rustin P, et al. Neonatal and delayed-onset liver involvement in disorders of oxidative phosphorylation. J Pediatr 1997;130:817–822.
152. Robinson BH. Human complex I deficiency: clinical spectrum and involvement of oxygen free radicals in the pathogenicity of the defect. Biochim Biophys Acta 1998;1364:271–286.
153. Trijbels JM, Ruitenbeek W, Sengers RC, et al. Benign mitochondrial encephalomyopathy in a patient with complex I deficiency. J Inherit Metab Dis 1996;19:149–152.
154. van den Heuvel L, Ruitenbeek W, Smeets R, et al. Demonstration of a new pathogenic mutation in human complex I deficiency: a 5-bp duplication in the nuclear gene encoding the 18-kD (AQDQ) subunit. Am J Hum Genet 1998;62:262–268.
155. Mourmans J, Wendel U, Bentlage HA, et al. Clinical heterogeneity in respiratory chain complex III deficiency in childhood. J Neurol Sci 1997;149:111–117.
156. Caruso U, Adami A, Bertini E, et al. Respiratory-chain and pyruvate metabolism defects: Italian collaborative survey on 72 patients. J Inherit Metab Dis 1996;19:143–148.
157. Haller RG, Lewis SF, Estabrook RW, et al. Exercise intolerance, lactic acidosis, and abnormal cardiopulmonary regulation in exercise associated with adult skeletal muscle cytochrome c oxidase deficiency. J Clin Invest 1989;84:155–161.
158. DiMauro S, Hirano M, Bonilla E, et al. Cytochrome Oxidase Deficiency: Progress and Problems. In AHV Schapira, S DiMauro (eds), Mitochondrial Disorders in Neurology. Oxford, UK: Butterworth–Heinemann, 1994;91–115.
159. Van Biervliet JP, Bruinvis L, Ketting D, et al. Hereditary mitochondrial myopathy with lactic acidemia, a De Toni-Fanconi-Debre syndrome, and a defective respiratory chain in voluntary striated muscles. Pediatr Res 1977;11:1088–1093.
160. DiMauro S, Nicholson JF, Hays AP, et al. Benign infantile mitochondrial myopathy due to reversible cytochrome c oxidase deficiency. Ann Neurol 1983;14:226–234.
161. Tritschler HJ, Bonilla E, Lombes A, et al. Differential diagnosis of fatal and benign cytochrome c oxidase-deficient myopathies of infancy: an immunohistochemical approach. Neurology 1991;41:300–305.
162. Rimoldi M, Bottacchi E, Rossi L, et al. Cytochrome-C-oxidase deficiency in muscles of a floppy infant without mitochondrial myopathy. J Neurol 1982;227:201–207.
163. Tatuch Y, Robinson BH. The mitochondrial DNA mutation at 8993 associated with NARP slows the rate of ATP synthesis in isolated lymphoblast mitochondria. Biochem Biophys Res Commun 1993;192:124–128.
164. Holme E, Greter J, Jacobson CE, et al. Mitochondrial ATP-synthase deficiency in a child with 3-methylglutaconic aciduria. Pediatr Res 1992;32:731–735.
165. Bentlage HA, Wendel U, Schagger H, et al. Lethal infantile mitochondrial disease with isolated complex I deficiency in fibroblasts but with combined complex I and IV deficiencies in muscle. Neurology 1996;47:243–248.
166. Sperl W, Ruitenbeek W, Sengers RC, et al. Combined deficiencies of the pyruvate dehydrogenase complex and enzymes of the respiratory chain in mitochondrial myopathies. Eur J Pediatr 1992;151:192–195.
167. Robinson BH, Chow W, Petrova Benedict R, et al. Fatal combined defects in mitochondrial multienzyme complexes in two siblings. Eur J Pediatr 1992;151:347–352.
168. Ogasahara S, Engel AG, Frens D, et al. Muscle coenzyme Q deficiency in familial mitochondrial encephalomyopathy. Proc Natl Acad Sci U S A 1989;86:2379–2382.

169. Sobreira C, Hirano M, Shanske S, et al. Mitochondrial encephalomyopathy with coenzyme Q_{10} deficiency. Neurology 1997;48:1238–1243.
170. Nyhan WL. Abnormalities of fatty acid oxidation. N Engl J Med 1988;319:1344–1346.
171. Waber LJ, Valle D, Neill C, et al. Carnitine deficiency presenting as familial cardiomyopathy: a treatable defect in carnitine transport. J Pediatr 1982;101:700–705.
172. Treem WR, Stanley CA, Finegold DN, et al. Primary carnitine deficiency due to a failure of carnitine transport in kidney, muscle, and fibroblasts. N Engl J Med 1988;319:1331–1336.
173. Rinaldo P, Stanley CA, Hsu BY, et al. Sudden neonatal death in carnitine transporter deficiency. J Pediatr 1997;131:304–305.
174. Shoji Y, Koizumi A, Kayo T, et al. Evidence for linkage of human primary systemic carnitine deficiency with D5S436: a novel gene locus on chromosome 5q. Am J Hum Genet 1998;63:101–108.
175. Lamhonwah AM, Tein I. Carnitine uptake defect: frameshift mutations in the human plasmalemmal carnitine transporter gene. Biochem Biophys Res Commun 1998;2:396–401.
176. Nezu J, Tamai I, Oku A, et al. Primary systemic carnitine deficiency is caused by mutations in a gene encoding sodium ion-dependent carnitine transporter. Nat Genet 1999;1:91–94.
177. Wang Y, Ye J, Ganapathy V, Longo N. Mutations in the organic cation/carnitine transporter OCTN2 in primary carnitine deficiency. Proc Natl Acad Sci U S A 1999;5:2356–2360.
178. Tang NLS, Ganapathy V, Wu X, et al. Mutations of OCTN2, an organic caton/carnitine transporter, lead to deficient cellular carnitine uptake in primary carnitine deficiency. Hum Mol Genet 1999;4:655–660.
179. Bougneres PF, Saudubray JM, Marsac C, et al. Fasting hypoglycemia resulting from hepatic carnitine palmitoyl transferase deficiency. J Pediatr 1981;98:742–746.
180. Britton CH, Schultz RA, Zhang B, et al. Human liver mitochondrial carnitine palmitoyltransferase I: characterization of its cDNA and chromosomal localization and partial analysis of the gene. Proc Natl Acad Sci U S A 1995;92:1984–1988.
181. DiMauro S, DiMauro PM. Muscle carnitine palmityltransferase deficiency and myoglobinuria. Science 1973;182:929–931.
182. Taroni F, Verderio E, Dworzak F, et al. Identification of a common mutation in the carnitine palmitoyltransferase II gene in familial recurrent myoglobinuria patients. Nat Genet 1993;4:314–320.
183. Stanley CA, Hale DE, Berry GT, et al. Brief report: a deficiency of carnitine-acylcarnitine translocase in the inner mitochondrial membrane. N Engl J Med 1992;327:19–23.
184. Pande SV, Brivet M, Slama A, et al. Carnitine-acylcarnitine translocase deficiency with severe hypoglycemia and auriculo ventricular block. Translocase assay in permeabilized fibroblasts. J Clin Invest 1993;91:1247–1252.
185. Chalmers RA, Stanley CA, English N, et al. Mitochondrial carnitine-acylcarnitine translocase deficiency presenting as sudden neonatal death. J Pediatr 1997;131:220–225.
186. Morris AA, Olpin SE, Brivet M, et al. A patient with carnitine-acylcarnitine translocase deficiency with a mild phenotype. J Pediatr 1998;132:514–516.
187. Indiveri C, Iacobazzi V, Giangregorio N, et al. The mitochondrial carnitine carrier protein: cDNA cloning, primary structure and comparison with other mitochondrial transport proteins. Biochem J 1997;321:713–719.
188. Huizing M, Iacobazzi V, Ijlst L, et al. Cloning of the human carnitine-acylcarnitine carrier cDNA and identification of the molecular defect in a patient. Am J Hum Genet 1997;61:1239–1245.
189. Coates PM, Hale DE, Finocchiaro G, et al. Genetic deficiency of short-chain acyl-coenzyme A dehydrogenase in cultured fibroblasts from a patient with muscle carnitine deficiency and severe skeletal muscle weakness. J Clin Invest 1988;81:171–175.
190. Stanley CA. Dissecting the spectrum of fatty acid oxidation disorders. J Pediatr 1998;132:384–386.
191. Naito E, Indo Y, Tanaka K. Identification of two variant short chain acyl-coenzyme A dehydrogenase alleles, each containing a different point mutation in a patient with short chain acyl-coenzyme A dehydrogenase deficiency. J Clin Invest 1990;85:1575–1582.
192. Tein I, De Vivo DC, Hale DE, et al. Short-chain L-3-hydroxyacyl-CoA dehydrogenase deficiency in muscle: a new cause for recurrent myoglobinuria and encephalopathy. Ann Neurol 1991;30:415–419.
193. Bennett MJ, Weinberger MJ, Kobori JA, et al. Mitochondrial short-chain L-3-hydroxyacyl-coenzyme A dehydrogenase deficiency: a new defect of fatty acid oxidation. Pediatr Res 1996;39:185–188.
194. Vredendaal PJ, van den Berg IE, Malingre HE, et al. Human short-chain L-3-hydroxyacyl-CoA dehydrogenase: cloning and characterization of the coding sequence. Biochem Biophys Res Commun 1996;223:718–723.
195. Roe CR, Coates PM. Mitochondrial Fatty Acid Oxidation Disorders. In CR Scriver, AL Beaudet, WS Sly, D Valle (eds), The Metabolic and Molecular Bases of Inherited Disease (7th ed). New York: McGraw-Hill, 1995;1501–1534.

196. Yokota I, Indo Y, Coates PM, et al. Molecular basis of medium chain acyl-coenzyme A dehydrogenase deficiency. An A to G transition at position 985 that causes a lysine-304 to glutamate substitution in the mature protein is the single prevalent mutation. J Clin Invest 1990;86:1000–1003.
197. Hale DE, Batshaw ML, Coates PM, et al. Long-chain acyl coenzyme A dehydrogenase deficiency: an inherited cause of nonketotic hypoglycemia. Pediatr Res 1985;19:666–671.
198. Yamaguchi S, Indo Y, Coates PM, et al. Identification of very-long-chain acyl-CoA dehydrogenase deficiency in three patients previously diagnosed with long-chain acyl-CoA dehydrogenase deficiency. Pediatr Res 1993;34:111–113.
199. Indo Y, Yang-Feng T, Glassberg R, et al. Molecular cloning and nucleotide sequence of cDNAs encoding human long-chain acyl-CoA dehydrogenase and assignment of the location of its gene (ACADL) to chromosome 2. Genomics 1991;11:609–620. [Published erratum appears in Genomics 1992;12:626.]
200. Glasgow AM, Engel AG, Bier DM, et al. Hypoglycemia, hepatic dysfunction, muscle weakness, cardiomyopathy, free carnitine deficiency and long-chain acylcarnitine excess responsive to medium chain triglyceride diet. Pediatr Res 1983;17:319–326.
201. Rocchiccioli F, Wanders RJ, Aubourg P, et al. Deficiency of long-chain 3-hydroxyacyl-CoA dehydrogenase: a cause of lethal myopathy and cardiomyopathy in early childhood. Pediatr Res 1990;28:657–662.
202. Wanders RJ, Duran M, Ijlst L, et al. Sudden infant death and long-chain 3-hydroxyacyl-CoA dehydrogenase. Lancet 1989;2:52–53.
203. Ijlst L, Wanders RJ, Ushikubo S, et al. Molecular basis of long-chain 3-hydroxyacyl-CoA dehydrogenase deficiency: identification of the major disease-causing mutation in the alpha-subunit of the mitochondrial trifunctional protein. Biochim Biophys Acta 1994;1215:347–350.
204. Treem WR, Rinaldo P, Hale DE, et al. Acute fatty liver of pregnancy and long-chain 3-hydroxyacyl-coenzyme A dehydrogenase deficiency. Hepatology 1994;19:339–345.
205. Aoyama T, Uchida Y, Kelley RI, et al. A novel disease with deficiency of mitochondrial very-long-chain acyl-CoA dehydrogenase. Biochem Biophys Res Commun 1993;191:1369–1372.
206. Bertrand C, Largilliere C, Zabot MT, et al. Very long chain acyl-CoA dehydrogenase deficiency: identification of a new inborn error of mitochondrial fatty acid oxidation in fibroblasts. Biochim Biophys Acta 1993;1180:327–329.
207. Ogilvie I, Pourfarzam M, Jackson S, et al. Very long-chain acyl coenzyme A dehydrogenase deficiency presenting with exercise-induced myoglobinuria. Neurology 1994;44:467–473.
208. Smelt AH, Poorthuis BJ, Onkenhout W, et al. Very long chain acyl-coenzyme A dehydrogenase deficiency with adult onset. Ann Neurol 1998;43:540–544.
209. Andresen BS, Bross P, Vianey Saban C, et al. Cloning and characterization of human very-long-chain acyl-CoA dehydrogenase cDNA, chromosomal assignment of the gene and identification in four patients of nine different mutations within the VLCAD gene. Hum Mol Genet 1996;5:461–472. [Published erratum appears in Hum Mol Genet 1996;5:1390.]
210. Frerman FE, Goodman SI. Nuclear-Encoded Defects of the Mitochondrial Respiratory Chain, Including Glutaric Acidemia Type II. In CR Scriver, AL Beaudet, WS Sly, D Valle (eds), The Metabolic and Molecular Bases of Inherited Disease (7th ed). New York: McGraw-Hill, 1995;1611–1629.
211. Brown GK, Otero LJ, LeGris M, et al. Pyruvate dehydrogenase deficiency. J Med Genet 1994;31:875–879.
212. Kerr DS. Lactic acidosis and mitochondrial disorders. Clin Biochem 1991;24:331–336.
213. Robinson BH, MacMillan H, Petrova-Benedict R, et al. Variable clinical presentation in patients with defective E1 component of pyruvate dehydrogenase complex. J Pediatr 1987;111:525–533.
214. Robinson BH, Taylor J, Sherwood WG. Deficiency of dihydrolipoyl dehydrogenase (a component of the pyruvate and alpha-ketoglutarate dehydrogenase complexes): a cause of congenital chronic lactic acidosis in infancy. Pediatr Res 1977;11:1198–1202.
215. Robinson BH, Sherwood WG, Kahler S, et al. Lipoamide dehydrogenase deficiency. N Engl J Med 1981;304:53–54.
216. Munnich A, Saudubray JM, Taylor J, et al. Congenital lactic acidosis, alpha-ketoglutaric aciduria and variant form of maple syrup urine disease due to a single enzyme defect: dihydrolipoyl dehydrogenase deficiency. Acta Paediatr 1982;71:167–171.
217. Matalon R, Stumpf DA, Michals K, et al. Lipoamide dehydrogenase deficiency with primary lactic acidosis: favorable response to treatment with oral lipoic acid. J Pediatr 1984;104:65–69.
218. Sakaguchi Y, Yoshino M, Aramaki S, et al. Dihydrolipoyl dehydrogenase deficiency: a therapeutic trial with branched-chain amino acid restriction. Eur J Pediatr 1986;145:271–274.
219. Elpeleg ON, Ruitenbeek W, Jakobs C, et al. Congenital lacticacidemia caused by lipoamide dehydrogenase deficiency with favorable outcome. J Pediatr 1995;126:72–74.

220. Craigen WJ. Leigh disease with deficiency of lipoamide dehydrogenase: treatment failure with dichloroacetate. Pediatr Neurol 1996;14:69–71.

221. Hong YS, Kerr DS, Craigen WJ, et al. Identification of two mutations in a compound heterozygous child with dihydrolipoamide dehydrogenase deficiency. Hum Mol Genet 1996;5:1925–1930.

222. Elpeleg ON, Saada AB, Shaag A, et al. Lipoamide dehydrogenase deficiency: a new cause for recurrent myoglobinuria. Muscle Nerve 1997;20:238–240.

223. Robinson BH, MacKay N, Chun K, et al. Disorders of pyruvate carboxylase and the pyruvate dehydrogenase complex. J Inherit Metab Dis 1996;19:452–462.

224. Kohlschutter A, Behbehani A, Langenbeck U, et al. A familial progressive neurodegenerative disease with 2-oxoglutaric aciduria. Eur J Pediatr 1982;138:32–37.

225. Whelan DT, Hill RE, McClorry S. Fumaric aciduria: a new organic aciduria, associated with mental retardation and speech impairment. Clin Chim Acta 1983;132:301–308.

226. Hall RE, Henriksson KG, Lewis SF, et al. Mitochondrial myopathy with succinate dehydrogenase and aconitase deficiency. Abnormalities of several iron-sulfur proteins. J Clin Invest 1993;92:2660–2666.

227. Bonnefont JP, Chretien D, Rustin P, et al. Alpha-ketoglutarate dehydrogenase deficiency presenting as congenital lactic acidosis. J Pediatr 1992;121:255–258.

228. Guffon N, Lopez Mediavilla C, Dumoulin R, et al. 2-Ketoglutarate dehydrogenase deficiency, a rare cause of primary hyperlactataemia: report of a new case. J Inherit Metab Dis 1993;16:821–830.

229. Zinn AB, Kerr DS, Hoppel CL. Fumarase deficiency: a new cause of mitochondrial encephalomyopathy. N Engl J Med 1986;315:469–475.

230. Petrova Benedict R, Robinson BH, Stacey TE, et al. Deficient fumarase activity in an infant with fumaricacidemia and its distribution between the different forms of the enzyme seen on isoelectric focusing. Am J Hum Genet 1987;40:257–266.

231. Walker V, Mills GA, Hall MA, et al. A fourth case of fumarase deficiency. J Inherit Metab Dis 1989;12:331–332.

232. Gellera C, Uziel G, Rimoldi M, et al. Fumarase deficiency is an autosomal recessive encephalopathy affecting both the mitochondrial and the cytosolic enzymes. Neurology 1990;40:495–499.

233. Remes AM, Rantala H, Hiltunen JK, et al. Fumarase deficiency: two siblings with enlarged cerebral ventricles and polyhydramnios in utero. Pediatrics 1992;89:730–734.

234. Bourgeron T, Chretien D, Poggi Bach J, et al. Mutation of the fumarase gene in two siblings with progressive encephalopathy and fumarase deficiency. J Clin Invest 1994;93:2514–2518.

235. Narayanan V, Diven W, Ahdab Barmada M. Congenital fumarase deficiency presenting with hypotonia and areflexia. J Child Neurol 1996;11:252–255.

236. Coughlin EM, Christensen E, Kunz PL, et al. Molecular analysis and prenatal diagnosis of human fumarase deficiency. Mol Genet Metab 1998;63:254–262.

237. King MP, Attardi G. Human cells lacking mtDNA: repopulation with exogenous mitochondria by complementation. Science 1989;246:500–503.

238. Lertrit P, Kapsa RM, Jean-Francois MJ, et al. Mitochondrial DNA polymorphism in disease: a possible contributor to respiratory dysfunction. Hum Mol Genet 1994;3:1973–1981.

239. Holt IJ, Dunbar DR, Jacobs HT. Behaviour of a population of partially duplicated mitochondrial DNA molecules in cell culture: segregation, maintenance and recombination dependent upon nuclear background. Hum Mol Genet 1997;6:1251–1260.

240. Prezant TR, Agapian JV, Bohlman MC, et al. Mitochondrial ribosomal RNA mutation associated with both antibiotic-induced and non-syndromic deafness. Nat Genet 1993;4:289–294.

241. Holt IJ, Harding AE, Morgan-Hughes JA. Deletions of muscle mitochondrial DNA in mitochondrial myopathies: sequence analysis and possible mechanisms. Nucleic Acids Res 1989;17:4465–4469.

242. Schon EA, Rizzuto R, Moraes CT, et al. A direct repeat is a hotspot for large-scale deletion of human mitochondrial DNA. Science 1989;244:346–349.

243. Mita S, Rizzuto R, Moraes CT, et al. Recombination via flanking direct repeats is a major cause of large-scale deletions of human mitochondrial DNA. Nucleic Acids Res 1990;18:561–567.

244. Chen X, Prosser R, Simonetti S, et al. Rearranged mitochondrial genomes are present in human oocytes. Am J Hum Genet 1995;57:239–247.

245. Hayashi J, Ohta S, Kikuchi A, et al. Introduction of disease-related mitochondrial DNA deletions into HeLa cells lacking mitochondrial DNA results in mitochondrial dysfunction. Proc Natl Acad Sci U S A 1991;88:10614–10618.

246. Mita S, Schmidt B, Schon EA, et al. Detection of "deleted" mitochondrial genomes in cytochrome-c oxidase-deficient muscle fibers of a patient with Kearns-Sayre syndrome. Proc Natl Acad Sci U S A 1989;86:9509–9513.

247. Poulton J, Deadman ME, Gardiner RM. Duplications of mitochondrial DNA in mitochondrial myopathy. Lancet 1989;1:236–240.

248. Superti-Furga A, Schoenle E, Tuchschmid P, et al. Pearson bone marrow-pancreas syndrome with insulin-dependent diabetes, progressive renal tubulopathy, organic aciduria and elevated fetal haemoglobin caused by deletion and duplication of mitochondrial DNA. Eur J Pediatr 1993;152:44–50.

249. Dunbar DR, Moonie PA, Swingler RJ, et al. Maternally transmitted partial direct tandem duplication of mitochondrial DNA associated with diabetes mellitus. Hum Mol Genet 1993;2:1619–1624.

250. Brockington M, Sweeney MG, Hammans SR, et al. A tandem duplication in the D-loop of human mitochondrial DNA is associated with deletions in mitochondrial myopathies. Nat Genet 1993;4:67–71.

251. Poulton J, Deadman ME, Bindoff L, et al. Families of mtDNA re-arrangements can be detected in patients with mtDNA deletions: duplications may be a transient intermediate form. Hum Mol Genet 1993;2:23–30.

252. Rotig A, Bessis JL, Romero N, et al. Maternally inherited duplication of the mitochondrial genome in a syndrome of proximal tubulopathy, diabetes mellitus, and cerebellar ataxia. Am J Hum Genet 1992;50:364–370.

253. Manfredi G, Vu T, Bonilla E, et al. Association of myopathy with large-scale mitochondrial DNA duplications and deletions: which is pathogenic? Ann Neurol 1997;42:180–188.

254. Boulet L, Karpati G, Shoubridge EA. Distribution and threshold expression of the tRNA(Lys) mutation in skeletal muscle of patients with myoclonic epilepsy and ragged-red fibers (MERRF). Am J Hum Genet 1992;51:1187–1200.

255. Chomyn A, Meola G, Bresolin N, et al. In vitro genetic transfer of protein synthesis and respiration defects to mitochondrial DNA-less cells with myopathy-patient mitochondria. Mol Cell Biol 1991;11:2236–2244.

256. Masucci JP, Schon EA. tRNA processing in human mitochondrial disorders. Mol Biol Rep 1995;22:187–193.

257. Enriquez JA, Chomyn A, Attardi G. MtDNA mutation in MERRF syndrome causes defective aminoacylation of tRNA(Lys) and premature translation termination. Nat Genet 1995;10:47–55.

258. King MP, Koga Y, Davidson M, et al. Defects in mitochondrial protein synthesis and respiratory chain activity segregate with the tRNA(Leu(UUR)) mutation associated with mitochondrial myopathy, encephalopathy, lactic acidosis, and strokelike episodes. Mol Cell Biol 1992;12:480–490.

259. Koga Y, Davidson M, Schon EA, et al. Analysis of cybrids harboring MELAS mutations in the mitochondrial tRNA (Leu(UUR)) gene. Muscle Nerve 1995;3:S119–S123.

260. Kaufmann P, Koga Y, Shanske S, et al. Mitochondrial DNA and RNA processing in MELAS. Ann Neurol 1996;40:172–180.

261. Hess JF, Parisi MA, Bennett JL, et al. Impairment of mitochondrial transcription termination by a point mutation associated with the MELAS subgroup of mitochondrial encephalomyopathies. Nature 1991;351:236–239.

262. Hammans SR, Sweeney MG, Wicks DA, et al. A molecular genetic study of focal histochemical defects in mitochondrial encephalomyopathies. Brain 1992;115:343–365. [Published erratum appears in Brain 1993;116(Pt 1):following 306.]

263. Moraes CT, Ricci E, Bonilla E, et al. The mitochondrial tRNA(Leu(UUR)) mutation in mitochondrial encephalomyopathy, lactic acidosis, and strokelike episodes (MELAS): genetic, biochemical, and morphological correlations in skeletal muscle. Am J Hum Genet 1992;50:934–949.

264. Moraes CT, Ciacci F, Bonilla E, et al. Two novel pathogenic mitochondrial DNA mutations affecting organelle number and protein synthesis. Is the tRNA(Leu(UUR)) gene an etiologic hot spot? J Clin Invest 1993;92:2906–2915.

265. Santorelli FM, Tanji K, Kulikova R, et al. Identification of a novel mutation in the mtDNA ND5 gene associated with MELAS. Biochem Biophys Res Commun 1997;238:326–328.

266. Trounce I, Neill S, Wallace DC. Cytoplasmic transfer of the mtDNA nt 8993 T→G (ATP6) point mutation associated with Leigh syndrome into mtDNA-less cells demonstrates cosegregation with a decrease in state III respiration and ADP/O ratio. Proc Natl Acad Sci U S A 1994;91:8334–8338.

267. Manfredi G, Schon EA, Moraes CT, et al. A new mutation associated with MELAS is located in a mitochondrial DNA polypeptide-coding gene. Neuromuscul Disord 1995;5:391–398.

268. Hanna MG, Nelson IP, Rahman S, et al. Cytochrome c oxidase deficiency associated with the first stop-codon point mutation in human mtDNA. Am J Hum Genet 1998;63:29–36.

269. Comi GP, Bordoni A, Salani S, et al. Cytochrome c oxidase subunit I microdeletion in a patient with motor neuron disease. Ann Neurol 1998;43:110–116.

270. Rahman S, Hanna MG, Leonard JV, et al. Cytochrome *c* oxidase (COX) deficiency caused by a novel point mutation in the COX subunit II gene [abstract]. Muscle Nerve 1998;7:S177.

271. Brown RM, Brown GK. Complementation analysis of systemic cytochrome oxidase deficiency presenting as Leigh syndrome. J Inherit Metab Dis 1996;19:752–760.

272. Munaro M, Tiranti V, Sandona D, et al. A single cell complementation class is common to several cases of cytochrome c oxidase-defective Leigh's syndrome. Hum Mol Genet 1997;6:221–228.

273. Adams PL, Lightowlers RN, Turnbull DM. Molecular analysis of cytochrome c oxidase deficiency in Leigh's syndrome. Ann Neurol 1997;41:268–270.

274. Lee N, Morin C, Mitchell G, et al. Saguenay Lac Saint Jean cytochrome oxidase deficiency: sequence analysis of nuclear encoded COX subunits, chromosomal localization and a sequence anomaly in subunit VIc. Biochim Biophys Acta 1998;1406:1–4.

275. Nashef L, Lane RJ. Screening for mitochondrial cytopathies: the sub-anaerobic threshold exercise test (SATET). J Neurol Neurosurg Psychiatry 1989;52:1090–1094.

276. Jackson MJ, Schaefer JA, Johnson MA, et al. Presentation and clinical investigation of mitochondrial respiratory chain disease. A study of 51 patients. Brain 1995;118:339–357.

277. Schwartz WJ, Hutchison HT, Berg BO. Computerized tomography in subacute necrotizing encephalomyelopathy (Leigh disease). Ann Neurol 1981;10:268–271.

278. Koch TK, Yee MH, Hutchinson HT, et al. Magnetic resonance imaging in subacute necrotizing encephalomyelopathy (Leigh's disease). Ann Neurol 1986;19:605–607.

279. Wray SH, Provenzale JM, Johns DR, et al. MRI of the brain in mitochondrial myopathy. AJNR Am J Neuroradiol 1995;16:1167–1173.

280. Valanne L, Ketonen L, Majander A, et al. Neuroradiologic findings in children with mitochondrial disorders. AJNR Am J Neuroradiol 1998;19:369–377.

281. Matthews PM, Allaire C, Shoubridge EA, et al. In vivo muscle magnetic resonance spectroscopy in the clinical investigation of mitochondrial disease. Neurology 1991;41:114–120.

282. Barkovich AJ, Good WV, Koch TK, et al. Mitochondrial disorders: analysis of their clinical and imaging characteristics. Am J Neuroradiol 1993;14:1119–1137.

283. Tulinius MH, Hagne I. EEG findings in children and adolescents with mitochondrial encephalomyopathies: a study of 25 cases. Brain Dev 1991;13:167–173.

284. Chu CC, Huang CC, Fang W, et al. Peripheral neuropathy in mitochondrial encephalomyopathies. Eur Neurol 1997;37:110–115.

285. Rosing HS, Hopkins LC, Wallace DC, et al. Maternally inherited mitochondrial myopathy and myoclonic epilepsy. Ann Neurol 1985;17:228–237.

286. Müller-Höcker J. Cytochrome c oxidase deficient fibres in the limb muscle and diaphragm in man without muscular disease: an age related alteration. J Neurol Sci 1990;100:14–21.

287. Berkovic SF, Carpenter S, Evans A, et al. Myoclonus epilepsy and ragged-red fibres (MERFF) 1. A clinical, pathological, biochemical, magnetic resonance spectrographic and positron emission tomographic study. Brain 1989;112:1231–1260.

288. Stadhouders A, Jap P, Wallimann T. Biochemical nature of mitochondrial crystals. J Neurol Sci 1990;98:304.

289. Moraes CT, Andreetta F, Bonilla E, et al. Replication-competent human mitochondrial DNA lacking the heavy-strand promoter region. Mol Cell Biol 1991;11:1631–1642.

290. Moraes CT, Ricci E, Petruzzella V, et al. Molecular analysis of the muscle pathology associated the mitochondrial DNA deletions. Nat Genet 1992;1:359–367.

291. Shoubridge AE, Karpati G, Hastings KEM. Deletion mutants are functionally dominant over wild-type mitochondrial genomes in skeletal muscle fiber segments in mitochondrial disease. Cell 1990;62:43.

292. Larsson NG, Tulinius MH, Holme E, et al. Segregation and manifestations of the mtDNA tRNA(Lys) A→G(8344) mutation of myoclonus epilepsy and ragged-red fibers (MERRF) syndrome. Am J Hum Genet 1992;51:1201–1212.

293. Harding AE, Sweeney MG, Govan GG, et al. Pedigree analysis in Leber hereditary optic neuropathy families with a pathogenic mtDNA mutation. Am J Hum Genet 1995;57:77–86.

294. Harding AE, Holt IJ, Sweeney MG, et al. Prenatal diagnosis of mitochondrial DNA8993T→G disease. Am J Hum Genet 1992;50:629–633.

295. Lam CW, Lau CH, Williams JC, et al. Mitochondrial myopathy, encephalopathy, lactic acidosis and stroke-like episodes (MELAS) triggered by valproate therapy. Eur J Pediatr 1997;156:562–564.

296. Grattan-Smith PJ, Shield LK, Hopkins IJ, et al. Acute respiratory failure precipitated by general anesthesia in Leigh's syndrome. J Child Neurol 1990;5:137–141.

297. Ogle RF, Christodoulou J, Fagan E, et al. Mitochondrial myopathy with tRNA(Leu(UUR)) mutation and complex I deficiency responsive to riboflavin. J Pediatr 1997;130:138–145.

298. Takanashi J, Sugita K, Tanabe Y, et al. Dichloroacetate treatment in Leigh syndrome caused by mitochondrial DNA mutation. J Neurol Sci 1997;145:83–86.

299. Saitoh S, Momoi MY, Yamagata T, et al. Effects of dichloroacetate in three patients with MELAS. Neurology 1998;50:531–534.

300. Bresolin N, Doriguzzi C, Ponzetto C, et al. Ubidecarenone in the treatment of mitochondrial myopathies: a multi-center double-blind trial. J Neurol Sci 1990;100:70–78.
301. Matthews PM, Ford B, Dandurand RJ, et al. Coenzyme Q10 with multiple vitamins is generally ineffective in treatment of mitochondrial disease. Neurology 1993;43:884–890.
302. Stacpoole PW, Wright EC, Baumgartner TG, et al. A controlled clinical trial of dichloroacetate for treatment of lactic acidosis in adults. The Dichloroacetate-Lactic Acidosis Study Group. N Engl J Med 1992;327:1564–1569.
303. De Stefano N, Matthews PM, Ford B, et al. Short-term dichloroacetate treatment improves indices of cerebral metabolism in patients with mitochondrial disorders. Neurology 1995;45:1193–1198.
304. Taylor RW, Chinnery PF, Clark KM, et al. Treatment of mitochondrial disease. J Bioenerg Biomembr 1997;29:195–205.
305. Clark KM, Bindoff LA, Lightowlers RN, et al. Reversal of a mitochondrial DNA defect in human skeletal muscle. Nat Genet 1997;16:222–224.
306. Shoubridge EA, Johns T, Karpati G. Complete restoration of a wild-type mtDNA genotype in regenerating muscle fibres in a patient with a tRNA point mutation and mitochondrial encephalomyopathy. Hum Mol Genet 1997;6:2239–2242.
307. Sweeney MG, Bundey S, Brockington M, et al. Mitochondrial myopathy associated with sudden death in young adults and a novel mutation in the mitochondrial DNA leucine transfer RNA(UUR) gene. QJM 1993;86:709–713.
308. Chinnery PF, Johnson MA, Taylor RW, et al. A novel mitochondrial tRNA isoleucine gene mutation causing chronic progressive external ophthalmoplegia. Neurology 1997;49:1166–1168.
309. Silvestri G, Servidei S, Rana M, et al. A novel mitochondrial DNA point mutation in the tRNA(Ile) gene is associated with progressive external ophthalmoplegia. Biochem Biophys Res Commun 1996;220:623–627.
310. Taylor RW, Chinnery PF, Bates MJ, et al. A novel mitochondrial DNA point mutation in the tRNA(Ile) gene: studies in a patient presenting with chronic progressive external ophthalmoplegia and multiple sclerosis. Biochem Biophys Res Commun 1998;243:47–51.
311. Seibel P, Lauber J, Klopstock T, et al. Chronic progressive external ophthalmoplegia is associated with a novel mutation in the mitochondrial tRNA(Asn) gene. Biochem Biophys Res Commun 1994;204:482–489.
312. Hattori Y, Goto Y, Sakuta R, et al. Point mutations in mitochondrial tRNA genes: sequence analysis of chronic progressive external ophthalmoplegia (CPEO). J Neurol Sci 1994;125:50–55.
313. Fu K, Hartlen R, Johns T, et al. A novel heteroplasmic tRNAleu(CUN) mtDNA point mutation in a sporadic patient with mitochondrial encephalomyopathy segregates rapidly in skeletal muscle and suggests an approach to therapy. Hum Mol Genet 1996;5:1835–1840.
314. Taylor RW, Chinnery PF, Haldane F, et al. MELAS associated with a mutation in the valine transfer RNA gene of mitochondrial DNA. Ann Neurol 1996;40:459–462.
315. Morten KJ, Cooper JM, Brown GK, et al. A new point mutation associated with mitochondrial encephalomyopathy. Hum Mol Genet 1993;2:2081–2087.
316. Nishino I, Komatsu M, Kodama S, et al. The 3260 mutation in mitochondrial DNA can cause mitochondrial myopathy, encephalopathy, lactic acidosis, and strokelike episodes (MELAS). Muscle Nerve 1996;19:1603–1604.
317. Goto Y, Nonaka I, Horai S. A new mtDNA mutation associated with mitochondrial myopathy, encephalopathy, lactic acidosis and stroke-like episodes (MELAS). Biochim Biophys Acta 1991;1097: 238–240.
318. Goto Y, Tsugane K, Tanabe Y, et al. A new point mutation at nucleotide pair 3291 of the mitochondrial tRNA(Leu(UUR)) gene in a patient with mitochondrial myopathy, encephalopathy, lactic acidosis, and stroke-like episodes (MELAS). Biochem Biophys Res Commun 1994;202:1624–1630.
319. Manfredi G, Schon EA, Bonilla E, et al. Identification of a mutation in the mitochondrial tRNA(Cys) gene associated with mitochondrial encephalopathy. Hum Mutat 1996;7:158–163.
320. Kawarai T, Kawakami H, Kozuka K, et al. A new mitochondrial DNA mutation associated with mitochondrial myopathy: tRNAleu(UUR) 3254C-to-G. Neurology 1997;49:598–600.
321. Zeviani M, Gellera C, Antozzi C, et al. Maternally inherited myopathy and cardiomyopathy: association with mutation in mitochondrial DNA tRNA(Leu)(UUR). Lancet 1991;338:143–147.
322. Silvestri G, Santorelli FM, Shanske S, et al. A new mtDNA mutation in the tRNA(Leu(UUR)) gene associated with maternally inherited cardiomyopathy. Hum Mutat 1994;3:37–43.
323. Taniike M, Fukushima H, Yanagihara I, et al. Mitochondrial tRNAile mutation in fatal cardiomyopathy. Biochem Biophys Res Commun 1992;186:47–53.
324. Merante F, Myint T, Tein I, et al. An additional mitochondrial tRNA(Ile) point mutation (A-to-G at nucleotide 4295) causing hypertrophic cardiomyopathy. Hum Mutat 1996;8:216–222.

325. Casali C, Santorelli FM, D'Amati G, et al. A novel mtDNA point mutation in maternally inherited cardiomyopathy. Biochem Biophys Res Commun 1995;213:588–593.
326. Tanaka M, Ino H, Ohno K, et al. Mitochondrial mutation in fatal infantile cardiomyopathy. Lancet 1990;336:1452.
327. Santorelli FM, Mak SC, Vazquez Acevedo M, et al. A novel mitochondrial DNA point mutation associated with mitochondrial encephalocardiomyopathy. Biochem Biophys Res Commun 1995;216:835–840.
328. Santorelli FM, Mak SC, El Schahawi M, et al. Maternally inherited cardiomyopathy and hearing loss associated with a novel mutation in the mitochondrial tRNA(Lys) gene (G8363A). Am J Hum Genet 1996;58:933–939.
329. Merante F, Tein I, Benson L, et al. Maternally inherited hypertrophic cardiomyopathy due to a novel T-to-C transition at nucleotide 9997 in the mitochondrial tRNA(glycine) gene. Am J Hum Genet 1994;55:437–446.

8
Metabolic Myopathies: Substrate Use Defects

Salvatore DiMauro and Ronald G. Haller

The major energy sources for muscle contraction are glycogen, glucose, and fatty acids, with metabolic pathways that converge into acetyl coenzyme A (acetyl-CoA) for final intramitochondrial oxidation through the Krebs cycle and the respiratory chain (Figure 8.1). Defects of substrate use in muscle cause two main clinical presentations (Figure 8.2): (1) acute, recurrent, reversible muscle dysfunction, manifesting as exercise intolerance or myalgia with or without painful cramps (contractures), and often culminating in muscle breakdown and myoglobinuria; or (2) fixed, often progressive, weakness, sometimes simulating dystrophic or neurogenic processes. Figure 8.2 is an updated version of a similar scheme published in 1985 [1]. Only one new glycogenosis (aldolase deficiency) has been discovered in the intervening 13 years, whereas several specific defects of fatty acid oxidation have been added, two of them (very-long-chain acyl-CoA dehydrogenase [VLCAD] and trifunctional protein [TP] deficiencies) affecting enzymes that were not even known in 1985 [1]. The list of substrate use defects causing fixed weakness has not changed very much, except for the addition of a few β-oxidation defects.

There are several detailed descriptions of both glycogenoses [2, 3] and lipid disorders [4]. We therefore briefly recap typical clinical presentations and muscle morphology and biochemistry. Our focus is on developments in molecular genetics (discussing genotype-phenotype correlations whenever possible) and in the physiopathology of exercise intolerance, cramps, and myoglobinuria. The physiopathology of weakness remains largely obscure, as reflected by the suggestion that it might be due to mechanical disruption of the contractile apparatus by the storage material, a rather simplistic explanation not always justified by morphologic evidence.

DISORDERS CAUSING EXERCISE INTOLERANCE AND MYOGLOBINURIA

In general, there is a good correlation between the circumstances leading to clinical problems and what we know about the different roles of glycogen and lipid

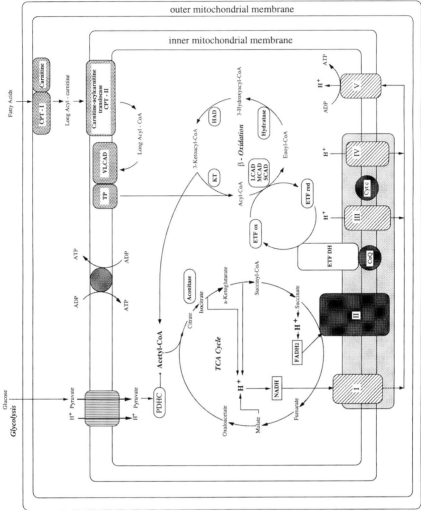

Figure 8.1 Schematic representation of mitochondrial metabolism. For details, see text. Respiratory chain components or complexes encoded exclusively by the nuclear DNA are solid; complexes containing some subunits encoded by the nuclear genome and others encoded by mtDNA are crosshatched. (PDHC = pyruvate dehydrogenase complex; ADP = adenosine diphosphate; ATP = adenosine triphosphate; TCA = tricarboxylic acid; NADH = reduced form of nicotinamide-adenine dinucleotide; FADH$_2$ = reduced form of flavin adenine dinucleotide; CPT = carnitine palmitoyltransferase; VLCAD = very-long-chain acyl coenzyme A (acyl-CoA) dehydrogenase; TP = trifunctional protein; LCAD = long-chain acyl-CoA dehydrogenase; MCAD = medium-chain acyl-CoA dehydrogenase; SCAD = short-chain acyl-CoA dehydrogenase; HAD = 3-hydroxyacyl-CoA dehydrogenase; KT = 3-ketothiolase; ETF ox = oxidized form of electron transfer flavoprotein; ETF red = reduced form of electron transfer flavoprotein; ETF DH = ETF–coenzyme Q oxidoreductase.) (Modified from S DiMauro, E Bonilla. Mitochondrial Encephalomyopathies. In RN Rosenberg, SB Prusiner, S DiMauro, RL Barchi [eds], The Molecular and Genetic Basis of Neurological Disease. Boston: Butterworth–Heinemann, 1997;201.)

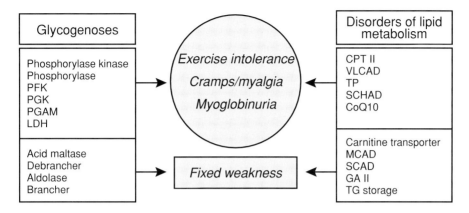

Figure 8.2 The two major clinical syndromes associated with defects of muscle substrate use. (PFK = phosphofructokinase; PGK = phosphoglycerate kinase; PGAM = phosphoglycerate mutase; LDH = lactate dehydrogenase; CPT = carnitine palmitoyltransferase; VLCAD = very-long-chain acyl coenzyme A (acyl-CoA) dehydrogenase; TP = trifunctional protein; SCHAD = short-chain 3-hydroxyacyl-CoA dehydrogenase; CoQ10 = coenzyme Q10 [ubiquinone]; MCAD = medium-chain acyl-CoA dehydrogenase; SCAD = short-chain acyl-CoA dehydrogenase; GA II = glutaric aciduria type II; TG = triglyceride.)

metabolism in the provision of energy to contracting muscles. In turn, standardized exercise studies in patients with known metabolic defects have contributed greatly to our understanding of normal muscle exercise physiology.

The fuel used by muscle depends on several factors, most importantly the type, intensity, and duration of exercise, but also diet and physical conditioning. At rest, muscle uses predominantly fatty acids, whereas the energy for intense aerobic exercise (close to one's maximum oxygen uptake, or $\dot{V}o_2max$) in dynamic exercise derives from the oxidation of carbohydrate. The energy for maximal force generation in intense isometric exercise or when there is a burst of activity with rapid acceleration to maximal exercise derives from anaerobic metabolism, particularly anaerobic glycogenolysis. During submaximal dynamic (aerobic) exercise, the type of fuel used by muscle depends on the relative intensity and duration of exercise. At low intensity (below $50\%\dot{V}o_2max$), the initial oxidative fuel is glycogen, with increasing proportions of oxidative energy supplied by blood glucose and free fatty acids (FFAs) as exercise duration increases. The type of circulating substrate used during mild exercise varies with time, and there is a gradual increase in the use of FFA over glucose until, a few hours into exercise, lipid oxidation becomes the major source of energy. Because the availability of FFA from adipose tissue is virtually unlimited, a healthy person can perform moderate dynamic exercise for many hours. At higher intensities of aerobic exercise, the proportion of energy derived from carbohydrate oxidation increases, and glycogen becomes an important fuel. At $70-80\%\dot{V}o_2max$, aerobic metabolism of glycogen is the crucial source of energy, and fatigue appears to set in when glycogen is exhausted. Maximal rates of muscle oxidative phosphorylation are fueled virtually exclusively by glycogen.

In agreement with the concept that glycogen metabolism is crucial for anaerobic or intense aerobic exercise, the symptoms of patients with glycogenoses are almost invariably related to an identifiable—and usually strenuous—bout of exertion, be it shoveling snow by a sedentary suburban dweller or darting to reach a bus by a sedentary urban dweller. Also, the muscles that hurt, swell, or cramp up are those that have been engaged in that particular type of exercise.

In contrast, patients with disorders of lipid metabolism, such as carnitine palmitoyltransferase (CPT) II deficiency, usually have little difficulty with short-term intense exercise. Their muscle symptoms follow prolonged moderate exercise, especially if associated with missing a meal. Impending myoglobinuria may be heralded by aching of exercising muscles but is never accompanied by actual shortening of muscles in the painful cramps that are typical of muscle glycolytic defects. In addition, prolonged fasting per se may cause myoglobinuria, in which case any muscle group can be affected, including respiratory muscles—a few patients with CPT II deficiency have been taken to the emergency room in respiratory distress during an episode of myoglobinuria [5].

The precipitating features of myalgia and myoglobinuria in CPT II deficiency were best illustrated by a young Orthodox Jewish patient, who, while serving in the Israeli army, became well known among his comrades for two reasons: his remarkable physical strength and his peculiar habit of filling his pockets with bread before long marches in an attempt to counteract the diffuse myalgia and weakness that would overcome him after walking for a few hours. When asked about his first episode of diffuse myalgia, he unhesitatingly traced it back to age 13, when he had to observe the 25-hour Yom Kippur fast for the first time [6]. The deleterious effect of fasting in CPT II deficiency is easily explained by the increased dependence of muscle on FFA oxidation, which is virtually blocked. Conversely, some patients with myophosphorylase deficiency note a beneficial effect of fasting on their exercise ability, which is explained by the mobilization of FFA, which facilitates the physiologic switch from carbohydrate to lipid use.

Glycogenoses

In reviewing the glycogenoses causing exercise intolerance and myoglobinuria, we follow the metabolic flow in the glycogenolytic and glycolytic pathways rather than the historical numeration (Figure 8.3).

Phosphorylase Kinase Deficiency (Glycogenosis Type VIII)

Phosphorylase kinase (PhK) is a key regulatory enzyme in glycogen metabolism, because it activates glycogen phosphorylase in response to neuronal or hormonal stimuli. PhK deficiency has been associated with four distinct clinical presentations, which are distinguished on the basis of tissue involvement (liver, muscle, heart, or liver and muscle) and mode of inheritance (autosomal or X-linked). This clinical and genetic heterogeneity is explained by the complexity of the enzyme, a decahexameric protein composed of four subunits $(\alpha\beta\gamma\delta)_4$: The α and β subunits are regulatory, the γ is catalytic, and the δ is identical to calmodulin and confers calcium sensitivity to the enzyme. In addition, there are two iso-

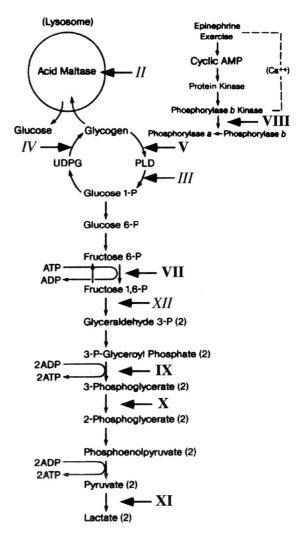

Figure 8.3 Scheme of glycogen metabolism and glycolysis. Roman numerals indicate enzymes with deficiencies that are associated with muscle glycogenoses: II = acid maltase; III = debrancher; IV = brancher; V = myophosphorylase; VII = phosphofructokinase; VIII = phosphorylase kinase; IX = phosphoglycerate kinase; X = phosphoglycerate mutase; XI = lactate dehydrogenase; XII = aldolase A. Bold numerals indicate glycogenoses causing exercise intolerance, cramps, and myoglobinuria. Italic numerals indicate glycogenoses causing fixed weakness. (AMP = adenosine monophosphate; UDPG = uridine diphosphate glucose; PLD = phosphorylase limit dextrin; ATP = adenosine triphosphate; ADP = adenosine diphosphate.)

forms for the α subunit (muscle and liver, α_M and α_L), both encoded by genes on the X chromosome, and two isoforms for the γ subunit (muscle and testis, γ_M and γ_T). Both γ isozymes and the β subunit are encoded by autosomal genes.

The purely myopathic variant of PhK deficiency usually manifests as a milder form of myophosphorylase deficiency (McArdle disease), with exercise intolerance, cramps, and, infrequently, myoglobinuria. One distinguishing laboratory feature is the lactate response to the forearm ischemic exercise—it is usually flat in McArdle patients, whereas it is normal or blunted in patients with PhK deficiency. Only approximately 15 patients with myopathic PhK deficiency have been reported [2], most of whom were men, suggesting the involvement of an X-linked gene. In agreement with this concept, the two molecular defects identified thus far—one in a 58-year-old man with progressive, predominantly distal limb weakness, the other in a 28-year-old man with more typical clinical presentation (exercise intolerance and myoglobinuria)—are both in the α_M gene, a nonsense mutation (G3334&) [7] and a splice junction mutation causing skipping of an exon [8].

The liver and muscle variant of PhK is an autosomal recessive condition dominated by hepatomegaly and fasting hypoglycemia with minimal muscle involvement. In one female and four male patients, five distinct nonsense mutations have been identified in the β subunit gene [9].

Myophosphorylase Deficiency (Glycogenosis Type V; McArdle Disease)

Although McArdle did not identify the biochemical defect, never was an eponym more appropriate than in this case. In 1951, on the basis of clinical observation and a few critical lab tests, Brian McArdle gave a remarkably precise description of the metabolic problem [10]. He noted that ischemic exercise resulted in painful cramps of forearm muscles, and that no electrical activity was recorded from the shortened muscles, indicating that they were in a state of contracture. He also noted that oxygen consumption and ventilation were normal at rest but increased more than normal with exercise. The astute observation that venous lactate and pyruvate did not increase after exercise made McArdle conclude that his patient's disorder was "characterized by a gross failure of the breakdown of glycogen to lactic acid." Nor was the specific involvement of muscle lost on McArdle, who noted that epinephrine elicited a normal rise of blood glucose, indicating intact hepatic glycogenolysis, and that "shed blood" in vitro accumulated lactate normally, leading him to conclude that "the disorder of carbohydrate metabolism affected chiefly if not entirely the skeletal muscles" [10].

The clinical picture of McArdle disease is rather stereotypical. It is dominated by exercise intolerance manifested by myalgia, premature fatigue, and stiffness or weakness of exercising muscles, which is relieved by rest. The type and amount of exercise needed to precipitate these symptoms vary somewhat from patient to patient, possibly in relation to training and diet, but two types of exertion are likely to cause problems: brief intense isometric exercise, such as lifting heavy weights, or less intense but sustained dynamic exercise, such as walking uphill. In the transition from rest to activity, even moderate exercise, such as walking on level ground, may initially cause fatigue, although after an adaptation phase, during which the delivery of extramuscular fuels is increased, such activity is usually easily tolerated. On the other hand, strenuous exercise invariably causes rapid fatigue and often results in painful cramps and muscle swelling, which can last for hours. Myoglobinuria was not a feature of McArdle's original patient, but it is seen in approximately one-half of the patients with myophosphorylase deficiency. However, as McArdle disease is the most common of the glycogenoses associated with exercise intolerance, it is also a common metabolic cause of recurrent myoglobinuria in adults, second only to CPT II deficiency [11]. An interesting phenomenon, almost invariably described or recognized by McArdle patients, is the second wind that they experience when, at the first appearance of exercise-induced fatigue, they rest briefly before resuming their activity.

Resting serum creatine kinase (CK) is consistently elevated in McArdle patients, indicating that individual fiber necrosis occurs even with everyday activities, a concept supported by morphologic observations and muscle imaging. The cumulative effect of this recurring muscle damage along the years may explain the appearance of fixed weakness in older individuals. We found that 28 of 52 patients had fixed weakness, and their mean age was 41.5 years, whereas the mean age of nonweak patients was 28.1 years [12]. However, there is no explanation for the severe and rapidly fatal weakness affecting a few infants with apparently isolated myophosphorylase deficiency. A 1997 occurrence of sudden and unexpected death in an infant with McArdle disease has raised the question of whether myophosphorylase deficiency (or other glycogenoses) may have a place among the heterogeneous etiologic factors of the sudden infant death syndrome (SIDS) [13].

In contrast to the relative clinical and biochemical homogeneity of McArdle disease, genetic heterogeneity was apparent from the first description of three mutations [14], which have rapidly escalated to 16 (according to our last estimate). These include missense, nonsense, and splice junction mutations, but by far the most common mutation in Europe and North America is the Arg49Stop mutation, which accounts for 81% of the alleles in British patients [15] and 63% of the alleles in U.S. patients [16]. The high frequency of this mutation, on at least one allele, has made the molecular diagnosis feasible in blood from patients with suspected McArdle disease [16]. However, it is prudent to remember that the frequency of different mutations varies in different ethnic groups. For example, the Arg49Stop mutation has never been found in Japan, and its frequency in Europe seems to decline with a North-South gradient, from 81% of alleles in the United Kingdom [15] to 56% in Germany [17] to 32% in Italy [18] and in Spain [19]. A useful addition to our diagnostic armamentarium has been a revision of the genomic structure of the myophosphorylase gene, which has clarified not only the full coding sequence but also the adjacent splice sites of the 20 exons [20].

The genotype to phenotype correlation in McArdle disease remains fuzzy. The most common genetic defect in patients with the typical presentation (homozygous Arg49Stop mutation) was also present in an infant with the fatal myopathic variant [21] and in the child who died of SIDS [13]. Of course, we cannot exclude that these unusual presentations may be due to additional gene defects. Unlikely as this situation may appear, it has been verified in two children with McArdle disease (both homozygous for the common mutation), who were also homozygous for the most common mutation associated with adenylate deaminase (AMPD) deficiency [22, 23]. One patient had onset of myoglobinuria at the unusually early age of 2 years [22]; the other was a young man with multiple episodes of myoglobinuria and early onset of weakness [23]. Although AMPD deficiency per se is an inconsistent cause of mild myopathy, it might have worsened the phenotypic expression of myophosphorylase deficiency. This concept is bolstered by a similar "double trouble" involving AMPD deficiency and phosphofructokinase deficiency: This patient also had an episode of myoglobinuria at 2 years of age [24].

Studies of the pathophysiology of McArdle disease have advanced understanding of the cellular and biochemical mechanisms of exercise intolerance in this condition and, at the same time, have provided new insights into the role of glycogen as a muscle energy source. Blocked glycogen breakdown impairs the production of adenosine triphosphate (ATP) via both substrate-level (anaerobic) and oxidative phosphorylation. In addition, by preventing the normal fall in muscle pH during exercise that is due to blocked lactate production, impaired glycogenolysis alters the equilibrium of the CK reaction, thus retarding the hydrolysis of phosphocreatine and resulting in an exaggerated rise in cellular levels of adenosine diphosphate (ADP) during exercise [25]. High levels of ADP promote a cascade of reactions that results in increased production of adenosine monophosphate, inosine monophosphate, and ammonia, as well as adenine nucleotide degradation products, including inosine, hypoxanthine, and uric acid. An exercise-related increase in uric acid via this mechanism has been termed *myogenic hyperuricemia* [26].

The limitations in energy availability from glycogenolysis ultimately lead to muscle dysfunction by impairing the operation of the ATPases—including Na^+K^+ ATPase, Ca^{++}ATPase, and myosin-ATPase—that couple the hydrolysis of ATP to cellular work. The interplay between deficient glycogenolytic energy production and deficits in ATPase function is complex. Membrane ATPases may be selectively dependent on ATP generated in substrate-level phosphorylation because of close structural and functional relationships with sites of glycolytic ATP production [27]. Also, the exaggerated increases in ADP that accompany glycolytic blocks may inhibit these ATPases. High levels of ADP and alkalosis result in exaggerated levels of intramuscular $[Ca^{++}]$ in exercise, consistent with ADP-mediated inhibition of Ca^{++}ATPase [28]. In addition, these metabolic conditions cause increased calcium sensitivity of contractile proteins [29]. High levels of ADP also may be inhibitory to Na^+K^+ ATPase. Furthermore, data from 1998 indicate that Na^+K^+ pump numbers are reduced in McArdle disease [30]. Resulting limitations in Na^+K^+ pump function likely promote the exaggerated increases in blood and extracellular potassium that are typical of exercise in McArdle disease [30]. High levels of extracellular potassium promote sarcolemmal inexcitability, which is a typical feature of muscle fatigue during repetitive neural stimulation [31].

The central role of glycogen in oxidative metabolism has been illuminated by studies of McArdle disease. Blocked glycogen breakdown limits the availability of substrate for oxidative phosphorylation. The biochemical mechanism is a lack of glycogen-derived pyruvate for incorporation in the tricarboxylic acid (TCA) cycle as acetyl-CoA and as malate and related TCA cycle intermediates via pyruvate-dependent anaplerosis [32, 33]. As a result, the rate of TCA cycle flux is restricted, the rate of generation of the reduced form of nicotinamide-adenine dinucleotide by the TCA cycle is attenuated, NADH-dependent electron transport is limited, and the peak rate of oxidative phosphorylation is low. The physiologic consequence is a low capacity for aerobic exercise that is most marked in the transition from rest to the first 5–8 minutes of exercise, until circulatory adjustments increase extramuscular fuel availability. The block in pyruvate-dependent oxidative phosphorylation accounts for the fact that oxidative metabolism is dependent on and fluctuates according to the availability of blood-borne fuels, particularly glucose and FFAs [34]. Increased cellular availability of these fuels produces the boost in exercise and muscle oxidative capacity that underlies the characteristic second-wind phenomenon [35].

Impaired muscle oxidative metabolism in McArdle disease causes exaggerated cardiopulmonary responses to exercise that result in tachycardia [36] and hyperventilation [37] at low-exercise workloads: These may be misinterpreted as indicating that exercise limitations are due to underlying cardiopulmonary disease.

The increase in muscle oxidative metabolism in exercise is normally coupled to the regulated delivery of oxygen and blood-borne fuel. This exercise response is mediated in part by regulatory metabolites released from working muscle, which activate sympathetic neural afferents and ultimately engage brainstem cardiovascular and related reflexes that increase the delivery of oxygen and blood-borne fuels. The responsible regulatory muscle metabolites are not known with certainty, but they likely include extracellular potassium, which is both a potent vasodilator and activator of cardiopulmonary reflexes [38]. Exaggerated sympathetic and endocrine responses during exercise are characteristic of muscle oxidative defects and presumably relate to the fact that muscle oxidative demand in exercise is not able to be met by increased oxygen delivery because of impaired muscle oxidative phosphorylation. The result is exaggerated oxygen delivery relative to oxygen use, as demonstrated by direct measurement of cardiac output and oxygen use [36] and by near infrared spectroscopy monitoring of oxygen uptake [39].

Exaggerated sympathetic responses to exercise also are responsible for a greater than normal increase in the mobilization of glucose from glycogen stores in the liver and fatty acids from triglyceride stores in adipose tissue [40]. The second wind represents the transition from a low to a higher muscle oxidative capacity. This results from an increase in cellular availability of glucose and fatty acids, which is promoted by increased rates of mobilization of these fuels and by an increased rate of fuel delivery attributable to exaggerated heart rate, cardiac output, and blood-flow responses to exercise. The higher capacity for muscle oxidative phosphorylation results in the ability to perform a given level of exercise more easily, at a substantially lower heart rate, and at a more normal level of cardiac output relative to oxygen use.

Therapy in McArdle disease has been based on a high-protein diet on the premise that branched-chain amino acids may represent alternative fuels to glycogen [41]. Although this dietary regimen in conjunction with aerobic exercise has been reasonably successful, direct administration of branched-chain amino acids to six patients resulted in impairment rather than improvement of bicycle exercise capacity, possibly because of an FFA-lowering effect of the amino acids [42]. In contrast, aerobic training of four McArdle disease patients improved peak cycle exercise capacity, circulatory capacity, and oxygen uptake [43].

Another therapeutic agent that has been used in McArdle disease is vitamin B_6. The rationale is that muscle levels of pyridoxal phosphate are reduced by approximately 80% in this disorder because of the usual lack of enzyme protein (to which PLP is bound) [44]. Some patients do not improve after B_6 supplementation [44]. But in one McArdle disease patient, after a brief (and blinded) discontinuation of vitamin B_6, symptoms of exercise intolerance returned, and the patient's ability to recover after ischemic fatiguing stimulation of the adductor pollicis muscle worsened markedly [45].

Phosphofructokinase Deficiency (Tarui Disease)

In its typical presentation, phosphofructokinase (PFK) deficiency (Tarui disease)—first described by Tarui et al. in a Japanese family [46] and soon thereafter by Layzer et al. in an Ashkenazi Jewish American patient [47]—is clinically indistinguishable from McArdle disease. Minor clinical differences that we have noted but that are not very helpful in the differential diagnosis include less common description of a second-wind phenomenon; more common report of nausea and vomiting accompanying the exercise-induced crises of myalgia, cramps, and weakness; and a lesser frequency of myoglobinuria attacks. Much more useful in distinguishing PFK deficiency from McArdle disease are some simple laboratory tests, such as increased bilirubin concentration and reticulocyte count (reflecting compensated hemolytic anemia).

The reason for the hemolytic trait in PFK deficiency is that PFK is a tetrameric enzyme under the control of three autosomal loci: A locus on chromosome 1 encodes the muscle (M) subunit; a locus on chromosome 21 encodes the liver (L) subunit; and a locus on chromosome 10 encodes the platelet (P) isozyme [2]. The three subunits are variably expressed in different tissues. Mature human muscle expresses only the M subunit and contains only the homotetramer M4, whereas erythrocytes express both the M and L subunits and contain five isozymes, the two homotetramers M4 and L4, and three hybrid isoforms. In patients with typical PFK deficiency, genetic defects of the M subunit cause total lack of activity in muscle but only partial PFK deficiency in red blood cells, where the residual activity (approximately 50% of normal) is accounted for by the L4 isozyme.

One clinical variant of PFK deficiency is characterized by fixed weakness, which brings patients to medical attention late in life, but this usually only overshadows their exercise intolerance in younger years. A more striking, and possibly heterogeneous, variant of PFK deficiency affects infants or very young children, who may present with arthrogryposis congenita and generalized weakness with respiratory insufficiency, but who also have diverse signs of multisystem involvement, including seizures, cortical blindness, corneal opacifications, and cardiopathy [2]. Curiously, none of the infantile cases had evidence of hemolytic anemia. Although the lack of red blood cell involvement is odd, the involvement of brain and heart might be explained by the high proportion of the M subunit in normal brain and heart PFK [48]. This, however, begs the question of why these tissues are spared in patients with the typical presentation.

In a peculiar kind of historical symmetry, the first molecular defect in PFK deficiency (a splice junction mutation resulting in a large deletion [49]) was identified in the Japanese family originally described by Tarui et al. [46], and soon thereafter, Raben et al. described two mutations, a splicing defect and a nucleotide deletion, which are common among Ashkenazi Jewish patients [50, 51]. Distinct mutations were then identified in patients of different ethnic origins [52, 53], and, by 1996, a total of 16 mutations had been described—a genetic heterogeneity comparable to that of myophosphorylase deficiency. The molecular basis of PFK deficiency in patients with infantile or childhood onset remains unknown.

The clinical similarities between McArdle disease and PFK deficiency are paralleled by metabolic and physiologic similarities. PFK deficiency impairs both anaerobic and aerobic glycogenolysis and blocks the fall in muscle pH that normally accompanies heavy exercise; results in high levels of ADP and increased adenine nucleotide degradation with exaggerated production of ammonia and myogenic hyperuricemia in exercise [26]; causes substrate-limited oxidative metabolism with fluctuations in exercise and oxidative capacity according to the availability of blood-borne fuels [54]; and causes exaggerated sympathetic neural responses to exercise associated with enhanced mobilization of extramuscular fuels [55] and with exaggerated heart rate, cardiac output, and blood flow relative to the capacity of muscle to use oxygen [39, 56].

These similarities suggest that the inability to use muscle glycogen as a fuel, which is common to both conditions, is the major energy limitation responsible for these clinical and metabolic features. However, the location of the metabolic block in PFK deficiency results in some characteristic differences. One that is useful in diagnosis is the fact that exercise causes the accumulation of sugar phosphates behind the metabolic block that can be detected as a phosphomonoester peak by [31]phosphorous magnetic spectroscopy [57]. An important clinical difference relates to the fact that because PFK deficiency blocks the metabolism of glucose, patients experience a substantial drop in exercise capacity in response to glucose infusion or a high-carbohydrate meal [54]. This response, which has been termed the "out of wind" phenomenon, relates to the fact that PFK deficient muscle is highly dependent on the availability of fatty acids and ketones for oxidative metabolism. Glucose causes an insulin-mediated inhibition of triglyceride hydrolysis and a fall in blood levels of fatty acids and ketones and thus deprives muscle of oxidative fuel and lowers the capacity for muscle oxidative phosphorylation.

Therapeutic attempts at bypassing the metabolic block are more difficult than in McArdle disease, because glucose is not an alternative substrate in PFK deficiency. In fact, the "out of wind" phenomenon suggests that patients should avoid high-carbohydrate meals. A 2-year-old boy with the infantile (and usually rapidly fatal) form of PFK deficiency—including arthrogryposis multiplex congenita, respiratory insufficiency, slowed motor nerve conductions, and abnormal electroencephalogram—seemed to benefit remarkably from a ketogenic diet [58]. There was clear improvement in strength, electromyographic features, and EEG pattern. Unfortunately, the child worsened suddenly at 35 months and died of complications of pneumonia. Still, a ketogenic diet ought to be considered, at least in children with the more severe variant of PFK deficiency.

Phosphoglycerate Kinase Deficiency (Glycogenosis Type IX)

Primary myopathy is not a common presentation of phosphoglycerate kinase (PGK) deficiency (glycogenosis type IX), an X-linked recessive disorder more commonly associated with nonspherocytic hemolytic anemia and central nervous system dysfunction. However, myopathy has been reported in four patients [59–62], and in 1998 we studied a fifth one. All five patients reported exercise intolerance with cramps and myoglobinuria. A sixth patient, an 11-year-old Japanese boy, had both exercise intolerance and mild mental retardation [63]. Molecular defects have been documented only in two of these patients. They consisted of a splice junction mutation in a man with pure myopathy [62] and of a single amino acid substitution in the child with myopathy and mental retardation [64].

The wide spectrum of clinical phenotypes in PGK deficiency is difficult to explain, because PGK is a monomeric enzyme encoded by a single gene on Xq13 and expressed in all tissues except the testis (a testicular isozyme, PGK2, is encoded by a gene on chromosome 19). Different amounts of residual activities in different tissues do not fully explain the clinical heterogeneity [65]. Although lack of myoglobinuria in patients with severe hemolytic anemia and brain dysfunction may be attributed to their inability to exercise, it is more difficult to explain the converse situation: lack of blood dyscrasia or brain disease in patients with myopathy.

Exercise evaluation of two patients with the myopathic form of PGK deficiency indicated substantial differences in exercise capacity and in susceptibility to exertional myoglobinuria, presumably attributable to differences in residual enzyme activity or to related structure-function alterations of the enzyme with different mutations [66].

Phosphoglycerate Mutase Deficiency (Glycogenosis Type X)

In contrast to PGK deficiency, phosphoglycerate mutase (PGAM) deficiency affects only muscle, causing exercise intolerance, cramps, and recurrent myoglobinuria. This is because PGAM is a dimeric enzyme composed of a muscle-specific (M) and a brain-specific (B) subunit, and normal muscle contains predominantly the MM homodimer, which accounts for 95% of the total activity. The only other tissues containing substantial amounts of the M subunit are heart and sperm, but there is no evidence of cardiopathy or male infertility in PGAM deficiency. Twelve patients have been reported, most of them from the United States. All U.S. patients have been black, and three distinct molecular defects in the PGAM-M gene (encoded by a gene on chromosome 7) have been identified so far among them [21]. A different mutation was found in the only affected white family [21, 67]. Despite the abundance of PGAM in muscle, heterozygous relatives of PGAM-deficient patients have reported exercise intolerance.

PGAM deficiency, like muscle lactate dehydrogenase (LDH) deficiency, retains some (usually approximately 5%) residual enzyme activity attributable to the presence in muscle of a small amount of the BB isoform. Thus, the block in glycolysis is incomplete, and lactate levels may increase two- to threefold with ischemic exercise in contrast to the flat lactate responses typical of complete glycolytic blocks. Also, such partial glycolytic defects—by preserving the capacity to generate pyruvate for oxidative metabolism—are generally not associated with the severe limitations of oxidative metabolism and major fluctuations in exercise capacity related to changes in extramuscular fuel availability that are typical of muscle phosphorylase and muscle PFK deficiencies [68].

Lactate Dehydrogenase Deficiency (Glycogenosis Type XI)

The discovery of glycogenosis type XI (LDH deficiency) was due to the astute observation that a patient with myoglobinuria had predictably high values of serum CK but extremely low values of LDH [69]. LDH is a tetrameric enzyme composed of various proportions of a muscle-specific subunit (LDH-A) and a cardiac subunit (LDH-B). LDH-A is encoded by a gene on chromosome 11, and three different mutations have been identified in Japanese patients [70–72], whereas the only two described white patients had two distinct mutations [73]. In addition to muscle symptoms, three affected Japanese women experienced dystocia necessitating cesarean section, and a few patients had dermatologic problems [74].

Disorders of Lipid Metabolism

Carnitine Palmitoyltransferase II Deficiency

This enzyme defect (or, to be precise, CPT deficiency, because at the time, CPT I and CPT II activities were not distinguishable) was identified in 1973 in two brothers with recurrent exercise-induced myoglobinuria whose muscle biopsies had shown normal phosphorylase and PFK activities and no glycogen storage [75]. A hindsight re-evaluation of their clinical histories revealed interesting differences from patients with glycogenoses: (1) Neither brother had any weakness nor any problem with brief intense exercise; (2) Neither reported cramps, but rather described muscle tenderness preceding myoglobinuria; (3) Both had problems with prolonged and not necessarily strenuous exercise: One brother had myoglobinuria after long hikes in the wilderness, the other after long hours of dancing; (4) Both identified fasting as a precipitating factor, usually in combination with exercise. Their histories illustrate perfectly the main clinical features of CPT II deficiency, except that additional precipitating factors may also include emotional stress, lack of sleep, and cold exposure. An important laboratory difference from patients with glycogenoses is the usually normal level of resting serum CK.

CPT II is a key enzyme in the rather elaborate system needed for the transport of long-chain fatty acids from the cytosol into the mitochondrion, a system requiring four elements: (1) CPT I, on the inner aspect of the outer mitochondrial membrane, which catalyzes the esterification of palmitoyl-CoA to palmitoyl-carnitine; (2) the carrier molecule L-carnitine; (3) CPT II, on the inner aspect of the inner mitochondrial membrane, which catalyzes the reverse reaction of CPT I, regenerating palmitoyl-CoA and liberating carnitine; and (4) a carnitine-acylcarnitine translocase, capable of exchanging acylcarnitine and carnitine across the inner mitochondrial membrane (see Figure 8.1).

Although the existence of two CPT enzymes—one outside and the other inside the inner mitochondrial membrane—was never questioned, for many years it was uncertain whether the two enzymes were distinct proteins under separate genetic control or a single protein with different milieus. We now know that CPT I and CPT II are different proteins: CPT I is encoded by a gene on chromosome 11q [76], and CPT II is encoded by a gene on chromosome 1p32 [77].

Although by 1990 it was apparent that CPT deficiency was an important cause of recurrent myoglobinuria [11], a vexing question was why the defect of such a key enzyme in lipid metabolism affected skeletal muscle selectively, especially when there was no evidence for the existence of tissue-specific CPT isozymes. The situation is now somewhat more clear. CPT I deficiency does, in fact, cause life-threatening hypoketotic hypoglycemia of infancy induced by fasting and is often accompanied by lethargy, coma, and seizures [4]. CPT II deficiency can also cause two different and severe infantile phenotypes: (1) a rapidly lethal neonatal form with hypoketotic hypoglycemia, generalized steatosis, and multiple malformations; and (2) an infantile hepatomuscular form characterized by episodes of hypoketotic hypoglycemia, lethargy, seizures, hepatomegaly, cardiomegaly, and cardiac arrhythmias. However, these variants are rare compared with the adult myopathic phenotype. Molecular genetic analysis has revealed distinct mutations in the different variants of CPT II deficiency, but genotype to phenotype correlations remain unclear. In the myopathic form, four mutations have been identified in European patients [78, 79], one of which (Ser113Leu) was far more common than the others. We have confirmed the common occurrence of the Ser113Leu mutation in North American patients [80]; screening genomic DNA from blood cells for this mutation in suspected patients may eliminate the need for a muscle biopsy. The large predominance of affected men in CPT II deficiency has been perplexing and has suggested a hormonal influence [81]; it is, therefore, interesting that studies of the CPT II promoter region do, in fact, suggest that gene expression may be hormonally regulated [82].

The physiologic consequences of a selective defect in long-chain fatty acid oxidation related to CPT II deficiency are remarkably subtle. Work and oxidative capacity are comparable to healthy subjects, and heart rate, cardiac output, and blood-flow responses are normal [39, 56, 83]. These results emphasize the fact that carbohydrate is the fuel essential for maximal aerobic and anaerobic exercise and that any gap in energy availability related to impaired fatty acid metabolism is able to be met as long as carbohydrate is readily available.

Defects of β-Oxidation

An increasing number of patients with recurrent myoglobinuria and the telltale precipitating circumstances of CPT II deficiency (prolonged exercise, prolonged fasting, intercurrent illnesses, cold exposure, and emotional stress) did not have this enzyme defect, and it soon became apparent that defects of β-oxidation could closely mimic the clinical phenotype of CPT II deficiency.

The 1992 documentation of a higher degree of complexity of the β-oxidation pathway has revealed two new important potential causes of recurrent myoglobinuria: VLCAD and TP deficiencies. In addition to the four classical concerted β-oxidation reactions in the mitochondrial matrix (flavin adenine dinucleotide–dependent dehydrogenation of acyl-CoAs; hydration of 2-enoyl-CoAs; NAD-dependent oxidation of 3-hydroxyacyl-CoAs; and CoA-SH-dependent thiolysis of 3-hydroxyacyl-CoAs), two additional enzymes bound to the inner mitochondrial membrane, VLCAD and TP, prepare long-chain fatty acids for β-oxidation in the matrix (see Figure 8.1). Jointly, VLCAD and TP act on long-chain fatty acyl-CoAs, while the matrix system acts on medium- and short-chain acyl-CoAs. Although both VLCAD and TP deficiencies are typically associated with devastating infantile syndromes characterized by hypoglycemia with Reye-like episodes, cardiopathy, and SIDS [4], they have also been increasingly reported in both children and adults with recurrent myoglobinuria simulating CPT II deficiency [84–87]. Complementary DNAs for VLCAD and for both α and β subunits of TP have been obtained, and increasing numbers of mutations are being reported in patients.

Recurrent myoglobinuria has also been associated with defects of enzymes in the cytosolic β-oxidation spiral, including long-chain acyl-CoA dehydrogenase and short-chain 3-hydroxyacyl-CoA dehydrogenase. It is likely that patients reported in the past as affected with long-chain acyl-CoA dehydrogenase deficiency actually had VLCAD deficiency. Short-chain 3-hydroxyacyl-CoA deficiency was documented in muscle (but not in fibroblasts) from a 16-year-old girl, who had, since age 13, recurrent encephalopathy and myoglobinuria triggered by fasting, together with hypertrophic and dilatative cardiomyopathy, and who died of cardiac failure [88].

Coenzyme Q_{10} (CoQ_{10}) Deficiency

Strictly speaking, CoQ_{10} deficiency belongs to the defects of the respiratory chain rather than to defects of substrate use (see Figure 8.1) and is considered in Chapter 7. However, CoQ_{10} is the final acceptor of electrons derived from β-oxidation via the electron transfer flavoprotein (ETF) and the ETF-dehydrogenase (see Figure 8.1) and, in this sense, it is part of lipid metabolism. The coexistence of ragged red fibers (RRF) and lipid storage in the muscle biopsies from patients with muscle CoQ_{10} deficiency underscores the dual metabolic nature of this disorder. Also, CoQ_{10} deficiency, although first described in 1989 [89], has been rediscovered in the late 1990s [90, 91] and may have been underestimated as a cause of recurrent myoglobinuria. In the five patients described thus far, primary CoQ_{10} deficiency in muscle was characterized by this triad: (1) exercise intolerance and recurrent myoglobinuria; (2) central nervous system dysfunction, with seizures or mental retardation; and (3) RRF and markedly increased lipid droplets in the muscle biopsy. Biochemical analysis of muscle shows a partial block at the level of complex III and variably severe deficiency of CoQ_{10}.

The metabolic and physiologic consequences of CoQ_{10} deficiency are similar to those of other respiratory chain defects [39, 92, 93]: Peak muscle oxidative capacity is severely reduced related to dramatically limited capacity of working muscle to extract available oxygen; cardiac output is greatly exaggerated relative to muscle metabolic rate; and blood lactate and lactate/pyruvate levels are high at rest and increase dramatically at low levels of exercise [90].

DISORDERS CAUSING WEAKNESS

As mentioned, we only briefly review disorders causing weakness, because the relationship between defective substrate use and muscle dysfunction—which is so dramatically illustrated by intermittent exercise intolerance, contractures, and myoglobinuria—is much less clear in patients with fixed weakness. In fact, chronic weakness is not a specific manifestation of metabolic derangement and is seen in hereditary defects of structural muscle proteins (e.g., dystrophinopathies), in neurogenic disorders, and in inflammatory myopathies.

Glycogenoses

In looking at Figure 8.2, two considerations come to mind. First, all but one of the glycogenoses causing exercise intolerance and myoglobinuria are due to muscle-specific enzyme defects, whereas all but one of those causing weakness are due to generalized enzyme defects. This suggests the possibility that factors other than defective substrate use may play a role in the etiology of weakness. One such obvious factor is the severe involvement of spinal motoneurons in the infantile form of acid maltase deficiency (Pompe disease) [94, 95]. A more subtle neurogenic involvement may occur in debrancher deficiency, in which glycogen storage has been documented in both intramuscular nerves [96] and in both Schwann cells and axons of sural nerve biopsies [97, 98]. Subclinical cardiopathy may contribute to weakness in both debrancher [99] and, possibly brancher deficiencies. Similarly, liver dysfunction with hypoglycemia in debrancher deficiency and with chronic hepatic failure in brancher deficiency undoubtedly contributes to the lack of stamina of these patients.

Second, the degree of glycogen storage is mild (sometimes hardly detectable) in the glycogenoses associated with exercise intolerance, whereas it tends to be more severe in the glycogenoses associated with weakness, especially in the infantile and juvenile forms of acid maltase deficiency and in debrancher deficiency. This raises the question of whether mechanical disruption of the contractile system may contribute to weakness, a possibility that seems bolstered in acid maltase deficiency by the lysosomal nature of the defective enzyme, which plays no clear role in energy generation. A similar parallel may be drawn for the disorders of lipid metabolism: Intramuscular lipid storage is minimal or absent in the adult form of CPT II deficiency, which is characterized by recurrent myoglobinuria, but it is rather massive in primary carnitine deficiency, which is accompanied by weakness.

Patients with fixed weakness are less amenable to standardized bicycle ergometer tests, and virtually no information on possible derangements of muscle fuel use in these conditions exists. Yet, studies in subjects capable of participating in standardized exercise tests would be interesting, especially in patients with debrancher deficiency or β-oxidation defects.

Acid Maltase Deficiency (Glycogenosis Type II)

Acid maltase deficiency (AMD) causes three very different clinical presentations: (1) a generalized (cardiomegalic) infantile form, which is invariably fatal before age 2 years; (2) a juvenile variant affecting exclusively muscle, with onset in childhood and causing severe proximal, truncal, and respiratory muscle weakness, usually leading to death in the second or third decade; and (3) a much milder adult-onset variant simulating limb-girdle dystrophy or polymyositis. The defective lysosomal enzyme, α-glucosidase, is encoded by a gene on chromosome 17. In the past few years, a flurry of mutations has been identified in patients with the three variants, the total number presently hovering around 35. The genotype to phenotype correlation is hard to establish because of the frequency of compound heterozygotes, but good correlation between the severity of the mutation and the severity of the clinical phenotype exists. Thus, deletions or nonsense mutations are usually associated with the infantile variant, whereas "leaky" mutations, such as the IVS1(–13T>G) splice site mutation, are associated with the adult-onset variant. This is nicely illustrated by molecular studies of a grandfather with adult-onset AMD and his grandson with Pompe disease [100].

An extremely useful animal model of the generalized form of AMD was obtained by targeted disruption of the murine acid α-glucosidase gene in embryonic stem cells [101]. This knockout mouse holds great promise for a better understanding of the still puzzling pathogenetic mechanisms of AMD in the different human variants and for the investigation of different therapeutic modalities.

Debrancher Deficiency (Glycogenosis Type III)

Debrancher deficiency is usually a benign disease of childhood characterized by hepatomegaly, growth retardation, and fasting hypoglycemia, which tend to resolve around puberty. However, later in life (the third or fourth decade), a small proportion of patients develops a myopathy, which is often distal more than proximal. Wasting of leg muscles and intrinsic hand muscles often leads to the diagnosis of motor neuron disease or peripheral neuropathy. This clinical picture—the mixed myopathic and neurogenic electromyogram pattern and the often slowed nerve conduction velocity—reinforces the impression that weakness in these patients may have a neurogenic component. It is, however, surprising that an enzyme that acts hand in hand with muscle phosphorylase in the degradation of glycogen does not cause exercise intolerance and myoglobinuria, at least in those patients who are not severely weak. Standardized exercise studies in these patients would be of interest.

The debranching enzyme is a single protein that catalyzes two enzymatic reactions—an oligo-1,4-1,4-glucantransferase and an amylo-1,6-glucosidase—and is encoded by a gene on chromosome 1p21. There are three biochemical variants: a rare deficiency of the transferase activity alone (type IIId), a common deficiency of both enzyme activities in both muscle and liver (type IIIa), and a less frequent deficiency of both enzyme activities in liver but not in muscle (type IIIb). Numerous mutations have been identified. Although the molecular basis for the differential tissue involvement in patients with the IIIa and IIIb variants remains unclear, it is interesting that most patients with the IIIb variant (but none with the IIIa variant) have mutations in exon 3 of the debrancher gene that are expected to result in truncated proteins [102].

Brancher Deficiency (Glycogenosis Type IV)

Brancher deficiency has a surprising spectrum of clinical phenotypes, considering that the branching enzyme is a single polypeptide (encoded by a gene on chromosome 3). The enzyme defect can be silent or can predominantly affect the liver, heart, skeletal muscle, or brain [2]. The typical presentation is in infancy with hepatosplenomegaly, progressive cirrhosis, and chronic hepatic failure. Cardiopathy dominates the clinical picture in a few older children. Isolated myopathy was reported in five patients: three siblings with delayed motor development and chronic proximal weakness and two adults in whom proximal weakness had started at 26 and 49 years of age. Brain involvement (adult polyglucosan body disease, APBD) is manifested by late-onset progressive upper and lower motor neuron symptoms, sensory loss, sphincter problems, and dementia. Although APBD is seen in various ethnic groups, branching deficiency has been documented only in Ashkenazi Jewish patients.

Several distinct mutations have identified in patients with various phenotypes [103], and one of these (Tyr329Ser) has also been found in seven patients with APBD [104].

Aldolase A Deficiency (Glycogenosis Type XII)

Aldolase A deficiency is the newest member of the glycogenoses, having been identified in 1996 [105]. Aldolase A is the isozyme that predominates in erythrocytes and skeletal muscle, and its deficiency had been recognized previously in patients with isolated nonspherocytic hemolytic anemia. The patient of Kreuder et al. was a 4.5-year-old boy who had episodes of exercise intoler-ance and weakness after febrile illnesses [105]. Although these were called episodes of rhabdomyolysis, the highest serum CK was only 6,480 U/liter (normal is <60; during attacks of myoglobinuria, CK levels tyically surpass 20,000) and no pigmenturia was described. Because of the presence of proxi-mal muscle wasting and weakness together with episodic exacerbations, this new glycogenosis seems to straddle the two clinical syndromes in Figure 8.2. Interestingly, the clinical crises apparently triggered by fever have been attrib-uted to the abnormal thermolability conferred to the enzyme by the mutation, which changes a negatively charged glutamic acid to a positively charged lysine at residue 206.

Disorders of Lipid Metabolism

The report in 1973 of a young woman with progressive, corticosteroid-responsive lipid-storage myopathy and carnitine deficiency in muscle [106] was followed by a flurry of papers describing patients with muscle carnitine deficiency. However, it was soon recognized that lipid-storage myopathy and carnitine deficiency could be secondary to several defects in lipid metabolism, which led to the dis-tinction of *primary* from *secondary* carnitine deficiencies. In fact, isolated lipid-storage myopathy with normal serum and low muscle carnitine, the hallmark features of the patient in the first report of muscle carnitine deficiency, are not seen frequently and were reported only in a few patients with short-chain acyl-CoA dehydrogenase (SCAD) deficiency [107, 108].

Although muscle weakness or hypotonia is reported in many patients with dis-orders of lipid metabolism, lipid-storage myopathy was an important and some-times the predominant feature in patients with the following conditions: primary carnitine deficiency (carnitine transporter defect), medium-chain acyl-CoA dehy-drogenase (MCAD), SCAD, glutaric aciduria type II (GA II), and Chanarin dis-ease (multisystem triglyceride storage disease).

Primary Carnitine Deficiency

Primary carnitine deficiency is an autosomal recessive trait that is due to a defect of the cell membrane transporter that carries carnitine against its concentration gradient from blood into heart and muscle. Its primary manifestation is progres-sive cardiomyopathy with heart failure presenting in childhood and progressing inexorably to heart failure unless L-carnitine is supplemented. Myopathy rarely presents in isolation and is usually associated with cardiomyopathy or encephalopathy; it also improves dramatically on L-carnitine administration, although the concentration of carnitine in muscle may not return to normal. The defect of carnitine uptake has been documented not only in cultured skin fibro-blasts [109, 110] but also in muscle culture from one patient [111]. The gene encoding the carnitine transporter has been cloned and localized to chromosome 5q31 [112]. Several pathogenic mutations in this gene have been identified in patients with primary carnitine deficiency [113, 114].

Medium-Chain Acyl-CoA Dehydrogenase Deficiency

MCAD deficiency is a common metabolic error that causes a variety of clinical phenotypes—including recurrent Reye syndrome, SIDS, and chronic neurodevelopmental disabilities—among whites of Northwestern European origin. Several patients initially described with systemic carnitine deficiency (including lipid-storage myopathy) were later diagnosed as having MCAD deficiency. The gene for MCAD is located on chromosome 1p31. Numerous mutations have been identified, the most common being an A to G transition at nt 985.

Short-Chain Acyl-CoA Dehydrogenase Deficiency

SCAD deficiency is especially interesting in this context because, as mentioned previously, it caused isolated myopathy with lipid storage and muscle carnitine deficiency in two patients [82, 83].

Glutaric Aciduria Type II

GA II gives rise to three major clinical phenotypes: (1) a severe neonatal form with hypotonia, hepatomegaly, hypoglycemia, multiple congenital anomalies, and early death; (2) a slightly milder form without congenital anomalies and with longer survival, but frequently accompanied by cardiomyopathy; and (3) a later-onset form with vomiting, hypoglycemia, hepatomegaly, and lipid-storage myopathy. GA II can be due to defects in ETF or in ETF-dehydrogenase, which result in *multiple acyl-CoA dehydrogenase deficiency* (another name for the disease). An 8-year-old boy with ETF-dehydrogenase deficiency had a limb-girdle syndrome in addition to hepatomegaly and episodic hypoketotic hypoglycemia. Postmortem examination showed massive lipid-storage myopathy and muscle carnitine deficiency [115].

Of considerable practical interest is the riboflavin-responsive form of GA II, which has been seen in adults with lipid-storage myopathy: In these patients, riboflavin administration improved wasting and weakness in a matter of weeks, and lipid storage in muscle was clearly decreased after a few months of therapy [116, 117].

Multisystem Triglyceride Storage (Chanarin Disease)

Chanarin disease was first reported by Chanarin in a Ugandan woman [118], and was then recognized in several patients from the Mediterranean area [119–121]. Patients suffer from ichthyosis, steatorrhea, and a neurologic syndrome that includes ataxia, nystagmus, neurosensory hearing loss, and slowly progressive proximal limb weakness. The pathologic hallmark is massive triglyceride storage in all tissues, including muscle, liver, gastrointestinal epithelium, endometrium, skin, bone marrow, and both fibroblast and muscle cells in culture [4]. The biochemical basis of this condition appears to be an inability of cells to degrade endogenously synthesized triglycerides, whereas use of exogenous triglycerides and phospholipids is normal [121, 122].

CONCLUSION

Inherited defects of muscle metabolism can interfere with muscle function—that is, with motion—in a specialized or generic way.

Impairments of specialized muscle function result in acute, intermittent, and reversible crises only when muscle is called to perform certain types of exercise, be it sprinting or marathon running. These problems have been related to specific enzyme defects in glycogen or fatty acid metabolism. Because patients with these diseases usually have normal strength between their energy crises, they have been recruited for sophisticated exercise physiology tests that have greatly enriched our understanding of normal muscle function. It used to be said that more doctors had lived off McArdle disease than patients had died from it. A less cynical point of view is that we have learned more about normal muscle physiology from the study of McArdle disease patients (or patients with other rare metabolic diseases) than we would have learned from the study of many control individuals.

Generic impairment of muscle function is fixed weakness, which represents the common final pathway of multiple insults, including, probably, chronic defects of substrate use. Chronically weak patients with inborn errors of carbohydrate or lipid metabolism have provided less interesting physiologic data because they are not good subjects for standardized exercise tests, and they usually suffer from multisystem disorders that can affect muscle indirectly. However, a closer look at the mechanisms that lead to weakness in these patients with defined biochemical defects may help us to understand the pathogenesis of weakness in more complex neurologic disorders.

Acknowledgments

Supported by NIH grant NS 11766 and by grants from the Muscular Dystrophy Association.

REFERENCES

1. DiMauro S. Myoglobinuria and myopathies of storage disease. In RB Conn (ed), Current Diagnosis. Philadelphia: Saunders, 1985;1037–1042.
2. DiMauro S, Servidei S, Tsujino S. Disorders of Carbohydrate Metabolism: Glycogen Storage Diseases. In RN Rosenberg, SB Prusiner, S DiMauro, RL Barchi (eds), The Molecular and Genetic Basis of Neurological Disease. Boston: Butterworth–Heinemann, 1997:1067–1097.
3. Chen YT, Burchell A. Glycogen Storage Diseases. In CR Scriver, AL Beaudet, WS Sly, D Valle (eds), The Metabolic and Molecular Basis of Inherited Disease (7th ed). New York: McGraw-Hill, 1995:935–966.
4. DiDonato S. Diseases Associated with Defects of Beta-Oxidation. In RN Rosenberg, SB Prusiner, S DiMauro, RL Barchi (eds), The Molecular and Genetic Basis of Neurological Disease. Boston: Butterworth–Heinemann, 1997:939–956.
5. Bertorini T, Yeh Y-Y, Trevisan CP, et al. Carnitine palmityltransferase deficiency: myoglobinuria and respiratory failure. Neurology 1980;30:263–271.
6. Argov Z, DiMauro S. Recurrent exertional myalgia and myoglobinuria due to carnitine palmityltransferase deficiency. Isr J Med Sci 1983;19:552–554.
7. Wehner M, Clemens PR, Engel AG, Kilimann MW. Human muscle glycogenosis due to phosphorylase kinase deficiency associated with a nonsense mutation in the muscle isoform of the alpha subunit. Hum Mol Genet 1994;3:552–554.

8. Bruno C, Manfredi G, Andreu AL, et al. A splice junction mutation in the alpha(M) gene of phosphorylase kinase in a patient with myopathy. Biochem Biophys Res Comm 1998;249:648–651.
9. Burwinkel B, Maichele AJ, Aagenaes O, et al. Autosomal glycogenosis of liver and muscle due to phosphorylase kinase deficiency is caused by mutations in the phosphorylase kinase beta subunit (PHKB). Hum Mol Genet 1997;6:1109–1115.
10. McArdle B. Myopathy due to a defect in muscle glycogen breakdown. Clin Sci 1951;10:13–33.
11. Tonin P, Lewis P, Servidei S, DiMauro S. Metabolic causes of myoglobinuria. Ann Neurol 1990;27:181–185.
12. DiMauro S, Bresolin N. Phosphorylase Deficiency. In AE Engel, BQ Banker (eds), Myology (Vol 2). New York: McGraw-Hill, 1986:1585–1601.
13. El-Schahawi M, Bruno C, Tsujino S, et al. Sudden infant death syndrome (SIDS) in a family with myophosphorylase deficiency. Neuromuscul Disord 1997;7:81–83.
14. Tsujino S, Shanske S, DiMauro S. Molecular genetic heterogeneity of myophosphorylase deficiency (McArdle's disease). N Engl J Med 1993;329:241.
15. Bartram C, Edwards RH, Claque J, Beynon RJ. McArdle's disease: a nonsense mutation in exon 1 of the muscle glycogen phosphorylase gene explains some but not all cases. Hum Mol Genet 1993;2:1291–1293.
16. El-Schahawi M, Tsujino S, Shanske S, DiMauro S. Diagnosis of McArdle's disease by molecular genetic analysis of blood. Neurology 1996;47:579–580.
17. Vogerd M, Kubisch C, Burwinkel B, et al. Mutation analysis in myophosphorylase deficiency (McArdle's disease). Ann Neurol 1998;43:326–331.
18. Martinuzzi A, Tsujino S, Vergani L, et al. Molecular characterization of myophosphorylase deficiency in a group of patients from Northern Italy. J Neurol Sci 1996;137:14–19.
19. Andreu AL, Bruno C, Gamez J, et al. Molecular genetic analysis of McArdle's disease in Spanish patients. Neurology 1998;51:260–262.
20. Kubisch C, Wicklein EM, Jentach TJ. Molecular diagnosis of McArdle disease: revised genomic structure of the myophosphorylase gene and identification of a novel mutation. Hum Mut 1998;12:27–32.
21. Tsujino S, Shanske S, Sakoda S, et al. The molecular genetic basis of muscle phosphoglycerate mutase (PGAM) deficiency. Am J Hum Genet 1993;52:472–477.
22. Tsujino S, Shanske S, Carroll JE, et al. Double trouble: combined myophosphorylase and AMP deaminase deficiency in a child homozygous for nonsense mutations at both loci. Neuromuscul Disord 1995;5:263–266.
23. Rubio JC, Martin MA, Bautista J, et al. Association of genetically proven deficiencies of myophosphorylase and AMP deaminase: a second case of "double trouble." Neuromuscul Disord 1997;7:387–389.
24. Bruno C, Minetti C, Shanske S, et al. Combined defects of muscle phosphofructokinase and AMP deaminase in a child with myoglobinuria. Neurology 1998;50:296–298.
25. Radda GK. The use of NMR spectroscopy for the understanding of disease. Science 1986;233:640–645.
26. Mineo I, Kono N, Hara N, et al. Myogenic hyperuricemia: a common pathophysiologic feature of glycogenosis types III, V, and VII. N Engl J Med 1987;317:75–80.
27. James JH, Fang C-H, Schrantz SJ, et al. Linkage of aerobic glycolysis to sodium-potassium transport in rat skeletal muscle. J Clin Invest 1996;98:2388–2397.
28. Ruff RL, Weissman J. Iodoacetate-induced contracture in rat skeletal muscle: possible role of ADP. Am J Physiol 1991;261:C828–C836.
29. Ruff RL. Elevated intracellular Ca^{2+} and myofibrillar Ca^{2+} sensitivity cause iodoacetate-induced muscle contractures. J Appl Physiol 1996;81:1230–1239.
30. Haller RG, Clausen T, Vissing J. Reduced levels of skeletal muscle $Na^{+}K^{+}$-ATPase in McArdle disease. Neurology 1998;50:37–40.
31. Dyken M, Smith D, Peake R. An electromyographic diagnostic screening test in McArdle's disease and a case report. Neurology 1967;17:45–50.
32. Sahlin K, Areskog N-H, Haller RG, et al. Impaired oxidative metabolism increases adenine nucleotide breakdown in McArdle's disease. J Appl Physiol 1990;69:1231–1235.
33. Sahlin K, Jorfeldt L, Henriksson K-G, et al. Tricarboxylic acid cycle intermediates during incremental exercise: attenuated increase in McArdle's disease. Clin Sci 1995;88:687–693.
34. Lewis SF, Haller RG. Human Disorders of Muscle Glycogenolysis/Glycolysis: The Consequences of Substrate-Limited Oxidative Metabolism. In AW Taylor (ed), Biochemistry of Exercise VII. Champaign, IL: Human Kinetics, 1990;211–226.
35. Pearson C, Rimer D, Mommaerts WFHM. A metabolic myopathy due to absence of muscle phosphorylase. Am J Med 1961;30:502–517.

36. Lewis S, Haller R, Cook J, Blomqvist CG. Metabolic control of cardiac output response to exercise in McArdle's disease. J Appl Physiol 1984;57:1749–1753.
37. Haller RG, Lewis SF. Abnormal ventilatory response to exercise in McArdle's disease: modulation by availability of substrate. Neurology 1986;36:716–719.
38. Haller RG, Vissing J. Circulatory Regulation in Muscle Disease. In B Saltin, N Secker (eds), Circulatory Regulation. Champaign, IL: Human Kinetics, 1999;in press.
39. Bank W, Chance B. An oxidative defect in metabolic myopathies: diagnosis by non-invasive tissue oxymetry. Ann Neurol 1994;36:830–837.
40. Vissing J, Lewis SF, Galbo H, Haller RG. Effect of deficient muscular glycogenolysis on extra-muscular fuel production in exercise. J Appl Physiol 1992;72:1773–1779.
41. Slonim A, Goans P. Myopathy in McArdle's syndrome. Improvement with a high-protein diet. N Engl J Med 1985;312:355–359.
42. MacLean D, Vissing J, Vissing SF, Haller RG. Oral branched-chain amino acids do not improve exercise capacity in McArdle's disease. Neurology 1998;51:1456–1459.
43. Haller RG, Wyrick P, Cavender D, et al. Aerobic conditioning: an effective therapy in McArdle's disease. Neurology 1998;50:A369.
44. Haller R, Dempsey W, Feit H, et al. Low muscle levels of pyridoxine in McArdle's syndrome. Am J Med 1983;74:217–220.
45. Phoenix J, Hopkins P, Bartram C, et al. Effect of vitamin B_6 supplementation in McArdle's disease: a strategic case study. Neuromuscul Disord 1998;8:210–212.
46. Tarui S, Okuno G, Ikura Y, et al. Phosphofructokinase deficiency in skeletal muscle. A new type of glycogenosis. Biochem Biophys Res Commun 1965;34:77–83.
47. Layzer R, Rowland L, Ranney H. Muscle phosphofructokinase deficiency. Arch Neurol 1967;17:512–523.
48. Dunaway GA, Kasten TP, Sebo T, Trapp R. Analysis of the phosphofructokinase subunits and isoenzymes in human tissues. Biochem J 1988;251:677–683.
49. Nakajima H, Kono N, Yamasaki T, et al. Genetic defect in muscle phosphofructokinase deficiency. Abnormal splicing of the muscle phosphofructokinase gene due to a point mutation at the 5'-splice site. J Biol Chem 1990;265:9392–9395.
50. Raben N, Sherman J, Miller F, et al. A 5' splice junction mutations leading to exon deletion in an Ashkenazi Jewish family with phosphofructokinase deficiency (Tarui disease). J Biol Chem 1993;268:4963–4967.
51. Sherman JB, Raben N, Nicastri C, et al. Common mutations in the phosphofructokinase-M gene in Ashkenazi Jewish patients with glycogenosis VII and their population frequency. Am J Hum Gen 1994;55:305–313.
52. Tsujino S, Servidei S, Tonin P, et al. Identification of three novel mutations in non-Ashkenazi Italian patients with muscle phosphofructokinase deficiency. Am J Hum Genet 1994;54:812–819.
53. Raben N, Sherman JB, Adams E, et al. Various classes of mutations in patients with phosphofructokinase deficiency (Tarui's disease). Muscle Nerve 1995;3(suppl):S35–S38.
54. Haller RG, Lewis SF. Glucose-induced exertional fatigue in muscle phosphofructokinase deficiency. N Engl J Med 1991;324:364–369.
55. Vissing J, Galbo H, Haller RG. Paradoxically enhanced glucose production during exercise in humans with blocked glycolysis due to muscle phosphofructokinase deficiency. Neurology 1996;47:766–771.
56. Lewis SF, Vora S, Haller RG. Abnormal oxidative metabolism and O_2 transport in muscle phosphofructokinase deficiency. J Appl Physiol 1991;70:391–398.
57. Bertocci LA, Haller RG, Lewis SF, et al. Altered high energy phosphate metabolism during exercise in muscle phosphofructokinase deficiency. J Appl Physiol 1991;70:1201–1207.
58. Swoboda KJ, Specht L, Jones HR, et al. Infantile phosphofructokinase deficiency with arthrogryposis: clinical benefit of a ketogenic diet. J Pediatr 1997;131:932–934.
59. Rosa R, George C, Fardeau M, et al. A new case of phosphoglycerate kinase deficiency: PFK creiteil associated with rhabdomyolysis and lacking hemolytic anemia. Blood 1982;182:84–91.
60. DiMauro S, Dalakas M, Miranda AF. Phosphoglycerate kinase deficiency: another cause of recurrent myoglobinuria. Ann Neurol 1983;13:11–19.
61. Tonin P, Shanske S, Miranda AF, et al. Phosphoglycerate kinase deficiency: biochemical and molecular genetic studies in a new myopathic variant (PGK Alberta). Neurology 1993;43:387–391.
62. Tsujino A, Tonin P, Shanske S, et al. A splice junction mutation in a new myopathic variant of phosphoglycerate kinase deficiency (PGK North Carolina). Ann Neurol 1994;35:349–353.
63. Sugie H, Sugie Y, Nishida M, et al. Recurrent myoglobinuria in a child with mental retardation: phosphoglycerate kinase deficiency. J Child Neurol 1989;4:95–99.

64. Sugie H, Sugie Y, Ito M, Fukuda T. A novel missense mutation (837T->C) in the phosphoglycerate kinase gene of a patient with a myopathic form of phosphoglycerate kinase deficiency. J Child Neurol 1998;13:95–97.

65. Tsujino S, Shanske S, DiMauro S. Molecular genetic heterogeneity of phosphoglycerate kinase (PGK) deficiency. Muscle Nerve 1995;3(suppl):S45–S49.

66. Haller RG, Fleckenstein JL, Taivassalo T, et al. Widely varying exercise capacity in two patients with phosphoglycerate kinase deficiency-metabolic mechanisms. Ann Neurol 1998;44:477.

67. Toscano A, Tsujino S, Vita G, et al. Molecular basis of muscle phosphoglycerate mutase (PGAM-M) deficiency in the Italian kindred. Muscle Nerve 1996;19:1134–1137.

68. Kissel JT, Beam W, Bresolin N, et al. Physiologic assessment of phosphoglycerate mutase deficiency. Neurology 1985;35:828–833.

69. Kanno T, Sudo K, Takeuchi I, et al. Hereditary deficiency of lactate dehydrogenase M-subunit. Clin Chim Acta 1980;108:267–276.

70. Maekawa M, Sudo K, Kanno T, Li S. Molecular characterization of genetic mutation in human lactate dehydrogenase-A (M) deficiency. Biochem Biophys Res Comm 1990;168:677–682.

71. Maekawa M, Sudo K, Li S, Kanno T. Analysis of genetic mutation in human lactate dehydrogenase-A (M) deficiency using DNA conformation polymorphism in combination with polyacrylamide gradient gel and silver staining. Biochem Biophys Res Comm 1991;180:1083–1090.

72. Maekawa M, Sudo K, Kanno T, et al. A novel mutation of lactate dehydrogenase A (M) gene in the fifth family with the enzyme deficiency. Hum Mol Genet 1994;3:825–826.

73. Tsujino S, Shanske S, Brownell AKW, et al. Molecular genetic studies of muscle lactate dehydrogenase deficiency in white patients. Ann Neurol 1994;36:661–665.

74. Kanno T, Maekawa M. Lactate dehydrogenase M-subunit deficiency: clinical features, metabolic background, and genetic heterogeneities. Muscle Nerve 1995;3(suppl):S54–S60.

75. DiMauro S, DiMauro-Melis PM. Muscle carnitine palmityltransferase deficiency and myoglobinuria. Science 1973;182:929–931.

76. Britton CH, Schultz RA, Zhang B, et al. Human liver mitochondrial carnitine palmitoyltransferase. I: Characterization of its cDNA and chromosomal localization and partial analysis of the gene. Proc Natl Acad Sci U S A 1995;92:1984–1988.

77. Gellera C, Verderio E, Floridia G, et al. Assignment of the human carnitine palmitoyltransferase II gene (CPT II) to chromosome 1p32. Genomics 1994;24:195–197.

78. Taroni F, Verderio E, Dworzak F, et al. Identification of a common mutation in the carnitine palmitoyltransferase II gene in familial recurrent myoglobinuria patients. Nat Genet 1993;4:314–320.

79. Verderio E, Cavadini P, Montermini L, et al. Carnitine palmitoyltransferase II deficiency: structure of the gene and characterization of two novel disease-causing mutations. Hum Mol Genet 1995;4:19–29.

80. Kaufmann P, El-Schahawi M, DiMauro S. Carnitine palmitoyltransferase II deficiency: diagnosis by molecular analysis of blood. Mol Cell Biochem 1997;174:237–239.

81. DiMauro S, Papadimitriou A. Carnitine Palmitoyltransferase Deficiency. In AG Engel, BQ Banker (eds), Myology. New York: McGraw-Hill, 1986:1697–1708.

82. Montermini L, Wang H, Verderio E, et al. Identification of 5' regulatory regions of the human carnitine palmitoyltransferase II gene. Biochim Biophys Acta 1994;1219:237–240.

83. Carroll JE, Brooke MH, DeVivo DC, et al. Biochemical and physiologic consequences of carnitine palmitoyl transferase deficiency. Muscle Nerve 1979;1:103–110.

84. Schaefer J, Jackson S, Dick DJ, Turnbull DM. Trifunctional enzyme deficiency: adult presentation of a usually fatal β-oxidation defect. Ann Neurol 1996;40:597–602.

85. Miyajima H, Orii KE, Shindo Y, et al. Mitochondrial trifunctional protein deficiency associated with recurrent myoglobinuria in adolescence. Neurology 1997;49:833–837.

86. Smelt AH, Poorthuis BJ, Onkenhout W, et al. Very long chain acyl-coenzyme A dehydrogenase deficiency with adult onset. Ann Neurol 1998;43:540–544.

87. Minetti C, Garavaglia B, Bado M, et al. Very-long-chain acyl-coenzyme A dehydrogenase deficiency in a child with recurrent myoglobinuria. Neuromuscul Disord 1998;8:3–6.

88. Tein I, De Vivo DC, Hale DE, et al. Short-chain L-3-hydroxyacyl-CoA dehydrogenase deficiency in muscle: a new cause for recurrent myoglobinuria and encephalopathy. Ann Neurol 1991;30:415–419.

89. Ogasahara S, Engel AG, Frens D, Mack D. Muscle coenzyme Q deficiency in familial mitochondrial encephalomyopathy. Proc Natl Acad Sci U S A 1989;86:2379–2382.

90. Sobreira C, Hirano M, Shanske S, et al. Mitochondrial encephalomyopathy with coenzyme Q_{10} deficiency. Neurology 1997;48:1238–1243.

91. Servidei S, Spinazzola A, Crociani P, et al. Replacement therapy is effective in familial mitochondrial encephalomyopathy with muscle CoQ_{10} deficiency. Neurology 1996;46:A420.

92. Haller RG, Bertocci LA. Exercise Evaluation of Metabolic Myopathies. In AG Engel, C Franzini-Armstrong (eds), Myology (Vol 1). New York: McGraw-Hill, 1994:807–821.
93. Vissing J, Galbo H, Haller RG. Exercise fuel mobilization in mitochondrial myopathy: a metabolic dilemma. Ann Neurol 1996;40:655–662.
94. Gambetti PL, DiMauro S, Baker L. Nervous system in Pompe's disease. Ultrastructure and biochemistry. J Neuropathol Exp Neurol 1971;30:412–430.
95. Martin JJ, DeBarsy T, Van Hoof F. Pompe's disease: an inborn lysosomal disorder with storage of glycogen. A study of brain and striated muscle. J Neuropathol Exp Neurol 1973;23:229–244.
96. Powell HC, Haas R, Hall CL, et al. Peripheral nerve in type III glycogenosis: selective involvement of unmyelinated fiber Schwann cells. Muscle Nerve 1985;8:667–671.
97. Moses SW, Gadoth N, Ben-David E, et al. Neuromuscular involvement in glycogen storage disease type III. Acta Paediatr 1986;7:289–296.
98. Ugawa Y, Inoue K, Takemura T, Iwamasa T. Accumulation of glycogen in sural nerve axons in adult-onset type III glycogenosis. Ann Neurol 1986;19:294–297.
99. Moses SW, Wanderman KL, Myroz A, Frydman M. Cardiac involvement in glycogen storage disease type III. Eur J Pediatr 1989;148:764–766.
100. Kroos MA, Van der Kraan M, Van Diggelen OP, et al. Two extremes of the clinical spectrum of glycogen storage disease type II in one family: a matter of genotype. Hum Mutat 1997;9:17–22.
101. Bijvoet AGA, van de Kamp EHM, Kroos MA, et al. Generalized glycogen storage and cardiomegaly in a knockout mouse model of Pompe disease. Hum Mol Genet 1998;7:53–62.
102. Shen J, Bao Y, Liu HM, et al. Mutations in exon 3 of the glycogen debranching enzyme gene are associated with glycogen storage disease type III that is differentially expressed in liver and muscle. J Clin Invest 1996;98:352–357.
103. Bao Y, Kishnani P, Wu J-Y, Chen Y-T. Hepatic and neuromuscular forms of glycogen storage disease type iv caused by mutations in the same glycogen-branching enzyme gene. J Clin Invest 1996;97:941–948.
104. Lossos A, Meiner Z, Barash V, et al. Adult polyglucosan body disease caused by the Tyr329Ser mutation in the glycogen branching enzyme gene in Ashkenazi Jews. Ann Neurol 1998;42:987.
105. Kreuder J, Borkhardt A, Repp R, et al. Inherited metabolic myopathy and hemolysis due to a mutation in aldolase a. N Engl J Med 1996;334:1100–1104.
106. Engel AG, Angelini C. Carnitine deficiency of human skeletal muscle with associated lipid storage myopathy: a new syndrome. Science 1973;179:899–902.
107. Turnbull DM, Bartlett K, Stevens DL, et al. Short-chain acyl-CoA dehydrogenase deficiency associated with a lipid-storage myopathy and secondary carnitine deficiency. New Engl J Med 1984;311:1232–1236.
108. Coates PM, Hale DE, Foinocchiaro G, et al. Genetic deficiency of short-chain acyl-coenzyme A dehydrogenase in cultured fibroblasts from a patient with muscle carnitine deficiency and severe skeletal muscle weakness. J Clin Invest 1988;81:171–175.
109. Treem WR, Stanley CA, Finegold DN, et al. Primary carnitine deficiency due to a failure of carnitine transport in kidney, muscle, and fibroblasts. N Engl J Med 1988;319:1331–1336.
110. Tein I, DeVivo DC, Bierman F, et al. Impaired skin fibroblast carnitine uptake in primary systemic carnitine deficiency manifested by childhood carnitine-responsive cardiomyopathy. Pediatr Res 1990;28:583–587.
111. Pons R, Carrozzo R, Tein I, et al. Deficient muscle carnitine transport in primary carnitine deficiency. Pediatr Res 1997;42:583–587.
112. Shoji Y, Koizumi A, Kayo T, et al. Evidence for linkage of human primary systemic carnitine deficiency with D5S436: a novel gene locus on chromosome 59. Am J Hum Genet 1998;63:101–108.
113. Lamhonwah A-M, Tein I. Carnitine uptake defect: frameshift mutations in the human plasmalemmal carnitine transporter gene. Biochem Biophys Res Comm 1998;252:396–401.
114. Nezu J-I, Tamai I, Oku A, et al. Primary systemic carnitine deficiency is caused by mutations in a gene encoding sodium ion-dependent carnitine transporter. Nat Genet 1999;21:91–94.
115. DiDonato S, Frerman FE, Rimoldi M, et al. Systemic carnitine deficiency due to lack of electron transfer flavoprotein: ubiquinone oxidoreductase. Neurology 1986;36:367–372.
116. DeVisser M, Scholte HR, Schutgens RBH, et al. Riboflavin-responsive lipid-storage myopathy and glutaric aciduria type II of early adult onset. Neurology 1986;36:367–372.
117. DiDonato S, Gellera C, Peluchetti D, et al. Normalization of short-chain acylcoenzyme A dehydrogenase after riboflavin treatment in a girl with multiple acylcoenzyme A deficiency myopathy. Ann Neurol 1989;25:479–484.
118. Chanarin L, Patel A, Slavin G, et al. Neutral-lipid storage disease: a new disorder of lipid metabolism. BMJ 1975;1:553–555.

119. Miranda AF, DiMauro S, Eastwood AB, et al. Lipid storage, ichthyosis, and steatorrhea. Muscle Nerve 1979;2:1–13.
120. Angelini C, Philippart M, Borrone C, et al. Multisystem triglyceride storage disease is due to a specific defect in the degradation of endocellularly synthesized triglycerides. Ann Neurol 1988;7:5–10.
121. DiDonato S, Garavaglia B, Strisciuglio P, et al. Multisystem triglyceride storage disease is due to a specific defect in the degradation of endocellularly synthesized triglycerides. Neurology 1988;38:1107–1110.
122. Radom J, Salvayre R, Negre A, et al. Metabolism of neutral lipids in cultured fibroblasts from multisystemic (or type 3) lipid storage myopathy. Eur J Biochem 1987;164:703–708.

9
Disorders of the Neuromuscular Junction

Lefkos T. Middleton

Disorders affecting the neuromuscular junction (NMJ), otherwise known as *myasthenias* (Table 9.1), are mainly characterized by fluctuating muscle weakness and abnormal fatigability of extraocular, bulbar, and limb muscles. The most frequent and best understood NMJ disease is acquired myasthenia gravis (MG), an autoimmune postsynaptic disease, related to the presence of antibodies against the acetylcholine receptor (AChR). The Lambert-Eaton myasthenic syndrome (LEMS) is a rare autoimmune presynaptic disorder, the autoantibodies being directed against the voltage-gated calcium channels (VGCC). NMJ disorders may also be secondary to toxic disorders due to agents such as bacterial toxins (e.g., botulism, tetanus), venom toxins, organophosphates, and drugs. Hereditary myasthenic syndromes (HMS) have been traditionally termed *congenital myasthenic syndromes.*

A series of breakthroughs have considerably enhanced our understanding of the physiology and microstructure of the junction and its synaptic mechanisms. The physiopathogenic mechanisms of the acquired autoimmune disorders have been delineated, and effective therapeutic approaches are now available. In HMS, advances in gene mapping and identification have defined the genetic mechanisms in many patients and families.

STRUCTURE AND FUNCTION
OF THE NEUROMUSCULAR JUNCTION

The NMJ is a highly specialized organ, which consists of presynaptic and postsynaptic regions separated by the synaptic space. Each presynaptic region consists of the nerve terminal (NT), which is the site of storage and release of ACh.

ACh molecules are stored in membrane-enclosed synaptic vesicles. A *quantum* is the amount of ACh released from a single vesicle—in other words,

Table 9.1   Disorders of neuromuscular junction

Acquired disorders
  Autoimmune disorders
    Myasthenia gravis
    Lambert-Eaton myasthenic syndromes
  Toxic disorders
    Bacterium toxin
    Botulism
    Tetanus
    Venom poisoning
    Drugs with adverse effects on neuromuscular transmission
    Hypermagnesemia
Inherited myasthenic disorders
  Autosomal recessive forms
  Autosomal dominant form: slow-channel syndrome
  Sporadic cases

6,000–10,000 ACh molecules per vesicle [1]. The ACh release sites are lined up within active zones, located opposite specialized regions of the postsynaptic muscle membrane, the primary junctional folds that contain the AChRs. The AChR molecules are aggregated on the terminal crests of the junctional folds [2, 3], connected by rapsyn, a 43K postsynaptic protein [4, 5]. Rapsyn also connects the clusters of AChRs to the dystrophin-glycoprotein complex (DGC), in association with other postsynaptic proteins, such as agrin and MuSK [6–8]. The DGC contains transmembrane and submembrane proteins. The former include α- and β-dystroglycan and the sarcoglycan complex of α-, β-, γ-, δ-, and ε-sarcoglycan; submembrane proteins are dystrophin, utrophin, the $\alpha 1$- and $\beta 1$-syntrophins, and the 87-kd dystrobrevin [9–11]. The laminin complex and merosin are located within the extracellular matrix, being attached to the DGC via the α-dystroglycan [12]. β-spectrin and -dystrophin may also play a role of anchoring AChRs to the cytoskeleton [3, 13].

The high concentration of AChRs at the peaks of the junctional folds is associated with an increased presence of messenger RNA (mRNA) [13]. This suggests enhanced gene transcription of AChR subunits, in particular the ε subunit, in these synaptic regions [14]. AChRs have a half-life of 8–11 days [15], and they are not recycled. The mechanism of their turnover is based on internalization, and receptor molecules are degraded and replaced by new AChRs [16]. The aggregation of AChRs in postsynaptic membrane and their virtual absence from extrajunctional cell membrane may be explained by nerve-derived factors affecting gene transcription of AChR subunits [2], such as agrin [17] and neuregulins [18]. In 1997, agrin was shown to slow the metabolic degradation of the receptors by significantly inducing the rapsyn-dependent clustering of AChRs [19].

The arrival of a nerve impulse leads to calcium influx into the NT through VGCC. Ca^{++} entry triggers the release of ACh through fusion of the vesicle with the presynaptic membrane (exocytosis) at the active zones, where the VGCCs are also located. The interaction of ACh with postsynaptic AChRs causes the opening of the ion channel, the passage of cations, and the depolarization of the end-

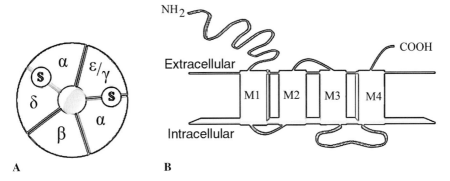

Figure 9.1   (**A**) Schematic drawing of acetylcholine receptor (AChR). AChR is a transmembrane pentamer glycoprotein composed of four homologous subunits that are made up of subunits α (two copies), β, δ, and ε. In the fetal isoform, the ε subunit is replaced by the γ subunit, which confers reduced conductance and prolonged open-time duration of the AChR channel. S indicates the α/δ and α/ε or α/γ ACh binding sites. (**B**) AChR subunit with its four transmembrane domains, M1–M4. Both the N-terminal and C-terminal portions are extracellular, with one extracellular loop (between M2 and M3) and two intracellular loops (a short one between M1 and M2 and a long cytoplasmic loop between M3 and M4.)

plate (EP), generating an EP potential (EPP). The effect is enhanced by the concomitant activation of voltage-gated sodium channels (VGSCs), which permits Na^{++} entry into the cell. VGSCs are concentrated over the lateral aspects and the depths of the secondary synaptic folds [3, 5] and may be attached to the cytoskeleton by ankyrin [3]. Spontaneous release of single quanta of ACh results in an unpropagated potential (miniature EPP, MEPP). The arrival of a propagated motor nerve action potential, releasing a larger number of vesicles, results in the generation of the EPP. When the EPP exceeds threshold levels, a propagated muscle action potential (MAP) of the muscle fiber is generated. The action of ACh is terminated by its hydrolysis by acetylcholinesterase (AChE)—located in the postsynaptic basal laminae—into choline and acetate. The former is recuperated by the NT for the resynthesis of ACh by choline acetyltransferase. The NT potential is reinstated after closure of the VGSC and the simultaneous opening of the voltage-gated K^+ channels.

The AChR is a transmembrane pentameric glucoprotein of a molecular weight of 290,000, comprising four highly homologous subunits encoded by different genes. Two AChR isoforms have been identified (Figure 9.1). The adult form is composed of subunits α (two copies), β, δ, and ε. In the fetal isoform, the γ subunit is normally expressed instead of the γ subunit until the thirty-first week of gestation [20]. The γ subunit is characterized by reduced conductance and prolonged open-time duration of the AChR channel [21]. Both the N-terminal and C-terminal portions of each subunit are extracellular. Each subunit is composed of four transmembrane domains (M1–M4), the M2 and M3 domains of each contributing to the formation of the central pore of the channel. There is one extracellular loop between M2 and M3, and two intracytoplasmic loops between M1,

M2, and M3–M4. The two ACh binding sites and the main immunogenic region of the AChR are located at the extracellular portions. The central pore of the AChR channel allows for the passage of cations through the channel, after binding of two ACh molecules to the ACh binding sites. In contrast to the voltage-gated channels, which are highly selective for specific cations—such as sodium, calcium, and potassium—the AChR channel is relatively nonselective among cations, and the size of its selectivity filter is much larger than that of voltage-gated ion channels [22].

A nerve action potential leads to the release of 50–300 synaptic vesicles [23], and the resulting EPP exceeds, normally, the threshold needed to generate a MAP. The difference between the actual EPP amplitude and the EPP amplitude required to activate an MAP represents the safety factor or safety margin. The safety margin is increased in fast-twitch fibers compared with slow-twitch fibers [24]. This is mainly due to the higher concentration of synaptic vesicles in the NTs and of VGSCs in the postsynaptic folds [25], as well as to an increased agonist sensitivity of AChRs [26] in fast-twitch fibers. Neuromuscular transmission is highly sensitive to structural or functional abnormalities of the junction affecting the safety margin, mainly in fast-twitch fibers.

Sophisticated morphologic and in vitro neurophysiologic techniques allow for the accurate elucidation of the components of NMS and the factors affecting the safety margin in normal and diseased muscle [27]. Light microscopic studies permit the cytochemical and immunocytochemical localization of AChE, AChR, and its subunits—as well as immune complexes—at the junction. Quantitative electron microscopy and electron cytochemistry allow for the evaluation of the size and density of synaptic vesicles and the morphology of synaptic membranes; the numbers of AChR binding sites may be measured through ultrastructural localization of peroxidase-labeled α-bungarotoxin (α-BuTx). In vitro neurophysiologic studies, including microelectrode techniques, noise analysis, and patch clamp recordings, permit the ascertainment of parameters of quantal release and kinetic abnormalities of AChR channels. Although vastly informative, these techniques have not become clinically relevant, because they require highly specialized equipment and expertise. In the clinical context, the most widely used neurophysiologic tools are repetitive stimulation studies (RSSs) and single-fiber electromyography (SFEMG), which allow for the in vivo ascertainment of abnormalities of neuromuscular transmission in individual patients.

ACQUIRED MYASTHENIA GRAVIS

The classic syndrome of fluctuating weakness and fatigability selectively involving ocular and other cranial muscles, with worsening of symptoms during the day, was initially described in the late nineteenth century by Wilks [28], Erb [29], and Goldflam [30]. Jolly [31] introduced the term *myasthenia gravis pseudoparalytica* to underline the severity of the disease in untreated patients and the absence of anatomic abnormalities of junctions. The author remarkably demonstrated that symptoms could be reproduced by repetitive faradic stimulation of the relevant motor nerve and improved with rest, and he advocated the use of physostigmine for the treatment of MG.

Campbell and Bramwell [32] in 1900 reported 60 patients with MG and suggested that the disease was caused by a circulating "toxin" that acted "selectively upon the lower motor neuron, so as to modify its functional activity." The relationship between MG and the thymus gland was demonstrated by Buzzard, who observed lymphocytic infiltrates in muscle and other organs and noted lymphoid hyperplasia in the thymus gland. He proposed the hypothesis of a common autotoxic agent as the cause of the muscle weakness, the lymphocytic infiltration in the muscle, and the thymic hyperplasia [33]. Furthermore, he commented on similarities of MG to Graves disease and Addison disease, which are now known to be of autoimmune etiology.

Physostigmine was proposed in the treatment of MG in 1934 by Walker [34], and Dale and Feldberg [35] subsequently demonstrated the role of ACh in neuromuscular transmission. Blalock initially reported the beneficial effect of thymectomy for thymoma in a patient with MG [36, 37]. The autoimmune hypothesis of MG was advocated by two independent reports in 1960 [38, 39]. Simpson suggested that antibodies directed against the AChR in skeletal muscle competitively blocked neuromuscular transmission [38]. The first direct proof of this hypothesis came from the work of Patrick and Lindstrom (1973) [40], who developed an animal model of experimental autoimmune MG by immunizing rabbits and rats with AChR of electric eel organ. The animals developed weakness and respiratory failure. In 1973, Fambrough et al. [41] applied α-BuTx, a specific neuromuscular toxin isolated from snakes, to motor EPs of patients with MG and were able to demonstrate a resulting marked AChR deficiency. Subsequently, AChR antibodies (AChR-Ab) were found in the majority of MG patients [42].

The identification of the autoimmune nature of MG led to the introduction of plasma exchange and immunosuppressants [43, 44] and the corticosteroids [45] in the treatment of MG. In the following years, the functional and structural postjunctional abnormalities, resulting from the autoimmune attack against the ACh receptors, were unveiled. The primary pathologic event was identified as an antibody-triggered acceleration of AChR internalization and progressive loss of AChR [46] associated with a complement-mediated degeneration of synaptic folds. The loss of AChRs results in decreased postsynaptic sensitivity to ACh [46]. Furthermore, there is progressive loss of EP VGSCs that is due to the degradation of synaptic folds [47]. This results in an increase of action potential thresholds near the EP [48], which further reduces the safety margin in MG.

Genetic factors do not play a major role in the pathogenesis of autoimmune MG, but a predisposing role may be inferred from the association of different types of MG with specific human leucocyte antigen haplotypes, immunoglobulin and T-cell antigen-receptor gene polymorphisms, and other studies [49].

Clinical Aspects

Epidemiology

Epidemiologic surveys on MG have shown considerable variation of the prevalence of the disease, from 1.2 per 100,000 in Japan [50] to 17.5 per 100,000 in Cyprus [51]. A prevalence of 14.2 per 100,000 was reported in West Virginia [52], with a trend toward a rising prevalence [53]. The same variation was noted in the

Table 9.2 Drugs adversely affecting neuromuscular transmission

Drugs with proven adverse effects
    Neuromuscular blocking agents
    Aminoglycoside antibiotics
    Quinine-quinidine-chloroquine
    Magnesium-containing drugs
    Radioimaging contrast agents
    Ciprofloxacin, perfloxacin, norfloxacin
    Lincomycin, clindamycin
Drugs with potential side effects
    Ampicillin, other antibiotics
    Beta-adrenergic blockers
    Calcium channel blockers
    Procainamide
    Diphenylhydantoin, trimethadione
    Morphine, other opiates
    Estrogens
    Chlorpromazine
    Lithium carbonate
    Carnitine
    Amantadine

incidence of the disease, ranging from 3.1 per million [54] to 9.1 per million [53]. The overall female-to-male ratio varies from 3 to 2 [55] to 1.6 to 1.0 [56].

MG may occur at any age. In a 1998 reported series, approximately 30% of MG patients were older than age 60 years at onset [57], and approximately 10% of myasthenic patients had their onset in childhood [52, 55]. In the Chinese and Japanese populations, more than 40% of MG patients manifest the disease before the age of 20 [58–61]. Younger than age 40, females are more commonly affected, with the incidence in males being higher when older than age 50 [62].

Clinical Features

The cardinal clinical features of MG are fluctuating weakness and abnormal fatigability. This can affect all voluntary muscles, with a predilection for extraocular, bulbar, and proximal limb muscles. The onset of the disease is typically insidious, but there are rare instances of acute onset, sometimes precipitated by events such as a febrile or systemic illness, pregnancy, or the puerperium. The disease may also manifest itself after general anesthesia or after the patient receives medication (e.g., aminoglycoside antibiotics, muscle relaxants; Table 9.2).

Initial symptoms involve the external ocular muscles in approximately 50% of cases [63], but bulbar and, more rarely, limb muscles may also be affected initially. The proximal limb muscles are usually more affected than the distal ones, but in rare instances, symptoms may predominate distally in the limbs [64]. Muscle weakness tends to be worse with repeated or prolonged exercise and typically exhibits diurnal fluctuation, worsening toward the evening hours. The symptoms may fluctuate daily or from week to week, with possible remissions for a variable period of time, although complete spontaneous remissions remain rare.

The predilection of certain muscles is characteristic of the disease. The extraocular muscles are affected in almost all MG patients and are most commonly the presenting symptoms. Papillary responses are normal. Eyelid ptosis, as a result of weakness of the levator palpebrae, is usually bilateral but asymmetric and is accompanied by some weakness of eyelid closure. After sustained upward gaze, ptosis may be exacerbated by the slow return of gaze to the horizontal position. Variable diplopia is the most common subjective symptom. The typical pattern of oculomotor weakness is asymmetric, fluctuating, and does not conform to a specific innervation. The susceptibility of extraocular muscles may be related to their functional properties [65], such as the high firing frequencies of their motor neurons and the tonic mode of contraction of subsets of multi-innervated muscle fibers, which lack significant safety margins [66]. It was postulated that a prominent expression of fetal AChR-γ isoform in extraocular muscles [65] and the presence of specific anti-AChR-γ antibodies [67] may also be incriminated, but the latter finding was not confirmed in subsequent studies [68].

Muscles of the face are frequently affected. The face may appear expressionless, and the head may be held slightly extended to compensate for ptosis [69]. The smile may have a characteristic snarling appearance. Speech may have a nasal quality with hoarseness associated with prolonged speaking. Regurgitation of liquids may occur. Laryngeal weakness may result in dysphonia. Chewing and swallowing of food may be particularly difficult, with possible nasal regurgitation or choking. Breathlessness may occur spontaneously or after exertion. Weakness of tensor tympani muscles may cause hypoacusia to low frequencies, but weakness of the stapedius muscles may result in hyperacusis [38]. Weakness of the muscles of the neck occurs frequently, usually affecting the neck flexor muscles, although weakness of neck extensors may, sometimes, be more prominent. Among skeletal muscle groups, truncal muscles and proximal muscles in the upper limbs are more frequently affected, but the patterns of limb weakness may be fluctuating, unpredictable, and multifocal.

Clinical Course

In untreated patients, the natural course of the illness is usually characterized by progressive deterioration. Important clues to the natural history of MG derived from the extensive studies of Grob and colleagues [62, 63] on more than 1,400 patients between 1940 and 1985. Fifty-three percent of patients had ocular symptoms, mainly diplopia or ptosis, at onset. Bulbar symptoms were present in 16%; marked fatigability and weakness were present in the extremities, face, neck, or trunk in 20%. Generalized fatigue was noted in 9%. Progressive deterioration was noted in most patients. Within 1 year from onset, the disease remained purely ocular in 40%, generalized in 35%, confined to the extremities in 10%, and bulbar or oculobulbar in 15%. Within 2 years after onset, myasthenic symptoms remained restricted to the extraocular muscles in only 14% of patients whose initial manifestations were only ocular, whereas 86% developed generalized manifestations. In untreated patients, progression of the disease was associated with fluctuations and significant relapses, the latter sometimes occurring under precipitating circumstances.

In the 1990s, the introduction of more effective therapies resulted in a better prognosis for the disease. In 78 treated patients with ocular myasthenia studied retrospectively over a mean period of 8 years [70], only 30% progressed to generalized MG. In the remaining patients, symptoms and signs remained confined to the extraocular muscles. The mortality of MG has also been reduced dramatically [71]. Between 1940 and 1957, the mortality rate for MG was 25% [54] and 31% [62], whereas between 1966 and 1985, the mortality rate was reduced to 7% [63]. No deaths directly related to MG were noted in the series of 100 MG patients of Beekman et al. [56] or in our own unpublished observations of 135 patients in the years 1990–1998. In childhood MG, no deaths were reported in two independent studies [72, 73]. However, episodes of respiratory distress can occur, usually under precipitating circumstances and mainly in patients with prominent bulbar involvement (myasthenic crisis). A series of 53 patients with history of myasthenic crisis was reported in 1997 [74], demonstrating the potential severity of the condition. Seventy-five percent of the patients were extubated within a month. Three patients died during crisis, and four patients died after extubation. More than one-half of those who survived remained functionally dependent at discharge. Three independent factors of poor prognosis for prolonged intubation were identified: (1) preintubation serum bicarbonate higher than 30 mg/dl; (2) peak vital capacity of less than 25 ml/kg in days 1–6 postintubation; and (3) age older than 50 years. The proportion of patients intubated longer than 2 weeks was 0% among those with no risk factors, 21% with one risk factor, 46% with two risk factors, and 88% with three risk factors. Four medical complications were found to be independently associated with prolonged intubation: (1) atelectasis, (2) anemia treated with transfusion, (3) *Clostridium difficile* infection, and (4) congestive heart failure.

Clinical Classification

A clinical classification of MG was initially proposed by Osserman in 1958 [75] and was subsequently modified [55] in an effort to better define the severity of disease and the long-term prognosis (Table 9.3).

In group I, myasthenic symptoms are confined to the extraocular muscles. However, there may be subtle clinical or neurophysiologic findings of the disease in other muscle groups, indicating a potential risk of developing generalized MG. Category IIA groups cases of generalized myasthenia that are slow to

Table 9.3   Classification of myasthenia gravis (MG)

I. Ocular myasthenia
II. Chronic, generalized MG
   IIA. Mild generalized
   IIB. Moderate generalized
III. Acute fulminating MG
   Late, severe MG

Source: Modified from KE Osserman, G Genkins. Studies in myasthenia gravis: review of a twenty-year experience in over 1200 patients. Mt Sinai J Med 1971;38:497–537.

progress, drug responsive, and have no risk for crisis; group IIB includes moderately severe, poorly responsive cases. Patients usually present significant diplopia, ptosis, bulbar symptoms, and fluctuating muscle weakness in the limbs. In group III, patients present with fulminating disease, often at onset, with rapid progression within 6 months. There is a high risk of myasthenic crisis and increased incidence of thymoma. Group IV includes patients with severe myasthenia after having a milder form of the disease for 2 or more years.

Other Clinical Forms

Neonatal Myasthenia Gravis

Neonatal MG, initially identified in 1942 by Strickroot et al. as a transient myasthenic disorder of infants born to mothers with MG [76], develops in approximately 12% of infants born to myasthenic mothers [77]. Myasthenic symptoms result from the transplacental transfer of AChR antibodies to the fetus [78]. Symptoms usually appear within the first few hours after birth with a mean duration of the disease of 18 days. The cardinal features are feeding difficulties, generalized weakness, respiratory distress, and poor cry. The disease is transient, with complete recovery if appropriately treated. Anti-AChR antibodies are detected in affected newborns, and their titers correlate with the severity of the neonatal disease [79]; they progressively disappear after clinical improvement.

Iatrogenic Autoimmune Myasthenia Gravis

Three types of systemic therapies have been incriminated in the etiology of acquired autoimmune MG: D-penicillamine, interferon, and bone marrow transplantation.

D-Penicillamine

Patients receiving D-penicillamine—for the treatment of disorders including rheumatoid arthritis and other chronic autoimmune diseases, cystinuria, Wilson disease, primary biliary cirrhosis, and eosinophilic fascitis—may develop a variety of autoimmune disorders, including MG [80–84]. Usually, patients develop mild, predominantly extraocular myasthenic symptoms, and the disease may be indistinguishable from idiopathic MG [85–87]. The mechanism of this drug effect has not been established, but events may be triggered by immune responses to D-penicillamine itself [88]. After the discontinuation of the drug, the majority of patients progressively recover over a period of several months.

Interferon Therapy

MG was reported in patients receiving α-interferon for the treatment of leukemia and other malignancies [89, 90], as well as in patients with chronic active hepatitis [91,

92]. A similar phenomenon was observed in 1997 in a patient with multiple sclerosis during treatment with β-interferon Ib [93]. The mode of action is unclear, but symptoms usually regress within months after the discontinuation of the drug.

Bone Marrow Transplantation

Autoimmune MG is an uncommon neurologic complication of bone marrow transplantation [94–99], occurring in approximately 0.5% of cases of chronic graft-versus-host disease [95, 97, 100].

Associated Diseases

The coexistence of MG and other autoimmune diseases was initially suggested by Simpson (1960) [38] and subsequently confirmed by other workers. The frequency of such associations varies from 4% [101] to 15% [56] of patients with MG. Autoimmune diseases most commonly associated with MG are hyperthyroidism, rheumatoid arthritis, and lupus erythematosus, but other disorders have also been reported, including Sjögren syndrome, mixed connective tissue disease, sarcoidosis and polymyositis. In one study, 30% of MG patients had a family history of one of these autoimmune disorders, suggesting the presence of a genetic susceptibility factor(s) to autoimmune disease in patients with MG [102].

A rare association of MG with giant cell polymyositis has been reported, also combining thymoma and cardiomyopathy [101, 103, 104]. Inflammatory foci have been noted in muscle and heart in autopsies of patients with MG [105, 106].

The risk of extrathymic malignancies is significantly higher in MG patients with thymoma [107–109], suggesting an indication for diagnostic screening for cancer in these patients.

Diagnostic Procedures

The clinical diagnosis is based on the typical clinical features of fluctuating weakness and abnormal fatigability of the extraocular muscles or the bulbar and limb muscles. The following investigations help to confirm diagnosis and to provide therapeutic guidelines.

Edrophonium Chloride (Tensilon) Test

The aim of the test is to demonstrate unequivocally the reversal of myasthenic symptoms and signs by anticholinesterase medication. Thus, this test may prove useful only in a patient with a significant degree of fatigable weakness that can be measured by the examiner and is of no value in a patient with nonmeasurable subjective symptoms, such as mild diplopia or minimal and variable proximal weakness.

The procedure is usually the following: Edrophonium (Tensilon) is injected intravenously. Initially, the amount of 2 mg is injected; if this dose is tolerated and no definite improvement occurs after 60 seconds, 6–8 mg is slowly given, and the patient is clinically re-evaluated to assess the clinical status and improvement of myasthenic features. The improvement is transient, lasting for 5–10 minutes. The usual side effects of the drug include fasciculations, sweating, nausea, and abdominal cramps. In patients with cardiac disease, the heart rate should be monitored for the presence of bradycardia. Injectable atropine (0.5 mg) may be given before edrophonium or be available at the time of the test for the rare occurrence of vagal bradycardia or hypotension. The injection may be preceded by a placebo injection of saline for comparison. Improvement after edrophonium is not specific of MG and may be noted in other disorders of neuromuscular transmission, such as LEMS and certain forms of inherited myasthenias. Furthermore, a positive response to edrophonium has been reported in disorders of the anterior horn, including poliomyelitis [110] and amyotrophic lateral sclerosis [111].

When the edrophonium test and other diagnostic investigations do not provide unequivocal results, another anticholinesterase with a longer action may be used, such as neostigmine (prostigmine), 1.5 mg intramuscularly, with an onset of action in 15–20 minutes, lasting for 2–3 hours. Alternatively, oral pyridostigmine may be used for several days as a therapeutic trial.

In a 1997 report, the edrophonium or neostigmine test was positive in 84% of patients with generalized MG and in 60% of patients with ocular myasthenia [56].

Clinical Neurophysiologic Testing

Routine nerve conduction studies and needle electromyography (EMG) do not provide direct diagnostic evidence in diseases of the NMJ, but they may be useful in the differential diagnosis of other neuromuscular disorders that may present with a variable degree of weakness. Such disorders include motor neuron disease, acquired neuropathies, and myopathies. RSSs and SFEMG are the essential tools of the neurophysiologic evaluation of the NMJ. Both techniques aim at evaluating the degree and causes of decrease of the safety margin of neuromuscular transmission.

Repetitive Stimulation Studies

RRS is the most commonly used electrophysiologic test of neuromuscular transmission. In MG, the major physiologic defect is the decremental response of the compound muscle action potential (CMAP) to a train of supramaximal stimuli of a nerve innervating the affected muscle, which is due to decreased postsynaptic sensitivity to ACh. This decremental response to repetitive stimulation can be measured by calculating the decrease in amplitude and area between the first CMAP and each successive CMAP. The recording is made with an active surface electrode over the motor point and the referential electrode distally over the tendon of the same muscle. The presence of a sharp negative deflection of the CMAP response is indicative of the correct positioning of the active electrode over the motor point of the muscle. Temperature should be controlled at 34°C or less, especially in the case of distal muscles.

Supramaximal stimulation is performed with surface electrodes, which need to be kept immobilized. Stimulation rates, which are most likely to produce a decremental response in MG, usually range between 2 and 5 Hz. Higher stimulation rates may produce artifacts or an increase of CMAP amplitude (potentiation). Furthermore, high frequency rates of stimulation or voluntary contraction of the muscle during stimulation may produce facilitation (due to an increase in the number of activated muscle fibers) or pseudofacilitation (i.e., an increase in CMAP amplitude with a reduction of the potential duration, without a change in the negative peak area). In control subjects, high rates of stimulation may produce mild facilitation or pseudo-facilitation, whereas no abnormalities are usually noted with slow rates (2–5 Hz). Modern EMG equipment now provides automatic measurements of the CMAP parameters (amplitude, duration, area). However, quality control measures should be taken on a regular basis to verify the results provided by automatic analysis.

Activation procedures are commonly used to increase the diagnostic yield of the technique. The most commonly used is muscle activation—which may be voluntary—in which the patient maximally contracts the muscle for 30–60 seconds. A similar response may be obtained through a train of tetanic stimuli. Both techniques result in an accumulation of calcium in the NT and may produce an increase of CMAP amplitude, termed *postactivation facilitation* (PAF). In LEMS, characterized by poor release of ACh vesicles, postactivation facilitation may be prominent, whereas in MG, the phenomenon may be limited to a transient regression of the decremental response previously obtained at low rate of stimulation. Prolonged exercise (≥1 minute) may result in an enhanced decremental response termed *postexercise exhaustion* (PEE).

Muscle selection is critical to increase the diagnostic yield of the test. The muscle should be clinically affected, and complete mobilization both of the recording and stimulating electrodes should be ensured, with minimal discomfort and maximum cooperation of the patient. Facial muscles, which are more commonly weak, may be more difficult to study, because repetitive stimulation of facial muscles is usually too uncomfortable for the patient to cooperate; similarly, proximal limb muscles (i.e., deltoid, biceps) may be difficult to study because of difficulties in limb immobilization. On the other hand, distal hand muscles are the most convenient to immobilize but are seldom clinically involved. In our laboratory, we routinely perform RSSs over the abductor digiti minimi muscle stimulating the ulnar nerve and the trapezius muscle stimulating the spinal accessory nerve. The study of this muscle is well tolerated, stabilization of the muscle is usually ensured with the patient in sitting position, and the muscle is frequently affected in mild-moderate generalized MG. The active electrode is placed at a midpoint between the C7 vertebra and the tip of the acromion over the trapezius muscle, and the reference electrode is placed over the acromion. The spinal accessory nerve is stimulated behind the ear, over the posterior border of the sternocleidomastoid muscle, where the nerve lies superficially.

For each muscle, the following protocol is used: Individual supramaximal stimuli are delivered to obtain a baseline CMAP. A very low CMAP amplitude at baseline may suggest Lambert-Eaton syndrome, and a double CMAP response may be diagnostic of two forms of inherited congenital myasthenic syndromes (slow-channel and cholinesterase deficiency syndromes). Then, trains of 10 supramaximal stimuli are delivered at 2 Hz and 5 Hz, separated by a 3-minute interval, and the CMAP responses are recorded. The amplitude and area of the first response are compared with the fifth and ninth responses. Any decrement or increment is expressed in percentages. In case of abnormalities, the same test (at 2 and 5 Hz) is repeated twice, at 3-minute intervals, to confirm the results.

Then, the patient is asked to exercise the muscle maximally for 1 minute. RSSs are repeated at 2 Hz at 10 seconds and postexercise at 1, 2, 3, and 4 minutes. A decrement that only appears after exercise suggests PEE. If PEE is observed, the patient is asked to exercise for 10 seconds, and RSSs at 2 Hz are performed. Improvement of decrement indicates postexercise facilitation.

The diagnostic yield of RSSs has not been clearly established, perhaps because of the lack of a universally followed protocol. In a large series of patients in generalized MG, a decremental response was obtained in distal muscles in 66% and in proximal muscles in 83% [112]. In ocular myasthenia, the test was less sensitive, with a decrement in distal muscles in 35% and in proximal muscles in 45%.

Single-Fiber Electromyography

As the name implies, SFEMG allows for the study of action potentials from individual muscle fibers. The monograph of Stalberg and Trontelj (1994) [113], who pioneered the technique, is an excellent reference for a more detailed description. Only a brief description of the techniques is outlined here. A concentric needle electrode is used to record single-fiber potentials from an active surface of 25 μm of diameter, localized on the side of the needle. Filtering is essential, with a low frequency filter set at 500 Hz. Two criteria for inclusion have been generally adopted to identify potentials generated from muscle fibers within a distance of 300 microns from the tip of the electrode: a rising time of 200 μm per second and an amplitude of 300 μV. The individual single-fiber potential is generated by a single muscle fiber and represents a suprathreshold EPP. Normally, within the motor unit, a propagated MAP is generated within all muscle fibers at approximately the same time. Abnormal variability of the latency from stimulus to response (in stimulated SFEMG) or between two adjacent muscle fibers (in conventional SFEMG) is termed *jitter*. The jitter is expressed as the mean value of consecutive differences of successive discharges (mean consecutive difference, or MCD). Any process altering the safety margin of neuromuscular transmission may result in an abnormally increased jitter. In cases of severe defect of neuromuscular transmission, the EPP may not reach the threshold for a propagated action potential, producing blocking.

SFEMG is the most sensitive technique for the neurophysiologic evaluation of neuromuscular transmission because it may detect abnormalities in clinically normal muscles before weakness becomes clinically overt. RSSs, on the other hand, usually require clinically evident weakness for the abnormalities to be detected. However, abnormalities of jitter are not specific for a myasthenic disorder; any disease that can alter the nerve action potential at the motor neurons or the motor peripheral fibers or any myopathic process may also result in an abnormal jitter. Thus, it is imperative for SFEMG studies to be performed after a careful neurologic examination—and in certain cases, nerve conduction studies and needle EMG—to rule out a neurogenic or myopathic process. On the other hand, a normal SFEMG study in a clinically weak muscle rules out the diagnosis of a myasthenic disorder.

Cholinesterase inhibitors may affect SFEMG findings mainly in mild MG cases and may need to be discontinued for at least 24 hours before repeating the study [114].

SFEMG can be performed using voluntary activation or electrical stimulation. The former requires active cooperation of the patient, whereas the latter is prone to more technical pitfalls. In both techniques, 20 single-fiber potentials are sampled, and the mean jitter is measured. The extensor digitorum communis biceps, frontalis, and orbicularis oculi are most widely used. Stimulated SFEMG (SSFEMG) is gaining increasing attention, because it requires little cooperation from the patient. It thus allows for the study of muscles that are commonly affected but in which controlled motor recruitment may be difficult, such as the orbicularis oculi muscle. Furthermore, several single-fiber potentials can be simultaneously recorded in one train of stimuli of a distal motor nerve, thus significantly reducing the duration of the test. However, extreme caution is required to identify pseudoabnormal single-fiber potentials, with increased MCD that is due to infra-maximal stimulation. Such single-fiber potentials should be excluded from the study even if they fulfill the criteria of rising time and amplitude. As a general rule, the normal jitter values for SSFEMG are slightly shorter compared with conventional SFEMG performed under voluntary contraction. In this technique, the patient is required to produce a minimal but constant voluntary effort. The single-fiber needle is positioned so that two time-locked fibers from the same motor unit adjacent to the needle tip can be recorded. A trigger is placed on one potential, and the variation of the interpotential interval is measured. The difference in interpotential intervals is then calculated for each successive discharge, and the MCD for the particular single-fiber potential is calculated. Modern commercial EMG machines offer the capability of automatically measuring the parameters of both the single-fiber potentials and potential pairs, as well as the mean values of all single-fiber potentials accepted in the study.

Normal values for individual potentials, as well as mean values per muscle, have been reported for several muscles [113, 115]. A study is abnormal if at least one of two criteria is met: (1) The mean MCD of all single-fiber potentials recorded is higher than the upper limit of the mean MCD established for the muscle, or (2) more than 10% of single-fiber potentials (i.e., >3/20) have individual mean MCD or blocking that exceeds the upper limit of normal for individual single-fiber potentials in that muscle.

Measurements of fiber density may help to differentiate a disorder of NMJ from other neuromuscular disorders causing abnormalities of jitter, such as neurogenic or myopathic processes. This technique involves moving the needle in search of single-fiber potentials that meet the inclusion criteria of amplitude and rise time to be counted at each site during minimal voluntary contraction. The mean fiber density is measured for 10–20 sites and usually remains at or below 1.5 in healthy young adults; however, the technique is highly prone to subjective interpretations, and its use is limited.

SFEMG and SSFEMG are gaining increasing acceptance internationally, mainly because of the availability of modern, user-friendly EMG equipment that provides automatic analysis of SFEMG parameters. Nevertheless, the techniques remain highly technical, and it requires a significant degree of experience and expertise to collect and accurately analyze electrophysiologic data.

Serologic Autoimmune Tests

Anti–AChR-Ab are found in the majority of patients with MG, confirming the autoimmune nature of the disease. However, the test may be positive in rare patients with other disorders, and the diagnosis of MG cannot rely solely on a positive antibody test.

The AChR binding antibody radioimmunoassays measure the amount of AChR bound to immunoglobulin in the presence of ^{125}I-labeled α-BuTx as developed by Lindstrom [42] and Lennon [116]. They are the most widely used radioimmunoassays.

Furthermore, AChR binding antibodies were detected in patients with other diseases, such as in patients with autoimmune liver disorders [117, 118], in 13% of patients with Lambert-Eaton syndrome, and in 3% of patients with primary lung cancer not associated with neurologic autoimmunity [119].

Overall, the test is positive in approximately 84% of MG patients [120], varying from 74% [121] to 94% [56]. In juvenile MG, the positivity of the assay is significantly lower, varying from 50% to 70% in prepubertal patients and at approximately 70% in peripubertal MG [122]. In purely ocular myasthenia, the test is negative in approximately 30–40% [56, 121, 123, 124], and the values of the antibody titers are also lower [123]. Anti-AChR-Ab levels vary among patients with similar clinical involvement, thus correlating poorly with the severity of the disease in studies of groups of patients [120]. In individual patients, there have been conflicting reports of no correlation [125] and strong correlation of anti-AChR antibody titers with the severity of the disease, decreasing with long-term clinical improvement after thymectomy [126] and during immunosuppressant therapy [123]. A transient decrease in titers may be observed after plasmapheresis associated with transient clinical improvement [127, 128].

Sanders et al. [121] studied the clinical features of seronegative compared with seropositive MG patients. Seronegative patients exhibited similar clinical features, although they had a less severe disease, and a greater proportion of them manifested purely ocular manifestations. In contrast to seropositive patients, the disease incidence in seronegative patients was equal in males and females, but disease severity differed significantly. Males were less severely affected compared with females; disease severity in females with seronegative myasthenia was similar before and after menopause, in contrast to seropositive myasthenia. The authors postulated that predisposing host factors in the pathogenesis of MG may offer important clues for better defined therapeutic strategies in the two categories of patients. The primary pathogenic event in seronegative patients is an autoimmune attack directed against AChR [129, 130] by a pathogenic agent that has not yet been identified.

In patients suspected of having MG who have negative binding assay, two additional assays may be considered. AChR-modulating antibody assays measure the loss of α-BuTx AChR binding sites. AChR-modulating antibodies are more common in generalized MG and in particular those patients with thymoma, who frequently exhibit a greater than 90% AChR loss [123]. However, in studies published in 1997, modulating AChR-Ab were increased only in 6% of patients in whom binding AChR-Ab was not elevated [121], thus conferring only a marginal increase in the diagnostic yield. AChR blocking antibodies are positive in only 1% of MG patients with no detectable binding antibodies [131]. Therefore, this is not indicated as a screening diagnostic test.

Antistriated muscle antibody (StrAb) assays are positive in approximately 30% of adult patients with MG, their frequency rising to 55% at older than age 61 [131]. They are detected in 85% of MG patients with thymoma and in approximately 24% of patients who have thymoma without signs of MG [132]. A progressive rise in StrAb titers after thymectomy may indicate tumor recurrence [133]. Titin, a giant filamentous protein representing 10% of the total protein mass of striated muscle, has been identified as the primary autoantigen [134].

StrAbs are frequently positive in patients with autoimmune liver diseases [118], in 6% of patients with LEMS with or without cancer, and in approximately 3% of patients with primary lung cancer [119]. Approximately 50% of MG patients with thymoma also have antibodies against ryanodine receptor [134, 135], a Ca++-release channel located in the sarcoplasmic reticulum of striated muscle.

Calcium Channel Binding Antibodies

Autoantibodies reactive with P/Q and N-type calcium channels are commonly found in patients with LEMS and not in MG. Thus, measurements of these antibodies are useful in differentiating between these two acquired autoimmune NMJ diseases.

Other Autoantibodies

Autoantibodies against thyroid peroxidase, thyroglobulin, and gastric parietal cells are found more frequently in patients with MG, particularly those with ocular myasthenia, compared with patients with control neurologic disorders [136].

Treatment

Several therapeutic options are now available, considerably ameliorating the prognosis of MG. These include—in addition to the cholinesterase inhibitors for symptomatic relief—immunosuppressant medications, thymectomy, plasma exchange, and intravenous immunoglobulin (IVIG) treatment. Treatment of MG is often a lifelong commitment, and the choice of therapeutic strategies in each patient needs to be designed based on the individual's condition, the severity and distribution of symptoms, the rate of progression, and the presence of other factors that may affect the clinical presentation of the patient (i.e., a concomitant disease) or the long-term therapy itself. Furthermore, therapeutic regimens may need to be modified or altered in the course of this typically variable disease. To ensure maximum compliance and cooperation, patients need to be adequately informed of the nature of their illness and the rationale of therapy. The easy access of patients to a specialized center with experienced staff and facilities for adequate and effective diagnosis and treatment provides the best framework for the management of MG.

Cholinesterase Inhibitors

Pyridostigmine (Mestinon) is the first-line treatment for symptomatic relief of MG. Cholinesterase inhibitors prolong the action of ACh on AChRs by inhibiting its degradation at the NMJ.

Pyridostigmine bromide (Mestinon) is the most widely used of these agents. The onset of action is usually noticed within 15–30 minutes, and the effect can last 3–4 hours. The initial dose is 15–60 mg four times a day. Neostigmine bromide (7.5–45.0 mg every 2–6 hours with a shorter half-life) is also available for intramuscular administration and may be used for symptomatic relief in more acute situations. The most common side effects of cholinesterase inhibitors are of muscarinic nature and include gastrointestinal cramps and diarrhea, upper respiratory secretions, and, more rarely, bradycardia. Occasionally, muscle weakness may be noted, which is a nicotinic side effect. These side effects may limit the total dose of pyridostigmine tolerated by the patient. In the past, oral atropine was used to treat or prevent these side effects. However, with the current trend for the use of immunosuppressants in the management of MG, anticholinesterases are usually prescribed in smaller doses, mostly adjuvant to other therapies, and their side effects become less prominent.

Thymectomy

The role of the thymus gland in the etiology of MG is not yet fully understood, but there is indirect evidence of the primary role of the gland in the pathogenesis of the disease [137–139]. The beneficial effect of thymectomy in MG patients with or without thymoma further supports the role of thymus in the pathogenesis of MG [140].

In thymomatous MG patients, resection of the gland is indicated in all patients at all ages [141]. Therefore, the diagnostic screening of every MG patient should include imaging studies of the mediastinum and measurements of StrAb. Routine chest radiographs may miss more than 25% of thymic masses, thus their diagnostic yield is limited. Computed tomography usually provides an adequate definition of the thymic tumor, but new-generation magnetic resonance imaging offers optimal information regarding the gland and possible thymic invasion of adjoining vascular and other structures [142].

In nonthymomatous MG, thymectomy is usually recommended for patients with generalized MG early in the disease [143]. Thymectomy was also shown to be effective in ocular MG and to prevent generalization of the disease, but it had no apparent advantage over immunosuppressants in a 1997 comparative study [70]. In many centers, an additional criterion for the operation is age younger than 60, but the operation may be considered in older patients whose general condition permits the procedure [144].

In juvenile MG, thymectomy performed within 2 years from onset was shown to be associated with increased remission [73, 145–147] for peripubertal MG patients. In patients with prepubertal onset [72]—as well as in Chinese [59] and Japanese children [61] more likely to have spontaneous remissions—the beneficial effect of thymectomy is less evident. Furthermore, thymectomy was not found to be associated with increased risk of malignancies or other complications in children, adolescent [73], and adult myasthenic patients [108].

The goal of thymectomy is complete removal of all thymic tissue. The transcervical-transsternal maximal thymectomy was shown to produce the highest remission rates: 81% [148]. A less invasive procedure, termed *video-assisted thoracoscopic thymectomy*, has been introduced, and it seems to be a promising surgical technique [149, 150]. Its benefits have not been fully documented.

Response to thymectomy is not immediate, and a remission may be observed within the first 3 years. Rarely, remission may be delayed for a much longer period [151].

Immunosuppressive Medication

The primary goal of treatment of MG is directed toward the autoimmune attack of AChR antibodies against the receptor. There is a range of *nonselective* immuno-suppressant drugs—including corticosteroids, azathioprine, cyclosporin, and cyclophosphamide—as well as short-term immunotherapies, including plasma exchange and human IVIG. The development of *selective* immunosuppressants aiming at the specific autoimmune response to AChR without interfering with the immune system may offer optimal therapeutic solutions in the future management of MG [152, 153].

Corticosteroids

Corticosteroids were the first immunosuppressant drugs used, and they remain the cornerstone of immunotherapy in the treatment of MG. Among corticosteroids, prednisone is the drug of first choice. There are two therapeutic protocols for the use of prednisone in MG. The first approach is to initiate treatment at high doses of 60–100 mg per day or 1.0–1.5 mg/kg. In most adults, a high dose of 100 mg daily is used, switching progressively to an alternate-day dosage [154]. Clinical improvement usually occurs within 2–3 weeks. However, transient worsening may be observed in 50% of patients after the introduction of treatment [155], and it has been reported that 8% of patients who experience worsening may need intubation [156]. Therefore, it is recommended to use this therapeutic scheme with severe MG patients and to admit them during the period of the introduction of high doses of prednisone therapy.

In patients with mild or moderate symptomatology or ocular myasthenia, the alternative therapeutic regime is to initiate prednisone in small doses, at 5–15 mg per day, and slowly increase the dose to therapeutic levels. Improvement may be delayed, but the risk of side effects is significantly reduced. Treatment may be initiated on an outpatient basis, provided that the patient is fully informed of the goal and risks of treatment and has easy and immediate access to the hospital in case of any deterioration.

In one large series of patients, prednisone treatment resulted in complete remission of symptoms in 88% of patients and in marked improvement (allowing for resumption of daily activities) in 52% of patients; moderate improvement was noted in 15%, and no improvement was noted in 5% of patients [156]. After maximal and persistent improvement of symptoms is noted for at least 3–4 months, tapering of prednisone may be initiated. The dose is slowly reduced, and the patient's clinical status is closely monitored. The majority of patients requires maintenance low-dose prednisone treatment for many years or indefinitely.

The usual side effects of chronic steroid treatment may occur, and preventive measures need to be taken. Alternate-day therapy reduces the risk of side effects, and patients are asked to follow a low-sodium, low-carbohydrate, and calorie-restricted diet. Patients are frequently screened for early signs of infection, diabetes mellitus, hypertension, osteoporosis, and cataracts.

Azathioprine

Azathioprine is a purine antimetabolite with a known inhibitory effect on T-lymphocytes. Although a randomized clinical European study [157] showed that azathioprine increases treatment response compared with prednisone monotherapy, the drug is usually considered as a second-line medication for MG. It is mainly reserved for the replacement of prednisone in the unresponsive patient or as adjuvant therapy, allowing for an optimal response at a lower dose of prednisone [158]. The gradual increase of medication—starting with 50 mg daily and slowly increasing to the therapeutic dose (2–3 mg/kg per day)—is recommended, under close monitoring for leukopenia and hepatotoxicity, which represent the most frequent side effects. Onset of improvement is noted within 3–12 months. Ten percent to 20% of patients may develop an idiosyncratic reaction of a flulike syndrome, including fever, nausea, vomiting, diarrhea, or thrush, within the first few weeks of treatment. This reaction suggests intolerance of the individual patient to the drug, which needs to be immediately discontinued. In the majority of patients who receive azathioprine in monoimmunotherapy, the drug is well tolerated, although toxic manifestations have been noted [159]. Malignancies have been reported as a potential side effect of long-term use (for a period of more than 10 years) in patients with multiple sclerosis [160], and a very small risk of lymphoma was found in patients treated with azathioprine for rheumatoid arthritis [161].

Cyclosporin

Cyclosporin has a potent, relatively selective immunosuppressive and immunomodulatory effect, inhibiting the activation of helper T lymphocytes and their production of interleukin-2 while relatively sparing suppressor T cells. Its beneficial effect in MG was shown in a 1993 study based on a prospective double-blinded, randomized, placebo-controlled trial [162] with improvement within 1–4 months. The dose of cyclosporin is 4–6 mg/kg per day, usually in two daily doses. Monitoring of blood levels is indicated, and a therapeutic range of 100–150 μg/liter usually correlates with clinical response. Renal function and blood pressure are the main limitations to therapy and should be regularly assessed. Combination with azathioprine may cause an increased risk of malignancies and infection. The drug is mostly used in combination with corticosteroids, which may increase plasma cyclosporin levels. The dose of steroids could be reduced in combination with cyclosporin [162]. The cost of the drug represents the most significant limiting factor for the use of cyclosporin as a first-line immunosuppressive therapy.

Short-Term Immunotherapies

The use of plasmapheresis and human IVIG in short-term immunotherapies has considerably improved the management of MG patients during acute exacerbations.

Plasma Exchange

The mode of action of plasmapheresis is the presumed depletion of circulating AChR antibodies through plasma exchange. Plasmapheresis has been used as a short-term immunosuppressant therapy in MG patients with or without severe weakness, even in the absence of detectable AChR antibodies [163]. A course of plasmapheresis consists in plasma exchange treatments of 3–4 liters of plasma each. The number, frequency, and duration of each exchange treatment during a course vary among centers; the usual course consists of 4–6 exchanges in 1 or 2 weeks. The onset of improvement is usually noted after the third exchange and is usually maximal at the end of the course, lasting for up to 2 months. In seropositive patients, improvement may be correlated with a reduction of circulating AChR titers [164].

In addition to its major indication for acute relapses (myasthenic crisis), plasmapheresis is frequently used in weak patients before thymectomy or during the initial period of steroid therapy. On rare occasions, repetitive courses of plasma exchange may be required in patients who do not respond to immunosuppressants.

Side effects are noted in fewer than 10% of patients and are generally mild, including hypotension, headaches, hypocalcemia, hypoalbuminemia, and gastrointestinal symptoms. Exceptionally, more severe complications have been reported, including pneumothorax or pulmonary embolism. The main limitations of plasmapheresis are related to difficulties in intravenous access and the high cost of treatment.

New techniques for semiselective removal of AChR antibodies with immunoadsorption plasmapheresis [165], such as protein A immunoadsorption, are now being evaluated [166].

Intravenous Immunoglobulin

IVIG was shown by several authors to have a short-term beneficial effect in MG exacerbations, mostly based on nonrandomized studies [167–169]. In a prospective study comparing IVIG with plasmapheresis, the usual regimen of 0.4 mg/kg per day for 3 and 5 consecutive days was applied. This treatment was shown to be as effective as plasmapheresis, with fewer side effects [170]; no significant difference between the 3-day and 5-day regimens was observed.

In these and other studies, the improvement was noted within 2 weeks after the initiation of treatment; it may persist for as long as 2 months in almost 60% of patients [171]. Although IVIG is usually well tolerated, there have been anecdotal reports of severe side effects, including renal failure (in patients with underlying renal disease [172]) and cerebral infarction [173].

Because of its high cost, this short-term treatment is usually reserved for patients with significant weakness who cannot undergo plasma exchange [174]. The mechanism of action in MG is still unclear.

Therapeutic Considerations in Specific Categories of Patients

Juvenile Myasthenia Gravis

Onset in childhood and adolescence of MG has been reported in 10–15% of white MG patients [52] and in more than 40% among Chinese [58, 59] and Japanese patients [60, 61]. In Asian populations, the disease appears more benign, with a higher portion of ocular myasthenia and remissions [59, 61]. In contrast, 90% of juvenile German MG patients had generalized symptoms at onset [175]. The diagnosis of autoimmune MG may be problematic in children with a higher proportion of seronegativity, mainly in the prepubertal period [122]. The use of short-term plasma exchange therapy or IVIG has been advocated as a therapeutic trial in seronegative juvenile MG patients with significant weakness [176]. With respect to treatment, sufficient evidence supports the indication of early thymectomy (preferably within the first year from onset) for producing an increased remission rate and clinical improvement in juvenile MG, mainly in peripubertal juvenile MG [73, 176]. Thymectomy is not indicated in patients with an increased rate of spontaneous remissions—such as prepubertal white patients [72] and Chinese or Japanese children [59, 61]—except those with severe generalized myasthenia. Chronic corticosteroid treatment was shown to produce significant improvement in approximately 60% of patients with juvenile myasthenia [177] compared with approximately 80% in adults [156]. The indication for chronic corticosteroid therapy should outweigh the significant side effects of growth retardation and bone demineralization, predisposing to later osteoporosis [176]. An alternate-day regimen is recommended to reduce these and other side effects of chronic corticosteroid treatment. The beneficial effects of azathioprine in juvenile MG are similar to those observed in adults, and the drug seems to be relatively well tolerated.

Myasthenic Crisis

Acute myasthenic exacerbations are becoming less frequent because of the response of the majority of patients to the range of available therapies. Nevertheless, myasthenic crisis may still occur and requires the immediate admission to an intensive treatment unit for management, including respiratory assistance. Prognostic factors for prolonged intubation include age greater than 50 years, preintubation serum bicarbonate 30 mg/dl or greater, and vital capacity less than 25 ml/kg [74]. In addition to general intensive care measures, plasmapheresis and IVIG therapy result in short-term improvement in the majority of patients. The overall mortality of myasthenic crisis has dropped dramatically.

Pregnancy

The effect of pregnancy on myasthenic symptoms is variable, and approximately 30% of women may experience worsening of their symptoms during this period [178]. Myasthenic female patients need to be fully informed of this risk and the possible side effects of the various drugs. When planning of pregnancy is possible, periods of persistent remission not requiring immunosuppressants should be chosen to avoid potential teratogenic effects, in particular with azathioprine. During pregnancy, patients should be regularly monitored for possible aggravation of myasthenic symptoms, which may be adequately controlled with plasmapheresis [179] in addition to cholinesterase inhibitors. The use of immunosuppressants during pregnancy requires extreme caution. Azathioprine is usually avoided because of the potential risks of skeletal teratogenicity, even in the absence of definite evidence for such a risk [180].

Labor and delivery are usually uneventful and, in the absence of other obstetric indications, cesarean delivery is not indicated. However, neonatal exacerbations of myasthenic symptoms are relatively common and warrant preventive measures for the mother and the newborn [178, 181].

Neonatal Myasthenia

The necessary precautions should be taken at birth for all infants of myasthenic mothers. The disorder may be recognized within the first hours, and anticholinesterases may be used intravenously (neostigmine bromide). Alternatively, pyridostigmine bromide may be used orally or by nasal-gastric tube (4–10 mg every 4 hours). To prevent overmedication, affected infants should be continuously monitored for vital signs, need of respiratory support, and the occurrence of cholinergic symptoms.

LAMBERT-EATON MYASTHENIC SYNDROME

The first report of an association of a myasthenic syndrome with pulmonary malignancies came from Lambert, Eaton, and Rooke in 1956 [182] and Eaton and Lambert in 1957 [183]. Their patients had myasthenic symptoms of fatigable weakness on exertion but differed from MG patients in the distribution of weakness, in the associated clinical features of loss of tendon reflexes and autonomic dysfunction, and in their neurophysiologic profiles.

LEMS is due to an impaired release of ACh at the motor NT [184]. Fukunaga et al. (1982) described ultrastructural abnormalities of the NT in LEMS—including marked reduction of the density of the active zones and active zones particles corresponding to VGCCs—and suggested that the presynaptic loss of VGCCs is the primary pathologic event of this disorder [185]. They postulated that the calcium channels were the target of autoantibodies. The autoantibodies directed against the VGCC were then identified [186–189]. This autoimmune attack depletes the calcium channels, and as a consequence, the influx of calcium into the NT is impaired, resulting in a decreased quantal release of ACh. Repetitive stimulation—raising the external calcium concentration—helps to increase calcium entry into the NT, thus enhancing the ACh release and improving neuromuscular transmission. LEMS autoantibodies were shown to inhibit calcium influx in small-cell lung cancer cell lines [187] and to bind to ^{125}I-ω-conotoxin (CmTx)–labeled VGCCs of small-cell carcinoma [188] and neuroblastoma cells [189].

Two independent studies demonstrated that more than 92% of LEMS patients, with and without associated neoplasms, had antibodies directed against the P/Q-type VGCCs [190, 191]. N-type VGCC antibodies were detected in 40–49% of all early LEMS and in approximately 70% of those with associated malignancies [191]. Thus, the primary target of LEMS antibodies is the P/Q-type VGCC predominantly at the NT, but they are also directed against postganglionic sympathetic and parasympathetic cells [192].

Clinical Aspects

Epidemiology

LEMS is relatively rare, occurring more frequently in men than women with a ratio of 4.7 to 1.0 [193]. A malignancy is present in approximately 60% of LEMS patients, being more frequently present in those older than age 40. Seventy percent of males and 25% of females have an associated malignancy, which is most frequently a small-cell carcinoma of the lung [194]; more rarely, LEMS has been reported in association with renal cell carcinoma and hematologic tumors. However, only a small fraction of patients with small cell carcinoma of the lung develops LEMS [195]. LEMS may be the presenting manifestation of a malignancy, which may become clinically overt several months later. Non-neoplastic causes, mostly in younger patients and females, mainly include autoimmune diseases, such as thyroid disorders, Sjögren syndrome, celiac disease, vitiligo, juvenile-onset diabetes mellitus [196], and MG (the last on the basis of seropositivity of AChR antibodies in LEMS patients) [197].

Clinical Features

In its classic presentation, the syndrome is characterized by weakness and fatigability, mostly affecting the proximal limb muscles, with minimal or moderate extraocular involvement or bulbar symptoms. Onset of symptoms usually occurs in the proximal lower limb muscles, which remain more predominantly involved. Symptoms may be worse on awakening and improve toward the evening hours. Respiratory muscle involvement is uncommon in LEMS, often related to the use of paralytic agents or coexisting pulmonary diseases [198]. Reflexes are reduced or may be absent. Autonomic symptoms and signs are usually prominent, typically including dry mouth and eyes, impotence, orthostatic hypotension, and hyperhidrosis. Papillary light reflexes may be reduced or absent. Clinical muscle facilitation (i.e., transient improvement of strength after a short period of maximum voluntary contraction) is seldom noted, although the corresponding neurophysiologic phenomenon remains the diagnostic landmark of the disease. However, a transient improvement of tendon reflexes after prolonged voluntary contraction of the muscles may be noted [194].

Diagnosis

Clinical Diagnosis

The clinical diagnosis is based on the triad of fatigable weakness predominantly in proximal limb muscles, reduced or absent reflexes, and autonomic features. Muscle weakness is unresponsive or partially responsive to the edrophonium test.

Clinical Neurophysiologic Testing

Nerve conduction studies and needle EMG may be helpful to differentiate LEMS from neurogenic or myopathic processes presenting with proximal limb weakness and hyporeflexia. SFEMG and SSFEMG cannot differentiate between MG and LEMS [199].

RSSs represent the most specific diagnostic tool, aiming to demonstrate the characteristic neurophysiologic features of this presynaptic disorder (i.e., reduced CMAP amplitude and postactivation facilitation after exercise or tetanic stimulation).

Initially, single stimuli are delivered to obtain a supramaximal response and exclude technical pitfalls. Temperature should be controlled ($\geq 34^\circ$C). The baseline CMAP is established, typically showing the characteristic reduced CMAP amplitude. Then, trains of supramaximal stimuli are delivered at 2 Hz, at 3-minute intervals, usually showing no abnormalities or a decremental response.

PAF requires voluntary exercise of 10 seconds or tetanic stimulation. The patient is asked to maximally exercise the muscle for 10 seconds, and the test is immediately repeated, showing an increment of the amplitude of the first CMAP response of at least 100%. Subsequent trains of stimuli may produce less or no PAF. The same procedure may be repeated, provided that the muscle is rested for at least 3 minutes.

Tetanic stimulation at 20–50 Hz is more painful and thus is indicated only if no PAF is observed after voluntary activation after the same procedure. PAF is frequently noted in hand muscles [200]. Although characteristic of LEMS, PAF is not pathognomonic of the disorder but may rarely be observed in patients with MG. In healthy individuals, an incremental response of as much as 40% may be recorded [201].

The decremental responses obtained at slow rates of stimulation are due to the corresponding depletion of calcium at the NT. PAF results from the accumulation of calcium and the consequent increased quantal release of ACh after voluntary maximal contraction or tetanic stimulation.

Autoimmune Serologic Testing

Several types of VGCCs have been identified in different types of neuronal and neuroendocrine cells. The P/Q-type VGCCs, which are the primary targets of LEMS autoantibodies [190, 192], are mostly expressed in motor NTs and the central nervous system, whereas N-type VGCCs are involved in cerebrocortical, cerebellar, spinal, and autonomic transmissions [123]. Small-cell lung cancer cells express both P/Q- and N-type calcium channels [202]. Immunoprecipitation radioassays for VGCC binding antibodies against the P/Q-type I-ω-CmTx-labeled channels and the ^{125}I-ω-CgTx-labeled N-type VGCCs became available in the late 1990s [119]. P/Q-type antibodies are detected in almost all LEMS patients with lung malignancies and in 91% of LEMS patients without malignancies. N-type antibodies are detected in 70% of patients with LEMS associated to neoplasms and in 40% of LEMS patients without associated malignancies [190, 191].

Treatment

The diagnosis of LEMS warrants the immediate search for the primary neoplasm, and its symptoms and signs may regress if the tumor is identified and responds to treatment [203]. If no neoplasm is identified, repeated investigations should be performed in search of a primary tumor in high-risk patients, such as heavy smokers. Autoimmune screenings should be performed as well, mainly for younger patients.

The symptomatic drug of choice is 3,4-diaminopyridine (3,4-DAP) [204, 205]. 3,4-DAP was shown to improve muscle strength and autonomic functions in the majority of patients. The usual therapeutic dose is 25–60 mg; pyridostigmine used as adjuvant therapy may produce additional symptomatic relief [206]. In this therapeutic range, the drug is well tolerated, with minimal side effects of transient perioral or peripheral paresthesias when the daily dose exceeds 40 mg. Other minor symptoms may include palpitations, sleeplessness, cough, and diarrhea. Rarely, seizures may occur in doses exceeding 60 mg; therefore, such doses are not usually recommended [205].

Other agents increasing the release of the ACh, such as guanidine hydrochloride, may also improve symptoms [207], albeit with more severe side effects, such as bone marrow depression, renal tubular necrosis and failure, hypotension, cardiac arrhythmias, hepatic toxicity, ataxia, and behavioral changes. [208].

The use of immunosuppressant agents has been advocated by a number of authors, mainly for LEMS patients without known associated malignancies. However, none of the studies were controlled and randomized, usually relying on anecdotal information, perhaps because of the rarity of the condition. The use of plasma exchange and immunosuppressants, including corticosteroids and azathioprine, was shown to be effective in a small number of patients with carcinomatous and noncarcinomatous LEMS [209]. Corticosteroids and azathioprine can be used independently or in combination, the latter repeatedly representing the optimal treatment of noncarcinomatous LEMS [196]. IVIG was shown to result in a temporary remission that lasted for several weeks [210–212].

Toxic Disorders of the Junction

Botulism

Botulism is caused by the exotoxin of the anaerobic bacterium *Clostridium botulinum*, an extremely powerful pathogenic organism able to proliferate in anaerobic environments and generate spores, thus securing its survival in extreme weather conditions [213]. Botulinum toxin (BTX) is the most potent neurotoxin, which blocks the presynaptic release of ACh by cleaving synaptic membrane proteins at specific peptide bonds [214, 215] at NMJs and autonomic synapses. Botulism may result from food poisoning and wound injuries. There are seven distinct types of toxins that are potent neuroparalytic agents, but only types A, B, E, and F cause the disease in humans. Most cases usually result from ingestion of poorly sterilized canned or bottled foods, type E being found mostly in seafood.

The disease is potentially fatal but is usually reversible. In infants and young children, *C. botulinum* bacteria colonize the gastrointestinal tract and produce toxin in the intestinal tract [216]. In adults, the toxin is released into the food containing the bacteria in food poisoning. In wound botulism, the anaerobic bacteria grow in deep wounds, such as compound fractures, or sites of subcutaneous tissue injections in drug addicts [213].

In adults, symptoms usually occur within 2–72 hours of exposure. Prodromal symptoms may include nausea, vomiting, diarrhea, and abdominal pain. Early neurologic signs can occur, including blurred vision, diplopia, dilated pupils, and dysarthria, followed by the fulminating disease. Usually, the extraocular and other cranial muscles are affected early and selectively, with a rapidly progressive massive descending quadriparesis, which may also involve the respiratory muscles. The deep tendon reflexes are usually abolished. Parasympathetic dysfunction is prominent, with pupil dilatation, decreased salivation, ileus, or constipation. The illness may progress for 1–2 weeks, followed with slow progressive recovery over several months.

In infants, the clinical presentation is usually less dramatic, mainly characterized by muscle hypotonia and descending muscle weakness with constipation. Cranial nerve palsies and—more rarely—respiratory distress may occur [216].

The neurophysiologic findings of botulism are similar to the ones observed in LEMS. In routine studies, sensory conduction studies are usually normal. In motor conduction studies, CMAP amplitudes are decreased in affected muscles, with normal latencies and conduction velocities. Needle EMG may show abnormalities at rest, with fibrillations and positive waves. Under voluntary contraction, the recruited motor unit action potentials are, typically, of small amplitude and short duration. SFEMG and SSFEMG show abnormalities suggesting neuromuscular dysfunction, such as jitter and blocking. RSSs may show decrement at slow rates of stimulation, with the characteristic increment after brief exercise or titanic stimulation. However, in severe forms of botulism characterized by massive blockage of ACh release, the phenomenon of facilitation may not be possible, and increment may not occur.

The diagnosis is confirmed by detection of the neurotoxin in the patient's serum or feces, the latter having a better diagnostic yield in infants. Polymerase-chain-reaction–based techniques are now being used for the identification of the organism in biological specimens and foods.

Over the last decade, BTX type A has emerged as an effective therapy in the treatment of patients with focal and segmental dystonia as well as other related movement disorders. In parallel to the increasing popularity of this mode of therapy, an increasing number of complications have been reported, both at the site of the injection and at a distance [217].

Patients receiving injections for spasmodic dysphonia frequently develop transient dysphagia [218]. In patients under treatment for spasmodic torticollis, dysphagia was noted in approximately one-third of patients, and 50% of patients may develop radiologic signs of peristaltic abnormalities [219].

Effects in muscles at a distance from the site of BTX treatment have been reported using SFEMG with abnormal jitter, suggesting impaired neuromuscular transmission [220, 221]. In addition, mild abnormalities of cardiovascular reflexes were shown to be indicative of autonomic dysfunction [217].

Extreme caution in the use of BTX treatment is required in patients with coexisting disorders of NMJ, as well as in patients also receiving aminoglycoside antibiotics or other drugs that may interfere with neuromuscular transmission [222]. In one patient with blepharospasm, BTX injections unmasked a subclinical LEMS [223].

Tetanus

The cause of tetanus is a potent neurotoxin released by the anaerobic bacterium *Clostridium tetani.* The toxin blocks the exocytosis of neurotransmitters—mainly γ-aminobutyric acid (GABA) and ACh—by cleaving surface proteins of the synaptic vesicles. Its effects are generalized, predominantly affecting the motor neurons of the spinal cord and brain stem, the cerebral cortex, and the sympathetic nervous system in the hypothalamus. Its selective blockage of GABA and other inhibitory neurotransmitters in the brain stem and spinal cord result in massive activation of neurons, producing local or generalized muscle spasms and rigidity, which are characteristic of the disease. Thus, the clinical symptoms and signs associated with the blockade of ACh release in NMJs are masked by the more powerful effects on the central nervous system and the motor neurons.

Venom Poisoning

The NMJ may be the primary site of action of rarer forms of poisoning, such as venoms of certain species of snakes, lizards, spiders, and scorpions. These contain potent neurotoxins that have a selective curare-like effect on the NMJ. Albeit rare, venom poisoning usually produces severe respiratory distress and may be fatal; thus, early diagnosis and management are critical.

Drug Toxicity on Neuromuscular Transmission

The NMJ is highly sensitive to anesthetics, in particular the nondepolarizing agents (see Table 9.2). The effects of these drugs on ACh release and neuromuscular transmission and the resulting severe paralysis of myasthenic patients have been known since 1939 [224]. Occasionally, prolonged paralysis may be noted in patients without preexisting disease of NMJ, in particular in critically ill patients under intensive care [225].

The effects of neuromuscular blocking depolarizing drugs on neuromuscular transmission are less dramatic, and patients with pre-existing neuromuscular disorders may show less intolerance to these drugs. However, the use of these agents in patients with and without a pre-existing disorder of NMJ requires caution, extensive knowledge of potential side effects, and predisposing factors to complications of neuromuscular blockade.

Antibiotics

The deleterious effects of aminoglycosides on neuromuscular transmission have been well established for practically all agents of this family of antibiotics, which are contraindicated in patients with MG and other NMJ disorders. Most aminoglycosides, including tobramycin and neomycin, exert their effect through reducing the number of ACh quanta released at the NT, after the arrival of the propagated nerve action potential [226]. Other antibiotics have been incriminated in myasthenic exacerbations, including ampicillin [227], ciprofloxacin [228], perfloxacin [229], and norfloxacin [230]. Clindamycin and lincomycin may produce a neuromuscular blockade not reversible with anticholinesterases, although the effect of the latter drug may be reversed with calcium and 3,4-aminopyridine [231, 232].

Magnesium Derivate

Hypermagnesemia is a rare disorder, associated with the use of drugs containing magnesium, such as antacids and laxatives, in patients with predisposing conditions, such as renal failure. Magnesium sulfate ($MgSO_4$) is used in the treatment of pre-eclampsia/eclampsia and for hemodynamic control during anesthesia and the immediate postoperative period.

The mode of action of magnesium is similar to LEMS. It blocks calcium entry into the NT, thus inhibiting ACh release. Magnesium can potentiate the action of neuromuscular blocking agents [233], and patients with NMJ disorders, such as MG and LEMS, may experience exacerbations with magnesium treatment [234, 235].

In mild and moderate forms, discontinuation of magnesium may be sufficient, but some patients may also require intravenous administration of calcium gluconate. In severe forms, hemodialysis may be indicated. Patients with pre-existing myasthenic disorders may also require anticholinesterases.

Other Drugs

β-Adrenergic blockers have been shown to produce increased symptoms of fatigable weakness in patients with MG [236, 237], although a 1996 report failed to produce any aggravation of symptoms after intravenous injections of propranolol and calcium channel antagonists in myasthenic patients [238]. Quinidine and quinine can produce worsening of weakness in patients with MG [239, 240], acting at the NT by inhibiting ACh synthesis or release. In 1996, quinine, quinidine, and chloroquine were shown to impair neuromuscular transmission—both at the presynaptic and postsynaptic levels—in microelectrode and patch clamp studies [241]. MG may be unmasked by quinidine [239] and procainamide [242].

Other drugs with potential side effects on myasthenic patients include morphine [243], chlorpromazine [244], lithium carbonate [245], carnitine [246], diphenylhydantoin [247], trimethadione [248], oral contraceptives [249], and amantadine [250].

Radiographic contrast agents were also shown to produce worsening of symptoms or even a myasthenic crisis in a small number of myasthenic patients [251, 252]. A similar effect was observed after intravenous administration of gadolinium–diethylenetriamine penta–acetic acid, used as a contrast agent for magnetic resonance imaging [253]. Therefore, contrast radiographic and magnetic resonance agents should be used with caution in patients with MG and other disorders of NMJ.

Organophosphate Poisoning

Organophosphorus compounds, mainly used as insecticides, inhibit AChE. They block ACh hydrolysis at central and ganglionic synapses and at the NMJ, resulting in excessive amounts of ACh in the synaptic cleft [254]. The acute clinical syndrome occurs within a few minutes or hours. It is characterized by a massive cholinergic crisis and may last for several days [255]. Signs of autonomic and central nervous system muscarinic (inhibitory) dysfunction include abdominal cramps, hypersalivation, hyperhidrosis, miosis, vomiting, agitation, confusion, tremor, and convulsions associated with nicotinic effects (excitatory), mainly at the NMJ (muscle weakness, fasciculations, and cramps), and paralysis may occur within 24 hours. Intercostal muscle biopsies of patients in the acute stage showed signs of necrotizing myopathy [256]. An intermediate syndrome may occur— usually after exposure to parathion and malathion—within the first 24–96 hours after exposure and may last as long as 6 weeks after recovery from the acute syndrome, resembling severe generalized MG with weakness of cranial respiratory and limb muscles [257]. A late syndrome may occur in 2–5 weeks after recovery from the acute phase in the form of a predominantly motor distal polyneuropathy [255].

In the acute and intermediate stages, the neurophysiologic findings are diagnostic of this condition [254, 258]. RSSs show a repetitive CMAP after single supramaximal stimuli and a decremental response, both at low and high frequencies, which persists for 4–12 days.

HEREDITARY MYASTHENIC DISORDERS

Hereditary myasthenic syndromes (HMSs) were initially termed *congenital MG* by Bowman [259] and Levin [260] to differentiate them from *neonatal MG,* a transient disease of infants born to mothers with MG [76]. Subsequently, the term *congenital myasthenic syndromes* has been adopted to group all familial forms of myasthenic syndromes, although an onset at birth is not found in the majority of these patients.

HMSs are relatively uncommon, with an estimated prevalence of less than 1 to 500,000. However, an increasing number of patients have been reported, mainly with autosomal recessive HMS, and this prevalence rate may be grossly underestimated.

The first clinical report of HMS came from Rothbart (1937) [261], of four siblings presenting with myasthenic symptomatology since early infancy. In 1960, Greer and Schotland reported a young female infant with neonatal episodes of respiratory distress associated with generalized myasthenic features responsive to treatment with significant remissions, last seen at the age of 12 weeks [262]. Her sister had a similar neonatal history and died during an apneic episode at the age of 3 months. Familial cases of myasthenia in infancy and childhood were reported by Namba et al. in 1971 [263] and Conomy et al. in 1975 [264], who introduced the terms *familial infantile MG* and *familial infantile myasthenia.*

The first of a series of publications from the Mayo group on HMS was of a boy with endplate AChE deficiency [265]. A syndrome "attributed to a prolonged open-time of the acetylcholine-induced ion channel" was subsequently reported [266] with a description of morphologic and kinetic observations of the channel, obtained through conventional microelectrode techniques. This autosomal dominant syndrome was subsequently termed *slow-channel syndrome* (SCS) [267]. Over the next 20 years, the development of sophisticated morphologic and in vitro electrophysiologic techniques by the Mayo group permitted remarkably detailed observations of individual patients with inherited myasthenic syndromes, mainly with respect to ultrastructural abnormalities of the junction, as well as kinetic properties of the receptor channel [27]. These studies require the presence of adequate numbers of NMJs, usually obtained from a muscle biopsy of the external intercostal [268] or the anconeus muscle [269]. Light microscopic studies involve—in addition to muscle histochemical staining—cytochemical and immunocytochemical localizations of AChE, AChRs, and their subunits, as well as immune complexes at the junction. Quantitative electron microscopy and electron-cytochemistry allow for the evaluation of the size and density of synaptic vesicles and for the study of the morphology of synaptic membranes and the perisynaptic region, whereas the numbers of AChR binding sites can be quantified through ultrastructural localization of peroxidase-labeled α-BuTx. In vitro neurophysiologic studies were further developed to include noise analysis techniques and investigations of the kinetic properties of the channel at voltage-clamped EPs of patients, such as the mean open duration of channel events and channel conductance. In the early 1990s, the properties of the receptor channels could be further elucidated by techniques of patch-clamp analysis [27].

An unparalleled series of reports on well-characterized HMS patients and syndromes, with detailed descriptions of morphologic and kinetic abnormalities as well as their genetic profiles, emanated from the Mayo Group in the 1990s. A classification of the inherited myasthenic syndromes was proposed by Engel in 1994 [270, 271] (Table 9.4), differentiating syndromes to (1) presynaptic defects, (2) synaptic defects, and (3) postsynaptic defects. In each of these groups, HMSs were subclassified according to their recognized ultrastructural and kinetic abnormalities. A separate category was reserved for syndromes that were described as "partially characterized" if their published reports contained incomplete morphologic or neurophysiologic data.

A second classification of HMS was proposed by the 34th International Workshop of the European Neuromuscular Center (ENMC), based on the mode of inheritance, the clinical symptomatology, and investigations commonly available in neuromuscular centers [272] (Table 9.5). Syndromes were divided into autosomal recessive myasthenic syndrome (ARMS) forms (Type I); the autosomal dominant myasthenic syndrome forms (Type II), corresponding to the SCS; and Type III, which includes sporadic cases with no family history, excluding MG and other acquired disorders of the junction.

Both classifications of inherited myasthenic syndromes present advantages and limitations. The classification of Engel is based on sophisticated techniques only available at the Mayo Clinics and *splits* patients, sometimes presenting with a

Table 9.4   Classification of congenital myasthenic syndromes

Presynaptic defects
   Defect in ACh resynthesis or packaging (familial infantile myasthenia)
   Paucity of synaptic vesicles and reduced quantal release
Synaptic defects
   Endplate AChE deficiency
Postsynaptic defects
   Kinetic abnormalities of AChR with AChR deficiency
      Slow-channel syndromes
         Due to delayed channel closure
         Due to repeated channel reopenings
      AChR deficiency and short channel open time
   Kinetic abnormalities of AChR without AChR deficiency
      Low-affinity fast-channel syndrome
      High-conductance fast-channel syndrome
   Severe AChR deficiency without a primary kinetic abnormality of AChR
Partially characterized syndromes
   CMS resembling LEMS
   AChR deficiency with paucity of secondary synaptic clefts
   Miscellaneous partially characterized AChR deficiencies
   Familial limb-girdle myasthenia
   Benign CMS with facial malformations

ACh = acetylcholine; AChE = acetylcholinesterase; AChR = acetylcholine receptor; LEMS = Lambert-Eaton myasthenic syndrome; CMS = congenital myasthenic syndrome.

Source: Modified from AG Engel, K Ohno, M Milone, et al. Congenital myasthenic syndromes caused by mutations in acetylcholine receptor genes. Neurology 1997;48(suppl 5):28–35; and AG Engel. Congenital myasthenic syndromes. Neurol Clin 1994;12:401–437.

Table 9.5   European Neuromuscular Center classification of congenital myasthenic syndromes (modified)

Type I	Autosomal recessive
Ia	Familial infantile myasthenia
Ib	Limb-girdle myasthenia
Ic	Acetylcholinesterase deficiency
Id	Acetylcholine receptor deficiency
Ie	Benign congenital myasthenic syndrome with facial dysmorphism
Type II	Autosomal dominant
IIa	Slow-channel syndrome
Type III	Sporadic
	Cases with no family history, excluding myasthenia gravis

Source: Modified from LT Middleton. Report of the 34th European Neuromuscular Center International Workshop: Congenital myasthenia syndromes. Neuromuscul Disord 1996;6:133–136.

similar phenotype, based on in vitro neurophysiologic and morphologic observations. The ENMC classification tends to *lump* patients who may harbor different pathophysiologic mechanisms and molecular defects. The identification of the gene(s) and the specific mutations in each HMS family and affected individuals, and the results of correlation studies with the onset, distribution, and severity of myasthenic and other symptoms and signs are necessary steps for their reconciliation into a more clinically relevant classification of HMS [273].

Autosomal Dominant Disorder: Slow-Channel Syndrome

SCS has an autosomal dominant mode of inheritance, with complete penetrance and variable expressivity in the majority of patients. Sporadic cases may occur, however, suggesting new mutations or possible genetic heterogeneity [270]. The age at onset is variable, ranging from infancy to adult life. There is selective involvement of cranial and scapular muscles and the extensors of hands and fingers, although all muscles may be affected. Progression may be gradual or intermittent and stepwise; there may be increasing characteristic weakness and atrophy of affected muscles due to progressive EP myopathy, which results from the cationic overloading of the postjunctional region [266]. The tendon reflexes may remain normal but may become hypoactive or absent in severely affected muscles. A consistent neurophysiologic finding is a double CMAP-evoked response to single-nerve stimulus. The landmark pathophysiologic abnormality was identified in the initial description of SCS as "a prolonged open time of the acetylcholine-induced ion channel," associated with ultrastructural evidence of focal EP myopathy, resulting from calcium overloading of the post-synaptic region [266]. Several physiopathogenic mechanisms may impair the safety margin, such as the progressive destruction of the postjunctional folds and the resulting loss of AChRs; the persistent depolarization that is due to temporal summation of prolonged EP potentials leading to inactivation of VGSC; and, for certain SCS mutations, the desensitization of some AChR, even in the resting state [271, 274, 275]. In vitro microelectrode studies demonstrated prolonged decay of MEPPs and currents [266] (Figure 9.2).

The first identified mutation was the T264P of the ε-AChR subunit, occurring in the pore-lining M2 transmembrane domain [275]. Six distinct mutations have been found in the ε-AChR subunit. Three mutations were reported by the Mayo Group: mutation G153S, located in the extracellular domain near the agonist binding site [276]; N217K in the M1 domain [277]; and V249F in the M2 domain [274]. In 1997, Croxen et al. reported three additional mutations in the gene encoding the ε-AChR subunit [278]: T254I in the pore-lining M2 domain; S269I in the short extracellular loop between M2-M3; and V156M, which lies in proximity to the G153S, in the extracellular domain. The two mutations identified in the ε subunit gene (V266M [277] and L262M [279]) are both located within the M2 domain. A second ε-AChR subunit mutation (L269F) was also reported [277, 280]. All SCS mutations are autosomal dominant, causing a pathogenic gain of function.

A number of interesting observations was made correlating the specific mutations and results of expression studies on one hand, and the clinical phenotype and in vitro neurophysiologic abnormalities on the other [271, 281]. Clinically,

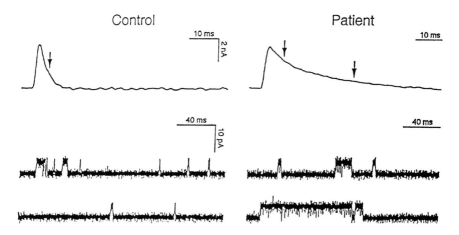

Figure 9.2 Comparison of miniature endplate currents (MEPCs) (upper traces) and channel events (lower traces) recorded from control (left) and slow-channel myasthenic syndrome endplate of a patient with the αG153S mutation (right). The MEPC decay is prolonged and associated with markedly prolonged channel events in the patient. The MEPC decay is best fitted by the sum of two exponentials. Vertical arrows indicate MEPC decay time constants. The prolonged channel events consist of bursts of normal-duration channel openings. (Reprinted from SM Sine, K Ohno, C Bouzat, et al. Mutation of the acetylcholine receptor α subunit causes a slow-channel myasthenic syndrome by enhancing agonist binding affinity. Neuron 1995;15:229–239, by permission of Cell Press.)

mutations in the extracellular domain are associated with a more benign disease, whereas mutations in the M2 domain result in a more severe phenotype. Expression studies of genetically engineered mutant AChRs in human embryonic kidney fibroblasts showed that the SCS mutations produce either normal [277] or slightly reduced [275] amounts of AChRs. Therefore, the EP AChR deficiency may represent a secondary consequence of the EP myopathy and not an abnormally reduced translation of the mutant subunit. [277]. Furthermore, the landmark neurophysiologic abnormality of a prolonged decay of EP current potential is associated with all SCS mutations but is more pronounced in M2 mutations that introduce a phenylalanine residue into the M2 domain [281]. The M2 mutations are associated with spontaneous openings of the AChR channel in the resting state, causing partial depolarization of the EP and inactivation of the postsynaptic junctional sodium channels, further reducing the safety margin of neuromuscular transmission [274, 277]. The persistent depolarization at rest enhances the cationic overloading of the postjunctional region, further aggravating the EP myopathy and the consequent progressive loss of AChRs. All M2 pore-lining mutations slow the rate of channel closure, resulting in longer opening events. The effect of M1 mutations is similar, but to a lesser extent, and one M1 mutation (αN217K) slows the rate of ACh dissociation from the binding site [282]. The extracellular mutation αG153S decreases the rate of ACh dissociation from the binding site without affecting the rate of channel closing, resulting in repeated reopenings of the channel during each ACh occupancy [276]. All mutations result in enhanced affinity of ACh binding at equilibrium through different mechanisms for each mutation [281].

In 1998, quinidine sulfate was shown to have a beneficial effect on muscle strength and the decremental response [283] in SCS. Quinidine sulfate was previously shown to have properties of an open-channel blocker of AChR, by reducing the duration of opening episodes of either wild-type or SCS mutant AChRs at concentrations lower than those that would compromise the safety margin of neuromuscular transmission [241, 284]. Potential side effects may occur, such as drug allergy and exacerbation of weakness—mainly at concentrations higher than 5 μg/ml—and possible respiratory failure in patients with borderline respiratory functions [283].

Autosomal Recessive Syndromes

In the ENMC classification, ARMS were grouped as Type I and were subdivided into four clinical syndromes [272]. HMSIa encompasses cases of *familial infantile myasthenia*, mainly characterized by its temporal clinical profile. The onset is at birth or early infancy, with initial symptoms of fluctuating ptosis, poor cry and suck, feeding difficulties, and possible episodes of respiratory distress, sometimes leading to early death. In early childhood, symptoms may be variable, mainly affecting ocular movements and eyelids and including mild to moderate fatigue-induced weakness. Episodic exacerbations may occur, usually under precipitating circumstances. Later in life, patients present with ophthalmoparesis without diplopia, associated with fluctuating ptosis and mild to moderate fatigable weakness of bulbar and limb muscles. Symptoms usually improve with anticholinesterases. Tendon reflexes remain normal, without signs of muscle atrophy. Sensation and coordination are normal. A decremental response is observed at 2- to 3-Hz stimulation in affected muscles, with the proviso that a decremental response may require prolonged exercise or repetitive stimulation at slow rate for 3 minutes to produce the exhaustion phenomenon. Several previously reported ARMS may correspond to Type Ia. *Familial infantile myasthenia* was a term initially introduced to describe familial cases of onset in early infancy presenting mild to moderate myasthenic symptoms with prominent oculomotor involvement [263] and patients with more severe symptoms, without marked ophthalmoparesis, requiring chronic treatment [264, 285, 286]. Other workers reserved the term for infants with sudden severe episodes of generalized myasthenia and respiratory distress, occurring acutely, early in life (as in the case of Greer and Schotland [262]) and adolescence [287] without significant intercurrent myasthenic symptoms or oculomotor manifestations. In three patients with this phenotype studied by Mora et al. [288], there was evidence of presynaptic defect in ACh resynthesis or packaging. Patients with the syndrome "associated with high conductance and fast closure of the acetylcholine receptor channel" [289], and "deficiency and short opening time of the acetylcholine receptor" [290] may also be compatible with HMSIa. Furthermore, in the reported series of 22 cases of AChR deficiency syndrome, [291] five patients were reported as having a family history of muscle weakness or perinatal respiratory failure in siblings.

HMS Type Id (corresponding to AChR deficiency syndrome) includes patients with a static benign form of myasthenia, mainly affecting extraocular muscles associated with mild generalized fatigable weakness in the limbs. Exacerbations and episodes of respiratory distress do not occur. Myasthenic symptoms respond to anticholinesterases.

HMSIb (limb-girdle myasthenic syndrome) is characterized by symmetric fatigue-induced weakness of limb-girdle muscles, occurring usually in childhood [292]. A decremental response at 2–3 Hz is noted, and muscle histochemistry may show presence of tubular aggregates with no significant morphologic abnormalities of NMJ [293, 294].

HMS Ic corresponds to AChE deficiency, initially recognized in 1977 by Engel et al. [265]. Clinically, the manifesting symptoms are initially fatigue-induced weakness of facial ocular and bulbar muscles at an early onset, to age 2 years. Motor milestones are delayed. There is progressive selective involvement of cervical and axial muscles, leading to fixed scoliosis. Ophthalmoparesis may also be present. Slow papillary responses to light are typical of this disorder. Symptoms are refractory to anticholinesterase medication. Tendon reflexes may be normal or reduced. A double CMAP-evoked response to single nerve stimuli is the typical clinical neurophysiologic sign. Morphologically, AChE deficiency is confirmed by enzyme histochemistry or immunocytochemical or double-staining techniques [295, 296]. On electron cytochemistry, AChE is severely reduced or absent in the synaptic basal lamina. Ultrastructural abnormalities include a significant decrease of the NT size and presynaptic membrane length and degeneration of the junctional folds and the underlying muscle fiber, being secondary effects to the deficiency of AChE. Mutational studies of genes encoding AChE failed to identify abnormalities [297]. Mutations were identified in the gene encoding the collagen-tail (ColQ) of AChE [298, 299], which plays an important role in triggering the synthesis and association of the catalytic subunits and in anchoring AChE molecules to the basal lamina.

A distinct form of ARMS was reported in Iraqi and Iranian Jews [300]. The age at onset is from birth to age 2 years, and the clinical symptomatology mainly includes marked fatigue-induced weakness mostly with ptosis, weakness of facial and masticatory muscles, and fatigable speech with associated facial malformations. These dysmorphic features include an elongated face, mandibular prognathism with malocclusion, and a high-arched palate. The course is mild and nonprogressive, and symptoms respond to anticholinesterase medication. This syndrome may be assigned as HMS type Ie [273]. Linkage studies were negative for the ε subunit locus, on chromosome 17p [301].

The forward genetics approach has been applied in studies of well-characterized ARMS patients and families. This approach was made possible by the detailed delineation of the morphologic and pathophysiologic mechanisms in selected ARMS patients, mainly by the Mayo Group and the available information on genes encoding AChR subunits. All mutations identified to date in ARMS (approximately 30 mutations) reside in the gene encoding the ε subunit; no mutations were identified in other AChR subunit genes. This may, perhaps, be due to the phenotypic rescue mechanisms of replacement of the ε subunit by the γ fetal isoform, allowing for the survival from null mutations, in contrast to mutations in other subunit genes, which, in the absence of such mechanisms, may be fatal.

In two patients with the low-affinity, fast-channel syndrome, two heteroallelic AChR ε subunit gene mutations were identified, causing a pathologic loss of function [302]. Expression studies in human embryonic kidney cells suggested that the syndrome stems from a common missense mutation εP121L, requiring a heteroallelic null mutation in the same gene to become clinically manifest [302]. AChR affinity to ACh was shown to be markedly reduced in the open-channel and desensitized states but not in the resting state, resulting in fewer and shorter AChR opening episodes with no EP AChR deficiency or myopathy [302]. In the severe endplate AChR deficiency syndrome, with presence of immature AChRs containing the fetal γ instead of the ε subunit, two nonsense mutations were initially identified at the level of the long intracellular loop between the M3 and M4 membrane domain [303]. In four additional patients with similar features, an association of heteroallelic nonsense/missense mutations in the ε subunit gene was shown, with expression of the fetal γ instead of the ε subunit [304, 305]. A single nucleotide deletion in the α subunit was identified in another group of patients [306]. Mutational screening by SSCP analysis of genes encoding other postjunctional proteins such as rapsyn [307] to date have failed to identify mutations in ARMS.

Reverse genetic techniques of linkage analysis were applied in mapping the gene of a large, clinically homogenous group of patients from the Eastern Mediterranean region, corresponding phenotypically to ARMS Type Ia to the telomeric region of chromosome 17p [308]. Two putative candidate genes (i.e., the gene encoding the presynaptic synaptobrevin-2 protein and the ε AChR subunit gene) already mapped to this region were analyzed. All patients were found to harbor mutations in the ε subunit gene, and a total of six homozygous mutations were identified [309]. Expression studies indicated reduced expression of each mutant AChR except for one single missense mutation identified in an Italian family (A411P). Four Gypsy families from Greece and Turkey had a common missense mutation (1267 del g). Further mutational studies in six Turkish kinships identified four additional ε subunit frame-shifting and splice-site null mutations [310, 311].

REFERENCES

1. Miledi R, Molenaar PC, Polak RL. Electrophysiological and chemical determination of acetylcholine release at the frog neuromuscular junction. J Physiol 1983;334:245–254.
2. Hall ZW, Sanes JR. Synaptic structure and development: the neuromuscular junction. Cell 1993;72:99–121.
3. Flucher BE, Daniels MP. Distribution of Na+ channels and ankyrin in neuromuscular junctions is complementary to that of acetylcholine receptors and the 43kD protein. Neuron 1989;3:163–175.
4. Froehner SC. The submembrane machinery for nicotonic acetylcholine receptor clustering. J Cell Biol 1991;114:1–7.
5. Apel ED, Roberds SL, Campbell KP, et al. Rapsyn may function as a link between the acetylcholine receptor and the agrin-binding dystrophin-associated glycoprotein complex. Neuron 1995;15:115–126.
6. Ferns M, Deiner M, Hall ZW. Agrin-induced acetylcholine receptor clustering in mammalian muscle requires tyrosine phosphorylation. J Cell Biol 1996;132:937–944.
7. Apel ED, Glass DJ, Moscoso LM, et al. Rapsyn is required for MuSK signaling and recruits synaptic components to a MuSK-containing scaffold. Neuron 1997;18:623–625.
8. Ohlendieck K. Towards an understanding of the dystrophin-glycoprotein complex: linkage between the extracellular matrix and the membrane cytoskeleton in muscle fibers. Eur J Cell Biol 1996;69:1–10.
9. Ohlendieck K, Ervasti JM, Matsumura SD, et al. Dystrophin-related protein is localized to neuromuscular junctions of adult skeletal muscle. Neuron 1991;7:499–508.
10. Bewick GS, Nicholson LV, Young C, et al. Different distributions of dystrophin and related proteins at nerve-muscle junctions. Neuroreport 1992;3:857–860.

11. Peters MF, Kramarcy NR, Sealock R, et al. β_2-syntrophin: localization at the neuromuscular junction in skeletal muscle. Neuroreport 1994;5:1577–1580.

12. Sanes JR, Apel ED, Gautam M et al. Agrin receptors at the skeletal neuromuscular junction. Ann N Y Acad Sci 1998;841:1–13.

13. Merlie JP, Sanes JR. Concentration of acetylcholine receptor mRNA in synaptic regions of adult muscle fibers. Nature 1985;317:66–68.

14. Martinou JC, Falls DI, Fischbeck GD, et al. Acetylcholine receptor-inducing activity stimulates expression of the epsilon-subunit gene of the muscle acetylcholine receptor. Proc Natl Acad Sci U S A 1991;88:7669–7673.

15. Salpeter MM, Loring RH. Nicotinic acetylcholine receptors in vertebrate muscle: properties, distribution, and neural control. Prog Neurobiol 1985;25:297–325.

16. Kaminski HJ, Suarez JI, Ruff RL. Neuromuscular junction physiology in myasthenia gravis: isoforms of the acetylcholine receptor in extraocular muscle and the contribution of sodium channels to the safety factor. Neurology 1997;48(suppl 5):8–17.

17. Reist NE, Werle MJ, McMahan UJ. Agrin released by motor neurons induces the aggregation of acetylcholine receptors at neuromuscular junctions. Neuron 1992;8:865–868.

18. Jo SA, Zhu X, Marchionni MA, et al. Neuregulins are concentrated at nerve-muscle synapses and activate ACh-receptor gene expression. Nature 1995;373:158–161.

19. Philips WD, Vladeta D, Han H, et al. Rapsyn and agrin slow the metabolic degradation of the acetylcholine receptor. Mol Cell Neurosci 1997;10:16–26.

20. Hesselmans LFGM, Jennekens FGI, Van Den Oord CJM, et al. Development of innervation of skeletal muscle fibers in man: relation to acetylcholine receptors. Anat Rec 1993;236:553–562.

21. Ruff RL, Spiegel P. Ca sensitivity and AChR currents of twitch and tonic snake muscle fibers. Am J Physiol 1990;259:911–919.

22. Dwyer TM, Adams DJ, Hille B. The permeability of the end plate channel to organic cations in frog muscle. J Gen Physiol 1980;75:469–492.

23. Katz B, Miledi R. Estimates of quantal content during chemical potentiation of transmitter release. Proc R Soc Lond B Biol Sci 1979;205:369–378.

24. Gertler RA, Robbins N. Differences in neuromuscular transmission in red and white muscles. Brain Res 1978;142:255–284.

25. Ruff RL, Whittlesey D. Comparison of Na+ currents from type IIa and IIb human intercostal muscle fibers. Am J Physiol 1993;265:171–177.

26. Storella RJ, Riker WF, Baker T. d-Tubocurarine sensitivities of fast and slow neuromuscular system of the rat. Eur J Pharmacol 1985;118:181–184.

27. Engel AG. The investigation of congenital myasthenic syndromes. Ann N Y Acad Sci 1993;681: 425–434.

28. Wilks S. On cerebritis, hysteria, and bulbar paralysis, as illustrative of arrest of function of the cerebrospinal centers. Guys Hospital Report 1877;22:7–55.

29. Erb W. Zur Casuistik der bulbaren Lahmungen. Arch Psychiatr Nervenkr 1879;9:325–350.

30. Goldflam S. Uber einen scheinbar heilbaren bulbarparalytischen Symptomen-complex mit Beteiligung der Extremitaten. Dtsch Z Nervenhlk 1893;4:312–352.

31. Jolly F. Uber Myasthenia gravis pseudoparalytica. Berl Klin Wochenschr 1895;32:1–7.

32. Campbell H, Bramwell E. Myasthenia gravis. Brain 1900;23:277–336.

33. Buzzard EF. The clinical history and post-mortem examination of five cases of myasthenia gravis. Brain 1905;28:438–451.

34. Walker MB. Treatment of myasthenia gravis with physostigmine (letter). Lancet 1934;1:1200–1201.

35. Dale HH, Feldberg W. Chemical transmission at motor nerve endings in voluntary muscle? J Physiol 1936;86:353–380.

36. Blalock A, Harvey AM, Ford FF, et al. The treatment of myasthenia gravis by removal of the thymus gland. JAMA 1941;117:1529–1533.

37. Blalock A. Thymectomy in the treatment of myasthenia gravis. Report of twenty cases. J Thorac Surg 1944;13:316–339.

38. Simpson JA. Myasthenia gravis: a new hypothesis. Scott Med J 1960;5:419–436.

39. Nastuk WL, Plescia OJ, Osserman KE. Changes in serum complement activity in patients with myasthenia gravis. Proc Soc Exp Biol Med 1960;105:177–184.

40. Patrick J, Lindstrom J. Autoimmune response to acetylcholine receptor. Science 1973;180:871–872.

41. Fambrough DM, Drachman DB, Satyamurti S. Neuromuscular junction in myasthenia gravis: decreased acetylcholine receptors. Science 1973;182:293–295.

42. Lindstrom JM, Seybold ME, Lennon VA, et al. Antibody to acetylcholine receptor in myasthenia gravis. Neurology 1976;26:1054–1059.

43. Pinching AJ, Peters DK, Newsom-Davis J. Remission of myasthenia gravis following plasma-exchange. Lancet 1976;2:1373.
44. Dau PC. Response to plasmapheresis and immunosuppressive drug therapy in sixty myasthenia gravis patients. Ann N Y Acad Sci 1981;377:700–708.
45. Mann JD, Johns TR, Campa JF. Long-term administration of corticosteroids in myasthenia gravis. Neurology 1976;26:729–740.
46. Drachman DB. Myasthenia gravis. N Engl J Med 1994;330:1797–1810.
47. Ruff RL, Lennon VA. End-plate voltage gated sodium channels are lost in clinical and experimental myasthenia gravis. Ann Neurol 1998;43:370–379.
48. Ruff RL. Action potential thresholds are elevated near the end-plate, but not elsewhere in myasthenia gravis and passive transfer experimental myasthenia gravis. Ann Neurol 1996;40:507–508.
49. Eymard B, Chillet P. Autoimmune myasthenia: recent physiopathological data. Presse Med 1997;26:872–879.
50. Okinaka S, Reese HH, Katsuki S, et al. The prevalence of multiple sclerosis and other neurological diseases in Japan. Acta Neurol Scand 1966;42(suppl 19):68–76.
51. Kyriallis K, Hristova AH, Middleton LT. What is the real epidemiology of myasthenia gravis [abstract]? Neurology 1995;45(suppl 4):351–352.
52. Philips LH, Torner JC, Anderson MS, et al. The epidemiology of myasthenia gravis in central and western Virginia. Neurology 1992;42:1888–1893.
53. Philips LH, Torner JC. Epidemiologic evidence for a changing natural history of myasthenia gravis. Neurology 1996;47:1233–1238.
54. Oosterhuis HJGH. The natural course of myasthenia gravis: a long term follow up study. J Neurol Neurosurg Psychiatry 1989;52:1121–1127.
55. Osserman KE, Genkins G. Studies in myasthenia gravis: review of a twenty-year experience in over 1200 patients. Mt Sinai J Med 1971;38:497–537.
56. Beekman R, Kuks JB, Oosterhuis HJ. Myasthenia gravis: diagnosis and follow-up of 100 consecutive patients. J Neurol 1997;224:112–118.
57. Slesak G, Melms A, Gerneth F et al. Late-onset myasthenia gravis. Follow-up of 113 patients diagnosed after age 60. Ann N Y Acad Sci 1998;841:777–780.
58. Chiu HC, Vincent A, Newsom-Davis J, et al. Myasthenia gravis: population differences in disease expression and acetylcholine receptor antibody titers between Chinese and Caucasians. Neurology 1987;37:1854–1857.
59. Wong V, Hawkins BR, Yu YL. Myasthenia gravis in Hong Kong Chinese. 2. Paediatric disease. Acta Neurol Scand 1992;86:68–72.
60. Uono M. Clinical statistics of myasthenia gravis in Japan. Int J Neurol 1980;14:87–99.
61. Fukuyama Y, Hirayama Y, Osawa M. Epidemiological and Clinical Features of Childhood Myasthenia Gravis in Japan. In E Satoyoshi (ed), Myasthenia Gravis—Pathogenesis and Treatment. Tokyo: University of Tokyo Press, 1981;19–27.
62. Grob D, Brunner NG, Namba T. The natural course of myasthenia gravis and effect of therapeutic measures. Ann N Y Acad Sci 1981;377:652–669.
63. Grob D, Asura EL, Brunner NG, et al. The course of myasthenia gravis and therapies affecting outcome. Ann N Y Acad Sci 1987;505:472–499.
64. Nations SP, Wolfe GI, Amato AA, et al. Clinical features of patients with distal myasthenia gravis [abstract]. Neurology 1997;48:64.
65. Horton RM, Manfredi AA, Conti-Tronconi BM. The "embryonic" gamma subunit of the nicotinic acetylcholine receptor is expressed in adult extraocular muscle. Neurology 1993;43:983–986.
66. Kaminski HJ, Maas E, Spiegel P, et al. Acetylcholine receptor expression in human extraocular muscles and their susceptibility to myasthenia gravis. Neurology 1990;40:1663–1669.
67. Missias AC, Chu GC, Klocke BJ, et al. Regulation of the acetylcholine receptor gamma subunit gene in developing skeletal muscle: analysis with subunit-specific antibodies, transgenic mice and cultured cells. Dev Biol 1996;179:223–238.
68. MacLennan C, Beeson D, Buijs AM, et al. Acetylcholine receptor expression in human extraocular muscles and their susceptibility to myasthenia gravis. Ann Neurol 1997;41:423–431.
69. Massey JM. Acquired myasthenia gravis. Neurol Clin 1997;15:577–595.
70. Sommer N, Sigg B, Melms A, et al. Ocular myasthenia gravis: response to long-term immunosuppressive treatment. J Neurol Neurosurg Psychiatry 1997;62:156–162.
71. Christensen PB, Jensen TS, Tsiropoulos I, et al. Mortality and survival in myasthenia gravis: a Danish population based study. J Neurol Neurosurg Psychiatry 1998;64:78–83.
72. Rodriguez M, Gomez MR, Howard FM, et al. Myasthenia gravis in children: long-term follow-up. Ann Neurol 1983;13:504–510.

73. Andrews PI, Massey JM, Howard JF, et al. Race, sex and puberty influence onset, severity and outcome in juvenile myasthenia gravis. Neurology 1994;44:1208–1214.
74. Thomas CE, Mayer SA, Gungor Y, et al. Myasthenic crisis: clinical features, mortality, complications, and risk factors for prolonged intubation. Neurology 1997;48:1253–1260.
75. Osserman KE. Myasthenia Gravis. New York: Grune & Stratton, 1958.
76. Strickroot FL, Schaeffer BL, Bergo HL. Myasthenia gravis occurring in an infant born of a myasthenic mother. JAMA 1942;120:1207.
77. Namba T, Brown SB, Grob D. Neonatal myasthenia gravis: report of two cases and a review of the literature. Paediatrics 1970;45:488.
78. Keesy J, Lindstrom J, Cokeley H, et al. Anti-acetylcholine receptor antibody in neonatal myasthenia gravis. N Engl J Med 1977;296:55.
79. Eymard B, Morel E, Dulac O, et al. Myasthenie et grossesse: une etude clinique et immunologique de 42 cas (21 myasthenies neonatales). Rev Neurol 1989;145:696–705.
80. Bucknall RC, Dixon A, Glick EN, et al. Myasthenia gravis associated with penicillamine treatment for rheumatoid arthritis. BMJ 1975;1:600–602.
81. Czlonkowska A. Myasthenia syndrome during penicillamine treatment. BMJ 1975;2:726.
82. Jaffe IA. Induction of auto-immune syndromes by penicillamine therapy in rheumatoid arthritis and other diseases. Springer Semin Immunopathol 1981;4:193–207.
83. Andonopoulos AP, Terzis E, Tsibri E, et al. D-Penicillamine induced myasthenia gravis in rheumatoid arthritis: an unpredictable common occurrence? Clin Rheumatol 1994;13:586–588.
84. Kato Y, Naito Y, Narita Y, et al. D-Penicillamine-induced myasthenia gravis in a case of eosinophilic fasciitis. J Neurol Sci 1997;146:85–86.
85. Kuncl RW, Pestronk A, Drachman DB, et al. The pathophysiology of penicillamine-induced myasthenia gravis. Ann Neurol 1986;20:740–744.
86. Tzartos SJ, Morel E, Efthimiadis A, et al. Fine antigenic specificities of antibodies in sera from patients with D-penicillamine-induced myasthenia gravis. Clin Exp Immunol 1988;74:80–86.
87. Drosos AA, Christou L, Galanopoulou V, et al. D-Penicillamine induced myasthenia gravis: clinical, serological and genetic findings. Clin Exp Rheumatol 1993;1:387–391.
88. Penn A, Low BW, Jaffe IA, et al. Drug-induced autoimmune myasthenia gravis. Ann N Y Acad Sci 1998;841:433–449.
89. Perez A, Perella M, Pastor E et al. Myasthenia gravis induced by alfa-interferon therapy. Am J Hematol 1995;49:365–366.
90. Batocchi AP, Evoli A, Servidei S, et al. Myasthenia gravis during interferon alfa therapy. Neurology 1995;45:382–383.
91. Picollo G, Franciotta D, Versino M, et al. Myasthenia gravis in a patient with chronic active hepatitis C during interferon-a treatment [letter]. J Neurol Neurosurg Psychiatry 1996;60:348.
92. Mase G, Zorzon M, Biasutti E, et al. Development of myasthenia gravis during interferon a treatment for anti-HCV positive chronic hepatitis. J Neurol Neurosurg Psychiatry 1996;60:348–349.
93. Blake G, Murphy S. Onset of myasthenia gravis in a patient with multiple sclerosis during interferon-1b treatment. Neurology 1997;49:1747–1748.
94. Nelson KR, McQuillen MP. Neurologic complications of graft-versus-host-disease. Neurol Clin 1988;6:389–403.
95. Seely E, Drachman D, Smith BR, et al. Post bone marrow transplantation (BMT) myasthenia gravis: evidence for acetylcholine receptor abnormality [abstract]. Blood 1984;64(suppl):221a.
96. Bolger GB, Sullivan KM, Spence AM, et al. Myasthenia gravis after allogeneic bone marrow transplantation: relationship to chronic graft-versus-host disease. Neurology 1986;36:1087–1091.
97. Lefvert AK, Bjorkholm M. Antibodies against the acetylcholine receptor in hematologic disorders: implications for the development of myasthenia gravis after bone marrow grafting. N Engl J Med 1987;317:170.
98. Grau JM, Casademont J, Monforte R, et al. Myasthenia gravis after allogeneic bone marrow transplantation: report of a new case and pathogenetic considerations. Bone Marrow Transplant 1990;5:435–437.
99. Adams C, August CS, Maguire H, et al. Neuromuscular complications of bone marrow transplantation. Pediatr Neurol 1995;12:58–61.
100. Hayashi M, Matsuda O, Ishida Y, et al. Change of immunological parameters in the clinical course of a myasthenia gravis patient with chronic graft-versus-host disease. Acta Paediatr Jpn 1996;38:151–155.
101. Penn AS, Schotland DL, Rowland LP. Immunology of muscle disease. Res Publ Assoc Res Nerv Ment Dis 1971;49:215.
102. Keezin-Storrar L, Metcalfe RA, Dyer PA, et al. Genetic factors in myasthenia gravis: a family study. Neurology 1988;38:38–42.

103. Namba T, Brunner NG, Grob D. Idiopathic giant cell polymyositis. Arch Neurol 1974;31:27.
104. Pascuzzi RM, Roos KL, Phillips LH. Granulomatous inflammatory myopathy associated with myasthenia gravis: a case report and review of the literature. Arch Neurol 1986;43:621.
105. Rowland LP, Hoefer PFA, Aranow H, et al. Fatalities in myasthenia gravis: a review of 39 cases with 26 autopsy reports. Neurology 1956;6:307–326.
106. Mendelow H. Pathology. In Osserman KE (ed), Myasthenia Gravis. New York: Grune & Stratton, 1958;10–43.
107. Monden Y. Extrathymic malignancy in patients with myasthenia gravis. Eur J Cancer 1991;27:745–747.
108. Masaoka A, Yamakawa Y, Niwa H, et al. Thymectomy and malignancy. Eur J Cardiothorac Surg 1994;8:251–253.
109. Evoli A, Batocchi AP, Tonali P, et al. Risk of cancer in patients with myasthenia gravis. Ann N Y Acad Sci 1998;841:742–745.
110. Hodes R. Electromyographic study of defects of neuromuscular transmission in human poliomyelitis. Arch Neurol Psych 1948;60:457–473.
111. Mulder DW, Lambert EH, Eaton LM. Myasthenic syndrome in patients with amyotrophic lateral sclerosis. Neurology 1959;9:627–629.
112. Oh SJ, Kim DE, Kuruoglu R, et al. Diagnostic sensitivity of the laboratory tests in myasthenia gravis. Muscle Nerve 1992;15:94–100.
113. Stalberg E, Trontelj J. Single Fiber Electromyography (2nd ed). New York: Raven Press, 1994.
114. Massey JM, Sanders DB, Howard JF, Jr. The effect of cholinesterase inhibitors on SFEMG in myasthenia gravis. Muscle Nerve 1989;12:154–155.
115. Gilchrist JM, Committee of the AAEM SFEMG special interest group. Single fiber EMG reference values: a collaborative effort. Muscle Nerve 1992;15:151–161.
116. Lennon VA. Myasthenia gravis. Diagnosis by assay of serum antibodies. Mayo Clin Proc 1982;57:723–724.
117. Sundevall AC, Lefvert AK, Olsson R. Anti-acetylcholine receptor antibodies in primary biliary cirrhosis. Acta Med Scand 1985;217:519–525.
118. Hay JE, Lennon VA, Czaja AJ, et al. High frequency of acetyl-choline receptor binding antibodies in autoimmune liver disease [abstract]. Clin Res 1989;37:538.
119. Griesmann GE, Lennon VA. Detection of Autoantibodies in Myasthenia Gravis and Lambert-Eaton Myasthenic Syndrome. In NR Rose, E Conway De Macario, et al. (eds), Manual of Clinical and Laboratory immunology (5th ed). Washington, DC: ASM Press, 1997;983–988.
120. Engel AG. Acquired Autoimmune Myasthenia Gravis. In AG Engel, C Franzini-Armstrong (eds), Myology. Basic and Clinical. New York: McGraw-Hill, 1994;1925–1954.
121. Sanders DB, Andrews PI, Howard JF, et al. Seronegative myasthenia gravis. Neurology 1997;48(suppl 5):40–45.
122. Andrews PI, Massey JM, Sanders DB. Acetylcholine receptor antibodies in juvenile myasthenia gravis. Neurology 1993;43:977–982.
123. Lennon VA. Serologic profile of myasthenia gravis and distribution from the Lambert-Eaton myasthenia syndrome. Neurology 1997;48(suppl 5):23–27.
124. Howard FM Jr, Lennon VA, Finley J, et al. Clinical correlations of antibodies that bind, block, or modulate human acetylcholine receptors in myasthenia gravis. Ann N Y Acad Sci 1987;505:526–538.
125. Roses AD, Olanow W, McAdams MW, et al. No direct correlation between antiacetylcholine receptor antibody levels and clinical state of individual patients with myasthenia gravis. Neurology 1981;31:220–224.
126. Cooks JBM, Oosterhuis HJGH, Limburg PC, et al. Anti-acetylcholine receptor antibodies decrease after thymectomy in patients with myasthenia gravis: clinical correlations. J Autoimmun 1991;4:197–200.
127. Newsom-Davis JW, Wilson SG, Vincent A, et al. Long term effects of repeated plasma exchange in myasthenia gravis. Lancet 1979;1:464.
128. Olarte MR, Schoenfeldt RS, Penn AS, et al. Effect of plasmapheresis in myasthenia gravis, 1978–1980. Ann N Y Acad Sci 1981;377:725–728.
129. Karni A, Zisman E, Katz Levy Y, et al. Reactivity of T cells from seronegative patients with myasthenia gravis to T cell epitopes of the human acetylcholine receptor. Neurology 1997;48:1638–1642.
130. Bufler J, Pitz R, Czep M, et al. Purified IgG from seropositive and seronegative patients with myasthenia gravis reversibly blocks current through nicotinic acetylcholine receptor channels. Ann Neurol 1998;43:458–464.
131. Lennon VA, Howard FM. Serological Diagnosis of Myasthenia Gravis. In RM Nakamura, MB O'Sullivan (eds), Clinical Laboratory Molecular Analysis: New Strategies in Autoimmunity, Cancer and Virology. New York: Grune & Stratton, 1985;29–44.

132. Aarli JA, Gilhus NE, Hofstad H. CA-antibody: an immunological marker of thymic neoplasia in myasthenia gravis? Acta Neurol Scand 1987;63:55–57.
133. Cikes N, Momoi MY, Williams CL, et al. Striational autoantibodies: quantitative detection by enzyme immunoassay in myasthenia gravis, thymoma and recipients of D-penicillamine and allogeneic bone marrow. Mayo Clin Proc 1988;63:474–481.
134. Aarli JA, Steffenson K, Marton SG, et al. Patients with myasthenia gravis and thymoma have in their sera IgG autoantibodies against titin. Clin Exp Immunol 1990;82:284–288.
135. Mygland A, Aarli AJ, Matre R. Ryanodine receptor auto-antibodies related to the severity of thymoma associated myasthenia gravis. J Neurol Neurosurg Psychiatry 1994;57:843–846.
136. Garlepp MJ, Dawkins RL, Christiansen FT, et al. Autoimmunity in ocular and generalized myasthenia gravis. J Neuroimmunol 1981;1:325–332.
137. Hohfeld R, Kalies I, Kohleisen B, et al. Myasthenia gravis: stimulation of antireceptor autoantibodies by autoreactive T cell lines. Neurology 1986;36:618–621.
138. Wekerle H. The thymus in myasthenia gravis. Ann N Y Acad Sci 1993;681:47–55.
139. Schonbeck S, Padberg F, Marx A, et al. Transplantation of myasthenia gravis thymus to SCID mice. Ann N Y Acad Sci 1993;681:66–73.
140. Penn AS, Jaretski A III, Wolff M, et al. Thymic abnormalities: antigen or antibody? Response to thymectomy in myasthenia gravis. Ann N Y Acad Sci 1981;377:786–803.
141. Lanska DJ. Indications for thymectomy in myasthenia gravis. Neurology 1990;40:1828–1829.
142. Batra P, Herrman C, Mulder O. Mediastinal imaging in myasthenia gravis: correlation of chest radiography, CT, MR, and surgical findings. Ann J Roentgenol 1987;148:515–519.
143. Bramis J, Pikoulis E, Lepponiemi A, et al. Benefits of early thymectomy in patients with myasthenia gravis. Eur J Surg 1997;163:897–902.
144. Evoli A, Batocchi AP, Tonali P, et al. Thymectomy for late-onset myasthenia gravis [abstract]. Neurology 1996;46:310.
145. Seybold ME, Howard FM, Duane DDJR, et al. Thymectomy in juvenile myasthenia gravis. Arch Neurol 1971;25:385–392.
146. Snead OC, Benton JW, Dwyer D, et al. Juvenile myasthenia gravis. Neurology 1980;30:732–739.
147. Adams C, Theodorescu D, Murphy EG, et al. Thymectomy in juvenile myasthenia gravis. J Child Neurol 1990;5:215–218.
148. Jaretzki A III, Penn AS, Younger DS, et al. "Maximal thymectomy" for myasthenia gravis. Results. J Thorac Cardiovasc Surg 1988;95:747–757.
149. Yim AP, Kay RL, Ho JK. Video-assisted thoracoscopic thymectomy for myasthenia gravis. Chest 1995;108:1440–1443.
150. Mantegazza R, Conflalonieri P, Antozzi C, et al. Video-assisted thoracoscopic extended thymectomy (VATET) in myasthenia gravis. Ann N Y Acad Sci 1998;841:749–752.
151. Mulder DG, Graves M, Herrmann C Jr. Thymectomy for myasthenia gravis: recent observation and comparisons with past experience. Ann Thorac Surg 1989;48:551–555.
152. Drachman DB. Immunotherapy in neuromuscular disorders: current and future strategies. Muscle Nerve 1996;19:1239–1251.
153. Yi Q, Lefvert AK. Current and future therapies for myasthenia gravis. Drugs Aging 1997;11:2: 132–139.
154. Warmolts JR, Engel WK. Benefit from alternate-day prednisone in myasthenia gravis. N Engl J Med 1972;286:17–20.
155. Miller RG, Milner-Brown S, Mirka A. Prednisone-induced worsening of neuromuscular function in myasthenia gravis. Neurology 1986;36:729–732.
156. Pascuzzi RM, Coslett HB, Johns TR. Long-term corticosteroid treatment of myasthenia gravis: report of 116 patients. Ann Neurol 1984;15:291–298.
157. Myasthenia Gravis Clinical Study Group. A randomized clinical trial comparing prednisone and azathioprine in myasthenia gravis. Results of the second interim analysis. J Neurol Neurosurg Psychiatry 1993;53:1157–1163.
158. Palace J, Newsom-Davis J, Lecky B, et al. A multicenter, randomized, double-blind trial of prednisolone plus azathioprine versus prednisolone plus placebo in myasthenia gravis. Neurology 1996;46:332–333.
159. Kissel JT, Levy RJ, Mendell JR, et al. Azathioprine toxicity in neuromuscular disease. Neurology 1986;36:35–39.
160. Confavreax C, Saddier P, Grimaud J, et al. Risk of cancer from azathioprine therapy in multiple sclerosis: a case-control study. Neurology 1996;46:1607–1612.
161. Silman AJ, Petrie JJ, Hazelman B, et al. Lymphoproliferative cancer and other malignancy in patients with rheumatoid arthritis treated with azathioprine: a 20-year follow-up study. Ann Rheum Dis 1988;47:988–992.

162. Tindall RSA, Phillips JT, Rollins JA, et al. A clinical therapeutic trial of cyclosporine in myasthenia gravis. Ann N Y Acad Sci 1993;681:539–551.
163. Massey JM. Treatment of acquired myasthenia gravis. Neurology 1997;48(suppl 5):46–51.
164. Newsom-Davis JW, Pinching AJ, Vincent A, et al. Function of circulating antibody to acetylcholine receptor in myasthenia gravis: investigation by plasma exchange. Neurology 1978;28:266.
165. Shibuya N, Sato T, Osama M, et al. Immunoadsorption therapy for myasthenia gravis. J Neurol Neurosurg Psychiatry 1994;57:578–581.
166. Cornelio F, Antozzi C, Confalonieri P, et al. Plasma treatment in diseases of the neuromuscular junction. Ann N Y Acad Sci 1998;841:803–810.
167. Arsura E, Bick A, Brunner NG, et al. High-dose intravenous immunoglobulin in the management of myasthenia gravis. Arch Intern Med 1986;146:1365–1368.
168. Van der Mech FG, Van Doorn PA. The current place of high-dose immunoglobulins in the treatment of neuromuscular disorders. Muscle Nerve 1997;20:136–147.
169. Gajdos PH, Chevret S, Clair B, et al. Plasma exchange and intravenous immunoglobulin in autoimmune myasthenia gravis. Ann N Y Acad Sci 1998;841:720–726.
170. Gajdos PH, Chevret S, Clair B, et al. Clinical trial of plasma exchange and high dose intravenous immunoglobulins in myasthenia gravis. Ann Neurol 1997;41:789–796.
171. Cosi V, Lombardi M, Piccalo G, et al. Treatment of myasthenia gravis with high dose intravenous immunoglobulin. Acta Neurol Scand 1991;84:81–84.
172. Tan E, Hadjinazarian M, Bay W, et al. Acute renal failure resulting from intravenous immunoglobulin therapy. Arch Neurol 1993;50:137–139.
173. Steg RE, Lefkowitz DM. Cerebral infarction following intravenous immunoglobulin therapy for myasthenia gravis. Neurology 1994;44:1180–1181.
174. Dalakas MC. Experience with IVIg in the treatment of patients with myasthenia gravis. Neurology 1997;48(suppl 5):64–69.
175. Lindner A, Schalke B, Toyka KV, et al. Outcome in juvenile-onset myasthenia gravis: a retrospective study with long-term follow-up of 79 patients. J Neurol 1997;244:515–520.
176. Andrews IP. A treatment algorithm for autoimmune myasthenia gravis in childhood. Ann N Y Acad Sci 1998;841:789–802.
177. Batocchi AP, Evoli A, Palmisani MT. Early-onset myasthenia gravis: clinical characteristics and response to therapy. Eur J Pediatr 1990;150:66–68.
178. Plauche WG. Myasthenia gravis in mothers and their newborns. Clin Obstet Gynecol 1991;34:82–99.
179. Levine SE, Keesey JC. Successful plasmapheresis for fulminant myasthenia gravis during pregnancy. Arch Neurol 1986;43:197–198.
180. Roubenoff R, Hoyt J, Petri M, et al. Effects of anti-inflammatory and immunosuppressive drugs on pregnancy and fertility. Semin Arthritis Rheum 1988;18:88–110.
181. Massey JM, Sanders DB. Single-fiber electromyography in myasthenia gravis during pregnancy. Muscle Nerve 1993;16:458–460.
182. Lambert EH, Eaton LM, Rooke ED. Defect of neuromuscular transmission associated with malignant neoplasm. Am J Physiol 1956;187:612.
183. Eaton LM, Lambert EH. Electromyography and electric stimulation of nerves and diseases of motor unit: Observations on myasthenic syndrome associated with malignant tumors. JAMA 1957;163:1117.
184. Lambert EH, Elmqvist D. Quantal components of end-plate potentials in the myasthenic syndrome. Ann N Y Acad Sci 1971;183:183–199.
185. Fukunaga H, Engel AG, Osame M, et al. Paucity and disorganization of presynaptic membrane active zones in the Lambert-Eaton myasthenic syndrome. Muscle Nerve 1982;5:686–697.
186. Kim Y, Neher E. IgG from patients with Lambert-Eaton syndrome blocks voltage-dependent calcium channels. Science 1988;239:405–408.
187. Lang B, Vincent A, Murray NMF, et al. Lambert-Eatson myasthenic syndrome: immunoglobulin inhibition of Ca^{2+} flux in tumor cells correlates with disease severity. Ann Neurol 1989;25:265–271.
188. Lennon VA, Lambert EH. Autoantibodies bind solubilized calcium-channel-omega-conotoxin complexes from small cell lung carcinoma: a diagnostic aid for Lambert-Eaton myasthenic syndrome. Mayo Clin Proc 1989;64:1498–1504.
189. Sher E, Gotti C, Canal N, et al. Specificity of calcium channel autoantibodies in Lambert-Eaton myasthenic syndrome. Lancet 1989;2:640–643.
190. Lennon VA, Kryzer TJ, Griermann G, et al. Calcium channel antibodies in Lambert-Eaton and other neuroplastic syndromes. N Engl J Med 1995;332:1467–1474.

191. Motomura M, Lang B, Johnston I, et al. Incidence of serum anti P/Q-type and anti N-type calcium channel autoantibodies in Lambert-Eaton myasthenic syndrome. J Neurol Sci 1997;147:35–42.
192. Lang B, Waterman S, Pinto A, et al. The role of autoantibodies in Lambert-Eaton myasthenic syndrome. Ann N Y Acad Sci 1998;841:596–605.
193. Elmqvist D, Lambert EH. Detailed analysis of neuromuscular transmission in a patient with the myasthenic syndrome sometimes associated with bronchogenic carcinoma. Mayo Clin Proc 1968;43:689–713.
194. O-Neill JH, Murray NM, Newsom-Davis J. The Lambert-Eaton myasthenic syndrome: a review of 50 cases. Brain 1988;111:577–596.
195. Elrington GM, Murray NM, Spiro SG, et al. Neurological paraneoplastic syndromes in patients with small cell lung cancer: a prospective survey of 150 patients. J Neurol Neurosurg Psychiatry 1991;54:764.
196. Engel AG. Myasthenic Syndromes. In AG Engel, C Franzini-Armstrong (eds), Myology. Basic and Clinical. New York: McGraw-Hill, 1994;1798–1853.
197. Lennon VA. Serological Diagnosis of Myasthenia Gravis and the Lambert-Eaton Myasthenic Syndrome. In R Lisak (ed), Handbook of Myasthenia Gravis. New York: Marcel Dekker, 1994;149–164.
198. Smith AG, Wald J. Acute ventilatory failure in Lambert-Eaton myasthenic syndrome and its response to 3,4-diaminopyridine. Neurology 1996;46:1143–1145.
199. Trontelj JV, Stalberg EV. Single motor end-plates in myasthenia gravis and LEMS at different firing rates. Muscle Nerve 1991;14:226–232.
200. Tim RW, Sanders DB. Repetitive nerve stimulation studies in the Lambert-Eaton syndrome. Muscle Nerve 1994;17:995–1001.
201. Oh SJ. Diverse electrophysiological spectrum of the Lambert Eaton myasthenic syndrome. Muscle Nerve 1989;12:464–469.
202. Oguro-Okano M, Griesmann GE, Wieben ED, et al. Molecular diversity of neuronal-type calcium channels identified in small cell lung carcinoma. Mayo Clin Proc 1992;67:1150–1159.
203. Jenkyn LR, Brooks PL, Forcier RJ, et al. Remission of the Lambert-Eaton syndrome and small cell anaplastic carcinoma of the lung induced by chemotherapy and radiotherapy. Cancer 1980;46:1123–1127.
204. McEvoy KM, Windebank AJ, Daube JR, et al. 3,4-Diaminopyridine in the treatment of Lambert-Eaton myasthenic syndrome. N Engl J Med 1989;321:1567–1571.
205. Sanders O, Howard JF, Massey JM. 3,4-Diaminopyridine in Lambert-Eaton myasthenic syndrome and myasthenia gravis. Ann N Y Acad Sci 1993;681:588–590.
206. Lundh HN, Nilsson O, Rosen I, et al. Practical aspects of 3,4-Diaminopyridine treatment of the Lambert-Eaton myasthenic syndrome. Acta Neurol Scand 1993;88:136–140.
207. Oh SJ, Kim DS, Head TC, et al. Low-dose guanidine and pyridostigmine: relatively safe and effective long-term symptomatic therapy in Lambert-Eaton myasthenic syndrome. Muscle Nerve 1997;20:1146–1152.
208. Cherington M. Guanidine and germine in Lambert-Eaton syndrome. Neurology 1976;26:944–946.
209. Newsom-Davis J, Murray NMF. Plasma exchange and immunosuppressive drug treatment in the Lambert-Eaton myasthenic syndrome. Neurology 1984;34:480–485.
210. Bird SJ. Clinical and electrophysiologic improvement in Lambert-Eaton myasthenic syndrome with intravenous immunoglobulin therapy. Neurology 1992;42:1422–1423.
211. Rich MM, Teener JW, Bird SJ. Treatment of Lambert-Eaton myasthenic syndrome with intravenous immunoglobulin. Muscle Nerve 1997;20:614–615.
212. Bain PG, Motomura M, Newsom-Davis J, et al. Effects of intravenous immunoglobulin on muscle weakness and calcium-channel autoantibodies in the Lambert-Eaton myasthenic syndrome. Neurology 1996;47:678–683.
213. Maselli RA. Pathogenesis of human botulism. Ann N Y Acad Sci 1998;841:122–140.
214. Sciavo G, Benefenati F, Poulain B, et al. Tetanus and botulinum-B neurotoxins block neurotransmitter release by a proteolytic cleavage of synaptobrevin. Nature 1992;359:832–835.
215. Blasi J, Chapman ER, Link E, et al. Botulinum neurotoxin A selectively cleaves the synaptic protein SNAP-25. Nature 1993;365:160–163.
216. Arnon SS, Midura TJ, Clay SA, et al. Infant botulism. Epidemiological, clinical and laboratory aspects. JAMA 1977;237:1946–1949.
217. Girlanda P, Vita G, Nicolosi C. Botulinum toxin therapy: distant effects on neuromuscular transmission and autonomic nervous system. J Neurol Neurosurg Psychiatry 1992;55:844–845.
218. Holzer SE, Ludlow CL. The swallowing side effect of botulinum toxin type A injection in spasmodic dysphonia. Laryngoscope 1996;106:86–92.

219. Cornella CL, Tanner CM, DeFoor-Hill L, et al. Dysphagia after botulinum toxin injections for spasmodic torticollis: clinical and radiographic findings. Neurology 1992;42:1307–1310.
220. Sanders DB, Massey EW, Buckley EG. Botulinum toxin for blepharospasm: single-fiber EMG studies. Neurology 1986;36:545–547.
221. Lange DJ. Systemic Effects of Botulinum Toxin. In J Jankovic, M Hallett (eds), Therapy with Botulinum Toxin. New York: Marcel Dekker, 1994;109–118.
222. Brin MF, Jankovic J, Cornella C, et al. Treatment of Dystonia Using Botulinum Toxin. In R Kurlan (ed), Treatment of Movement Disorders. Philadelphia: JB Lippincott, 1995;183–246.
223. Erbguth F, Claus D, Engelhard A, et al. Systemic effects of local botulinum toxin injections unmasks the subclinical Lambert-Eaton myasthenic syndrome. J Neurol Neurosurg Psychiatry 1993;56: 1235–1236.
224. Harvey AM. The actions of procaine on neuromuscular transmission. Bull Johns Hopkins Hosp 1939;65:223–228.
225. Hund EF. Neuromuscular complications in the ICU: the spectrum of critical illness-related conditions causing muscular weakness and weaning failure. J Neurol Sci 1996;136:10–16.
226. Elmqvist D, Josefsson JO. The nature of the neuromuscular block produced by neomycin. Acta Physiol Scand 1962;54:105–110.
227. Argov Z, Brenner T, Abramsky O. Ampicillin may aggravate clinical and experimental myasthenia gravis. Arch Neurol 1986;43:255–256.
228. Moore B, Safani M, Keesey J. Possible exacerbation of myasthenia gravis by ciprofloxacin. Lancet 1988;1:882.
229. Vial T, Chauplannaz G, Brunel P, et al. Exacerbation of myasthenia gravis by perfloxacin. Rev Neurol 1995;251:286–287.
230. Rauser EH, Ariano RE, Anderson BA. Exacerbation of myasthenia gravis by norfloxacin. Ann Pharmacother 1990;24:207–208.
231. Rubbo JT, Gergis SD, Sokoll MD. Comparative neuromuscular effects of lincomycin and clindamycin. Anesth Analg 1977;56:329–332.
232. Booij LHD, Miller RD, Crul JF. Neostigmine and 4-aminopyridine antagonism of lincomycin pancuronium neuromuscular blockade in man. Anesth Analg 1978;57:316–322.
233. Ghoneim MM, Long JP. The interaction between magnesium and other neuromuscular blocking agents. Anaesthesiology 1970;32:23–27.
234. George WK, Han CL. Calcium and magnesium administration in myasthenia gravis. Lancet 1962;2:561.
235. Gutmann L, Takamori M. Effect of magnesium on neuromuscular transmission in the Eaton-Lambert syndrome. Neurology 1973;23:977–980.
236. Herishanu Y, Rosenberg P. Beta blockers and myasthenia gravis. Ann Intern Med 1975;83:834–835.
237. Shaivitz SA. Timolol in myasthenia gravis. JAMA 1979;242:1611–1612.
238. Jonkers I, Swerup C, Pirskanen R, et al. Acute effects of intravenous injection of beta-adrenoreceptor- and calcium channel antagonists and agonists in myasthenia gravis. Muscle Nerve 1996;19: 959–965.
239. Weisman SJ. Masked myasthenia gravis. JAMA 1949;141:917–918.
240. Shy ME, Lange DJ, Howard JF, et al. Quinidine exacerbating myasthenia gravis: a case report and intracellular recordings. Ann Neurol 1985;18:120.
241. Sieb JP, Milone M, Engel AG. Effects of the quinoline derivatives quinine, quinidine and chloroquine on neuromuscular transmission. Brain Res 1996;712:179–189.
242. Kornfeld P, Horowich SH, Genkins G, et al. Myasthenia gravis unmasked by antiarrhythmic agents. Mt Sinai J Med 1976;43:10–14.
243. Kim YI, Howard JF, Sanders DB. Depressant effects of morphine and mipraradine (sp) on neuromuscular transmission in rat and human myasthenic muscles [abstract]. Soc Neurosci 1979;5:482.
244. McQuillen MP, Gross M, Johns RJ. Chlorpromazine-induced weakness in myasthenia gravis. Arch Neurol 1963;8:286–290.
245. Hill GE, Wong KC, Hodges MR. Potentiation of succinylcholine neuromuscular blockade by lithium carbonate. Anaesthesiology 1976;44:439–442.
246. Bazzato G, Coli U, Landini S, et al. Myasthenia-like syndrome after D,L- but not L-carnitine. Lancet 1981;1:209.
247. Brumlik J, Jacobs RS. Myasthenia gravis associated with diphenylhydantoin therapy for epilepsy. Can J Neurol Sci 1974;1:127–129.
248. Peterson HDC. Association of trimethadione therapy in myasthenia gravis. N Engl J Med 1966;274:506–507.

249. Bikerstaff ER. Neurological Complications of Oral Contraceptives. London: Oxford University Press, 1975.

250. Tsai MC, Mansour NA, Eldefrawi AT, et al. Mechanism of action of amantadine on neuromuscular transmission. Mol Pharmacol 1978;14:787–803.

251. Chagnac Y, Hadani M, Goldhammer Y. Myasthenic crisis after intravenous administration of iodinated contrast agent. Neurology 1985;35:1219–1220.

252. Frank JH, Cooper GW, Black WC, et al. Iodinated contrast agents in myasthenia gravis. Neurology 1987;37:1400–1402.

253. Nordenbo AM. Acute deterioration of myasthenia gravis after intravenous administration of gadolinium-DPTA. Lancet 1992;340:1168.

254. Besser R, Gutmann L, Dillmann U, et al. End-plate dysfunction in acute organophosphate intoxication. Neurology 1989;39:561–567.

255. Namba IT, Nolte CT, Jackrel J. Poisoning due to organophosphate insecticides: acute and chronic manifestations. Am J Med 1971;50:475.

256. Meschul CK, Boyne AF, Deshphande SS, et al. Comparison of the ultrastructural myopathy induced by anticholinesterase agents at the end-plates of rat soleus and extensor muscles. Exp Neurol 1985;89:96.

257. De Bleecker J. The intermediate syndrome in organophosphate poisoning: an overview of experimental and clinical observations. Clin Toxicol 1995;33:683–686.

258. Wadia RS, Chitra S, Amin RB, et al. Electrophysiological studies in acute organophosphate poisoning. J Neurol Neurosurg Psychiatry 1987;50:1442–1448.

259. Bowman JR. Myasthenia gravis in young children. Paediatrics 1948;1:472.

260. Levin PM. Congenital myasthenia in siblings. Arch Neurol Psych 1949;62:745.

261. Rothbart HB. Myasthenia gravis. Familial occurrence. JAMA 1937;108:715–717.

262. Greer M, Schotland M. Myasthenia gravis in the newborn. Paediatrics 1960;26:101–108.

263. Namba T, Brunner NG, Brown SB, et al. Familial myasthenia gravis: report of 27 patients in 12 families and review of 164 patients in 73 families. Arch Neurol 1971;25:49–60.

264. Conomy JP, Levinsohn M, Fanaroff A. Familial infantile myasthenia gravis: a cause of sudden death in young children. J Pediatr 1975;87:428–429.

265. Engel AG, Lambert EH, Gomez MR. A new myasthenic syndrome with end-plate acetylcholinesterase deficiency, small nerve terminals, and reduced acetylcholine release. Ann Neurol 1977;1:315–330.

266. Engel AG, Lambert EH, Mulder DM, et al. A newly recognized congenital myasthenic syndrome attributed to a prolonged open time of the acetylcholine-induced ion channel. Ann Neurol 1982;11: 553–569.

267. Oosterhuis HJ, Newsom-Davis J, Wokke JH, et al. The slow channel syndrome. Two new cases. Brain 1987;110:1061–1079.

268. Elmqvist D, Quastel DMJ. Presynaptic action of hemicholinium at the neuromuscular junction. J Physiol 1965;177:463–482.

269. Maselli RA, Mass DP, Distad BJ, et al. Anconeus muscle: a human muscle preparation suitable for in-vitro microelectrode studies. Muscle Nerve 1991;14:1189–1192.

270. Engel AG. Congenital myasthenic syndromes. Neurol Clin 1994;12:401–437.

271. Engel AG, Ohno K, Milone M, et al. Congenital myasthenic syndromes caused by mutations in acetylcholine receptor genes. Neurology 1997;48(suppl 5):28–35.

272. Middleton LT. Report of the 34th ENMC International Workshop—congenital myasthenia syndromes. Neuromuscul Disord 1996;6:133–136.

273. Middleton LT. Congenital Myasthenic Syndromes. In AEH Emery (ed), Neuromuscular Disorders: Clinical and Molecular Genetics. Chichester, UK: Wiley, 1998;469–485.

274. Milone M, Wang H-L, Ohno K, et al. Slow-channel syndrome caused by enhanced activation, desensitization, and agonist binding affinity due to mutation in the M2 domain of the acetylcholine receptor alpha subunit. J Neurosci 1997;17:5651–5665.

275. Ohno K, Hutchinson DO, Milone M, et al. Congenital myasthenic syndrome caused by prolonged acetylcholine receptor channel openings due to a mutation in the M2 domain of the epsilon subunit. Proc Natl Acad Sci U S A 1995;92:758–762.

276. Sine SM, Ohno K, Bouzat C, et al. Mutation of the acetylcholine receptor alpha subunit causes a slow-channel myasthenic syndrome by enhancing agonist binding affinity. Neuron 1995;15:229–239.

277. Engel AG, Ohno K, Milone M, et al. New mutations in acetylcholine receptor subunit genes reveal heterogeneity in the slow-channel congenital myasthenic syndrome. Hum Mol Genet 1996; 5:1217–1227.

278. Croxen R, Newland C, Beeson D, et al. Mutations in different functional domains of the human muscle acetylcholine receptor alpha subunit in patients with the slow-channel congenital myasthenic syndrome. Hum Mol Genet 1997;6:767–773.
279. Gomez CM, Maselli R, Gammack J, et al. A beta-subunit mutation in the acetylcholine receptor channel gate causes severe slow-channel syndrome. Ann Neurol 1996;39:712–723.
280. Gomez CM, Gammack JT. A leucine-to-phenylalanine substitution in the acetylcholine receptor ion channel in a family with the slow-channel syndrome. Neurology 1995;45:982–985.
281. Engel AG, Ohno K, Milone M, et al. Congenital myasthenic syndromes. New insights from molecular genetics and patch-clamp studies. Ann N Y Acad Sci 1998;841:140–156.
282. Wang H-L, Auerbach A, Bren N, et al. Mutation in the M1 domain of the acetylcholine receptor alpha subunit decreases the rate of agonist dissociation. J Gen Physiol 1997;109:757–766.
283. Harper CM, Engel AG. Quinidine sulfate therapy for the slow-channel congenital myasthenic syndrome. Ann Neurol 1998;43:480–484.
284. Fukudome T, Ohno K, Brengman JM, et al. Quinidine sulfate normalizes the open duration of slow channel congenital myasthenic syndrome acetylcholine receptor channels expressed in human embryonic kidney cells [abstract]. Neurology 1997;48:72.
285. Scoppetta C, Casali C, Piantalli M. Congenital myasthenia gravis. Muscle Nerve 1983;5:493.
286. Gieron MA, Korthals JK. Familial infantile myasthenia gravis. Report of three cases with follow-up until adult life. Arch Neurol 1985;42:143–144.
287. Robertson WC, Raymond WM, Chun MD, et al. Familial infantile myasthenia. Arch Neurol 1980;37:117–119.
288. Mora M, Lambert EH, Engel AG. Synaptic vesicle abnormality in familial infantile myasthenia. Neurology 1987;37:206–214.
289. Engel AG, Uchitel O, Walls TJ, et al. Newly recognized congenital myasthenic syndrome associated with high conductance and fast closure of the acetylcholine receptor channel. Ann Neurol 1993;34:38–47.
290. Engel AG, Nagel A, Walls TJ, et al. Congenital myasthenic syndromes. I: Deficiency and short open-time of the acetylcholine receptor. Muscle Nerve 1993;16:1284–1292.
291. Vincent A, Newsom-Davis J, Wray D, et al. Clinical and experimental observations in patients with congenital myasthenic syndromes. Ann N Y Acad Sci 1993;681:451–460.
292. McQuillen MP. Familial limb girdle myasthenia. Brain 1966;89:121–132.
293. Dobkin BH, Verity MA. Familial neuromuscular disease with type 1 fiber hypoplasia, tubular aggregates, cardiomyopathy, and myasthenic features. Neurology 1978;28:1135–1140.
294. Furui E, Fukushima K, Sakashita T, et al. Familial limb-girdle myasthenia with tubular aggregates. Muscle Nerve 1997;20:599–603.
295. Hutchinson DO, Walls TJ, Nakano S, et al. Congenital endplate acetylcholinesterase deficiency. Brain 1993;116:633–653.
296. Jennekens FGI, Hesselmans LFGM, Veldman H, et al. Deficiency of acetylcholine receptors in a case of end-plate acetylcholinesterase deficiency: a histochemical investigation. Muscle Nerve 1992;15:63–72.
297. Camp S, Bon S, Li Y, et al. Patients with congenital myasthenia associated with end-plate acetylcholinesterase deficiency show normal sequence, mRNA splicing, and assembly of catalytic subunits. J Clin Invest 1995;95:330–340.
298. Ohno K, Bzengman JM, Tsujino A, et al. Human endplate acetylcholinesterase deficiency caused by mutations in the collagen-like tail subunit (ColQ) of the asymmetric enzyme. Proc Natl Acad Sci U S A 1998;95:9654–9659.
299. Dougez C, Kzejci E, Sezzadell P, et al. Mutation in the human acetylcholinesterase–associated gene, CoLQ, is responsible for congenital myasthenic syndrome with end-plate acetylcholinesterase deficiency. Am J Hum Genet 1998;63:967–975.
300. Goldhammer Y, Blatt I, Sadeh M, et al. Congenital myasthenia associated with facial malformations in Iraqi and Iranian Jews. Brain 1990;113:1291–1306.
301. Menold MM, Lennon F, Sadeh M, et al. Evidence for genetic heterogeneity supports clinical differences in congenital myasthenic syndromes (CMS) [abstract]. Am J Hum Genet 1997;615:286.
302. Ohno K, Wang HL, Milone M, et al. Congenital myasthenic syndrome caused by decreased agonist binding affinity due to a mutation in the acetylcholine receptor epsilon subunit. Neuron 1996;17:157–170.
303. Engel AG, Ohno K, Bouzat C, et al. End-plate acetylcholine receptor deficiency due to nonsense mutations in the epsilon subunit. Ann Neurol 1996;40:810–817.
304. Ohno K, Quiram PA, Milone M, et al. Congenital myasthenic syndromes due to heteroallelic nonsense/missense mutations in the acetylcholine receptor epsilon subunit gene. Hum Mol Genet 1997;6:753–766.

305. Milone M, Ohno K, Fukudome T, et al. Congenital myasthenic syndrome caused by novel loss of function mutations in the human AChR epsilon subunit gene. Ann N Y Acad Sci 1998;841:184–188.
306. Croxen R, Beeson D, Newland C. A single nucleotide deletion in the epsilon subunit of the acetyl-choline receptor (AChR) in five congenital myasthenic syndrome patients with AChR deficiency. Ann N Y Acad Sci 1998;841:195–198.
307. Beeson D, Newland C, Croxen R. Congenital myasthenic syndromes. Studies of the AChR and other candidate genes. Ann N Y Acad Sci 1998;841:181–183.
308. Christodoulou K, Tsingis M, Deymeer F, et al. Mapping of the familial infantile myasthenia (con-genital myasthenic syndrome type Ia) gene to chromosome 17p with evidence of genetic homo-geneity. Hum Mol Genet 1997;16:635–640.
309. Middleton L, Ohno K, Christodoulou K, et al. Chromosone 17p linked myasthenias stem from defects in the acetylcholine receptor ε subunit gene. Neurology 1999 (in press).
310. Ohno K, Anlar B, Ozdimir E, et al. Frameshifting and splice-site mutations in the acetylcholine receptor epsilon subunit gene in three Turkish kinships with congenital myasthenic syndromes. Ann N Y Acad Sci 1998;841:189–194.
311. Ohno K, Anlar B, Ozdimir E, et al. Myasthenic syndromes in Turkish kinships due to mutations in the acetylcholine receptor. Ann Neurol 1998;44:234–241.

10
Inflammatory Myopathies: Dermatomyositis, Polymyositis, Inclusion Body Myositis, and Related Diseases

Anthony A. Amato and Richard J. Barohn

The three major categories of idiopathic inflammatory myopathy are dermatomyositis (DM), polymyositis (PM), and inclusion body myositis (IBM). These inflammatory myopathies are clinically, histologically, and pathogenically distinct (Table 10.1) [1–4]. The incidence of these disorders is approximately 1 in 100,000 [3, 5]. Although there are a few reports of DM, PM, and IBM occurring in parents and children and in siblings, including identical twins [6–12], the inflammatory myopathies are best considered as acquired diseases. Other forms of inflammatory myopathy include overlap syndromes with various connective tissue diseases, focal myositis, eosinophilic PM and fasciitis, sarcoidosis, Behçet syndrome, and granulomatous myositis. In this chapter, we review the characteristic features of these inflammatory myopathies, update the developments in this area, and provide a rationale for treatment.

COMMON IDIOPATHIC INFLAMMATORY MYOPATHIES

Dermatomyositis

Clinical Features

DM can present at any age and is common in childhood. Most childhood cases present between 5 and 14 years of age [5], but DM can even develop during infancy [13]. Although the pathogenesis of childhood and adult DM are presumably similar, there are important differences in some of the clinical features and associated disorders.

Women are affected more commonly than men in both the childhood and adult onset forms of DM. Onset of weakness is typically subacute (over several weeks), although it can develop abruptly (over days) or insidiously (over months) [1, 3, 14–18]. The earliest and most severely affected muscle groups are the

Table 10.1 Idiopathic inflammatory myopathies: clinical and laboratory features

	Sex	Typical age at onset	Rash	Pattern of weakness	Creatine kinase	Muscle biopsy	Cellular infiltrate	Response to immuno-suppressive therapy	Common associated conditions
Dermatomyositis	Female > male	Childhood and adult	Yes	Proximal > distal	Increased (up to 50× normal)	Perimysial and perivascular inflammation; membrane attack complex, immunoglobulin, complement deposition on vessels	CD4+ T cells; B cells	Yes	Myocarditis, interstitial lung disease, malignancy, vasculitis, other connective tissue diseases
Polymyositis	Female > male	Adult	No	Proximal > distal	Increased (up to 50× normal)	Endomysial inflammation	CD8+ T cells; macrophages	Yes	Myocarditis, interstitial lung disease, other connective tissue diseases
Inclusion body myositis	Male > female	Elderly (>50 yrs)	No	Proximal = distal; predilection for finger/wrist flexors and knee extensors	Normal or mildly increased (<10× normal)	Endomysial inflammation; rimmed vacuoles; amyloid deposits; electron microscopy: 15- to 18-nm tubulofilaments	CD8+ T cells; macrophages	None or minimal	Neuropathy, autoimmune disorders—uncommon

Source: Reprinted with permission from AA Amato and RJ Barohn. Idiopathic inflammatory myopathies. Neurol Clin 1997;15:615–648.

neck flexors, shoulder girdle, and pelvic girdle muscles. As a result, patients have difficulty lifting their arms over their heads, climbing steps, and rising from chairs. Distal extremity weakness can also often be demonstrated, although involvement is seldom as severe as the proximal muscle weakness [14]. Children are more likely to present with fatigue, low-grade fevers, and a rash followed by an insidious onset of muscle weakness and myalgias [2, 19]. Inflammation of oropharyngeal and esophageal muscles leads to dysphagia in approximately 30% of DM patients [3, 4, 15–18]. Rare patients have chewing difficulties secondary to masseter muscle involvement [19]. Dysarthria or speech delay occasionally occurs in children because of involvement of the pharyngeal and tongue muscles [19]. Sensation is normal, and muscle stretch reflexes are preserved until a severe degree of weakness has developed.

Early recognition and diagnosis of DM is facilitated because of the characteristic rash that may accompany or precede the onset of muscle weakness [1, 3, 4, 16, 17]. The classic skin manifestations include a heliotrope rash (purplish discoloration of the eyelids often associated with periorbital edema) and Gottron sign (papular, erythematous, scaly lesions over the knuckles). In addition, a flat, erythematous, sun-sensitive rash may appear on the face, neck, and anterior chest (V-sign); on the shoulders and upper back (shawl sign); and on the elbows, knees, and malleoli. The nail beds often have dilatated capillary loops, occasionally with thrombi or hemorrhage. *Amyopathic DM* refers to the rare patients who have the characteristic rash but never develop weakness [20].

Thirty to 70% of children develop subcutaneous calcifications, whereas they are an uncommon complication in adults [1, 2, 4, 16, 19, 21]. Cutaneous calcinosis tends to occur over pressure points (buttocks, knees, elbows) and presents as painful, hard nodules. In severe cases, ulceration of the overlying skin with extrusion of calcific debris can occur.

Associated Manifestations

Although cardiac symptoms are uncommon, electrocardiographic (ECG) abnormalities—including conduction defects and arrhythmias—occur frequently in childhood and adult DM [17, 18, 22–26]. Nevertheless, congestive heart failure, pericarditis, and myocarditis can complicate the myopathy [17, 24]. Echocardiography and radionucleotide scintigraphy may demonstrate ventricular and septal wall motion abnormalities and reduced ejection fractions [24].

Approximately 10% of DM patients develop interstitial lung disease (ILD) [4, 16, 17, 19, 27–30]. Symptoms of ILD (i.e., dyspnea, nonproductive cough) can develop abruptly or insidiously and often precede the development of the characteristic rash and muscle weakness. A diffuse reticulonodular pattern with a predilection for involvement at the lung bases is apparent on chest radiographs. A diffuse alveolar pattern or ground-glass appearance is seen in more fulminant abrupt-onset cases [16, 30]. Pulmonary function tests demonstrate restrictive defects and a decreased diffusion capacity, and hypoxemia is evident on arterial blood gases. In at least 50% of ILD cases associated with inflammatory myopathies, there are antibodies directed against t-histidyl transfer RNA (tRNA) synthetase, so-called Jo-1 antibodies [31–33]. One additional pulmonary complication is aspiration pneumonia, which can develop in patients with significant oropharyngeal and esophageal weakness [30].

Inflammation of the skeletal and smooth muscles of the gastrointestinal tract can lead to dysphagia and delayed gastric emptying [19]. Vasculitis of the gastrointestinal tract is a serious complication and can result in mucosal ulceration, perforation, and life-threatening hemorrhage [2, 4, 16, 19]. Vasculitis of the gastrointestinal tract is much more common in childhood DM compared with adult DM.

Arthralgias with or without arthritis are a frequent finding. Arthritis involves both the large and small joints and is typically symmetric. The arthralgias and myalgias often ease when the limbs are flexed, which unfortunately leads to the development of flexion contractures across the major joints [19]. Flexion contractures at the ankles, leading to toe-walking, is a common early finding in childhood DM [4].

In addition to the skin, muscle, and gastrointestinal system, necrotizing vasculitis may affect other tissues, including the eyes (retina and conjunctiva), kidneys, and lungs [16, 19]. Rarely, massive muscle necrosis can develop secondary to ischemia, leading to myoglobinuria and acute renal tubular necrosis.

There is an increased incidence of underlying malignancy in adult DM, ranging from 6% to 45% [3, 4, 15–18, 34–36]. A similar risk of cancer is not evident in childhood DM. Detection of an underlying neoplasm can precede or occur after the diagnosis of DM; the majority of malignancies are identified within 2 years of the presentation of the myositis. The risk of malignancy is similar in men and women and is greater in patients older than age 40 years. Patients with cutaneous vasculitis may have an increased risk of malignancy [37, 38]. The severity of the inflammatory myopathy does not appear to correlate with the presence or absence of a neoplasm [16]. Muscle strength may improve after treatment of the underlying malignancy [4].

The search for an underlying malignancy should include a comprehensive history and annual physical examinations, with breast and pelvic examinations for women and testicular and prostate examinations for men [1, 16, 35, 39]. Examiners should obtain a complete blood cell count (CBC), routine blood chemistries, urinalysis, and stool specimens for occult blood. Chest x-rays and mammograms are the only radiographic studies that should be routinely ordered.

Laboratory Features

Blood Tests (Including Autoantibodies)

Necrosis of muscle fibers results in elevations of serum creatine kinase (CK), aldolase, myoglobin, lactate dehydrogenase, aspartate aminotransferase (AST), and alanine aminotransferase (ALT). Serum CK is the most sensitive and specific marker for muscle destruction and is elevated in more than 90% of DM patients [1, 14, 17, 18, 39, 40]. Serum CK levels can be normal or as high as 50 times the normal value. Importantly, serum CK levels do not correlate with the severity of weakness and can be normal even in markedly weak individuals, particularly in childhood DM [2, 4, 16, 19]. Erythrocyte sedimentation rate (ESR) is usually normal or only mildly elevated and is not a reliable indicator of disease severity [4, 16, 40].

Antinuclear antibodies (ANA) can be detected in 24–62% of DM patients [17, 32, 33] (Table 10.2). The presence of these antibodies should lead to consideration of an overlap syndrome (discussed in the section Overlap Syndromes) [17, 32, 33]. Some have suggested that myositis-specific antibodies (MSAs) are useful in

Table 10.2   Autoantibodies in inflammatory myopathies

	Frequency	Conditions
Muscle-specific antibody		
Antisynthetase		
Jo-1	18–20%	Polymyositis and dermatomyositis with interstitial lung disease, arthritis, Raynaud phenomenon, "mechanic's hands," moderate response to therapy
Others (PL-7, PL-12, EJ, OJ)	≤3%	Same as Jo-1
Nonsynthetase		
Signal recognition particle	4%	Polymyositis with acute onset/severe weakness, poor response to therapy
Mi-2	15–20%	Dermatomyositis with good response to therapy
Mas	1%	Polymyositis with alcoholic rhabdomyolysis; chronic hepatitis
Associated with overlap syndromes		
Antinuclear antibodies	16–32%	All myositis groups
	24–62%	Dermatomyositis
	16–40%	Polymyositis
	72–77%	Overlap syndromes
	19–23%	Inclusion body myositis
Polymyositis-Scl	<8%	All myositis groups
	25%	Scleroderma-myositis (North America)
Anti-Ku	1%	Scleroderma-myositis (Japan)
		Systemic lupus erythematosus without myositis (North America)
U1 ribonuclear protein	12%	Mixed connective tissue disease, systemic lupus erythematosus
SS-A/SS-B	90%	Sjögren syndrome
	10%	Systemic lupus erythematosus

Source: Modified with permission from AA Amato and RJ Barohn. Idiopathic inflammatory myopathies. Neurol Clin 1997;15:615–648.

predicting response to therapy and prognosis [32, 33, 41–43]. The MSAs are interesting in that they are associated with specific HLA haplotypes, and each patient can have only one type of MSA. However, the MSAs are demonstrated in only a minority of patients with inflammatory myopathy and have not been studied prospectively in regard to their predictive value. Further, the pathogenic relationship of these antibodies to inflammatory myopathies is unknown; they may just represent an epiphenomenon [4].

The MSAs include (1) the cytoplasmic antibodies directed against translational proteins (i.e., various tRNA synthetases and the antisignal recognition particle), and (2) those directed against Mi-2 and Mas antigens [32, 33, 42, 43]. The most common of the antisynthetases are the Jo-1 antibodies, which are associated with ILD and arthritis and are demonstrated in as many as 20% of patients with inflammatory myopathy [31–33]. Jo-1 antibodies are more common in PM than

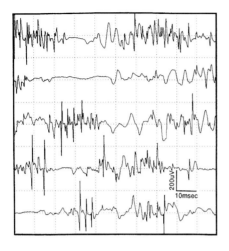

Figure 10.1   Needle electromyography in a patient with an inflammatory myositis demonstrates short-duration, small-amplitude motor unit potentials with early recruitment.

adult DM; there are only a few reports of these antibodies in childhood DM [19, 32, 33]. The presence of Jo-1 antibodies has been associated with only a moderate response to treatment and a poor long-term prognosis [41, 42]. This is not surprising, given the association of Jo-1 antibodies with ILD. No prospective study has demonstrated treatment outcomes of myositis-ILD patients with anti-Jo-1 antibodies compared with similar patients without these antibodies. The other antisynthetases (which are not as yet commercially available) are much less common and are each found in less than 2–3% of inflammatory myopathy patients [33]. Mi-2 antibodies are seen almost exclusively in DM and can be found in 15–20% of DM patients. Mi-2 is a 240 kd nuclear protein of unknown function. Most patients with anti-Mi-2 antibodies have an acute onset, a florid rash, a good response to therapy, and a favorable prognosis [32, 33, 41–43].

Electromyography

Electromyography (EMG) characteristically demonstrates (1) increased insertional and spontaneous activity with fibrillation potentials, positive sharp waves, and, occasionally, pseudomyotonic and complex repetitive discharges; (2) short-duration, small-amplitude, polyphasic motor unit potentials (MUPs); and (3) MUPs that recruit early but at normal frequencies (Figure 10.1). Decreased recruitment (fast-firing MUPs) can be seen in advanced disease secondary to the loss of muscle fibers of entire motor units. Late in the course of poorly responsive disease, insertional activity may be decreased secondary to fibrosis. In addition, long-duration, high-amplitude polyphasic MUPs may be seen later in the course, reflecting chronicity of the disease with muscle fiber splitting and regeneration rather than a superimposed neurogenic process. The amount of spontaneous EMG activity is reflective of ongoing disease activity.

   EMG is often helpful in determining which muscle to biopsy in patients with only mild weakness. EMG may also be useful in previously responsive myositis patients who become weaker by differentiating relapse from weakness secondary to type 2 muscle fiber atrophy from disuse or chronic steroid administration. Isolated type 2 muscle fiber atrophy is not associated with abnormal spontaneous activity on EMG.

Muscle Imaging

Magnetic resonance imaging (MRI) can provide information on the pattern of muscle [44–47]. MRI can reveal signal abnormalities in affected muscles secondary to inflammation and edema or to replacement by fibrotic tissue. Some have advocated MRI as a guide to which muscle to biopsy [47]. However, MRI adds little to a good clinical examination and EMG in defining the pattern of muscle involvement and determining which muscle to biopsy.

Histopathology

The pathologic process is multifocal, and the frequency and severity of histologic abnormalities can vary within the muscle biopsy specimens. Perifascicular atrophy is the characteristic histologic feature, occurring in as many as 90% of children and in at least 50% of adults with DM [1–4, 16] (Figure 10.2A). The perifascicular area contains small degenerating fibers and atrophic and non-atrophic fibers with microvacuolation and disrupted oxidative enzyme staining. Occasionally, microinfarcts of muscle fascicles are apparent. Scattered necrotic fibers may be present; however, in contrast to PM and IBM (discussed later), invasion of nonnecrotic fibers is not seen. Inflammation, when present, is predominantly perivascular and located in the perimysium rather than the endomysium (Figure 10.2B). The inflammatory infiltrate is composed primarily of macrophages, B cells, and CD4+ (T-helper) cells [48, 49].

The earliest demonstrable histologic abnormality on light microscopy in DM is deposition of the C5b-9 complement membrane attack complex on small blood vessels [50–52] (Figure 10.2C). This membrane attack complex deposition precedes inflammation and other structural abnormalities in the muscle and is specific for DM [50]. Other complement components (C3 and C9), immunoglobulin M (IgM), and, less often, IgG are deposited within the walls of intramuscular blood vessels [53]. The subsequent necrosis of vessels results in a reduction in the capillary density [50]. Electron microscopy reveals small intramuscular blood vessels (arterioles and capillaries) with endothelial hyperplasia, microvacuoles, and cytoplasmic inclusions; these abnormalities precede other structural abnormalities on electron microscopy [7, 54].

Pathogenesis

The immunologic studies and other histologic features on muscle biopsies suggest that DM is a humorally mediated microangiopathy. The etiology of this autoimmune disorder is unknown. The microangiopathy leads to ischemic damage of muscle fibers. The perifascicular atrophy is believed to be a reflection of hypoperfusion in the watershed region of muscle fascicles.

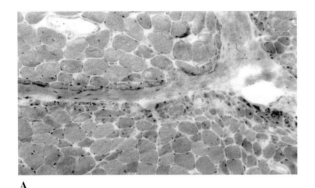

A

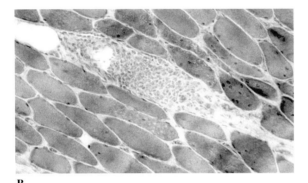

B

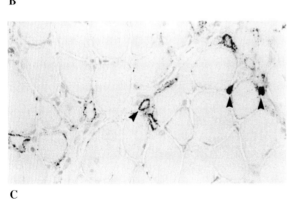

C

Figure 10.2 Dermato-myositis muscle biopsy. (**A**) Characteristic perifascicular atrophy (modified trichrome). (**B**) Prominent perivascular inflammation in a perimysial blood vessel (modified trichrome). (**C**) Membrane attack complex (MAC) deposit on small blood vessels (*arrowheads*) (immunoperoxidase stain using anti-MAC antibodies). (**A** and **B** reprinted with permission from AA Amato and RJ Barohn. Idiopathic inflammatory myopathies. Neurol Clin 1997;15: 615–648.)

Prognosis

In absence of malignancy, prognosis is favorable in patients with DM. Poor prognostic features are increased age, associated ILD, cardiac disease, and pre-vious inadequate or late treatment [17, 18, 41, 55, 56]. Five-year survival rates of adult DM range from 70% to 93% [57–59]. The mortality rate in children is very low [19]. More details regarding the response to therapy are discussed in the section Treatment of Inflammatory Myopathies.

Polymyositis

Clinical Features

PM generally presents in patients older than age 20 years. Like DM, it is more prevalent in women [1, 3–5, 14–18]. Although there are rare cases of myositis beginning in infancy [60, 61], it is likely that most of these cases are congenital muscular dystrophies with secondary inflammation [2, 62, 63]. Compared with DM, there is often a delay from onset of symptoms to diagnosis, perhaps because there is no associated rash, which serves as a red flag to patients and their physicians. As with DM, patients typically present with neck flexor and symmetric proximal arm and leg weakness developing over several weeks or months [14, 15]. Distal muscles may also become involved but are not as weak as the more proximal muscles [14, 16]. Myalgias and tenderness are common. Dysphagia occurs in approximately one-third of patients secondary to oropharyngeal and esophageal involvement [3, 4, 16–18]. Mild facial weakness may occasionally be evident on examination [14]. Sensation and muscle stretch reflexes are usually normal.

Associated Manifestations

The cardiac and pulmonary complications of PM are similar to those described with DM. Myositis resulting in secondary congestive heart failure or conduction abnormalities occurs in as many as one-third of patients [17, 18, 22–26, 64, 65]. At least 10% of PM patients develop ILD, one-half of whom have Jo-1 antibodies [17, 18, 27, 29, 30, 32, 33]. ILD can manifest before muscle weakness. As many as 45% of PM patients have polyarthritis at the time of diagnosis [18]. The risk of malignancy with PM is lower than with DM, but it may be slightly higher than that expected in the general population [18, 34–36].

Laboratory Features

Blood Tests (Including Autoantibodies)

Serum CK level is elevated five- to 50-fold in the majority of PM cases [1, 3, 4, 14, 16–18, 40]. Serum CK can be useful in monitoring response to therapy, but only in conjunction with the physical examination. As with DM, serum CK levels can be elevated in patients who have normal manual muscle and functional testing, whereas weak patients can have normal levels. Likewise, ESR is normal in at least one-half of the patients and does not correlate with disease activity or severity [4, 40].

Positive ANAs are detected in 16–40% of PM patients [17, 18, 32, 40] (see Table 10.2). The possible relationships of the MSAs to the inflammatory myopathies is discussed in the section on DM. The muscle-specific antibodies are more common in PM than DM, specifically Jo-1 and anti-signal recognition particle (SRP) antibodies [32, 33, 42]. Jo-1 antibodies are detected in approximately 20% of PM patients and are associated with ILD [31–33]. Approximately

4% of PM patients have antibodies to SRP [32, 33, 42]. Patients with SRP antibodies often have an acute onset of severe weakness, myalgias, and myocarditis. These patients usually are resistant to immunosuppressive therapy and have a very poor prognosis, with a 5-year survival rate of 25% [32, 33, 41, 42]. Anti-Mas antibodies are directed against a cytoplasmic tRNA and are evident in only 1% of PM [32].

Electromyography

Increased insertional and spontaneous activity, small polyphasic MUPs, and early recruitment are usually evident on EMG [1]. These findings are nonspecific and do not distinguish PM from other myopathies. The paraspinals—being the most proximal muscle group—are the earliest involved on EMG and should always be studied in patients suspected of having PM.

Muscle Imaging

As with DM, MRI can suggest areas of inflammation in affected muscles [44–47].

Histopathology

PM is histologically different from DM. Muscle biopsies are characterized by variability in fiber size, scattered necrotic and regenerating fibers, and endomysial inflammation with invasion of nonnecrotic muscle fibers (Figure 10.3). Major histocompatibility complex (MHC) class 1 antigen is expressed on all of the invaded and some of the noninvaded muscle fibers—a finding not normally present in the sarcolemma of muscle fibers [66]. The endomysial inflammatory cells consist primarily of activated CD8+ (cytotoxic), α, β T cells, and macrophages [4, 48, 49]. There is one report of PM with CD4−, CD8−, γ, δ T-cell inflammation [58].

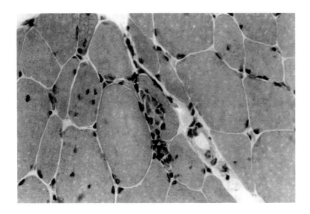

Figure 10.3 Polymyositis muscle biopsy. Endomysial mononuclear inflammatory cells invading nonnecrotic muscle fiber (modified trichrome).

The T-cell receptor repertoire of endomysial T cells in PM consists of an oligo-clonal pattern of gene rearrangements [67]. There is also a restricted motif in the CD3R region of the TCR. These findings suggest the immune response is antigen specific [67]. Finally, in contrast to DM, no evidence of a humorally mediated vasculopathy exists.

Pathogenesis

PM results from an HLA-restricted, antigen-specific, cell-mediated immune response directed against muscle fibers. The antigen to which this autoimmune attack is generated and the trigger of this response is not known. Some have speculated that the etiology is viral (i.e., enteroviruses), but no conclusive evidence exists to support this theory [3, 4, 68, 69]. Viral antigens and genomes have not been identified in the muscle fibers. Perhaps a viral infection could indirectly trigger an autoimmune response by secondary cross-reactivity with specific muscle antigens, altering the expression of self-antigens on muscle fibers, or by the loss of physiologic self-tolerance [4]. Interestingly, PM can develop in patients infected with human immunodeficiency virus (HIV) and human T-lymphocyte virus-1 (HTLV-1) [1, 3]. The myositis associated with HIV and HTLV-1 infections appears to be the result of such indirect triggering of the immune response against muscle fibers.

Prognosis

Most patients with PM improve with immunosuppressive therapies, although many require lifelong treatment [17, 18, 39, 41, 55–57]. Some retrospective studies suggest that the response in PM is not as favorable as in DM [14, 41]. Older age, ILD, cardiac disease, the presence of Jo-1 or SRP antibodies, and a delay in treatment or previous inadequate treatment are poor prognostic features [17, 18, 41, 55, 56].

Infantile Myositis/Congenital Inflammatory Myopathy

Myositis with perinatal onset was first described in Japan [70]. Subsequently, there have been several reports in the western hemisphere of so-called infantile myositis or congenital inflammatory myopathy [60, 61, 71–73]. The disorder is characterized by the perinatal onset of hypotonia and generalized weakness, elevated serum CKs, myopathic EMGs, and prominent inflammation on muscle biopsy. Careful review of these reported patients suggests that most of them had congenital muscular dystrophy [2]. Only one case—with perifascicular atrophy and immunoglobulin and complement deposition on the biopsy characteristic of DM, which improved with steroids—was strongly suggestive of a primary myositis [73]. Importantly, most of the reported children did not significantly improve with corticosteroids. Also, the biopsies had dystrophic features in addition to the inflammatory infiltrates. Inflammation is not specific for a primary inflammatory myopathy and can be demonstrated in Duchenne, facioscapulohumeral, and

Fukuyama-type muscular dystrophies [74]. There have been several reports of patients with the classic type of congenital muscular dystrophy with hypomyelination who had prominent inflammation and merosin (laminin α2) deficiency on muscle biopsy [62, 63, 75]. Mutations within the merosin gene have also been demonstrated in some cases [63, 75]. Thus, we presume that the majority of infants with inflammation on biopsy have a form of congenital muscular dystrophy rather than a primary myositis.

Overlap Syndromes

The overlap syndromes are a group of disorders in which an inflammatory condition occurs in association with another well-defined connective tissue disorder (CTD), such as scleroderma, mixed connective tissue disease, Sjögren syndrome, systemic lupus erythematosus (SLE), or rheumatoid arthritis (RA) [1, 3, 4, 16]. Clinical and histologic features of either DM or PM can develop. Some suggest that the myositis associated with overlap syndromes is more responsive to immunosuppressive treatment than DM and PM [17, 41]. In our experience, the prognoses are more related to the severity of the underlying CTD.

Scleroderma

Proximal muscle weakness is common in scleroderma; however, most patients have normal serum CK and EMG [4]. Mild variability in fiber size with atrophy of type 2 muscle fibers and perimysial fibrosis are evident on muscle biopsy [4, 16]. Myositis is uncommon, but it has been reported in 5–17% of patients with scleroderma and can occur in either of its two major forms: progressive systemic sclerosis or CREST syndrome (which consists of *c*alcinosis cutis, *R*aynaud phenomenon, *e*sophageal dysfunction, *s*clerodactyly, and *t*elangiectasia) [33, 38, 76–78]. Scleroderma-myositis should be expected in patients with increased serum CK levels and irritable and myopathic EMGs. Muscle biopsies can demonstrate features of either DM or PM.

Anticentromere antibodies are seen in the majority of patients with CREST syndrome, and anti-Scl-70 antibodies are common in patients with progressive systemic sclerosis. In addition, approximately 25% of North American patients with scleroderma-myositis have anti-PM-Scl (also called anti-PM-1) antibodies [33]. However, only 50% of patients with anti-PM-Scl antibodies have the scleroderma-myositis overlap syndrome. Therefore, these antibodies are not very specific [33]. In Japan, the scleroderma-myositis syndrome is associated with anti-Ku antibodies rather than anti-PM-Scl antibodies [33]. In North America, anti-Ku antibodies are not associated with myositis but can be demonstrated in some patients with SLE.

Sjögren Syndrome

Sjögren syndrome is characterized by dryness of the eyes and mouth (sicca syndrome) and other mucosal membranes. Muscle pain and weakness are common in

Sjögren syndrome; however, actual myositis is rare [4, 16]. Weakness is more often related to inactivity secondary to arthritis and pain, resulting in disuse atrophy. However, patients with Sjögren syndrome can develop either DM or PM [33, 43, 79–81]. Approximately 90% of patients have ANAs directed against ribonucleo-proteins, specifically SS-A (Ro) and, less commonly, SS-B (La) antibodies [4, 81].

Systemic Lupus Erythematosus

SLE is an autoimmune disorder affecting multiple organ systems. Patients with SLE often develop proximal weakness, which is most often the result of type 2 fiber atrophy secondary to disuse or chronic steroids [16]. Although inflammatory myopathies are uncommon in SLE, some series have reported that as many as 8% of DM and PM patients have SLE [33, 82].

Most patients with SLE have positive ANA titers, which are directed against native DNA (highly specific for SLE) and ribonuclear proteins (RNP). Anti-RNP antibodies are present in fewer than one-half of SLE patients and include anti-SS-A and anti-SS-B (also present in Sjögren syndrome), anti-U1 RNP (also present in mixed connective tissue disease), and anti-Sm (specific for SLE) [1].

Rheumatoid Arthritis

As many as 13% of patients with DM and PM have RA, although the incidence of inflammatory myopathy in patients with RA is much less [4, 16, 33]. The major cause of weakness in patients with RA is type 2 muscle fiber atrophy from chronic steroids or disuse secondary to severe arthralgias.

Mixed Connective Tissue Disease

Mixed connective tissue disease has clinical features of scleroderma, SLE, RA, and myositis [83]. Both DM and PM occur in association with mixed connective tissue disease, although DM is more common [3, 4, 16, 33, 83, 84]. High titers of anti-U1 RNP antibodies are common [4, 33, 84]. However, these antibodies are not specific, as they can also be detected in SLE.

Inclusion Body Myositis

Clinical Features

Sporadic IBM presents with an insidious onset of slowly progressive proximal and distal weakness [1, 3, 9, 14, 16, 85–89]. Although IBM is the most common inflammatory myopathy in patients older than age 50 years, it is frequently misdiagnosed. The slow evolution of the disease process probably accounts in part for the delay in diagnosis, averaging approximately 6 years from the onset of symptoms [14, 87, 89]. Unlike the female predominance seen with DM and PM, men are much more commonly affected than women in IBM. In addition, IBM

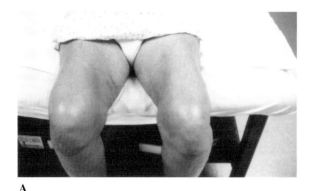

A

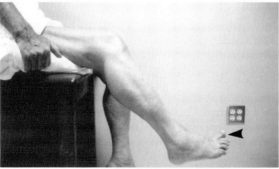

B

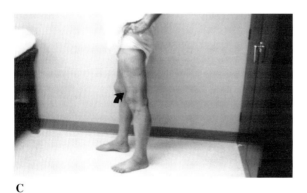

C

Figure 10.4   Inclusion body myositis patient exhibiting characteristic quadriceps involvement. (**A**) Quadriceps atrophy noted with patient seated. (**B**) Inability to completely extend the knee against gravity because of quadriceps weakness. Also, pseudo–Babinski sign with great toe extension because of weakness of toe flexors (*arrowhead*). (**C**) Genu recurvatum that is due to quadriceps atrophy and weakness (*arrow*).

patients have a unique pattern of weakness, with early weakness and atrophy of the quadriceps (Figure 10.4), volar forearm muscles (i.e., wrist and finger flexors), and ankle dorsiflexors [9, 14, 87, 89]. Weakness of toe flexors can produce chronic toe extension, a pseudo–Babinski sign (see Figure 10.4B). The quadriceps weakness can produce a genu recurvatum, or back knee, and lead to accelerated degenerative knee arthritis and pain (see Figure 10.4C). The manual muscle scores of the finger and wrist flexors (Figure 10.5) are usually lower than those of the shoulder abductors, and the muscle scores of the knee extensors are

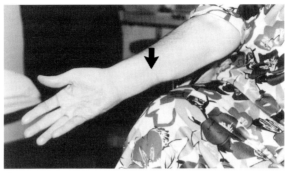

A

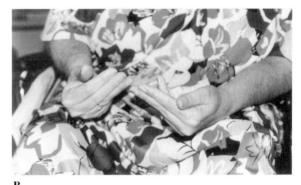

Figure 10.5 Inclusion body myositis patient with distal forearm and hand weakness. (**A**) Atrophy of forearm muscle (*arrow*). (**B**) Inability to flex fingers because of forearm muscle weakness. Patient's fingers are in chronic finger extension.

B

the same or lower than those of the hip flexors in patients with IBM [14]. The opposite relationship between muscle scores is present in DM and PM. In addition, muscle involvement in IBM is often asymmetric, in contrast to the symmetric involvement in DM and PM. The presence of slowly progressive, asymmetric, quadriceps and wrist/finger flexor weakness in a patient older than age 50 years strongly suggests the diagnosis of IBM [14].

As many as 40% of patients report dysphagia, which can be so severe that some require cricopharyngeal myotomy [87, 90, 91]. Approximately one-third of IBM patients have mild facial weakness on examination; however, this weakness is clinically insignificant [14, 87, 89]. Extraocular muscles are spared. Although most patients have no sensory symptoms, evidence for a generalized peripheral neuropathy can be detected in as many as 30% of patients on clinical examination and electrophysiologic testing [14]. Muscle stretch reflexes are normal or slightly decreased, particularly the patellar reflexes, which are lost early [87].

There are hereditary forms of inclusion body *myopathy,* but these are clinically and histologically distinct from the more common sporadic inclusion body *myositis.* Hereditary autosomal recessive inclusion body myopathy has no inflammation on muscle biopsy and spares the quadriceps muscle [92, 93]. This rare disorder is now considered to be the same entity as Nonaka distal myopathy, as both disorders have been linked to the same region on chromosome 9p1q1 [94–97].

Associated Manifestations

Unlike DM and PM, IBM is not associated with myocarditis or ILD, nor is there an increased risk of malignancy [35]. Autoimmune disorders, such as SLE, Sjö-gren syndrome, scleroderma, thrombocytopenia, and sarcoidosis, have been reported in as many as 15% of IBM patients [87, 89, 98, 99]. Lotz et al. reported diabetes mellitus in 20% of their IBM patients [87], but others have not reported a similar increased incidence [89].

Laboratory Features

Blood Tests

Unlike DM and PM, the serum CK is normal or only mildly elevated (less than 10-fold above normal) in patients with IBM [9, 14, 87, 89]. Autoantibodies are usually absent, except for the occasional patients with concurrent CTD, although some series have reported positive ANAs in approximately 20% of their IBM patients [32, 99]. There is a significant incidence of the HLA DR3 phenotype (*0301/0302) in IBM [100].

Electromyography

EMG demonstrates increased insertional and spontaneous activity, small polyphasic MUPs, and early recruitment [87]. In addition, large polyphasic MUPs, so-called neurogenic potentials, are also evident in one-third of patients [87, 101, 102]. However, similar large polyphasic MUPs can also be seen in DM, PM, and other muscle disorders (i.e., muscular dystrophies). This probably reflects chronicity of the disease process rather than a neurogenic etiology. Macro-EMG studies also support a myopathic etiology [103]. Nevertheless, nerve conduction studies reveal evidence of a mild axonal sensory neuropathy in as many as 30% of patients [14].

Muscle Imaging

MRI demonstrates atrophy and signal abnormalities in clinically affected muscle groups [47, 104].

Histopathology

Muscle biopsies characteristically demonstrate endomysial inflammation, small groups of atrophic fibers, eosinophilic cytoplasmic inclusions, and muscle fibers with one or more rimmed vacuoles lined with granular material [9, 87] (Figure 10.6). Amyloid deposition is evident on Congo red staining using polarized light or fluorescence techniques (Color Plate 9 and Color Plate 10) [105, 106]. We reported that the number of vacuolated and amyloid-positive fibers may increase

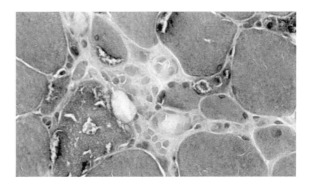

Figure 10.6   Inclusion body myositis muscle biopsy vacuoles within muscle fibers (modified trichrome).

with time in individual patients [107]. An increased number of ragged red fibers is also evident in IBM compared with DM and PM patients and age-matched controls [108]. Electron microscopy demonstrates 15- to 21-nm cytoplasmic and intranuclear tubulofilaments [87]. In addition, intermediate-sized, 6- to 10-nm tubulofilaments can also be found in the cytoplasm of vacuolated muscle fibers [9, 98]. Several muscle biopsies may be required to identify the rimmed vacuoles and abnormal tubulofilament or amyloid accumulation to histologically confirm the diagnosis of IBM [14].

The endomysial inflammation in IBM is composed of macrophages and CD8+ cytotoxic/suppressor T lymphocytes that invade nonnecrotic fibers, similar to PM [9, 49, 98]. In addition, as with PM, MHC class 1 antigens are expressed on necrotic and nonnecrotic muscle fibers [66], and there is an oligoclonal pattern of gene rearrangement of the TCR [9, 67, 109]. However, in contrast to PM, there is heterogeneity of the CDR3 domain. These immunologic features indicate that the T-cell response is not directed against a muscle-specific antigen, although the response could be triggered by a superantigen.

Pathogenesis

The pathogenesis of IBM is unknown. IBM may be a primary inflammatory myopathy like DM and PM. However, a primary degenerative myopathic disorder, such as a dystrophy with secondary inflammation, is also a possibility [9]. The prominent inflammatory response and immunohistochemical studies described in the previous section support the hypothesis that IBM is an autoimmune disorder mediated by cytotoxic T cells. In this regard, Pruitt et al. reported that the frequency of invaded fibers was greater than either necrotic or amyloidogenic fibers, suggesting that the inflammatory response plays a more important role than the accumulation of vacuoles or amyloidogenic filaments in the pathogenesis of IBM [110].

On the other hand, the poor clinical response to various immunosuppressive therapies argues against a primary autoimmune basis for IBM. We treated eight patients with IBM for 6–24 months with immunosuppressive medications, evaluated their responses to treatment, and analyzed their pre- and posttreatment muscle biopsies [107]. Despite lower serum CK levels and reduced inflammation on the posttreatment biopsies, none of the patients improved in strength or function. Interestingly, the amount of vacuolated muscle fibers and fibers with amyloid deposition were increased in the follow-up biopsies, suggesting that the accumulation of vacuoles and amyloid may have a role in the pathogenesis of IBM. Interestingly, Griggs et al. have documented the accumulation of Alzheimer-characteristic proteins in vacuolated muscle fibers in IBM [9]. The abnormal accumulation of B-amyloid, C- and N-terminal epitopes of B-amyloid precursor protein (B-APP), prion protein (PrP^c), apolipoprotein E, α1-antichymotrypsin, ubiquitin, hyperphosphorylated tau protein, and neurofilament heavy chain within IBM vacuolated fibers is similar to that observed in the brains of Alzheimer patients [9, 105, 106, 111–116]. Although one study of 14 IBM patients reported a significant increase in the apolipoprotein E ϵ4 frequency, as observed in Alzheimer patients [100], other studies found no significant increase in the frequency of that allele in IBM [117, 118]. In addition, increased acetylcholine receptor, PrP^c, and B-APP messenger RNAs in IBM-vacuolated fibers have also been described, suggesting that the increased prion and B-amyloid deposition in these muscle fibers probably result, in part, from increased transcription of the PrP^c and B-APP genes [9, 119]. Muscle fibers transfected in vitro with B-APP cDNA using a recombinant-deficient adenovirus vector result in Congo red–positive, vacuolated fibers with tubulofilaments and abnormal mitochondria typical of that observed in IBM [114]. Although intriguing, the pathogenic relationship of these Alzheimer-characteristic proteins to the pathogenesis of IBM is not clear, and they may be just an epiphenomenon rather than the primary pathogenic defect.

Mitochondrial abnormalities, as indicated by ragged red fibers and mitochondrial DNA mutations, are more frequent in IBM patients than in the other inflammatory myopathies and age-matched controls [9, 108, 120]. However, these mitochondrial abnormalities are felt to be secondary changes and not the primary cause of the myopathy.

Some have speculated a viral etiology in the pathogenesis of IBM. Chronic persistent mumps was previously suspected, based on immunostaining of inclusions by antimumps antibodies [121]. However, this theory was subsequently rejected after in situ hybridization and polymerase chain reaction studies failed to confirm mumps infection [68, 122–124]. Interestingly, histologic abnormalities similar to IBM have been reported in patients with retroviral infections and postpolio syndrome [89, 125, 126].

Prognosis

Unfortunately, patients with IBM do not significantly improve with immunosuppressive treatment [1, 3, 16, 89, 98, 108, 127, 128]. However, a few retrospective, unblinded studies report mild or transient improvement in IBM treated with prednisone [41, 129]. One group of researchers reported that 40–58% of their IBM patients partially responded to prednisone, although none had a complete remission [41, 129]. However, these were retrospective, unblinded studies, in which a positive response included *subjective* improvement or lower serum CK levels after treatment. The same researchers conducted a small (11 patients), unblinded, prospective, crossover-designed study comparing prednisone plus azathioprine and oral methotrexate with prednisone plus intravenous methotrexate [129]. They found no clinically significant improvement in strength. However, serum CK levels decreased in 66–70% of the patients, and there was no decline in strength over the 6-month treatment period in most of the patients in both study arms. They concluded that the combination of immunosuppressive medications stabilized the disease process. However, because IBM is a slowly progressive disorder, and the trial lasted only 6 months and was neither blinded nor placebo controlled, the assertion that immunosuppressive medications stabilize the course of IBM is premature.

Life expectancy does not appear to be significantly altered. In our experience, most patients remain ambulatory, although they frequently require or at least benefit from a cane or a wheelchair for long-distance movement. However, some patients become severely incapacitated and require a wheelchair within 10–15 years [87].

Many patients with so-called steroid resistant or refractory PM eventually have IBM. It is important to note that there are patients whose symptoms clinically resemble IBM, but in whom a definitive diagnosis cannot be confirmed on muscle biopsy [14]. We diagnose these patients with *possible* or *probable* IBM [9, 14]. We do not advocate immunosuppressive therapy in patients with IBM because of the side effects of the medications and the unlikelihood of significant clinical improvement [14].

OTHER IDIOPATHIC INFLAMMATORY MYOPATHIES

Eosinophilic Polymyositis

Clinical Features

Eosinophilic PM usually occurs as a part of the hypereosinophilic syndrome (HES) [130–132]. The diagnostic criteria of HES are (1) persistent eosinophilia of 1,500 eosinophils/mm^3 for at least 6 months, (2) no evidence of parasitic or other recognized causes of eosinophilia, and (3) signs and symptoms of organ system involvement related to infiltration of eosinophils. Eosinophilic PM is characterized by an insidious onset of muscle pain and proximal weakness. The myopathy is often accompanied by other systemic manifestations of HES, including encephalopathy; peripheral neuropathy; myocarditis/pericarditis (i.e., fibrosis, congestive heart failure, arrhythmia, conduction block); pulmonary (i.e., fibrosis, pleuritis, and asthma), renal, and gastrointestinal involvement; and skin changes (i.e., petechial rash, splinter hemorrhages of the nail beds, livedo reticularis, and Raynaud phenomenon [130–132]).

Laboratory Features

Hypereosinophilia, hypergammaglobulinemia, anemia, elevated serum CK, and rheumatoid factor are evident. ESR is elevated in less than 50% of cases, and ANA is usually negative. ECG may demonstrate cardiac arrhythmias or conduction block. Pulmonary infiltrates may be apparent on chest x-ray. EMG demonstrates increased insertional and spontaneous activity (i.e., fibrillation potentials, positive sharp waves, and early recruitment of small polyphasic MUPs).

Histopathology

Muscle biopsies demonstrate perivascular and endomysial inflammation predominantly composed of eosinophils. Necrotic, invaded, and regenerating muscle fibers are evident. Nodular granulomas may also be evident.

Pathogenesis

The etiology of eosinophilic PM and HES is unknown. Tissue destruction may be related to infiltration by eosinophils and the release of toxins contained within the eosinophilic granules.

Prognosis

Early reports suggested a poor prognosis for long-term survival, with fewer than 20% of patients surviving 3 years. However, these series may have been biased by the inclusion of autopsied cases. Response to corticosteroids has been inconsistent but effective in some patients in reducing the eosinophilia and end organ damage. Second-line cytotoxic agents should be tried if patients do not improve with steroids (see section Treatment of Inflammatory Myopathies).

Diffuse Fasciitis with Eosinophilia

Clinical Features

Diffuse fasciitis with eosinophilia, also known as *Shulman syndrome*, is characterized by sclerodermalike skin changes and peripheral eosinophilia [130, 133, 134]. Men are affected more commonly than women, with a 2 to 1 ratio. The majority of patients are between ages 30 and 60 years, but the disorder has been reported in children. Early symptoms include myalgias, muscle tenderness, arthralgias, and low-grade fever. Thickening of the skin with edema and dimpling (*peau d'orange*) develops in the extremities and, occasionally, the trunk. Joint contractures may develop in the hands, elbows, knees, and, less commonly, at the shoulders and hips secondary to immobilization because of severe pain. Proximal muscles may be weak, although quantification is difficult secondary to decreased effort because of the pain. Unlike HES with eosinophilic PM, the heart, lungs, kidneys, and other visceral organs are usually not involved. However, there does appear to be a disproportionate number of hematologic complications, including aplastic anemia, idiopathic thrombocytopenia, leukemia, lymphoma, and other lymphoproliferative disorders.

Laboratory Features

Peripheral eosinophilia (>7%) occurs in more than two-thirds of patients. Hypergammaglobulinemia and elevated ESR occur in at least one-third of patients [133]. Serum CK is usually normal, and ANA testing is positive in as many as

25.5%. EMG may demonstrate myopathic MUPs and muscle membrane instability in the superficial subfascial layers.

Histopathology

Full-thickness biopsy, extending from the skin to muscle, is required for diagnosis. Histologic sections demonstrate thickened fascia infiltrated by lymphocytes, macrophages, plasma cells, and eosinophils [130, 133, 134]. Inflammatory infiltrates may invade the adjacent subcutaneous tissue, perimysium, and endomysium. Scattered necrotic fibers and perifascicular atrophy have been described. Immunoglobulin and C3 deposition in the fascia have also been reported in some patients.

Pathogenesis

The etiology of diffuse fasciitis with eosinophilia is not known. Laboratory and histologic features suggest an autoimmune basis. The disorder shares many clinical and histologic features with the eosinophilic myalgia [135] and toxic oil syndromes [136], which are caused by the ingestion of tryptophan and denatured rapeseed, respectively. The similarity of these conditions suggests the possibility of a toxin-induced fasciitis; however, the majority of patients with eosinophilic fasciitis reports no known toxic exposures.

Prognosis

Patients usually respond rapidly to corticosteroid treatment, although spontaneous remission may also occur. Relapses have been reported in a minority of patients. The prognosis is not as favorable in cases with hematologic complications.

Granulomatous and Giant Cell Myositis

Clinical Features

An interesting variant of PM is granulomatous or giant cell PM [137, 138]. Most reported patients also had myasthenia gravis (MG) or thymoma. The thymoma can be benign or malignant. The myositis can develop before or after the clinical presentation of MG or the diagnosis of the thymoma. In addition to proximal weakness, patients with concurrent MG had diplopia, ptosis, and bulbar dysfunction. Importantly, a granulomatous myocarditis can also develop.

Laboratory Features

Serum CK is usually elevated. Acetylcholine receptor antibodies may be evident in patients with superimposed MG, as can a decrement of repetitive nerve stimulation. EMG may demonstrate myopathic MUPs and muscle membrane instability.

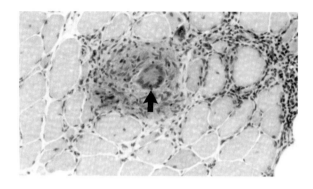

Figure 10.7 Granulomatous myositis. Endomysial inflammation and multinucleated giant cell (*arrow*) within a granuloma.

Histopathology

Muscle biopsy reveals granulomatous inflammation and multinucleated giant cells in skeletal and often cardiac muscle (Figure 10.7).

Pathogenesis

The myositis is an autoimmune disorder of unknown etiology. The granulomatous inflammation and giant cell formation suggest an abnormality in cell-mediated immunity; the frequent occurrence of MG supports aberrant humoral-mediated immunity as well.

Prognosis

Some patients improve with corticosteroids; however, the response does not seem to be as favorable as evident in the more common idiopathic PM. The poorer response is probably related to the frequent myocardial involvement and the superimposed MG and thymoma. More aggressive immunosuppressive therapy with high-dose corticosteroids and second-line agents, such as azathioprine and methotrexate, may be warranted.

Sarcoid Myopathy

Clinical Features

Sarcoidosis is more prevalent in blacks than in whites and in women than in men. Although uncommon, it has been reported in children. The majority of patients present with pulmonary symptoms and lymphadenopathy. Erythema nodosum and arthralgias are also early features. Many patients with sarcoidosis have granulomas in the muscle, although signs and symptoms of muscle involvement are present in the minority [130, 139, 140]. Muscle involvement can be focal, multifocal, or generalized. Patients may develop focal muscle pain, tenderness, and weakness, or generalized proximal weakness greater than distal weakness. There is atrophy of the involved muscles with chronic disease. Asymptomatic granulomas may be palpated within the muscle. Rarely, a superimposed neuropathy is also evident. There have been a few reports of patients with sarcoid myopathy who concomitantly have clinical and histologic features of either DM or IBM.

Laboratory Features

Serum angiotension–converting enzyme levels are often elevated. Patients are frequently anergic to antigen skin testing. Chest films usually demonstrate hilar lymphadenopathy and parenchymal involvement of the lungs. Serum CK is usually normal or only mildly elevated. EMG can be normal or show myopathic features. Mixed myopathic and neurogenic MUPs may be found in patients with a chronic myopathy or with a superimposed neuropathy.

Histopathology

The lesions predominate perivascularly in the connective tissue and take the form of noncaseous granulomas consisting of clusters of epithelioid cells, lymphocytes, and giant cells. Because of the multifocal involvement, several pieces of muscle and serial sections may be required to demonstrate the granulomas.

Pathogenesis

The exact pathogenic mechanism of sarcoidosis is unknown but involves abnormal cell-mediated immunity as reflected by the granulomas and T-cell anergy in vitro and in vivo.

Prognosis

Treatment of sarcoidosis is usually focused on other systemic manifestations, because the myositis is typically asymptomatic. Corticosteroids are effective in treating the myositis.

Behçet Disease

Clinical Features

Behçet disease is a multisystemic disorder with recurrent mucocutaneous and ocular manifestations (e.g., oral and genital ulcers, hypopyon, iritis). Other manifestations include erythema nodosum, thrombophlebitis, colitis, meningoencephalitis, and peripheral neuropathy. In addition, there are a few reports of myositis, as well as myocarditis, in Behçet disease [141–147]. Onset can be in childhood or late adult life. Patients frequently report focal myalgias with or without weakness, although symptoms can generalize. There is a predilection for involvement of the lower extremities, particularly the calves.

Laboratory Features

Leukocytosis, elevated ESR and c-reactive protein levels, and normal or mildly elevated serum CK levels are usually present. Approximately 50% of patients are HLA-B5 positive [146].

Histopathology

Light microscopy demonstrates granulocytic-monocytic inflammation with invasion of nonnecrotic muscle fibers. Immunocytochemistry predominantly reveals macrophages along with CD4+ and CD8+ lymphocytes [146]. MHC class 1 antigens are expressed on most muscle fibers. Deposits of complement factor C3 and immunoglobulins may be found in blood vessel walls [146].

Pathogenesis

The etiology of Behçet disease is unknown. The immunohistologic findings suggest a cell-mediated attack directed against muscle fibers. However, a 1996 study, demonstrating enhanced neutrophil migration and immune complex deposition on blood vessels, supports a leukocytoclastic vasculitis or vasculopathy in the pathogenesis of the disease [146].

Prognosis

The myositis is responsive to immunosuppressive therapy.

Focal Myositis

Clinical Features

Focal myositis is a rare disorder that can develop at any time from infancy to late adulthood [148–153]. It presents as a solitary, painful, and rapidly expanding skeletal muscle mass that often mimics a malignant soft-tissue tumor. The leg is the most common site of involvement, but it can also affect the upper extremities, abdomen, head, and neck. The disorder needs to be distinguished from sarcoidosis, Behçet syndrome, and vasculitis, which can begin focally and involve skeletal muscle and soft-tissue tumors (e.g., sarcoma). The lesions may resolve spontaneously or with corticosteroid treatment.

Laboratory Features

Serum CK and ESR are usually normal. MRI and computed tomography demonstrate edema within the affected muscle groups [148, 152, 153].

Histopathology

Mononuclear inflammatory cells composed of CD4+ and CD8+ T lymphocytes and macrophages are present in the endomysium [148]. Necrosis and phagocytosis of necrotic fibers are apparent. Nonspecific myopathic features, such as fiber-size variability, split fibers, increased centronuclei, and endomysial fibrosis, are also described. One report noted that MHC class 1 antigens were not expressed on muscle fibers, in contrast to PM, in which these antigens are typically abnormally expressed on the fibers [148].

Pathogenesis

The etiology is unknown. Immunologic studies suggest that the disorder is distinct from PM and not the result of a cell-mediated attack directed against a muscle-specific antigen [148].

Prognosis

The myositis usually resolves spontaneously or with treatment. There are rare cases of focal myositis generalizing to more typical PM [151].

TREATMENT OF INFLAMMATORY MYOPATHIES

The response of the inflammatory myopathies to immunomodulating therapies (Table 10.3) has been the subject of a large number of studies. Unfortunately, many of these studies grouped adult and childhood DM with PM and IBM patients. Further, most of these treatment trials were retrospective, unblinded, and lacked placebo controls. Only three published prospective, double-blinded, placebo-controlled trials exist in the treatment of inflammatory myopathy: One involved azathioprine in the treatment of PM [154], a second studied intravenous immunoglobulin (IVIG) in the treatment of DM [155], and the third investigated IVIG in IBM [156]. Finally, in several reports, patients with *subjective* improvement or lower serum CK levels were defined as positive responses rather than the more important *objective* improvement in muscle strength and function [41, 129]. Nevertheless, most experienced clinicians are convinced that immunotherapy can improve strength and function in DM and PM [1, 3, 14, 16, 39, 157, 158]. In contrast, IBM is believed to be refractory to immunosuppressive therapy [4, 6].

Corticosteroids

Prednisone is the usual treatment of choice for DM and PM [1, 3, 16, 157, 158]. High-dose prednisone reduces morbidity and improves muscle strength and function [14, 18, 41, 55–57, 158, 159]. Short courses of intravenous methylpred-

Table 10.3   Immunosuppressive therapy for inflammatory myopathies

Therapy	Route	Dose	Side effects	Monitor
Prednisone	PO	100 mg/day for 2–4 wks, then 100 mg every other day; single AM dose	Hypertension, fluid and weight gain, hyperglycemia, hypokalemia, cataracts, gastric irritation, osteoporosis, infection, aseptic femoral necrosis	Weight, blood pressure, serum glucose/potassium, cataract formation
Methylpred-nisolone	IV	1 g in 100 ml of normal saline over 1–2 hrs, daily or every other day for 3–6 doses	Arrhythmia, flushing, dysgeusia, anxiety, insomnia, fluid and weight gain, hyperglycemia, hypokalemia, infection	Heart rate, blood pressure, serum glucose/potassium
Azathioprine	PO	2–3 mg/kg/day; single AM dose	Flulike illness, hepatotoxicity, pancreatitis, leukopenia, macrocytosis, neoplasia, infection, teratogenicity	Monthly blood cell count, liver enzymes
Methotrexate	PO	7.5–20.0 mg weekly, single or divided doses; one-day-a-week dosing	Hepatotoxicity, pulmonary fibrosis, infection, neoplasia, infertility, leukopenia, alopecia, gastric irritation, stomatitis, teratogenicity	Monthly liver enzymes, blood cell count; consider liver biopsy at 2-gm accumulative dose
	IV/IM	20–50 mg; weekly one-day-a-week dosing	Same as PO	Same as PO
Cyclophos-phamide	PO	1.5–2.0 mg/kg/day; single AM dose	Bone marrow suppression, infertility, hemorrhagic cystitis, alopecia, infections, neoplasia, teratogenicity	Monthly blood cell count, urinalysis
	IV	1 g/m^2	Same as PO (more severe bone marrow suppression, nausea/vomiting, and alopecia, but hemorrhagic cystitis is less frequent)	Weekly blood cell count, urinalysis
Chloram-bucil	PO	4–6 mg/day, single AM dose	Bone marrow suppression, hepatotoxicity, neoplasia, infertility, teratogenicity, infection	Monthly blood cell count, liver enzymes
Cyclosporine	PO	4–6 mg/kg/day, split into two daily doses	Nephrotoxicity, hypertension, infection, hepatotoxicity, hirsutism, tremor, gum hyperplasia, teratogenicity	Blood pressure, monthly cyclosporine level, creatine/blood urea nitrogen, liver enzymes

Table 10.3 *(continued)*

Therapy	Route	Dose	Side effects	Monitor
Intravenous immuno- globulin	IV	2 g/kg over 2–5 days; then every 4–8 wks as needed	Hypotension, arrhythmia, diaphoresis, flushing, nephrotoxicity, head- ache, aseptic meningitis, anaphylaxis, stroke	Heart rate, blood pressure, cre- atine/blood urea nitrogen

Source: Reprinted with permission from AA Amato, RJ Barohn. Idiopathic inflammatory myopathies. Neurol Clin 1997;15:615–648.

nisolone sodium succinate (Solu-Medrol; 1 g daily for 3 days) may also be beneficial [157, 160]. Of DM patients, 58–100% at least partially improve, and
30–66% respond completely with prednisone therapy [14, 41]. More than 80%
of PM patients at least partially improve, and 10–33% completely respond to
prednisone [14, 41]. Objective clinical improvement is usually evident within 3–6
months of starting prednisone [14, 18, 39]. If no response is noted after an adequate trial of high-dose prednisone, other alternative diagnoses (i.e., IBM or an
inflammatory muscular dystrophy) need to be considered and a repeat muscle
biopsy performed.

Many authorities recommend starting prednisone at a high dose (1.0–2.0
mg/kg per day) [1, 3, 4, 16, 39, 157, 158]. We initiate treatment with prednisone
(1.5 mg/kg up to 100 mg) as a once-a-day dose every morning. After 2–4 weeks
of daily prednisone, we switch directly to alternate-day dosing (i.e., 100 mg
every other day). Some advocate slowly tapering to alternate-day dosing over a
2- to 3-month period [3, 39]. We monitor patients initially at least every 2–4
weeks. High-dose prednisone is maintained until patients are back to normal
strength or until improvement in strength has reached a plateau (usually after 4–6
months). At this point, we slowly taper the prednisone by 5 mg every 2–3 weeks.
Once the dose is reduced to 20 mg every other day, prednisone is tapered no faster
than 2.5 mg every 2 weeks. We add one of the second-line agents (azathioprine
or methotrexate) in patients who do not significantly improve after 4–6 months
of high-dose prednisone or if there is an exacerbation during the taper. In patients
who relapse during steroid taper, we double the dose of prednisone and give it
daily (no more than 100 mg per day) for at least 2 weeks before switching back
to every-other-day dosing. Once patients have regained strength, we resume the
prednisone taper at a slower rate while continuing the second-line agent.
Although we monitor serum CK levels, adjustments of prednisone and other
immunosuppressive agents are based on the objective clinical examination and
not the CK levels or patients' subjective responses. Serum CK may be elevated
in patients with no objective weakness or may be normal or only mildly elevated
in patients with active disease. An increasing serum CK can herald a relapse, but
without objective clinical deterioration, we would not increase the dose of the
immunosuppressive agent. However, we may hold the dose or slow the taper. A
maintenance dose of prednisone may be required to sustain the clinical response.

Some authorities maintain treatment with daily prednisone rather than switching to alternate-day therapy [158]. In addition, some split the daily dose of prednisone (two to three times a day) instead of consolidating the prednisone into a single morning dose. We have found no advantage in splitting the dose of prednisone or maintaining daily dosing. Further, studies have suggested that alternate-day dosing of prednisone is as effective as and is associated with fewer side effects than daily steroids [161, 162].

In patients who become weaker while on prednisone, relapse of the myositis needs to be distinguished from steroid myopathy or disuse atrophy. High-dose, long-term steroids and lack of physical activity can cause type 2 muscle fiber atrophy with proximal muscle weakness. In such cases, the serum CK is normal, and EMG does not usually demonstrate significant abnormalities. Neck flexor strength may remain relatively stable with type 2 muscle fiber atrophy, but it worsens when weakness is related to relapse of the myositis [39]. Patients who have increasing serum CK levels and abnormal spontaneous activity on EMG while the steroids are being tapered are more likely experiencing a flare of the myositis. In contrast, patients with normal serum CK and EMG and other evidence of steroid toxicity (i.e., Cushingoid appearance) may have type 2 muscle fiber atrophy and could benefit from physical therapy and a reduced dose of steroids.

Concurrent Management While on Corticosteroids

A chest x-ray and a purified protein derivative (PPD) skin test with controls are obtained on all patients before initiating immunosuppressive medications. Patients with a history of tuberculosis or a positive PPD may need to be treated prophylactically with isoniazid. We prescribe calcium supplementation (1 g daily) and vitamin D for prophylaxis against steroid-induced osteoporosis. Estrogen supplements should be given to postmenopausal women. Biphosphonates have been introduced for the treatment of osteoporosis [163–166]; we use biphosphonates when osteoporosis is present. This is usually demonstrated by assessing bone marrow density with dual-energy x-ray absorptiometry (DEXA). A DEXA should be obtained before initiating corticosteroids and then annually for the duration of therapy. If the DEXA becomes abnormal, either alendronate or etidronate is added. Alendronate (10 mg) is given daily, and etidronate is given for 14 days (400 mg per day) every 3 months. Both etidronate and alendronate are licensed for use in the United States, but only alendronate is U.S. Food and Drug Administration–approved for the treatment of osteoporosis. Alendronate (5 mg) has also been shown to be effective in prevention of osteoporosis in patients receiving corticosteroids [165].

Patients are not treated with histamine-H$_2$ receptor blockers unless they develop gastrointestinal discomfort or have a history of peptic ulcer disease. Patients are given a dietary consultation to instruct them on a low-sodium, low-carbohydrate, high-protein diet to prevent excessive weight gain. In addition, physical therapy and an aerobic exercise program are started. It is important to measure blood pressure and perform eye examinations for cataracts and glaucoma. Fasting blood glucose and serum potassium levels are periodically checked. Potassium supplementation may be required if the patient becomes hypokalemic.

Second-Line Therapies

Second-line therapies are used to treat patients who have been poorly responsive to prednisone or who relapse during prednisone taper, as well as for their potential steroid-sparing effect [1].

Azathioprine

Several retrospective studies suggested that azathioprine can be an effective therapy in DM and PM [18, 41, 158]. One study reported that 64% of DM and PM patients improved with azathioprine, although a complete response occurred in only 11% [41]. Patients who previously responded with prednisone were more likely to improve with the addition of azathioprine than previously prednisone-refractory patients. A prospective, double-blind study comparing azathioprine (2 mg/kg) in combination with prednisone to placebo plus prednisone demonstrated no significant difference in objective improvement at 3 months [154]. However, in the open-label follow-up period, patients on the combination of azathioprine and prednisone required lower doses of prednisone and did better than those on prednisone [167]. Azathioprine is also effective in childhood DM but is generally avoided, given its oncogenic potential with long-term use [2].

We start azathioprine at a dose of 50 mg per day in adults and gradually increase it over 2 months to a total dose of 2–3 mg/kg per day [1]. A systemic reaction, characterized by fever, abdominal pain, nausea, vomiting, and anorexia, occurs in 12% of patients, requiring discontinuation of the drug [168]. This systemic reaction generally occurs within the first few weeks of therapy and resolves within a few days of discontinuing the azathioprine. Rechallenge with azathioprine usually results in the recurrence of the systemic reaction. Other major complications of azathioprine are bone marrow suppression, hepatic toxicity, pancreatitis, teratogenicity, oncogenicity, and risk of infection. Allopurinol should be avoided, because combination with azathioprine increases the risk of bone marrow and liver toxicity. A major drawback of azathioprine is that it often takes 6 months or longer to see an effect from the medication.

We monitor CBC and liver function tests (LFTs)—AST, ALT, bilirubin, and γ-glutamyl transpeptidase—every 2 weeks until the patient is on a stable dose of azathioprine, then once a month. It is important to check the γ-glutamyl transpeptidase—as it is the most reliable indicator of hepatic dysfunction—because the AST and ALT can be elevated from muscle involvement. Azathioprine is decreased if the white blood cell count (WBC) falls below 4,000/mm^3 and held if the WBC declines to 2,500/mm^3 or the absolute neutrophil count falls to 1,000/mm^3. Leukopenia can develop as early as 1 week or as late as 2 years after initiating azathioprine [168]. The leukopenia is usually reversible within 1 month, and patients can be rechallenged with azathioprine without recurrence of the severe leukopenia. We stop azathioprine if the LFTs increase to more than twice the baseline values. Liver toxicity generally develops within the first several months of treatment and can take several months to resolve. Patients can occasionally be successfully rechallenged with azathioprine after LFTs return to baseline without recurrence of hepatic dysfunction [168].

Methotrexate

Methotrexate has been used to treat patients refractory to prednisone, although no prospective, blinded, controlled studies exist to support its benefit. Retrospective series have reported that 71–88% of DM and PM patients improve with the addition of methotrexate [41, 169–172]. One retrospective study suggested that methotrexate was more effective than azathioprine in men, patients with anti-synthetase antibodies, and those patients previously refractory to prednisone [171]. Methotrexate may reduce morbidity in refractory childhood DM [173, 174], although the potential side effects have limited its use in children.

   Methotrexate is administered only 1 day a week. We begin methotrexate orally at 7.5 mg per week, given in three divided doses 12 hours apart [1]. The dose is gradually increased by 2.5 mg each week, up to 20 mg per week. If there is no improvement after 1 month of 20 mg per week of oral methotrexate, we switch to weekly parenteral (intramuscular or intravenous) methotrexate and increase the dose by 5 mg every week, up to 60 mg per week. The major side effects of methotrexate are alopecia; stomatitis; ILD; teratogenicity; oncogenicity; risk of infection; and bone marrow, renal, and liver toxicity. Doses higher than 50 mg per week require leucovorin rescue, although we rarely use such high doses.

   Methotrexate can cause ILD; therefore, we avoid its use in patients with myositis who already have the associated ILD. Baseline and periodic pulmonary function tests are evaluated on patients treated with methotrexate. We monitor CBCs and LFTs once a month. Because liver toxicity is cumulative, patients receiving more than a 2-g total dose may need a liver biopsy if the medication is to be continued.

Cyclophosphamide

We reserve cyclophosphamide for patients refractory to prednisone, azathioprine, and methotrexate. Some studies have reported improvement in individual patients with oral and intravenous cyclophosphamide [18, 175–180]. However, other series have not found a similar beneficial response; rather, an increased morbidity with intravenous cyclophosphamide has been described [39, 181, 182]. Cyclophosphamide may be effective in patients with ILD and in children with DM and vasculitis [157, 183].

   We have had only limited success using cyclophosphamide in refractory myositis patients. Cyclophosphamide can be given orally at a dose of 1.0–2.0 mg/kg per day. We reserve pulsed intravenous cyclophosphamide at 1 g/M^2 per month for patients with severe refractory myositis and ILD. The major side effects are gastrointestinal upset, bone marrow toxicity, alopecia, hemorrhagic cystitis, teratogenicity, sterility, and increased risk of infections and secondary malignancies. A high fluid intake is important to avoid hemorrhagic cystitis. Urinalysis and CBCs are monitored closely (every 1–2 weeks at the onset of therapy and then at least monthly). Cyclophosphamide is decreased if the WBC falls below 4,000/mm^3. We hold the cyclophosphamide if the WBC falls below 3,000/mm^3, if the absolute neutrophil count falls below 1,000/mm^3, or if there is evidence of hematuria. Cyclophosphamide can be restarted at a lower dose once the leukopenia has resolved, but we discontinue the medication in patients with hematuria.

Chlorambucil

We have only rarely used chlorambucil because of its oncogenic potential and less predictable effect on the bone marrow. Other significant side effects include a hypersensitivity reaction with severe rash (Stevens-Johnson syndrome), gastrointestinal disturbance, infection, teratogenicity, and liver toxicity. Nevertheless, there are a few reports in the literature of PM and DM treated with this medication [158, 169, 180, 184, 185]. Five DM patients previously refractory to prednisone, azathioprine, and methotrexate improved within 4–6 weeks of starting oral chlorambucil (4 mg per day) [184]. Four patients were able to stop the chlorambucil and corticosteroids after 13–30 months with remission of their DM. Some studies report that chlorambucil in combination with methotrexate and prednisone may also be effective in refractory PM [158, 169, 180, 185]. The risks of secondary malignancies and liver and bone marrow toxicity are presumably increased using combination chemotherapy. Obviously, CBCs and LFTs need to be monitored closely in patients treated with chlorambucil.

Cyclosporine and Tacrolimus

Several small series report that cyclosporine (2.5–10.0 mg/kg per day) is an effective treatment of DM and PM, including childhood DM [88, 186–196]. Improvement in strength was noted within 2–6 weeks, and prednisone was able to be decreased or discontinued in the majority of patients. A pilot study of tacrolimus (FK506) reported improvement in a small number of refractory PM patients [197]. The cost and potential side effects of cyclosporine and tacrolimus have limited their use. Side effects of cyclosporine and tacrolimus are renal toxicity, hypertension, electrolyte imbalance, gastrointestinal upset, hypertrichosis, gingival hyperplasia, oncogenicity, tremor, and risk of infection.

We start cyclosporine at a dose of 3.0–4.0 mg/kg per day in two divided doses and gradually increase to 6.0 mg/kg per day as necessary. The cyclosporine dose should initially be titrated to maintain trough serum cyclosporine levels of 50–200 ng/ml. Blood pressure, electrolytes and renal function, and trough cyclosporine levels need to be monitored periodically. We have not used tacrolimus to treat myositis.

Intravenous Immunoglobulin

IVIG has been used in the treatment of many different autoimmune diseases and has become increasingly popular in the treatment of refractory myositis [198, 199]. Improvement following IVIG therapy has been reported in several small, uncontrolled series of DM and PM patients [198, 200–207]. Efficacy of IVIG has been most convincingly demonstrated for DM based on a prospective double-blind, placebo-controlled study of 15 patients with DM who demonstrated significant clinical improvement with IVIG [155]. Further, repeat biopsies in five of the responsive patients revealed an increase in muscle fiber diameter, an increase in the number and a decrease in the diameter of capillaries, a resolution of complement components on capillaries, and a reduction in the expression of intercellular adhesion molecule 1 and MHC class 1 antigens. A blinded study of IVIG in PM has not been performed, and we have been unimpressed with the results of IVIG treatment in refractory PM.

Regarding IBM, one study suggested a benefit in three of four patients treated with IVIG [208]. However, we were unable to document any significant clinical improvement in nine IBM patients treated with IVIG [127]. A 1997 prospective, double-blind, placebo-controlled study of IVIG in IBM revealed no significant improvement [128, 156]. Therefore, there is no compelling evidence indicating that IVIG should be used for IBM.

We initiate IVIG (2 g/kg) slowly over 2–5 days and repeat infusions at monthly intervals for at least 3 months. Before treatment, we obtain an IgA level. Patients with low IgA levels may have anti-IgA antibodies in their sera, a condition that predisposes them to anaphylactic reactions to IVIG, because IVIG contains small amounts of IgA. Patients should also have their blood urea nitrogen and creatine measured, especially those with diabetes mellitus, because of a risk of IVIG-induced renal failure. Flulike symptoms—headaches, myalgias, fever, chills, nausea, and vomiting—are common and occur in as many as one-half of the patients. Rash, aseptic meningitis, and stroke can also occur.

Plasmapheresis and Leukapheresis

Improvement following plasmapheresis or leukapheresis has been reported in a few uncontrolled series of DM, PM, and IBM patients [209–213]. However, a controlled trial of 36 patients with DM and PM, comparing plasmapheresis with leukapheresis and with sham apheresis, failed to demonstrate improvement with either plasmapheresis or leukapheresis [214].

Total Body Irradiation

A few case reports of refractory DM and PM patients suggest improvement after total body irradiation (TBI) [215–218]. However, others have not found TBI to be effective in PM [219]. TBI is not effective in IBM and may cause worsening in strength [220].

Thymectomy

A few patients with PM and DM have had thymectomy with a beneficial response [221, 222].

Treatment of Extramuscular Manifestation of Dermatomyositis

Rash

In most DM cases, the rash improves along with muscle strength with immuno-suppressive therapy. Dalakas et al. reported resolution of the rash, in addition to improved strength, with IVIG [155]. Hydroxychloroquine, chloroquine, topical steroids, and sunscreen have also been used to treat the rash [157, 223].

Subcutaneous Calcifications

Once calcinosis develops, it is extremely difficult to treat. Colchicine, probenecid, warfarin, and phosphate buffers have been tried but only with limited success [4, 16, 158]. Oral diltiazem has been reported to produce a dramatic reduction of calcinosis in some DM patients [224, 225]. We have not observed similar results, but we believe this may be a therapeutic option that deserves further study.

REFERENCES

1. Amato AA, Barohn RJ. Idiopathic inflammatory myopathies. Neurol Clin 1997;15:615–648.
2. Amato AA, Kissel JT. Inflammatory Myopathies. In KF Swaiman (ed), Pediatric Neurology (2nd ed). St Louis: Mosby (in press).
3. Dalakas MC. Polymyositis, dermatomyositis, and inclusion body myositis. N Engl J Med 1991;325: 1487–1498.
4. Engel AG, Hohlfeld B, Banker BQ. The polymyositis and dermatomyositis syndromes. In AG Engel, C Franzini-Armstrong (eds), Myology (2nd ed). New York: McGraw-Hill, 1994;1335–1383.
5. Medsger TA Jr, Dawson WN, Masi AT. The epidemiology of polymyositis. Am J Med 1970;48:715–723.
6. Amato AA, Shebert RT. Inclusion body myositis in twins. Neurology 1998;51:598–600.
7. Banker BQ. Dermatomyositis of childhood: ultrastructural alterations of muscle and intramuscular blood vessels. J Neuropathol Exp Neurol 1975;34:46–75.
8. Cook CD, Rosen FS, Banker BQ. Dermatomyositis and focal scleroderma. Pediatr Clin North Am 1963;10:979–1016.
9. Griggs RC, Askanas V, DiMauro S, et al. Inclusion body myositis and myopathies. Ann Neurol 1995;38:705–713.
10. Harati Y, Niakan E, Bergman EW. Childhood dermatomyositis in monozygotic twins. Neurology 1986;36:721–723.
11. Leukonia RM, Buxton PH. Myositis in father and daughter. J Neurol Neurosurg Psychiatry 1973;36:820–825.
12. Sivakumar K, Semino-Mora C, Dalakas MC. An inflammatory, familial, inclusion body myositis with autoimmune features and a phenotype identical to sporadic inclusion body myositis. Studies in three families. Brain 1997;120:653–661.
13. Bruguier A, Texier P, Clement MC, et al. Dermatomyosites infantiles: à propos de vingthuit observations. Arch Fr Pediatr 1984;41:9–14.
14. Amato AA, Gronseth GS, Jackson CE, et al. Inclusion body myositis: clinical and pathological boundaries. Ann Neurol 1996;40:581–586.
15. Bohan A, Peters JB. Polymyositis and dermatomyositis. Part 1. N Engl J Med 1975;292:344–347.
16. Griggs RC, Mendell JR, Miller RG. Inflammatory Myopathies. In Evaluation and Treatment of Myopathies. Philadelphia: FA Davis, 1995;154–210.
17. Hochberg MC, Feldman D, Stevens MB. Adult-onset polymyositis/dermatomyositis: analysis of clinical and laboratory features and survival in 76 cases with a review of the literature. Semin Arthritis Rheum 1986;15:168–178.
18. Tymms KE, Webb J. Dermatomyositis and other connective tissue diseases: a review of 105 cases. J Rheumatol 1985;12:1140–1148.
19. Pachman LM. Juvenile dermatomyositis. Pathophysiology and disease expression. Pediatr Rheumatol 1995;42:1071–1098.
20. Euwer RL, Sontheimer RD. Amyopathic dermatomyositis: a review. J Invest Dermatol 1993;100: 124S–127S.
21. Henriksson KG, Sandstedt P. Polymyositis-treatment and prognosis. A study of 107 patients. Acta Neurol Scand 1982;65:280–300.

22. Askari AD. Inflammatory disorders of muscle: cardiac abnormalities. Clin Rheum Dis 1984; 131–149.
23. Denbow CE, Lie JT, Tancredi RG, et al. Cardiac involvement in polymyositis. Arthritis Rheum 1979;22:1088–1092.
24. Gottdiener JS, Sherber HS, Hawley RJ, et al. Cardiac manifestations in polymyositis. Am J Cardiol 1978;41:1141–1149.
25. Haupt HM, Hutchins GM. The heart and conduction system in polymyositis-dermatomyositis. Am J Cardiol 1982;50:998–1006.
26. Strongwater SL, Annesley T, Schnitzer TJ. Myocardial involvement in polymyositis. J Rheumatol 1983;10:459–463.
27. Frazier RA, Miller RD. Interstitial pneumonitis in association with polymyositis and dermatomyositis. Chest 1974;65:403–407.
28. Park S, Nyhan WL. Fatal pulmonary involvement in dermatomyositis. Am J Dis Child 1975;129:727–728.
29. Schwartz MI, Matthay RA, Sahn SA, et al. Interstitial lung disease in polymyositis and dermatomyositis: analysis of six cases and review of the literature. Medicine (Baltimore) 1976;55:89–104.
30. Dickey BF, Myers AR. Pulmonary disease in polymyositis/dermatomyositis. Semin Arthritis Rheum 1984;14:60–76.
31. Hochberg MC, Feldman D, Stevens MB, et al. Antibody to Jo-1 in polymyositis/dermatomyositis: association with interstitial pulmonary disease. J Rheumatol 1984;11:663–665.
32. Love LA, Leff RL, Fraser DD, et al. A new approach to the classification of idiopathic inflammatory myopathy: myositis-specific autoantibodies define useful homogeneous patient groups. Medicine (Baltimore) 1991;70:360–374.
33. Targoff IN. Immune manifestations of inflammatory disease. Rheum Dis Clin North Am 1994;20: 857–880.
34. Bohan A, Peter JB, Bowman RL, et al. A computer-assisted analysis of 153 patients with polymyositis and dermatomyositis. Medicine (Baltimore) 1977;56:255–286.
35. Callen JP. Relationship of cancer to inflammatory muscle diseases: dermatomyositis, polymyositis, and inclusion body myositis. Rheum Dis Clin North Am 1994;20:943–953.
36. Sigurgeirsson B, Lindelöf B, Edhag O, et al. Risk of cancer in patient with dermatomyositis or polymyositis. N Engl J Med 1992;326:363–367.
37. Basset-Seguin N, Roujeau J-C, Gherardi R, et al. Prognostic factors and predictive signs of malignancy in adult dermatomyositis: a study of 32 cases. Arch Dermatol 1990;126:633–637.
38. Feldman D, Hochberg MC, Zizic TM, et al. Cutaneous vasculitis in adult polymyositis/dermatomyositis. J Rheumatol 1983;10:85–89.
39. Dalakas MC. How to diagnose and treat the inflammatory myopathies. Semin Neurol 1994;14: 137–145.
40. Bohan A, Peters JB. Polymyositis and dermatomyositis. Part 2. N Engl J Med 1975;292:403–407.
41. Joffe MM, Love LA, Leff RL. Drug therapy of idiopathic inflammatory myopathies: predictors of response to prednisone, azathioprine, and methotrexate and a comparison of their efficacy. Am J Med 1993;94:379–387.
42. Miller FW. Myositis-specific antibodies: touchstones for understanding the inflammatory myopathies. JAMA 1993;270:1846–1849.
43. Plotz PH, Rider LG, Targoff IN, et al. Myositis: immunologic contributions to understanding cause, pathogenesis, and therapy. Ann Intern Med 1995;122:715–724.
44. Fraser DD, Frank JA, Dalakas M, et al. Magnetic resonance imaging in idiopathic inflammatory myopathies. J Rheumatol 1991;18:1693–1700.
45. Hernandez RJ, Sullivan DB, Chenevert TL, et al. MR imaging in children with dermatomyositis: findings and correlations with clinical and laboratory findings. AJR Am J Roentgenol 1993;161:359–366.
46. Mastaglia FL, Laing NG. Investigation of muscle disease. J Neurol Neurosurg Psychiatry 1996;60:256–274.
47. Pitt AM, Fleckenstein JL, Greenlee RG Jr, et al. MRI-guided biopsy in inflammatory myopathy: initial results. Magn Reson Imaging 1993;11:1093–1099.
48. Arahata K, Engel AG. Monoclonal antibody analysis of mononuclear cells in myopathies. I: Quantitative of subsets according to diagnosis and sites of accumulation and demonstration and counts of muscle fibers invaded by T cells. Ann Neurol 1984;16:193–208.
49. Engel AG, Arahata K. Monoclonal antibody analysis of mononuclear cells in myopathies. II: Phenotypes of autoinvasive cells in polymyositis and inclusion body myositis. Ann Neurol 1984;16:209–215.
50. Emslie-Smith AM, Engel AG. Microvascular changes in early and advanced dermatomyositis: a quantitative study. Ann Neurol 1990;27:343–356.

51. Kissel JT, Halterman RK, Rammohan KW, Mendell JR. The relationship of complement-mediated microvasculopathy to the histologic features and clinical duration of disease in dermatomyositis. Arch Neurol 1991;48:26–30.
52. Kissel JT, Mendell JR, Rammohan KW. Microvascular deposition of complement membrane attack complex in dermatomyositis. N Engl J Med 1986;314:331–334.
53. Whitaker JN, Engel WK. Vascular deposits of immunoglobulin and complement in idiopathic inflammatory myopathy. N Engl J Med 1972;286:332–338.
54. DeVisser M, Emslie-Smith AM, Engel AG. Early ultrastructural alterations in dermatomyositis: capillary abnormalities precede other structural changes in muscle. J Neurol Sci 1989;94:181–192.
55. Chwalinska-Sadowska H, Madykowa H. Polymyositis-dermatomyositis: 25 year follow-up of 50 patients—disease course, treatment, prognostic factors. Mater Med Pol 1990;22:213.
56. Murayabashi K, Saito E, Okada S, et al. Prognosis and life in polymyositis/dermatomyositis. Ryumachi 1991;31:391.
57. Hochberg MC, Lopez-Acuna D, Gittleshon AM. Mortality from polymyositis and dermatomyositis in the United States, 1968-1978. Arthritis Rheum 1983;26:1465–1471.
58. Hohlfeld R, Engel AG, Ii K, et al. Polymyositis mediated by T lymphocytes that express the gamma-delta receptor. N Engl J Med 1991;324:877–881.
59. Zitnan D, Rovensky J, Lukac J, et al. Systemic connective tissue diseases-prognostic conclusions on a 30-year study. Vnitr Lek 1991;37:853.
60. Shevell M, Rosenblatt B, Silver K, et al. Congenital inflammatory myopathy. Neurology 1990;40:1111–1114.
61. Thompson CE. Infantile myositis. Dev Med Child Neurol 1982;24:307–313.
62. Morse RP, Kagan-Hallet K, Amato AA. Congenital inflammatory myopathy: a real entity [abstract]? J Child Neurol 1995;10:162.
63. Pegoraro E, Mancias P, Swerdlow SH, et al. Congenital muscular dystrophy with primary laminin 2 (merosin) deficiency presenting as inflammatory myopathy. Ann Neurol 1996;40:782–791.
64. Henderson A, Cumming WJK, Williams DO, et al. Cardiac complications of polymyositis. J Neurol Sci 1980;47:425–428.
65. Kehoe RF, Bauernfeind R, Tommaso C, et al. Cardiac conduction defects in polymyositis: electrophysiologic studies in four patients. Ann Intern Med 1981;94:41–43.
66. Emslie-Smith AM, Arahata K, Engel AG. Major histocompatibility complex 1 antigen expression, immunolocalization of interferon subtypes, and T cell-mediated cytotoxicity in myopathies. Hum Pathol 1989;20:224–231.
67. Mantegazza R, Andreetta F, Bernasconi P, et al. Analysis of T cell receptor of muscle-infiltrating T lymphocytes in polymyositis: restricted V/ rearrangements may indicate antigen-driven selection. J Clin Invest 1993 91:2880–2886.
68. Leff RL, Love LA, Miller FW, et al. Viruses in idiopathic inflammatory myopathies: absence of candidate viral genomes in muscle. Lancet 1992;339:1192–1195.
69. Ytterberg SR. The relationship of infectious agents to inflammatory myositis. Rheum Clin North Am 1994;20:995–1015.
70. Kinoshita M, Iwasaki Y, Wada F, et al. A case of congenital polymyositis: a possible pathogenesis of "Fukuyama type congenital muscular dystrophy." Clin Neurol 1980;20:911–916.
71. Kinoshita M, Nishina M, Koya N. Ten years follow-up study of steroid therapy for congenital encephalomyopathy. Brain Dev 1986;8:281–284.
72. Nagai T, Hasgawa T, Saito M, et al. Infantile polymyositis: a case report. Brain Dev 1992;14:167–169.
73. Roddy SM, Ashwal S, Peckham N, et al. Infantile myositis: a case diagnosed in the neonatal period. Pediatr Neurol 1986;2:241–244.
74. Olney RK, Miller RG. Inflammatory infiltration in Fukayama type congenital muscular dystrophy. Muscle Nerve 1983;6:75–76.
75. Mendell JT, Feng B, Sahenk Z, et al. Novel laminin-2 mutations in congenital muscular dystrophy [abstract]. Neurology 1997;48(suppl 2):A195.
76. Marguerie C, Bunn CC, Copier J, et al. The clinical and immunogenic features of patients with antibodies to the nucleolar antigen PM-Scl. Medicine (Baltimore) 1992;71:327–336.
77. Ringel RA, Brick JE, Brick JF, et al. Muscle involvement in the scleroderma syndromes. Arch Intern Med 1990;150:2550–2552.
78. Tuffanelli DL, Winkelman RK. Scleroderma: a clinical study of 727 cases. Arch Dermatol 1961;84:359–371.
79. Denko CW, Old JW. Myopathy in the sicca syndrome (Sjögren's syndrome). Am J Clin Pathol 1969;51:631–637.

80. Ponge T, Mussini JM, Ponge A, et al. Primary Gougerot-Sjögren syndrome with necrotizing polymyositis: improvement by hydroxychloroquine. Rev Neurol 1987;143:147–148.
81. Ringel SP, Forstot JZ, Tan EM, et al. Sjögren's syndrome and polymyositis or dermatomyositis. Arch Neurol 1982;1982:39:157–163.
82. Foote RA, Kimbrough SM, Stevens JC. Lupus myositis. Muscle Nerve 1982;5:65–68.
83. Sharp GC, Irvan WS, Tan E, et al. Mixed connective tissue disease—an apparently distinct rheumatic disease syndrome associated with a specific antibody to an extractable nuclear antigen (ENA). Am J Med 1972;52:148–159.
84. Lunberg I, Hedfors E. Clinical course of patients with anti-RNP antibodies: a prospective study of 32 patients. J Rheumatol 1991;18:1511–1519.
85. Carpenter S. Inclusion body myositis, a review. J Neuropathol Exp Neurol 1996;55:1105–1114.
86. Heffner RR. Inflammatory myopathies. A review. J Neuropathol Exp Neurol 1993;52:339–350.
87. Lotz BP, Engel AG, Nishino H, et al. Inclusion body myositis. Observations in 40 patients. Brain 1989;112:727–747.
88. Mehregan AL, Bohan A, Goldberg LS, et al. Cyclosporine treatment for dermatomyositis/polymyositis. Cutis 1993;51:59–61.
89. Sekul EA, Dalakas MC. Inclusion body myositis: new concepts. Semin Neurol 1993;13:256–263.
90. Darrow DH, Hoffman HT, Barnes GJ, et al. Management of dysphagia in inclusion body myositis. Arch Otolaryngol Head Neck Surg 1992;118:313–317.
91. Verma A, Bradley WG, Adensina AM, et al. Inclusion body myositis with cricopharyngeus muscle involvement and severe dysphagia. Muscle Nerve 1991;14:470–473.
92. Argov Z, Yarom R. "Rimmed vacuole myopathy" sparing the quadriceps: a unique disorder in Iranian Jews. J Neurol Sci 1984;64:33–43.
93. Sadeh M, Gadoth N, Hadar H, et al. Vacuolar myopathy sparing the quadriceps. Brain 1993;116:217–232.
94. Askanas V. New developments in hereditary inclusion body myopathies. Ann Neurol 1997;41:432–437.
95. Ikeuchi T, Asaka T, Saito M, et al. Gene localization for autosomal recessive distal myopathy with rimmed vacuoles maps to chromosome 9. Ann Neurol 1997;41:432–437.
96. Argov Z, Tiram E, Eisenberg I, et al. Hereditary inclusion body myopathy maps to chromosome 9p1-q1. Ann Neurol 1997;41:548–551.
97. Barohn RJ, Amato AA, Griggs RC. Overview of distal myopathies: from the clinical to the molecular. Neuromuscul Disord 1998;8;309–316.
98. Mikol J, Engel AG. Inclusion Body Myositis. In AG Engel, C Franzini-Armstrong (eds), Myology (2nd ed). New York: McGraw-Hill, 1994;1384–1398.
99. Koffman BM, Rugiero M, Dalakas MC. Immune-mediated conditions and antibodies associated with sporadic inclusion body myositis. Muscle Nerve 1998;27:115–117.
100. Garlepp MJ, Laing B, Zilko PJ, et al. HLA associations with inclusion body myositis. Clin Exp Immunol 1994;98:40–45.
101. Eisen A, Berry K, Gibson G. Inclusion body myositis (IBM): myopathy or neuropathy? Neurology 1983;33:1109–1114.
102. Joy JL, Oh SJ, Baysal AI. Electrophysiological spectrum of inclusion body myositis. Muscle Nerve 1990;13:949–951.
103. Luciano CA, Dalakas MC. Inclusion body myositis: no evidence of a neurogenic component. Neurology 1997;48:29–33.
104. Sekul EA, Chow C, Dalakas MC. Magnetic resonance imaging (MRI) of the forearm as a diagnostic aid in patients with inclusion body myositis. Neurology 1997;48:863–866.
105. Askanas V, Engel WK, Alvarez RB. Enhanced detection of amyloid deposits in muscle fibers of inclusion body myositis and brain of Alzheimer disease using fluorescence technique. Neurology 1993;43:1265–1267.
106. Mendell JR, Sahenk Z, Gales T, et al. Amyloid filaments in inclusion body myositis. Novel findings provide insight into nature of filaments. Arch Neurol 1991;48:1229–1234.
107. Barohn RJ, Amato AA, Sahenk Z, et al. Inclusion body myositis: explanation for poor response to therapy. Neurology 1995;45:1302–1304.
108. Rifai Z, Welle S, Kamp C, Thornton CA. Ragged red fibers in normal aging and inflammatory myopathy. Ann Neurol 1995;37:24–25.
109. O'Hanlon TP, Dalakas MC, Plotz PH, et al. The alpha-beta T-cell receptor repertoire in inclusion body myositis: diverse patterns of gene expression by infiltrating lymphocytes. J Autoimmun 1994;7:321–333.
110. Pruitt JN II, Showalter CJ, Engel AG. Sporadic inclusion body myositis: counts of different types of abnormal fibers. Ann Neurol 1996;39:139–143.
111. Askanas V, Alvarez RB, Engel WK. Beta-amyloid precursor epitopes in muscle fibers of inclusion body myositis. Ann Neurol 1993;34:551–560.

112. Askanas V, Engel WK. New advances in inclusion-body myositis. Curr Opin Rheumatol 1993;5:732–741.
113. Askanas V, Engel WK, Bilak M, et al. Twisted tubulofilaments of inclusion body myositis resemble paired helical filaments of Alzheimer brain and contain hyperphosphorylated tau. Am J Pathol 1994;144:177–187.
114. Askanas V, McFerrin J, Baque S, et al. Over expression of beta-amyloid precursor protein gene in cultured normal human muscle using adenovirus vector induces aspects of inclusion-body myositis phenotype [abstract]. Neurology 1995;45(suppl 4):A208.
115. Askanas V, Mirabella M, Engel WK, et al. Apolipoprotein E immunoreactive deposits in inclusion-body muscle. Lancet 1994;343:364–365.
116. Mirabella M, Askanas V, Bilak M, et al. Abnormal accumulation of phosphorylated neurofilament heavy-chain in sporadic inclusion-body myositis (S-IBM): differences between S-IBM and hereditary inclusion body myositis (h-IBM) [abstract]. Neurology 1995;45(suppl 4):A209.
117. Askanas V, Mirabella M, Engel WK, et al. Apolipoprotein E alleles in sporadic inclusion body myositis and hereditary inclusion body myopathy. Ann Neurol 1996;40:264.
118. Harrington CR, Anderson JR, Chan KK. Apolipoprotein E type 4 allele frequency is not increased in patients with sporadic inclusion-body myositis. Neurosci Lett 1995;183:35–38.
119. Sarkozi B, Askanas V, Engel WK. Abnormal accumulation of prion protein mRNA in muscle fibers of patients with sporadic inclusion body myositis and hereditary inclusion body myopathy. Am J Pathol 1994;160:1280–1284.
120. Oldfors A, Larsson NG, Lindberg C, et al. Mitochondria DNA deletions in inclusion body myositis. Brain 1993;116:325–336.
121. Chou SM. Inclusion body myositis: a chronic persistent mumps infection? Hum Pathol 1986;17:765–777.
122. Kallajoki M, Hyypiä T, Halonen P, et al. Inclusion body myositis and paramyxoviruses. Hum Pathol 1991;22:29–32.
123. Nishino H, Engle AG, Rima BK. Inclusion body myositis: the mumps virus hypothesis. Ann Neurol 1989;25:260–264.
124. Rammohan LW, Wolinsky J, Omerza J, et al. Mumps virus in IBM: studies implicating cross-reactivity accounting for antigen localization [abstract]. Neurology 1988;38:151.
125. Cupler EJ, Leon-Monzon M, Semino-Mora C, et al. Inclusion body myositis in HIV-1 and HTLV-1 infected patients. Brain 1996;199:1887–1893.
126. Semino-Mora C, Dalakas MC. Red rimmed vacuoles with B-amyloid deposition in the muscles of patients with post-polio syndrome: histopathologic similarities with inclusion body myositis [abstract]. Neurology 1996;46(suppl):116.
127. Amato AA, Barohn RJ, Jackson CE, et al. Inclusion body myositis: treatment with intravenous immunoglobulin. Neurology 1994;44:1516–1518.
128. Barohn RJ. The therapeutic dilemma of inclusion body myositis. Neurology 1997;48:567–568.
129. Leff RL, Miller FW, Hicks J, Fraser DD, Plotz PH. The treatment of inclusion body myositis: a retrospective review and a randomized, prospective trial of immunosuppressive therapy. Medicine (Baltimore) 1993;72:225–235.
130. Banker BQ. Other Inflammatory Myopathies. In AG Engel, C Franzini-Armstrong (eds), Myology (2nd ed). New York: McGraw-Hill, 1994;1461–1886.
131. Layzer RB, Shearn MA, Satya-Murti. Eosinophilic polymyositis. Ann Neurol 1977;1:65–71.
132. Moore PM, Harley JB, Fauci AS. Neurologic dysfunction in the idiopathic hypereosinophilia syndrome. Ann Intern Med 1985;102:109–114.
133. Lakhanpal S, Ginsbburg WW, Michet CJ, et al. Eosinophilic fasciitis: clinical spectrum and therapeutic response in 52 cases. Semin Arthritis Rheum 1988;17:221–231.
134. Shulman LE. Diffuse fasciitis with eosinophilia: a new syndrome? Trans Assoc Am Physicians 1975;88:70–86.
135. Hertzman PA, Blevins WL, Mayer J, et al. Association of the eosinophilia-myalgia syndrome with the ingestion of tryptophan. N Engl J Med 1990;322:869–873.
136. Kilbourne EH, Rigau-Perez J, Heath CW, et al. Clinical epidemiology of toxic-oil syndrome. Manifestations of a new disease. N Engl J Med 1983;309:1408–1414.
137. Namba T, Brunner NG, Grob D. Idiopathic giant cell polymyositis. Arch Neurol 1974;31:27–31.
138. Pazcuzzi RM, Roos KL, Phillips LH. Granulomatous inflammatory myopathy associated with myasthenia gravis. Arch Neurol 1986;43:621–623.
139. Silverstein A, Siltzbach LE. Muscle involvement in sarcoidosis. Asymptomatic myositis and myopathy. Arch Neurol 1969;21:235–241.
140. Stjernberg N, Cajander S, Truedsson H, Uddenfeldt P. Muscle involvement in sarcoidosis. Acta Med Scand 1981;209:213–216.

141. Afifi AK, Frayha RA, Bahuth N, Tekian A. The myopathology of Behçet's disease: histochemical, light and electron microscopic study. J Neurol Sci 1980;48:333–342.
142. Di Giacomo V, Carmini G, Meloni F, Valesini G. Myositis in Behçet's disease [letter]. Arthritis Rheum 1982;25:1025.
143. Finucane P, Dollye C, Ferris J, et al. Behçet's disease with myositis and glomerulonephritis. Br J Rheumatol 1985;24:372–375.
144. Lang BA, Laxer R, Thorner P, et al. Pediatric onset of Behçet's syndrome with myositis: case report and literature review illustrating unusual features. Arthritis Rheum 1990;33:418–425.
145. Lingenfelser T, Duerk H, Stevens A, et al. Generalized myositis in Behçet's disease: treatment with cyclosporine. Ann Intern Med 1992;116:651–653.
146. Worthmann F, Bruns J, Turker T, Gosztonyi G. Muscular involvement in Behçet's disease: case report and review of the literature. Neuromuscul Disord 1996;6:247–253.
147. Yazici H, Tzner N, Tzn Y, Yurdakul S. Localized myositis in Behçet's disease [letter]. Arthritis Rheum 1981;24:636.
148. Caldwell CJ, Swash M, Van der Walt JD, Geddes JF. Focal myositis: a clinicopathological study. Neuromuscul Disord 1995;5:317–321.
149. Colding-Jorgenson E, Laursen H, Lauritzen M. Acta Neurol Scand 1993;88:289–292.
150. Heffner RR, Armbrustmacher VW, Earle KM. Focal myositis. Cancer 1977;40:301–306.
151. Heffner RR, Barron SA. Polymyositis beginning as a focal process. Arch Neurol 1981;38:439–442.
152. Moreno-Lugris C, Gonzalez-Gay M, Sanchez-Andrade A, et al. Magnetic resonance imaging: a useful technique in the diagnosis and follow-up of focal myositis. Ann Rheum Dis 1996;55:856.
153. Moskowitz E, Fisher C, Westbury G, Parsons C. Focal myositis, a benign inflammatory pseudotumor: CT appearances. Br J Radiol 1991;64:489–493.
154. Bunch TW, Worthington JW, Combs JJ, et al. Azathioprine with prednisone for polymyositis. Ann Intern Med 1980;92:365–369.
155. Dalakas MC, Illa I, Dambrosia JM, et al. A controlled trial of high dose intravenous immunoglobulin infusions as treatment for dermatomyositis. N Engl J Med 1993;329:1993–2000.
156. Dalakas MC, Saries B, Dambrosia JM, et al. Treatment of inclusion body myositis with IVIg: a double-blind, placebo-controlled study. Neurology 1997;48:712–716.
157. Adams EM, Plotz PH. The treatment of myositis. How to approach resistant disease. Rheum Dis Clin North Am 1995;21:179–202.
158. Oddis CV. Therapy of inflammatory myopathy. Rheum Dis Clin North Am 1994;20:899–918.
159. Zhanuzakov MA, Vinogradova OM, Soleva AP. Effect of corticosteroids on survival of patients with idiopathic dermatomyositis. Ter Arkh 1986;58:102–105.
160. Laxer RM, Stein LD, Petty RE. Intravenous pulse methylprednisolone treatment of juvenile dermatomyositis. Arthritis Rheum 1987;30:328–334.
161. Cook JD, Fink CW, Henderson-Tilton AC. Comparison of the initial response of childhood dermatopolymyositis to daily versus alternate day corticosteroid administration: a retrospective study [abstract]. Ann Neurol 1984;16:400–401.
162. Uchino M, Araki S, Yoshida O, et al. High single dose alternate day corticosteroid regiments in treatment of polymyositis. J Neurol 1985;232:175–178.
163. Hurley DL, Khosla S. Update on primary osteoporosis. Mayo Clin Proc 1997;72:943–949.
164. Gourley MF. Reducing the risks of glucocorticoid-induced osteoporosis. Contemp Int Med 1998;10:34-43.
165. Saag KG, Emkey R, Schnitzer TJ, et al. Alendronate for the prevention and treatment of glucocorticoid-induced osteoporosis. N Engl J Med 1998;339:292–299.
166. Adachi JD, Bensen WG, Brown J, et al. Intermittent etidronate therapy to prevent corticosteroid-induced osteoporosis. N Engl J Med 1997;337:382–387.
167. Bunch TW. Prednisone and azathioprine for polymyositis: long-term follow-up. Arthritis Rheum 1981;24:45–48.
168. Kissel JT, Levy RJ, Mendell JR, Griggs RC. Azathioprine toxicity in neuromuscular disease. Neurology 1986;36:35–39.
169. Cagnoli M, Marchesoni A, Tosi S. Combined steroid, methotrexate, and chlorambucil therapy for steroid resistant dermatomyositis. Clin Exp Rheumatol 1991;9:658–659.
170. Giannini M, Callen JP. Treatment of dermatomyositis with methotrexate and prednisone. Arch Dermatol 1979;115:1251–1252.
171. Metzger AL, Bohan A, Goldberg LS, et al. Polymyositis and dermatomyositis: combined methotrexate and corticosteroid therapy. Ann Intern Med 1974;81:182–189.
172. Sokoloff MC, Goldberg LS, Pearson CM. Treatment of corticosteroid-resistant polymyositis with methotrexate. Lancet 1971;1:14–16.

173. Jacob JC. Methotrexate and azathioprine treatment of childhood dermatomyositis. Pediatrics 1977; 59:212–218.
174. Miller LC, Sisson BA, Tucker LB, et al. Methotrexate treatment of recalcitrant childhood dermatomyositis. Arthritis Rheum 1992;35:1143–1149.
175. Bombardieri S, Hughes GRV, Neri R, et al. Cyclophosphamide in severe polymyositis [letter]. Lancet 1988;1:1138–1139.
176. Haga HJ, D'Cruz D, Asherson R, et al. Short-term effects of intravenous pulses of cyclophosphamide in the treatment of connective tissue disease crisis. Ann Rheum Dis 1992;51:885–888.
177. Kono DW, Klashman DJ, Gilbert RC. Successful IV pulsed cyclophosphamide in refractory PM in 3 patients with SLE [letter]. J Rheumatol 1990;17:982–983.
178. Leroy JP, Drosos AA, Yiannopoulos DI, et al. Intravenous pulse cyclophosphamide therapy in myositis and Sjögren's syndrome. Arthritis Rheum 1990;33:1579–1581.
179. Niakan E, Pitner SE, Whitaker JN, et al. Immunosuppressive agents in corticosteroid-refractory childhood dermatomyositis. Neurology 1980;30:286–291.
180. Trotter D, McCarthy DJ, Csuka ME. Treatment of dermatomyositis/polymyositis with combination chemotherapy in early disease [abstract]. Arthritis Rheum 1991;34:S149.
181. Cronin ME, Miller FW, Hicks JE, et al. The failure of intravenous cyclophosphamide therapy in refractory idiopathic inflammatory myopathy. J Rheumatol 1989;16:1225–1228.
182. Fries JF, Sharp GC, McDevitt HO, et al. Cyclophosphamide therapy in systemic lupus erythematosus and polymyositis. Arthritis Rheum 1973;16:154–162.
183. Talesni KE, Lagomarsino E, Gayan A, et al. Chronic hemorrhagic cystitis induced by cyclophosphamide in dermatomyositis refractory to corticosteroid therapy. Rev Child Pediatr 1991;62:121–124.
184. Sinoway PA, Callen JP. Chlorambucil: an effective corticosteroid-sparing agent for patients with recalcitrant dermatomyositis. Arthritis Rheum 1993;36:319–324.
185. Wallace DJ, Metzger AL, White KK. Combination immunosuppressive treatment of steroid-resistant dermatomyositis/polymyositis. Arthritis Rheum 1985;28:590–592.
186. Borleffs JC. Cyclosporine as monotherapy for polymyositis? Transplant Proc 1988;20:333–334.
187. Correia O, Polonia J, Nunes JP, et al. Severe acute form of adult dermatomyositis treated with cyclosporine. Int J Dermatol 1992;31:517–519.
188. Girardin E, Drayer JM, Paunier L. Cyclosporine for juvenile dermatomyositis [letter]. J Pediatr 1988;112:165–166.
189. Goei HS, Jacobs P, Hoeben H. Cyclosporine in the treatment of intractable polymyositis [letter]. Arthritis Rheum 1985;28:1436–1437.
190. Heckmatt J, Hasson N, Saunders C, et al. Cyclosporine in juvenile dermatomyositis. Lancet 1989;1:1063–1066.
191. Jones DW, Snaith ML, Isenberg DA. Cyclosporine treatment for intractable polymyositis [letter]. Arthritis Rheum 1987;30:959–960.
192. Jongen PJH, Joosten EMG, Berden JHM, et al. Cyclosporine therapy in chronic slowly progressive polymyositis. Transplant Proc 1988;20(suppl 4):335–339.
193. Lueck CJ, Trend P, Swash M. Cyclosporine in the management of polymyositis and dermatomyositis. J Neurol Neurosurg Psychiatry 1991;54:1007–1008.
194. Pistoia V, Buoncompagni A, Scribanis R, et al. Cyclosporin A in the treatment of juvenile chronic arthritis and childhood polymyositis-dermatomyositis: results of a preliminary study. Clin Exp Rheumatol 1993;11:203–208.
195. Rawlings DJ, Richardson L, Szer IS, et al. Cyclosporine is safe and effective in refractory JRA and JDMS: results of an open trial [abstract]. Arthritis Rheum 1992;35:S188.
196. Reinert P, Hamberger C, Rahimy MC, et al. Value of cyclosporine A in dermatomyositis as a child. Arch Fr Pediatr 1988;45:201–203.
197. Oddis CV, Caroll P, Abu-Elmagd K, et al. FK506 in the treatment of polymyositis [abstract]. Arthritis Rheum 1994;37(suppl 6):R19.
198. Gelfand EW. The use of intravenous immune globulin in collagen vascular disorders: a potential new modality of therapy. J Allergy Clin Immunol 1989;84:613–616.
199. Thornton CA, Griggs RC. Plasma exchange and intravenous immunoglobulin treatment of neuromuscular disease. Ann Neurol 1994;35:260–268.
200. Barron KS, Sher MR, Silverman ED. Intravenous immunoglobulin therapy: magic or black magic. J Rheumatol 1992;33(suppl):94–97.
201. Bodemer C, Teillac D, LeBurgeois M, et al. Efficacy of intravenous globulins in sclerodermatomyositis. Br J Dermatol 1990;123:545–546.
202. Cherin P, Herson S, Wechsler B, et al. Efficacy of intravenous globulin therapy in chronic refractory polymyositis and dermatomyositis: an open study with 20 adult patients. Am J Med 1991;91:162–168.

203. Hanslik T, Jaccard A, Guillon JM, et al. Polymyositis and chronic graft-versus-host disease: efficacy of intravenous gammaglobulin. J Am Acad Dermatol 1993;28:492–493.
204. Jann S, Beretta S, Moggio M, et al. High-dose intravenous immunoglobulin in polymyositis resistant to treatment. J Neurol Neurosurg Psychiatry 1992;55:60–62.
205. Lang BA, Laxer RM, Murphy G, et al. Treatment of dermatomyositis with intravenous immunoglobulin. Am J Med 1991;91:169–172.
206. Roifman CM, Schaffer FM, Wachsmuth SE, et al. Reversal of chronic polymyositis following intravenous immune serum globulin therapy. JAMA 1987;258:513–515.
207. Stoll T, Michel BA, Neidhart M, et al. Polymyositis: disease course and therapy with intravenously administered immunoglobulins. Scheiz Med Wochenschr 1992;122:1458–1465.
208. Soueidan SA, Dalakas MC. Treatment of inclusion body myositis with high-dose intravenous immunoglobulin. Neurology 1993;43:876–879.
209. Anderson L, Ziter FA. Plasmapheresis via central catheter in dermatomyositis: a new method for selected pediatric patients. J Pediatr 1981;98:240–241.
210. Brewer EJ, Giannini EH, Rossen RD, et al. Plasma exchange therapy of a childhood onset dermatomyositis patient. Arthritis Rheum 1980;23:509–513.
211. Dau PC. Plasmapheresis in idiopathic inflammatory myopathy. Arch Neurol 1981;38:544–552.
212. Dau PC. Leukocytapheresis in inclusion body myositis. J Clin Apheresis 1987;3:167.
213. Herson S, Cherin P, Coutellier A. The association of plasma exchange synchronized with intravenous gamma globulin therapy in severe intractable polymyositis [letter]. J Rheumatol 1992;19:828–829.
214. Miller FW, Leitman SF, Cronin ME, et al. Controlled trial of plasma exchange and leukopheresis in polymyositis and dermatomyositis. N Engl J Med 1992;326:1380–1384.
215. Engel WK, Lichter AS, Galdi AP. Polymyositis: remarkable response to total body irradiation [letter]. Lancet 1981;1:658.
216. Hubbard WN, Walport MJ, Halnan KE, et al. Remission from polymyositis after total body irradiation. BMJ 1982;284:1915–1916.
217. Kelly JJ, Madoc-Jones H, Adelman LS, et al. Response to total body irradiation in dermatomyositis. Muscle Nerve 1988;11:120–123.
218. Morgan SH, Bernstein RM, Coppen J. Total body irradiation and the course of polymyositis. Arthritis Rheum 1985;28:831–835.
219. Cherin P, Herson S, Coutellier A, et al. Failure of total body irradiation in polymyositis: report of three cases. Br J Rheumatol 1992;31:282–283.
220. Kelly JJ, Madoc-Jones H, Adelman LS, et al. Total body irradiation not effective in inclusion body myositis. Neurology 1986;36:1264–1266.
221. Lane RJM, Hudgson P. Thymectomy in polymyositis [letter]. Lancet 1984;1:626.
222. Cumming WJK. Thymectomy in refractory dermatomyositis [letter]. Muscle Nerve 1989;12:424.
223. Woo TY, Callen JP, Voorhees JJ, et al. Cutaneous lesions of dermatomyositis are improved with hydroxychloroquine. J Am Acad Dermatol 1984;10:592–600.
224. Bertorini TE, Sebes JI, Genaro MA, et al. Diltiazem in the treatment of calcinosis in juvenile dermatomyositis [abstract]. Neurology 1998;50:A204–A205.
225. Olizeri MB, Palermo R, Mautalen C, Hübscher O. Regression of calcinosis during diltiazem treatment in juvenile dermatomyositis. J Rheumatol 1996;23:2152–2155.

11
Muscle Infection:
Viral, Parasitic, Bacterial, and Spirochetal

Noshir H. Wadia and Sarosh M. Katrak

Inflammatory disorders of muscle compose the largest group of acquired myopathies, but those that are due to infection form only a small part of that group. The majority of such infections occurs in populations of developing and tropical countries through parasitic infestations. Viral myositis is even less common, appearing universally in sporadic or epidemic form. Among these, muscle involvement is most evident with cysticercus cellulose, trichinella spiralis, and human immunodeficiency virus (HIV) (Table 11.1).

VIRAL MYOSITIS

Numerous viruses have been implicated, but only a few produce significant inflammatory myopathies.

Human Immunodeficiency Virus–Associated Myositis

Inflammatory myopathies are more common in HIV-infected patients than in the general population [1]. However, some studies have defined myopathy only on the basis of myalgia and elevated creatine kinase (CK), showing a higher incidence than other studies with more objective criteria of myopathy [2]. This is because the HIV-associated myopathies are not as well characterized as the peripheral neuropathies, and there is a wide spectrum of involvement, ranging from asymptomatic elevation of CK, to mild generalized fatigue, to severe proximal limb-girdle weakness. Berman et al. [1] found muscle involvement in 18% of 101 patients, of whom 10 had myalgia, six muscle atrophy, and two polymyositis (PM). The spectrum of muscle involvement includes (1) a PM-like myopathy with typical clinical/electromyographic (EMG) features but varying features on muscle biopsy, (2) zidovudine (AZT)-induced myopathy, (3) an ill-

Table 11.1   Clinical features of viral, parasitic, and bacterial infections of muscles

	Myalgia	Weakness	Focal swelling	Pseudo-hypertrophy	Cardiac	Rhabdomyolysis	Rash	Subcutaneous nodules	Central nervous system/peripheral nervous system
Human immunodeficiency virus									
Polymyositislike	++	++	–	–	–	–	–	–	++
Muscle wasting syndrome	±	±	–	–	–	–	–	–	++
Human T-lymphotrophic virus-1	±	++	–	–	–	–	–	–	+++
Coxsackie	++	+	–	–	–	+	+	–	–
Influenza	++	+	–	–	–	+	–	–	–
Echovirus	+	+	–	–	–	–	+	–	–
Cysticercosis	±	±	++	+++	+	–	–	++	++
Hydatidosis	–	–	++	–	–	–	–	–	+
Sparganosis	+	–	++	–	±	–	–	–	+
Coenurosis	±	–	++	–	–	–	–	+	+
Trichinosis	+++	++	+	–	++	–	++	–	+
Toxocariasis	±	–	±	–	–	–	+	–	+
Toxoplasmosis	+	+	–	–	+	–	–	–	++
Sarcosporidiosis	+	+	+	–	+	–	–	–	±
Trypanosomiasis	+	+	–	–	++	–	+	–	++
Tropical pyomyositis	+	–	+	–	–	++	–	–	–
Lyme disease	++	±	+	–	+	–	++	–	+
Leptospirosis	++	–	–	–	+	+	–	–	+

– = absent; ± = occasionally present; + = mild involvement; ++ = moderate involvement; +++ = severe involvement.

defined variety of muscle wasting syndrome, and (4) an infective myopathy of bacterial and protozoal origin that is due to immunosuppression.

Polymyositislike Myopathy

Inflammatory myositis was first reported in 1983 [3], and Dalakas et al. [4] described two patients with PM as the initial manifestation of the disease. The clinical features are a progressive, symmetric, proximal limb-girdle weakness affecting the lower extremities most often; occasionally, the distal muscles are also affected. Dysphagia, respiratory weakness, and skin rash do not occur. Most patients report myalgia, which is a nonspecific symptom in HIV-infected patients. Sensations and autonomic function are normal, and deep tendon reflexes are preserved. Serum muscle enzymes, including CK, lactic dehydrogenase, and serum glutamic-oxaloacetic transaminase are usually elevated. The rise in CK levels may be as much as 100 times normal values (range, 300–18,000 U/liter). EMG shows a myopathic pattern. The clinical and electrophysiologic picture is indistinguishable from PM in HIV-negative patients.

In cases with severe weakness and EMG changes, the muscle biopsy is invariably abnormal, although histologic features may be variable. Some muscles have disseminated, degenerating, and necrotic muscle fibers with mononuclear infiltrates in the perimysium and perivascular spaces. Immunohistochemical staining against HIVp24 antigen has been positive within mononuclear cells [5, 6]. In some muscle biopsies, there may be atypical features. There is a paucity of inflammatory infiltrate in the muscles. This may be explained by the profound B- and T-cell abnormalities in these patients. Also, many type 1 muscle fibers contain electron-dense nemaline rod bodies and selective loss of thick Z-band myofibrillar filaments [7, 8]. The presence of these rod bodies helps to differentiate HIV-associated inflammatory myopathy from PM in HIV-negative patients.

The pathogenesis of this myopathy is poorly understood, as the variable histologic findings suggest different pathogenetic mechanisms. In situ hybridization techniques reveal evidence of HIV nucleic acid in the lymphoid cells of the inflammatory infiltrate but not in the muscle fiber or cultured myotubules [6, 9]. However, an autoimmune basis is quite likely, because patients do respond to corticosteroid therapy (see following paragraph on prednisolone). The problem is further complicated because, even in asymptomatic patients, there is elevation of serum CK levels, and muscle histology may show evidence of an inflammatory myopathy.

HIV-associated PM must be differentiated from AZT-induced myopathy (see Chapter 12). In pure AZT-induced myopathy, muscle weakness is not a prominent feature, although myalgia and fatigability may be remarkable. Simpson et al. [2] found significant myopathy in only 5 of 360 patients receiving AZT. Elevation of CK levels is common in these patients, and EMG may show myopathic changes. Muscle biopsy shows mitochondrial abnormalities with ragged red fibers in the majority [10], differentiating it from HIV-associated myositis. In patients in whom these abnormalities are not present, the differentiation may be difficult, and clinical judgment must be exercised.

HIV-associated myositis is often complicated by the concurrent use of AZT. Affected patients should be clinically evaluated before deciding on therapeutic options. If there is no objective clinical evidence of weakness, but routine laboratory data show elevated CK levels, then AZT should be continued. If myalgia is a prominent symptom or there is objective evidence of muscle weakness with elevated CK levels, AZT should be discontinued. Myalgia and CK levels decrease first, followed by a delayed improvement in strength. Some patients may tolerate reintroduction of smaller doses of AZT, although the use of another retroviral therapy is preferable. Others, including a few with ragged red fibers on muscle biopsy, continue to deteriorate after cessation of AZT and respond only to steroid therapy [10].

Prednisolone has also been used with considerable success in patients with PM-like and nemaline rods myopathy. Prednisolone is usually started in a dose of 60–80 mg per day and is continued until there is clinical improvement. The dose is then given on alternate days over several months and stopped if there is no relapse. Steroids should be used with caution in such immunocompromised patients, particularly in developing countries, for fear of flaring up other latent opportunistic infections. Other modes of therapy include plasma exchange [11] and high doses of intravenous immunoglobulins [12]. Such patients must also be evaluated for other treatable bacterial and protozoan myositis (see following section, Infective Myositis: Bacterial and Protozoal) and concurrent spinal cord and peripheral nerve disorders.

Muscle Wasting Syndrome

Severe muscle wasting with significant weight loss (more than 10% of baseline weight) with normal muscle strength or mild weakness has been described in HIV-infected patients as the ill-defined *muscle wasting syndrome* [13, 14]. The specific cause of the cachexia is not known, but a generalized systemic infection, lack of ambulation, and poor nutrition may be contributory. Malabsorption was ruled out in one study [14]. Surprisingly, some of these patients have responded to corticosteroid therapy [14], stressing the importance of a specific diagnosis of this myopathy. Oxandrolone, an oral anabolic steroid, at a dose of 5 or 15 mg per day, increased weight and general well-being [15].

Infective Myositis: Bacterial and Protozoal

Because of their immunosuppressed state, HIV-infected individuals are particularly prone to focal muscle infection, especially after minor trauma or at intramuscular injection sites. In Africa, staphylococcal pyomyositis is a relatively common complication of HIV infection (see the following section, Bacterial Infections: Tropical Pyomyositis) [16] and has also been reported from other centers [17, 18]. Rare cases of inflammatory myositis that are due to *Mycobacterium tuberculosis,* microsporidian *Pleistophora*, and a newly described species, *Trachipleistophora hominis,* have been reported in patients with acquired immunodeficiency syndrome (AIDS) [19–23].

Human T-Lymphotrophic Virus-1–Associated Myositis

Although human T-lymphotrophic virus (HTLV)-1 retrovirus has been implicated in tropical spastic paraparesis or HTLV-1–associated myelopathy, peripheral neuropathy and myositis are more common than initially suspected. In a retrospective analysis of 276 cases from Martinique [24], eight patients had myositis, and a further 20 patients had a combination of peripheral neuropathy and myositis. By 1996, more than 60 cases of HTLV-1–associated myositis were reported [24–26].

The clinical picture is that of predominant proximal hip-girdle weakness, but involvement of distal muscles and proximal upper limbs is also known [25]. Occasionally, sensory signs and electrophysiologic abnormalities [25, 26] are detected that are due to concurrent peripheral neuropathy. Serum CK levels may be slightly elevated. The muscle biopsy may show evidence of PM or a noninflammatory myopathy [25–27] and may be associated with fiber type I atrophy. When muscle involvement is prominent, the clinical picture is that of dermatomyositis/polymyositis (DM/PM). However, the associated spastic gait and bladder and minor sensory involvement help to differentiate it from the classic DM/PM. The diagnosis is established by serologic studies and polymerase chain reaction (PCR) analysis of the muscle biopsy for proviral sequences.

In high HTLV-1–endemic areas of the world, HTLV-1 and PM have been clearly linked. This combination occurs in patients who have received infected blood transfusions and also in those coinfected with HIV type 1 retrovirus [28]. Although HTLV-1–like particles have never been identified in biopsied muscles, proviral sequences were found by PCR and immunohistochemistry [25, 27, 28]. Although PCR does not permit exact localization of these proviral sequences in the muscle fiber itself, these results support a possible viral etiopathogenesis.

Coxsackie Virus

Coxsackie virus mainly produces an acute myalgic syndrome and, uncommonly, a myositis with rhabdomyolysis and myoglobinuria [29].

In 1985–1986, there was an epidemic of a peculiar acute inflammatory myopathy in the Indian states of Maharashtra, Karnataka, and Gujarat. We are aware of a large number of individuals affected, including some under our care; apart from one published report [30], two others were unpublished communications [31, 32]. In these three studies, a total of 91 cases were well investigated. Young adult men were most affected. The onset was acute, with fever, myalgia, muscle weakness, and an erythematous macular rash. Generalized nonpitting swelling of the limbs, seen in the majority of these patients, was a prominent feature of this myositis. There was a high incidence of bulbar and respiratory involvement (50%) [30]. Myoglobinuria was not seen in any of these patients. Another peculiarity was the presence of subclinical sensorimotor neuropathy in 40–70% of patients [30–32]. Electron microscopy failed to show any viral inclusions in the muscle biopsies, but antiviral antibody titers in a few patients suggested Coxsackie B infection [30].

The majority of patients responded dramatically to corticosteroid therapy with reduction in the generalized swelling and improvement in muscle strength. The mortality rate varied from 10% to 38% and was mainly due to respiratory arrest and cardiac failure.

Influenza Virus

Influenza virus produces a benign myopathy and a generalized myopathy with rhabdomyolysis.

Benign Influenza Myopathy

An acute and transient but painful myopathy of the lower limbs may occur during the convalescence phase from influenza. Young children, particularly boys, are usually affected [33]. There is an acute onset of pain in the calf muscles, sometimes affecting other leg and thigh muscles, associated with swelling and tenderness. Weakness is not a prominent feature. The disorder is self-limiting, and recovery is usually rapid, the patients being ambulant in 7–10 days.

CK levels are usually elevated and at times approach 60 times normal values [34, 35]. EMG may show myopathic motor unit potentials [36]. Most of the cases of severe leg pain are due to influenza B, but influenza A, parainfluenza, mumps, measles viruses, and mycoplasma have all been implicated [35, 37]. Viral cultures of muscle have been negative except in one, in which the influenza B virus was isolated in a case of PM [38].

The precise etiopathogenesis of influenza myopathy is not well known. It is uncertain whether a direct infection by the virus or an immune-mediated reaction causes the myopathy in a minority of patients.

Generalized Myopathy with Rhabdomyolysis

In contrast to the restricted muscle involvement in benign influenza myopathy, a generalized myopathy with rhabdomyolysis and myoglobinuria may develop in the course of influenza [39, 40]. This is associated with transient renal insufficiency in approximately 50% of cases. Myalgia, muscle weakness, and dark urine may occur at the onset of the febrile illness or during the convalescent stage. Josselson et al. [41] reviewed 15 cases in adults, of which seven were due to influenza A infection and the others to Coxsackie, echovirus, and parainfluenza.

Echovirus

Patients with echovirus infection have myalgias but do not develop a myopathy unless they are immunocompromised. Several patients with X-linked agamma-globulinemia have developed a syndrome resembling DM [41–43]. In these patients, CK levels were markedly elevated, EMG showed myopathic potentials, and muscle biopsy revealed muscle fiber degeneration with perivascular lympho-cytic infiltration. One patient [42] was successfully treated with infusions of intravenous immunoglobulins.

Adenovirus

Very few cases of acute myositis associated with human adenovirus 21 have been documented [44].

PARASITIC INFECTIONS

Among the host of parasites that inhabit and invade the human body, three main groups infect muscles: cestodes, nematodes, and protozoa. The symptoms of myositis result from the presence and number of parasites, the inflammatory response, and the host's immune status. Often, the muscle involvement may remain silent.

Cestode Infection

Tapeworm infestation is endemic in many countries, and quite often it is asymptomatic. The symptoms are caused by larvae, which spread through the bloodstream to the central nervous system and, to a lesser extent, to the muscles, causing cysticercosis, hydatidosis, sparganosis, and coenurosis.

Cysticercosis

Once universal, this disease is now largely restricted to the non-Islamic tropical and developing countries. It affects 50 million people and causes 50,000 deaths annually. However, cases have been reported from certain parts of the United States among Hispanic immigrants and travelers from endemic areas [45–47].

The adult tapeworm, *Taenia solium,* is made up of several hundred segments (*proglottids*). Each proglottid contains a vast number of viable ova, which are discharged in the feces when it disintegrates. These are a potent source of infection for both humans and free-range pigs. In deprived rural parts of the world and urban slums, human excreta are perforce lodged in open fields and spaces. The free-range pigs swallow the ova with the excreta and become the natural intermediate host. Humans are an accidental intermediate host, infected through fecal contamination of water or soil or by consuming unwashed raw vegetables grown in these endemic areas. More important, spread of ova occurs through unclean hands or migrant domestic staff's and food handlers' harboring the taenia ova. This is the cause of the upsurge of cysticercosis in advanced countries like the United States [45–47] and among urban vegetarians in India [48]. Rarely, autoinfection can occur in a person carrying the tapeworm through unwashed hands or regurgitation of the proglottids or ova into the stomach by reverse peristalsis.

The swallowed ova in both humans and pigs convert into oncospheres (the immature larvae), penetrate the gut, enter the bloodstream, and lodge principally in the brain, muscles, subcuticular tissues, and eyes as mature larvae. The life cycle is completed when humans eat raw or undercooked infected (measly) pork.

The main disease manifestations are cerebral and vary depending on the number, type, location, and evolution of the parasite. The muscle invasion is mostly asymptomatic. The disease can present with seizures or symptoms and signs of raised intracranial pressure, mental disorder, chronic meningitis, and focal compression, or varying combinations of the five.

Involvement of the muscles has been recognized since the disease was first described. In early accounts it was considered rare, but MacArthur [49] and Morrison [50] described calcification in dying and dead cysticerci in the muscles of British soldiers stationed in India who suffered from epilepsy. The lodging of cysticerci in the muscles, especially in small numbers, is largely asymptomatic. Great stress should be laid on palpation of muscles, subcuticular tissues, and tongue in any person suspected to be suffering from cysticercosis, regardless of whether he or she reports subcutaneous swellings. Such palpable swellings are usually oval, vary in size, lie between muscle fibers, and appear singly or in crops.

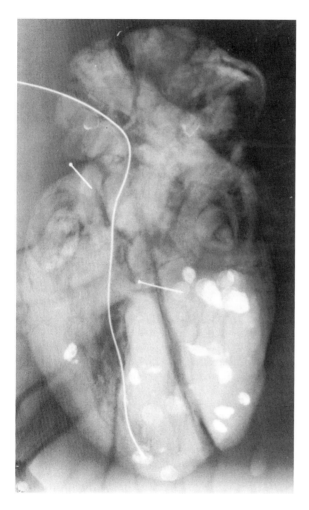

Figure 11.1   Radiograph of the autopsy specimen of the heart of a patient with cysticercosis. Note the calcified cysticerci and the pacemaker.

Myalgia is reported during the initial acute phase of parasitemia and invasion of muscles by the oncospheres. In children and some adults, there may be associated fever, headache, vomiting, and even seizures [49, 51]. There are occasions in which a single cysticercus enlarges to a great size, appearing as a swelling in a muscle that can be mistaken for a tumor [49, 52]. Cardiac muscle may be affected, producing varying electrocardiographic changes and arrhythmias, and very rarely requiring a pacemaker (Figure 11.1).

Pseudohypertrophy of Muscles (Disseminated Cysticercosis)

Disseminated cysticercosis is a dramatic but rare presentation of cysticercosis that has not yet found its proper place, even in the recent reviews and classifications

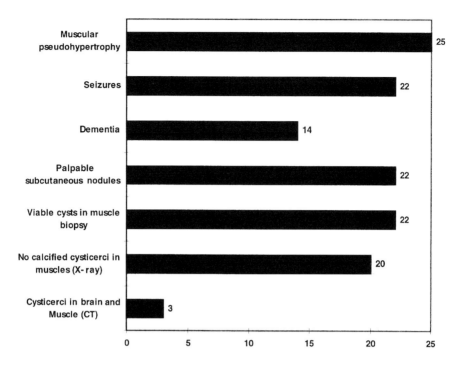

Figure 11.2   Data of 25 patients with disseminated cysticercosis. (CT = computed tomography.) (Data compiled from references 56–69, 72–74, and 76.)

of the disease [53–56]. Gang-Zhi et al. [57] found it in only 9 of 1,400 Chinese patients (0.6%). This pseudohypertrophy results from the dissemination of thousands of living cysticerci in the brain and throughout the musculature. It causes massive enlargement of muscles.

Krishnaswami [58] reported the first case in 1912 from Burma in a South Indian who presented with fatigue and myalgia on exertion, although the muscles were not appreciably enlarged. Trichinellosis was diagnosed, but on biopsy and autopsy, innumerable cysticerci were found in the skeletal muscles and other organs. Further reports followed from British Army officers in India [59–61]. The enlargement was so remarkable that these accounts vividly describe pseudohypertrophy as "Sandow-type" [59] swelling of muscles and describe the person as a "professional wrestler" [60] or "a veritable Hercules" [61]. Forty-eight similar cases have been mentioned in the world literature [57, 62–79]. Interestingly, except for a solitary case from Brazil [65], there are no other reports from South and Central America, where cysticercosis is rampant. Wadia et al. [79, 80] were able to analyze the clinical features in 25 such cases in which sufficient details were available—21 from India, three from China, and one from Brazil (Figure 11.2). Twenty-seven cases from China could not be analyzed for want of sufficient details [57, 73, 74, 77, 78].

The clinical features are fairly consistent and usually involve young adults. The duration of the illness varies from 1 to 5 years. The characteristic pseudohypertrophy is first noticed in the calves and thighs. Muscles of the pelvic and shoulder girdle can be equally prominent. Rarely, a striking hypertrophy of the nuchal and masseter muscles has been reported [64]. The enlargement of muscles usually takes weeks or months but has occurred in 2–3 weeks. Muscle strength does not increase in proportion to muscle size; hence the term *pseudohypertrophy*. In fact, in a few patients, mild weakness—especially of the limb-girdle muscles—was observed. Fatigue on exertion is an occasional report. Pain and tenderness are not prominent features.

Focal and generalized seizures frequently occur and may precede the pseudohypertrophy. Mild to severe cognitive dysfunction amounting to dementia is present in a little more than one-half of the analyzed cases. Signs of raised intracranial pressure or focal compression are uncommon.

Clinical diagnosis is easy, as no other human disease manifests with pseudohypertrophy of muscles without weakness and with seizures and dementia. The finding of visible and palpable nodules would clinch the diagnosis. There should be no diagnostic difficulty, even in those patients in whom pseudohypertrophy is the lone manifestation. The rapid muscular enlargement with no weakness or atrophy, the age of the patient, and the absence of family history distinguishes this condition from muscular dystrophy, idiopathic PM, primary amyloidosis, and hypothyroidism with dementia, in which pseudohypertrophy may also be seen. The absence of myalgia and weakness would exclude trichinosis.

The diagnosis can be confirmed by a biopsy of a subcutaneous nodule or the hypertrophied muscle, plain radiographs of the limbs, and computed tomography (CT) or magnetic resonance imaging (MRI) of the muscles and brain. In all but 3 of the reported 25 cases, subcutaneous nodules revealed the *cysticercus*. Disseminated cysticercosis being an unusual disease, muscle biopsy was performed in 22 patients. In these patients, larval cysts were seen to pour out like a bunch of grapes as soon as the muscle was incised (Color Plate 11). In the majority of cases, these were living cysticerci [79], although Jolly and Pallis [66] believed, on rather tenuous grounds, that there was "early larval death." Pericystic inflammatory reaction was uncommon. In only one case was myositis seen at some distance from the cyst [70].

Calcified cysticerci were not seen on radiographs of the soft tissue in any of the patients with pseudohypertrophy. However, fine mottling was noticed by McGill [61], and Jolly and Pallis [66] saw a few spotty opacities of less than 2 mm in diameter, which they considered to be scolices. The CT scan of limb muscles imaged the living cysticerci as well-defined, low-attenuation-density cysts with high-attenuation-density nubbins within them, indicating the scolices. No calcification or postcontrast pericystic inflammatory reaction was seen. The appearance of the cysticerci within the muscles was aptly described as "honeycomb" or "leopard spots" by Wadia et al. [79], who first described them (Figure 11.3A). The cysts were closely packed, numbering 3–4/cm^2. Similar numbers were seen on CT scan of the brain, but here the scolices were more prominent than the cysts. MRI of such patients showed even more vividly the cysticerci in the T2-weighted images (Figure 11.3B).

The diagnostic immunologic tests have never been performed in this entity, but considering the large number of cysticerci, the tests should be strongly positive. The creatine phosphokinase was not raised in these patients, and EMG results were largely normal in all those in whom EMG was performed.

The pathogenesis of this form of cysticercosis is not entirely clear, and some questions remain unanswered. No good explanation has been offered nor any

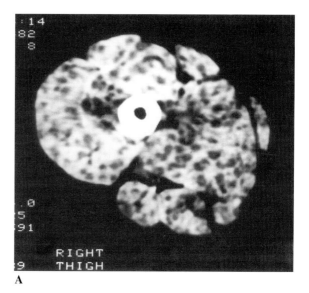

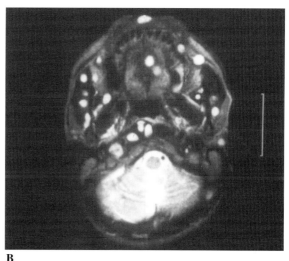

Figure 11.3 Computed tomography (CT) and magnetic resonance imaging (MRI) in disseminated cysticercosis. (**A**) CT scan of the thigh muscle. Note the large number of cysts. (**B**) T2-weighted MRI of the base of the skull. Note the hyperintense cysts in the soft tissue.

immunosuppressive mechanism shown to explain the dissemination of thousands of cysticerci all over the body in this as opposed to other forms of cysticercosis.

MacArthur [49] maintained that in the early stages of larval death, the cyst enlarges and becomes tense. Based on this observation, Jolly and Pallis [66] believed that the enlargement of muscles was due to the large numbers of cysticerci in "early larval death." Yet they did not demonstrate any dying cysticerci nor any inflammatory reaction in the muscles around the tense cysts of their patients. On the other hand, Wadia et al. [79] maintained that the muscles enlarged simply because of the space-occupying effect of a large number of viable cysticerci, demonstrated histologically in 22 of 25 of the reported cases (see Figure 11.2).

They also demonstrated live cysts with intact scolices without contrast enhancement on CT imaging of muscle and brain.

Finally, although mild pericystic inflammation has been shown in a few cases, significant primary inflammatory myositis was demonstrated only in the solitary case of Sawhney et al. [70]. Hence the terms *myositis* and *pseudohypertrophy*, although used conventionally, are in effect misnomers, and stress should be laid on the massive dissemination of living cysticerci in the pathogenesis of this condition.

Treatment is given essentially for the cerebral manifestation, and cysticidal drugs, praziquantel, and albendazole have been extensively prescribed. However, Wadia et al. [79, 80] have cautioned against their use, because rapid destruction of a large number of cysticerci is followed not only by a systemic reaction but also by an exaggerated inflammatory edema that can cause life-threatening cerebral symptoms. Indeed, in one of their patients, swelling of the limb and ocular muscles produced cyanosis of the feet bordering on gangrene and severe chemosis and proptosis.

Hydatidosis

Infection with hydatidosis is not uncommon in humans in countries like Australia, New Zealand, Argentina, and Chile, and in several other regions of the world where livestock is raised in association with dogs. Two forms of this tapeworm exist: *Echinococcus granulosus* and *Echinococcus multilocularis*. The larva in the cystic form is called the *hydatid cyst* and is responsible for the multiorgan disease hydatidosis.

The infection mostly spreads to humans through close contact with dogs that harbor the tapeworm, but in certain regions, the fox, wolf, or moose may act as the definitive host. The ova discharged in the feces are ingested by a variety of intermediate hosts, but the sheep is the most common in the domestic setting. Humans are accidental intermediate hosts when they ingest ova through food and water contaminated with dog feces. The external covering of the ova is digested in the duodenum, liberating hooked embryos—the oncospheres—which penetrate the intestinal wall, enter the bloodstream, and get lodged in various organs, principally the liver and lungs. Muscles are the third common site, where the embryo grows and is transformed into the hydatid cyst. The disease is endemic, because the cycle of infection continues when a dog eats infected meat.

The hydatid cyst presents as a muscle mass. It is usually a slow-growing, deep, lobular, painless mass of varying size but firm consistency [81]. Paravertebral and thigh muscles are the most frequent sites. There is no weakness or tenderness unless secondary infection occurs, when it presents as an abscess.

Diagnosis is made by serologic tests for echinococcosis. Cysts can be demonstrated by routine radiographs, especially when calcified. CT or ultrasonography may identify specific hydatid features [82]. A cure is effected by surgical excision.

Sparganosis

Sparganosis is the term applied to a rare infection caused by the migrating plerocercoid larvae—*sparganum*—of the parasite *Spirometra mansonoides* (or

Spirometra mansoni). Most cases of sparganosis have been reported from Japan, China, Korea, Vietnam, and other Southeast Asian countries [83], but rare cases have been documented from the United States [84] and India [85] (SMK, personal experience). Eggs of the worm excreted in the feces of the final carnivore host—dogs, cats, foxes—grow to coracidia in freshwater and are eaten by *Cyclops*, the first intermediate host, which in turn is eaten by the second intermediate host (frogs, snakes, freshwater fish, and, rarely, pigs), in which the larva burrows through the intestinal wall and lodges in the subdermal tissues and muscles and grows into plerocercoids—the spargana. When the second intermediate host is eaten by the final host, the life cycle is completed. Humans are usually infected by drinking contaminated water or eating uncooked flesh of frogs, snakes, fish, or, rarely, pork. In Thailand and Vietnam, raw flesh of frogs or snakes has been used as a poultice for infected eyes and accounts for cases of ocular sparganosis.

Humans are usually infected by the larvae and, very rarely, by the adult worm [86]. Sparganosis commonly involves the subcutaneous tissue and muscles; occasionally the kidneys, heart, and eyes; and, rarely, the central nervous system. The common presentation is that of a fluctuant subcutaneous or superficial intramuscular lump. Occasionally, the lump is tender with signs of inflammation. An unusual but characteristic feature is a downward migration of this lump. Nakamura et al. [87] have reported a rare proliferative form of sparganosis, in which the larval cestode of an unknown species proliferated in various organs of the body. Innumerable egglike 3-mm parasites were detected in the gluteal muscles and pelvic bones of the patient. Morphologic features were those of an ill-differentiated plerocercoid larvae, and serologic data confirmed it to be of the sparganum family. The therapy usually involves excision of this lump with histologic confirmation.

Coenurosis

Coenurosis, a rare infection of humans, is caused by the larval stage of dog tapeworm, *Taenia multiceps* or *Taenia serialis*. In parts of Africa, domestic dogs or foxes and jackals are infested with another species, the *Multiceps braunii*. As with cysticercosis, involvement of the central nervous system, the subcutaneous tissue, and muscles is most common. The coenuri are globular cysts containing several scolices. The cysts vary in size and produce palpable, tender, focal swellings of muscles, predominantly in the trunk and abdominal wall. Usually, there is no muscle weakness, and generalized myalgia is rare. Anthelmintic drugs are not effective. A positive diagnosis is only made after surgical excision, which is the treatment of choice.

Nematode Infections

Trichinosis

Trichinella spiralis, a nematode, produces an inflammatory myopathy in humans. Human infection is usually acquired by eating uncooked or undercooked pork, but it can also occur after the ingestion of bear, horse, wild boar, or walrus meat infected with encysted larvae. It has a worldwide distribution and is closely related to cultural and dietary habits. The incidence is high in Thailand, China, Japan, and Latin and South America [88, 89]. Outbreaks are still recognized in the United States, largely among immigrants or members of ethnic refugee groups who prefer raw or under-cooked pork [88]. Cases after travel to Mexico or Southeast Asian countries have also been reported [90]. Trichinosis has not yet been reported from Australia [91], and the incidence is low in Europe because of mandatory inspection of pork.

After ingestion of infected meat, the cyst is digested, and the larvae are released. These larvae lodge in the small intestines and burrow into the epithelial lining, producing the enteric phase of the illness seen in approximately one-third of cases. In 2–3 days, the larvae become sexually mature after four moults. The viviparous female begins to deposit newly formed larvae in another 4–5 days. These second-generation larvae migrate into the bloodstream and invade several organs, producing the acute systemic phase, termed *trichinellotic syndrome.*

The enteric phase is in the first 2 weeks after ingestion of infected meat. The predominant symptom is diarrhea, but abdominal pain and vomiting may also occur. The acute systemic phase occurs after a week to 10 days and may last for as long as 2 months. In this phase, some patients develop myositis, fever, myalgia, muscle swelling with focal or generalized tenderness, and muscular weakness. Periorbital and facial edema, a maculopapular rash, retinal or subconjunctival hemorrhages, and subungual splinter hemorrhages may occur, representing an allergic inflammatory reaction. The course may vary, and several organs may be involved. Lung involvement may be heralded by hemoptysis and pulmonary infiltrates. Cardiovascular features include tachycardia, arrhythmia, severe congestive heart failure, and nonspecific electrocardiographic changes. Central nervous system involvement occurs in 10–24% of symptomatic cases [92]. Symptoms and signs suggestive of encephalitis, with or without focal signs, have also been observed. The mortality is 5–10% and usually occurs in severe cases with congestive heart failure or encephalitis [92].

Severe leukocytosis and eosinophilia are seen in the acute phase of the illness. With myositis, the CK levels rise commensurate with the severity of the involvement. EMG shows both myopathic changes and fibrillatory potentials, as in PM. Specific serum antibodies are detected by complement fixation, enzyme-linked immunosorbent assay (ELISA), and the bentonite flocculation tests. These tests may be negative in the first 2 weeks after ingestion but subsequently become positive. A rising titer is particularly helpful.

From the third week on, the muscle biopsy is highly diagnostic. It should be performed in clinically affected muscles. The muscle biopsy shows multiple small foci of inflammatory cells in the endomysium and perivascular regions. Serial sections show *Trichinella* larvae in several muscle fibers (Color Plate 12). At times, the inflammatory reaction may be seen at a distance from the encysted larvae, raising the possibility of an immune-mediated inflammatory myopathy [92]. The diagnosis is not difficult in areas in which trichinosis is endemic. However, in sporadic cases, PM remains a close differential diagnosis. A relatively short history of myositis (3 months or less) with a severe eosinophilia should raise the possibility of trichinosis, even if the muscle biopsy shows nonspecific changes of inflammation.

Patients with active myositis show improvement with prednisolone in doses of 30–80 mg per day, depending on the severity. Therapeutic action against the encysted larvae is controversial. Thiabendazole, albendazole (400 mg, three times daily for 2 weeks), and mebendazole are usually administered and act against the adult worm. Most patients respond to therapy. Patients with cardiac failure or central nervous system involvement, or those who are immunocompromised, may succumb to the illness.

Toxocariasis

Toxocariasis is a common form of visceral larva migrans caused by the larvae of the canine ascarid *Toxocara canis* and, less commonly, the feline ascarid *Toxocara cati*. Human toxocariasis occurs when ova from the soil, contaminated with dog and cat feces, are swallowed by children. The ova hatch in the intestines and liberate the larvae. The larvae enter the circulation and usually lodge in the liver, but they sometimes go to the lungs, brain, eyes, and muscles. The larvae may remain actively motile in these tissues, provoking intense local eosinophilic granulomatous responses. The degree of clinical illness depends on the number of larvae, tissue distribution, and host's immunity. Mild infections are asymptomatic and only show eosinophilia. Systemic features may include fever, malaise, anorexia, weight loss, cough, wheezing, and rash. Lesions in muscles are less numerous, and muscle pain is an occasional feature [93]. The diagnosis is made by the evident eosinophilia with leukocytosis and ELISA for toxocaral antibodies. The vast majority of *Toxocara* infections are mild and self-limiting. Anthelmintics do not alter the course of the disease. Preventive measures with more hygienic habits in schoolchildren are more effective.

Protozoal Infections

Toxoplasmosis

Toxoplasma is a worldwide infection of many mammals, birds, and humans. The intracellular protozoon parasite has a three-stage life cycle: cyst, tachyzoite, and oocyst. Primary infection can occur by handling cat feces or eating undercooked meat, whereas congenital infection occurs by transplacental transfer. With an acute infection, there is a widespread distribution of tachyzoites, particularly in the lymph nodes, muscles, myocardium, and brain. In the immunocompetent host, most infections are asymptomatic; however, apparent infection can range from a febrile illness with or without myalgia, to fever with generalized lymphadenopathy, to hepatitis, pneumonitis, myocarditis, or meningoencephalitis. Myalgia and generalized weakness occasionally dominate, but clinical features resembling PM are also seen [94].

Despite adequate immunity, a few cysts can remain dormant in the host's tissues and have the potential for reactivation. In HIV infection or during immunosuppression therapy, reactivation of an inapparent infection is based on serologic tests or histologic demonstration in tissues. Because immunoglobulin (Ig) G titers may be high after a primary infection, high or rising titers of IgM would be a better indicator of acute infection. *Toxoplasma* is rarely recovered from muscle in presumed *Toxoplasma* myositis. Thus, Remington and Cavanaugh [95] found positive serology in 50% of autopsy cases, but *Toxoplasma* could be isolated from muscle in only 6% of seropositive patients. Infrequently, *Toxoplasma* has been identified in diseased muscle in immunocompetent and immunosuppressed patients [96, 97]. Although these findings imply a direct role of the parasite in the inflammatory myopathy, immune mechanisms do play a part in the evolution of the myositis. On reviewing the association of *Toxoplasma gondii* in inflammatory myopathy, Matsubara et al. [98] found that in six of the 20 cases reviewed, histologic demonstration of *Toxoplasma* in diseased muscle was negative, but major histocompatibility complex class I and II antigens were observed in the inflammatory cells and blood vessels.

It follows that individual case reports from the literature are inconclusive to support the belief that toxoplasmosis causes an inflammatory myopathy in the majority of cases, even in immunosuppressed individuals. High or rising titers of IgM antibodies would be a better indicator of an acute infection than elevated IgG levels, because the latter would only indicate past infection. Therapy with pyrimethamine, sulfadiazine, or clindamycin may result in rapid clinical improvement.

Sarcosporidiosis

The protozoal parasite, class Sporozoasida, with the generic name *Sarcocystis*, is found in muscles of many mammals but is rarely reported in humans. Carnivorousness is important in the transmission of this infection, as these parasites have an obligatory life cycle involving two hosts. Sporocysts passed in the feces of one vertebrate host—the *predator* (dog, cheetah, lynx)—are ingested by the other host—the *prey* (e.g., rodents and birds). Asexual multiplication occurs in the lymphoid cells of the prey. When the prey is eaten, sexual reproduction occurs in the intestines of the predator, and sporocysts are passed in the feces. Ingestion of fecally derived sporocysts can lead to cysts in striated and cardiac muscles in humans. Human sarcosporidiosis is generally an asymptomatic disorder. Some patients report myalgia and muscle swelling. These sarcocysts die, producing microscopic calcification in muscles [81]. Electron microscopic features in a solitary case have been described by Pamphlett and O'Donoghue [99]. No specific therapy for sarcosporidiosis exists.

Trypanosomiasis

Trypanosomiasis, caused by the flagellated protozoa, *Trypanosoma*, appears in two distinct varieties: American and African. There is more involvement of the muscle in the American variety.

American Trypanosomiasis (Chagas Disease)

First described by Chagas, this disease is caused by the protozoan *Trypanosoma cruzi*. It essentially affects populations of South and Central America and Mexico, but it also prevails in the southern United States [100]. In the endemic areas, 25% of the population are considered at risk of infection, and approximately 5 million people suffer from the chronic effects of the disease. This creates immense health care problems.

The parasite differs from the African *Trypanosoma brucei* in that it does not multiply in the bloodstream. The disease is transmitted by the reduviid bugs (Hemiptera). It is not injected directly by the bite but enters through the broken skin from the feces of the bug deposited on the nearby skin.

After the initial parasitemia, the trypanosomes enter various tissues, principally the lymph glands, cardiac and voluntary muscles, and the central nervous system in a nonflagellated (amastigotes) form. There, they multiply and enlarge the cell, causing it to rupture and triggering an inflammatory reaction and focal damage. Amastigotes can be seen in clusters among inflammatory cells and within histiocytes and muscle fibers [101]. Various stages of degeneration and regeneration follow. Remarkable inflammatory changes are seen in small and medium-sized arteries. The infection then becomes chronic in some patients, leading to cardiomyopathy. Chronic myositis is much rarer, despite the myotropism of *T. cruzi* and the finding of autoantibodies against skeletal muscles and endothelial cells in patients with Chagas disease [96].

The disease has three stages. In the acute stage of parasitemia, the patient reports fever and general malaise. The glands, liver, and spleen may be enlarged, and the site of the bite may be marked by a focal inflammatory swelling (chagoma). In a proportion of patients, signs of acute myocarditis leading to cardiomyopathy are evident. Muscle weakness, fatigue, myalgia, and superficial erythema suggestive of DM are not infrequently seen. Potentially fatal encephalitis, which is more severe in infants, may occur at this stage.

In approximately 10 weeks, the disease manifestations settle, and many patients are free of any symptoms. This phase may last several years or indefinitely [102]. Serum tests for trypanosomiasis become positive.

The chronic phase emerges insidiously after years in 30% of the patients, with cardiac, digestive, and, less frequently, neurologic symptoms [103]. Chronic PM is uncommonly seen. Dilated cardiomyopathy is the most common and most recognized disorder in Chagas disease and presents with a variety of arrhythmias [102]. It is a common source of cerebral embolism in endemic areas [104].

Diagnosis is established by demonstration of *Trypanosoma* in the peripheral blood or elevated titers of anti–*T. cruzi* IgM antibodies [103]. Parasites can be found in the muscles or lymph nodes in the acute phase.

African Trypanosomiasis

Trypanosomiasis has been recognized in Africa as *sleeping sickness* for 200 years. The disease is caused by *T. brucei,* and the transmitting vector is the tsetse fly. It affects populations as far apart as sub-Saharan Africa, Northern Angola, and Mozambique.

The dominating illness is an acute meningoencephalitis that moves into a chronic phase. Although myocarditis is known to occur in the acute systemic phase, cardiac signs are not an essential feature of the disease [105]. An infiltration of perimysium and endomysium by lymphocytes, plasma cells, and histiocytes at autopsy is witness to the usually silent presence of myocarditis and PM [101].

BACTERIAL INFECTIONS: TROPICAL PYOMYOSITIS

Spontaneous infection of muscles by pyogenic bacteria is commonly referred to as *tropical pyomyositis*. It accounts for approximately 3% of surgical admissions in Africa. It used to be an unusual infection in temperate zones, but with the advent of AIDS, its incidence is rising [17]. The clinical features of pyomyositis are the same in the tropical and temperate zones.

The clinical features can be divided into two syndromes: a subacute disorder that is usually due to staphylococcal infection, and a hyperacute one that is due to β-hemolytic streptococci.

The subacute syndrome begins insidiously, with pain, tenderness, swelling, and induration of muscles. Several large muscle groups are involved in 30–40% of cases [18]. Over the next 7–10 days, generalized cramping occurs with an increase in tenderness and a low-grade fever. The involved muscles have a characteristic rubbery or woody feel. There is no fluctuation, because the involvement is deep within the large muscles. However, ultrasonography-guided needle aspiration at this stage yields pus. By the end of the second week, the patient is toxic, develops local lymphadenopathy, and has an eosinophilic leukocytosis and high erythrocyte sedimentation rate. Surprisingly, CK is normal, and rhabdomyolysis has been rarely reported [18, 106]. In 95% of cases, *Staphylococcus aureus* is the causative organism, but catalase-positive gram-negative bacteria have also been incriminated [17, 18].

The etiopathogenesis of pyomyositis is rather intriguing. First, skeletal muscles are resistant to pyogenic infection, and muscle abscesses are uncommon in septicemia. Second, blood cultures are rarely positive in tropical pyomyositis, and other organs are not involved in the pyogenic process. The pathogenesis of tropical pyomyositis is not clearly established, but there are predisposing factors. In Africa, boils and furuncles coupled with trauma are the main predisposing factors. These factors, associated with HIV infection, increase the mortality and morbidity rate [16, 107]. Other recognized predisposing factors are diabetes mellitus; intravenous drug use; malignancy following chemotherapy, neutropenia and thrombocytopenia; poor socioeconomic conditions; and, rarely, a preceding viral infection [18]. Widrow et al. [18] have even mentioned minor trauma and vigorous exercise as predisposing factors in their HIV-infected patients. All of these factors indicate either an underlying asymptomatic muscle abnormality or a defective host B-cell function.

Ultrasonography and CT scans are very useful in localizing the deep-seated abscesses. The therapy consists of ultrasonography-guided needle aspiration of the abscess with appropriate antibiotic therapy. In the late stages, surgical drainage with débridement may be required.

Hyperacute streptococcal myositis is a rare disorder that begins acutely with focal muscle pain, tenderness, and swelling without generalized weakness or other features of myopathy. The patient rapidly deteriorates over the next 2–3 days, with toxemia, acute renal failure, cardiac arrhythmia, and circulatory shock. This syndrome frequently does not respond to antibiotic therapy. The source of streptococcal infection is not evident in most cases. A preceding or simultaneous viral infection has been implicated in some cases [108, 109].

SPIROCHETAL INFECTIONS

Lyme Disease

Lyme disease is a tick-borne spirochetal illness that was first recognized in the town of Lyme, Connecticut, in 1970. Since then, it has been seen in other parts of the United States, Europe, Russia, China, Japan, and Australia. More than 50,000 cases have been reported in the United States since 1989. The causative agent is the spirochete *Borrelia burgdorferi,* which is transmitted by a variety of ixodid ticks. The spirochete is injected into the skin by the bite of the tick, producing a characteristic local expanding lesion called *erythema migrans* (stage 1). It then disseminates hematogenously to many organs of the body, causing a systemic disease (stage 2). Finally, after a long interval, the infection becomes persistent in untreated patients (stage 3).

The systemic illness occurs days or weeks after the erythema migrans. Skin rash, fever, severe malaise, myalgia, and arthralgia are predominant. At least 10% of patients develop complications [110]. In stage 2 of the illness, cardiac and voluntary muscles are affected. A variety of cardiac abnormalities has been reported in 8% of patients. Skeletal muscle involvement is even less common, although myalgia is a frequent symptom (43%) in the early stage of the disease [96]. Characteristically, the infection is focal and localized near the skin lesions, arthritic joints, and affected nerves [111]. Rarely, a generalized painful weakness affecting limbs, neck, and bulbar muscles has been described, simulating DM [110, 112].

EMG often confirms the inflammatory myositis. Serum enzymes are elevated only when there is generalized PM. Histologically, degeneration and necrosis of muscle fibers with perivascular lymphocellular infiltration are seen [111, 113]. Immunohistologic examination of seven muscle biopsies of patients [111] revealed macrophages in the infiltrate and T helper or inducer cells.

Some patients improve with corticosteroid therapy, but this could be more because of improvement in arthralgia. Therapy with ceftriaxone has been effective in treating the muscle weakness caused by the spirochete itself.

Leptospirosis

Leptospirosis is an infectious disease produced by spirochetes of the genus *Leptospira.* The disease has a wide range of involvement, from a flulike illness to a severe disease with hepatorenal failure. *Leptospira* has two species: the pathogenic *Leptospira interrogans* and the free-living *Leptospira biflexa.* Rodents are the most common reservoir, but cattle, dogs, pigs, and birds may also harbor the microorganisms. Human infection can occur by contact with animal or rodent urine and usually occurs in rural or rainwater catchment areas or by handling animal tissues [114, 115]. Presence of cuts in the skin facilitate the entry of *Leptospira.*

The majority of patients usually have a relatively mild anicteric form of leptospirosis. Only 5–10% develop severe jaundice with hepatorenal failure (Weil syndrome). Leptospirosis may present with an acute flulike illness with fever, chills, headache, nausea, and vomiting—the phase of leptospiremia. Myalgia, particularly of the calves, low back, and abdomen, is a prominent feature in 80–100% of patients. Pulmonary involvement with cough and chest pain— and, occasionally, hemoptysis, aseptic meningitis, and conjunctival suffusion—are not uncommon. Muscle tenderness is a less common finding, but significant muscle weakness suggestive of myopathy does not occur. Most patients recover within 1 week, but the illness recurs in some after 1–2 weeks. This immune phase coincides with the formation of antibodies and lasts for a few days. Fever and myalgia are less pronounced than in the leptospiremic phase. Weil syndrome is the most severe form of leptospirosis and is characterized by severe jaundice, renal dysfunction, and a high mortality. Rhabdomyolysis, myocarditis, and cardiogenic shock have been described in this syndrome [114].

The diagnosis of leptospirosis is usually made by detecting IgM antibodies by the ELISA method and the microscopic agglutination test. CK levels are elevated in the leptospiremic phase. Myalgia and elevated CK levels have been considered reliable early diagnostic aids [116]. Most patients respond to either penicillin or doxycycline.

Acknowledgment

We sincerely thank Dr. Ahalya S. Katrak for all the help and cooperation that she has given us in the preparation of this manuscript.

REFERENCES

1. Berman A, Espinoza LR, Diaz JD, et al. Rheumatic manifestations of human immunodeficiency virus infection. Am J Med 1988;85:59–64.
2. Simpson DM, Slasor P, Dafni U, et al. Analysis of myopathy in a placebo controlled zidovudine trial. Muscle Nerve 1997;20:382–385.
3. Snider WD, Simpson DM, Nielsen S, et al. Neurological complications of acquired immune deficiency syndrome. Ann Neurol 1983;14:403–418.
4. Dalakas MC, Pezeshkpour GH, Gravell M, et al. Polymyositis associated with AIDS retrovirus. JAMA 1986;256:2381–2383.
5. Espinoza LR, Aguilar JL, Espinoza CG, et al. Characteristics and pathogenesis of myositis in human immunodeficiency virus infection—distinction from azidothymidine-induced myopathy. Rheum Dis Clin North Am 1991;17:117–129.
6. Chad DA, Smith TW, Blumenfeld A, et al. Human immunodeficiency virus (HIV)–associated myopathy: immunocytochemical identification of an HIV antigen (GP41) in muscle macrophages. Ann Neurol 1990;28:579–582.
7. Gonzales MF, Olney RK, So YT, et al. Subacute structural myopathy associated with human immunodeficiency virus infection. Arch Neurol 1988;45:585–587.
8. Simpson DM, Bender AN. Human immunodeficiency virus–associated myopathy: analysis of 11 patients. Ann Neurol 1988;24:79–84.
9. Leon-Monzon M, Lamperth L, Dalakas MC. Search for HIV proviral DNA and amplified sequences in the muscle biopsies of patients with HIV polymyositis. Muscle Nerve 1993;16:408–413.
10. Dalakas MC, Illa I, Pezeshkpour GH, et al. Mitochondrial myopathy caused by long-term zidovudine therapy. N Engl J Med 1990;322:1098–1105.
11. Chalmers AC, Greco CM, Miller RG. Prognosis in AZT myopathy. Neurology 1991;41:1181–1184.
12. Griggs RC, Mendell JR, Miller RG. Evaluation and Treatment of Myopathies. Philadelphia: FA Davis, 1995;154–210.

13. Miller RG, Carson PJ, Moussavi RS, et al. Fatigue and myalgia in AIDS patients. Neurology 1991;41:1603–1607.
14. Simpson DM, Citak KA, Godfrey E, et al. Myopathies associated with human immunodeficiency virus and zidovudine: can their effects be distinguished? Neurology 1993;43:971–976.
15. Berger JR, Pall L, Hall CD, et al. Oxandrolone in AIDS-wasting myopathy. AIDS 1996;10:1657–1662.
16. Pallangyo K, Hakanson A, Lema L, et al. High HIV seroprevalence and increased HIV associated mortality amongst hospitalised patients with deep bacterial infections in Dar-es-Salaam, Tanzania. AIDS 1992;6:971–976.
17. Patel SR, Olenginski TP, Perruquet JL, et al. Pyomyositis: clinical features and predisposing conditions. J Rheumatol 1997;24:1734–1738.
18. Widrow CA, Kellie SM, Saltzman BR, et al. Pyomyositis in patients with the human immunodeficiency virus: an unusual form of disseminated bacterial infection. Am J Med 1991;91:129–136.
19. Pouchot J, Vinceneux P, Barge J, et al. Tuberculous polymyositis in HIV infection. Am J Med 1990;89:250–251.
20. Ledford DK, Overman A, Gonzalo A, et al. Microsporidiosis myositis in a patient with acquired immunodeficiency syndrome. Ann Intern Med 1985;102:628–630.
21. Chupp GL, Alroy J, Adelman LS, et al. Myositis due to Pleistophora (Microsporidia) in a patient with AIDS. Clin Infect Dis 1993;16:15–21.
22. Grau A, Valls ME, Williams JE, et al. Myositis caused by Pleistophora in a patient with AIDS (Spanish). Med Clin (Barc) 1996;107:779–781.
23. Field AS, Marriott DJ, Miliken ST, et al. Myositis associated with a newly described Microsporidian, *Trachipleistophora hominis*, in a patient with AIDS. J Clin Microbiol 1996;34:2803–2811.
24. Vernant J-C. Viral Conditions: HTLV-1. In RA Shakir, PK Newman, CM Poser (eds), Tropical Neurology. London: Saunders, 1996;19–35.
25. Gabbai AA, Wiley CA, Oliveira ASB, et al. Skeletal muscle involvement in tropical spastic paraparesis/HTLV-1–associated myelopathy. Muscle Nerve 1994;17:923–930.
26. Inose M, Higuchi I, Yoshimine K, et al. Pathological changes in skeletal muscles in HTLV-1–associated myelopathy. J Neurol Sci 1992;101:73–78.
27. Dickoff DJ, Simpson DM, Wiley CA, et al. HTLV-1 in acquired adult myopathy. Muscle Nerve 1993;16:162–165.
28. Wiley CA, Neremberg M, Cros D, et al. HTLV-1 polymyositis in a patient also infected with the human immunodeficiency virus. N Engl J Med 1989;320:992–995.
29. Karpati G, Currie GS. The Inflammatory Myopathies. In J Walton, G Karpati, D Hilton-Jones (eds), Disorders of Voluntary Muscles. London: Churchill Livingstone, 1994;619–646.
30. Nagaraja D, Taly AB, Suresh TG, et al. Epidemic of acute inflammatory myopathy in Karnataka, South India: 30 cases. Acta Neurol Scand 1992;86:230–236.
31. Wadia RS. Epidemic myositis disorder in India. Pune experience. Presented at: Spine 1998 (meeting of the Hirabai Cowasji Jehangir Medical Research Institute); April 5, 1998; Pune, India.
32. Baheti M, Taori GM. Acute polymyositis—a clinical and electrophysiological study. Programs and abstracts of the XXVI Annual Conference of the Indian Association of Physiotherapists; Nagpur, India; 30–31 January 1988.
33. Farrell MK, Partin JC, Bove KE. Epidemic influenza myopathy in Cincinnati in 1977. J Pediatr 1980;96:545–551.
34. Friman G. Serum creatine phosphokinase in epidemic influenza. Scand J Infect Dis 1976;8:13–20.
35. Belardi C, Roberge R, Kelly M, et al. Myalgia cruris epidemica (benign acute childhood myositis) associated with a mycoplasma pneumonia infection. Ann Emerg Med 1987;16:579–581.
36. Ruff RL, Secrist D. Viral studies in benign acute childhood myositis. Arch Neurol 1982;39:261–263.
37. McKinlay IA, Mitchell I. Transient myositis in childhood. Arch Dis Child 1976;51:135–137.
38. Gamboa ET, Eastwood AB, Hays AP et al. Isolation of influenza virus from muscle in myoglobinuric polymyositis. Neurology 1979;29:1323–1325.
39. Berlin BS, Simon NM, Bovner RN. Myoglobinuria precipitated by viral infection. JAMA 1974;227:1414–1415.
40. Morgensen JL. Myoglobinuria and renal failure associated with influenza. Ann Intern Med 1974;80:362–363.
41. Josselson J, Pula T, Sadler JH. Acute rhabdomyolysis associated with an echovirus 9 infection. Arch Intern Med 1980;140:1671–1672.
42. Mease PJ, Ochs HD, Wedgwood RJ. Successful treatment of echovirus meningoencephalitis and myositis-fasciitis with intravenous immune globulin therapy in a patient with X-linked agammaglobulinemia. N Engl J Med 1981;304:1278–1281.

43. Jehn UW, Fink MK. Myositis, myoglobinaemia and myoglobinuria associated with enterovirus ECHO 9 infection. Arch Neurol 1980;37:457–458.
44. Wright J, Conconnai G, Hodges GR. Adenovirus type 21 infection: concurrence with pneumonia, rhabdomyolysis and myoglobinuria in an adult. JAMA 1979;241:2420–2421.
45. McCormick GF, Zee CS, Heiden J. Cysticercosis cerebri: review of 127 cases. Arch Neurol 1982;39:534–539.
46. Earnest MP, Barth Reller L, Filley CM et al. Neurocysticercosis in the United States: 35 cases. Rev Infect Dis 1987;9:961–979.
47. Shandera WX, White CA, Chen JC, et al. Cysticercosis in Houston, Texas: a report of 112 patients. Medicine (Baltimore) 1994;73:37–51.
48. Wadia NH. Neurocysticercosis. In RA Shakir, PK Newman, CM Poser (eds). Tropical Neurology. London: Saunders, 1996;247–273.
49. MacArthur WP. Cysticercosis as seen in the British army with special reference to the production of epilepsy. Trans R Soc Trop Med Hyg 1934;27:343–363.
50. Morrison, WK. Cysticercosis in twin brothers aged 13 years with radiological study of the calcified cysticercus in twelve cases. BMJ 1934;1:13–15.
51. Lopez-Hernandez A, Garaizar G. Childhood cerebral cysticercosis: clinical features and computed tomographic findings in 89 Mexican children. Can J Neurol Sci 1982;9:402–407.
52. Case records of the Massachusetts General Hospital: case number 26. N Engl J Med 1994;330: 1887–1893.
53. Sotelo J, Guerrero V, Rubio F. Neurocysticercosis: a new classification based on active and inactive forms. A study of 753 cases. Arch Intern Med 1985;142:442–445.
54. Estanol B, Corona T, Abad P. A prognostic classification of cerebral cysticercosis: therapeutic implications. J Neurol Neurosurg Psychiatry 1986;49:1131–1134.
55. Del Brutto OH, Sotelo J. Neurocysticercosis: an update. J Neurol Neurosurg Psychiatry 1988;10:1075–1087.
56. Davis LE, Kornfeld M. Neurocysticercosis: neurologic, pathogenic, diagnostic and therapeutic aspects. Eur Neurol 1991;31:229–240.
57. Gang-Zhi W, Gun-Jiang M, Ha-Mei M, et al. Cysticercosis of the central nervous system—a clinical study of 1400 cases. Chin Med J (Engl) 1988;101:493–500.
58. Krishnaswami CS. Case of cysticercosis cellulose. Indian Med Gazette 1912;47:43–44.
59. Priest R. A case of extensive somatic dissemination of cysticercus cellulose in man. BMJ 1926;2:471–472.
60. McRoberts GR. Somatic taeniasis (solium cysticercosis). Indian Med Gazette 1944;79:399–400.
61. McGill RJ. Cysticercosis resembling myopathy. Lancet 1948;2:728–730.
62. Singh A, Jolly SS. Cysticercosis: case report. Indian J Med Sci 1957;11:98–101.
63. Prakash C, Kumar R. Cysticercosis with taeniasis in a vegetarian. J Trop Med Hyg 1965;68:100–103.
64. Jacob JC, Mathew NT. Pseudohypertrophic myopathy in cysticercosis. Neurology 1968;18:767–771.
65. Armbrust-Figueiredo J, Speciali JG, Lison MP. Forma myopatic da cysticerosa. Arq Neuropsiquiatr 1970;28:385–390.
66. Jolly SS, Pallis C. Muscular pseudohypertrophy due to cysticercosis. J Neurol Sci 1971;12:155–162.
67. Rao CM, Sattar SA, Gopal PS, et al. Cysticercosis resembling myopathy: report of a case. Indian J Med Sci 1972;26:841–843.
68. Salgaokar SV, Watcha MF. Muscular hypertrophy in cysticercosis: a case report. J Postgrad Med 1974;20:148–152.
69. Vigg B, Rai V. Muscular involvement in cysticercosis with pseudohypertrophy of muscles. J Assoc Physicians India 1975;23:593–595.
70. Sawhney BB, Chopra JS, Banerji AK, et al. Pseudohypertrophic myopathy in cysticercosis. Neurology 1976;26:270–272.
71. Vijayan GP, Venkataraman S, Suri ML, et al. Neurological and related manifestations of cysticercosis. Trop Geogr Med 1977;29:271–278.
72. Dinakar I, Suvarna Kumari G, Alikhan MJ. Cysticercosis resembling myopathy. Neurology (India) 1979;27:41–43.
73. Yingkun F, Shan O, Xiuzhen Z, et al. Clinico-electroencephalographic studies of cerebral cysticercosis—158 cases. Chin Med J (Engl) 1979;92:770–786.
74. Zhiplao XB, Yvequing Z, Weiji C, et al. Muscular pseudohypertrophy due to cysticercus cellulosae: report of three cases. Chin Med J (Engl) 1980;93:48–53.
75. Venkataraman S, Rao SV, Singh N, et al. Unusual presentation of cysticercosis muscular pseudohypertrophy. Med J Armed Forces India 1981;37:130–133.
76. Venkataraman S, Vijayan GP. Uncommon manifestations of human cysticercosis with muscular pseudohypertrophy. Trop Geogr Med 1983;35:75–77.

77. Zhu D, Xu W. Effect of biltricide on cysticercosis cellulosae with muscular pseudohypertrophy—a report of three cases. Chi Sheng Chung Hsueh Yu Chi Sheng Chung Ping Tsa Chih 1983;1:185–186.
78. Xu Z, Chen W, Zong H, et al. Praziquantel in treatment of cysticercosis cellulosae. Report of 200 cases. Chin Med J (Engl) 1985;98:489–494.
79. Wadia NH, Desai SB, Bhatt MB. Disseminated cysticercosis—new observations including CT scan findings and experience with treatment with Praziquantal. Brain 1988;11:597–614.
80. Wadia NH. Disseminated Cysticercosis: Pseudohypertrophic Muscular Type. In F Clifford Rose (ed), Recent Advances in Tropical Neurology. Amsterdam, the Netherlands: Elsevier, 1995;119–130.
81. Pallis CA, Lewis PD. Involvement of Human Muscles by Parasites. In J Walton, G Karpati, D Hilton-Jones (eds), Disorders of Voluntary Muscles. London: Churchill Livingstone, 1994;743–759.
82. Hollander D, Munsat TL. Infections of Muscles. In SL Gorbach, JG Bartlett, NR Blacklow (eds), Infectious Diseases. Philadelphia: Saunders, 1992;1078–1079.
83. Yamashita K, Akimura T, Kawano K, et al. Cerebral Sparganosis mansoni: report of two cases. Surg Neurol 1990;33:28–34.
84. Sarma DP, Weilbaecher TG. Human sparganosis. J Am Acad Dermatol 1986;15:1145–1148.
85. Datta KK, Datta SP, Sharma LS, et al. Sparganosis. J Indian Med Assoc 1982;79:78–80.
86. Ali-Khan Z, Irving RT, Wingnall N, et al. Imported sparganosis in Canada. CMAJ 1973;108:590.
87. Nakamura T, Hara M, Matsuoka M, et al. Human proliferative sparganosis. A new Japanese case. Am J Clin Pathol 1990;94:224–228.
88. Taratuto AL, Venturiello SM. Trichinosis. Brain Pathol 1997;7:663–672.
89. Murrell KD, Bruschi F. Clinical trichinellosis. Prog Clin Parasitol 1994;4:117–148.
90. McAuley JB, Michelson MK, Schantz PM. Trichinella infections in travellers. J Infect Dis 1991;164:1013–1016.
91. Grove DI. Tissues Nematodes (Trichinosis). In GL Mandell, RG Douglas, JE Bennet (eds), Principles and Practice of Infectious Diseases. New York: Churchill Livingstone, 1990;2140–2141.
92. Kramer MD, Aita JF. Trichinosis: Infections of the Central Nervous System. In BJ Vinken, GW Bruyn (eds), Handbook of Clinical Neurology. Amsterdam, the Netherlands: North Holland Publishing, 1978;267–290.
93. Hunter GW, Swatzwelder JC, Clyde DE. Tropical Medicine (5th ed). Philadelphia: Saunders, 1976.
94. Pollock JL. Toxoplasmosis: appearing to be dermatomyositis. Arch Dermatol 1979;115:736–737.
95. Remington JS, Cavanaugh EN. Isolation of the encysted form of Toxoplasma gondii from human skeletal muscle and brain. N Engl J Med 1965;273:1308–1310.
96. Ytterberg SR. The relationship of infectious agents to inflammatory myositis. Rheum Dis Clin North Am 1994;20:995–1015.
97. Gherardi R, Baudrimont M, Lionnet F, et al. Skeletal muscle toxoplasmosis in patients with acquired immunodeficiency syndrome: a clinical and pathological study. Ann Neurol 1992;32:535–542.
98. Matsubara S, Takamori M, Adachi H, et al. Acute toxoplasma myositis: an immunohistochemical and ultrastructural study. Acta Neuropathol (Berl) 1990;81:223–227.
99. Pamphlett R, O'Donoghue P. Sarcocystis infection of human muscle. Austr N Z J Med 1990;20:705–707.
100. World Health Organisation. Control of Chagas disease. Report of the WHO expert committee. WHO Technical Report Series 811. Geneva, 1991.
101. Banker BQ. Parasitic Myositis. In AG Engel, BQ Banker (eds), Myology. New York: McGraw-Hill, 1986;1467–1500.
102. Sica REP. Peripheral Nervous System Involvement in Human Chronic American Trypanosomiasis. In F Clifford Rose (ed), Recent Advances in Tropical Neurology. Amsterdam, the Netherlands: Elsevier, 1995; 175–192.
103. Spina Franca A. American Trypanosomiasis. In RA Shakir, PK Newman, CM Poser (eds), Tropical Neurology. London: Saunders, 1996;287–294.
104. Rey RC, Monteverde DA, Sica REP. Cardiac source of cerebral embolism. Arch Neurol 1991;48:359–360.
105. Dumas M. African trypanosomiasis. In Shakir RA, Newman PK, Poser CM (eds). Tropical Neurology. London: Saunders, 1996;275–286.
106. Armstrong JH. Tropical pyomyositis and myoglobinuria. Arch Intern Med 1978;138:1145–1146.
107. Jellis JE. Orthopaedic surgery and HIV disease in Africa. Int Orthop 1996;20:253–256.
108. Porter CB, Hinthorn DR, Couchonnal G, et al. Simultaneous streptococcus and picornavirus infection. Muscle involvement in acute rhabdomyolysis. JAMA 1981;245:1545–1547.
109. Schattner A, Hay E, Lifschitz-Mercer B, et al. Fulminant streptococcal myositis. Ann Emerg Med 1989;18:320–322.
110. Schoenen J, Sianard-Gainko J, Carpentier M, et al. Myositis during *Borrelia burgdorferi* infection (Lyme disease). J Neurol Neurosurg Psychiatry 1989;52:1002–1005.

111. Reimer CD, de Koning J, Neubert U, et al. *Borrelia burgdorferi* myositis: report of eight patients. J Neurol 1993;240:278–283.
112. Horowitz HW, Sanghera K, Goldberg N, et al. Dermatomyositis associated with Lymes disease: case report and review of Lyme myositis. Clin Infect Dis 1994;18:166–171.
113. Muller-Felber W, Reimer CD, de Koning J, et al. Myositis in *Lymes borreliosis*: an immunohisto-chemical study of seven patients. J Neurol Sci 1993;118:207–212.
114. Farr RW. Leptospirosis. Clin Infect Dis 1995;21:1–6.
115. Muthusethupathi MA, Shivakumar S, Suguna R, et al. Leptospirosis in Madras—a clinical and serological study. J Assoc Physicians India 1995;43:456–458.
116. Pinn TG. Leptospirosis in the Seychelles. Med J Aust 1992;156:163–167.

12
Endocrine and Toxic Myopathies

Osama O. Zaidat, Robert L. Ruff,
and Henry J. Kaminski

Exogenous chemicals and imbalance of the endocrine system may have profound effects on skeletal muscle and produce a wide range of clinical presentations. Cushing disease, iatrogenic steroid myopathy, and disorders of the thyroid gland, including Graves ophthalmopathy, are emphasized in this chapter. Muscle disease associated with acromegaly and pituitary dysfunction is reviewed, and the effects of abnormalities of calcium metabolism on muscle are summarized.

Prescription medications, drug abuse, vitamin deficiency or overuse, and environmental exposure produce a wide range of neuromuscular complications. The incidence of toxic myopathies is not known and is likely to vary widely across the world based on regional variations in drug abuse, use of pharmaceuticals, industrialization, and socioeconomic factors. The best understood and most common endocrine and toxic myopathies are described.

TOXIC MYOPATHIES

A uniform classification of toxic myopathies is difficult to achieve. Most authors have used a mixture of clinical patterns, mechanisms, and individual agents to characterize toxin-induced muscle disease [1, 2]; this review is no different. The most frequent presentation is a necrotizing myopathy (Figure 12.1) that may be so severe as to produce myoglobinuria and renal failure. Toxins may produce inflammatory, mitochondrial, and lysosomal-type muscle diseases. A wide variety of agents produces isolated myoglobinuria without significant evidence of weakness. Myalgia or muscle cramping is reported with a number of medications (Table 12.1). We review a number of agents that may produce muscle disease (Table 12.2).

Necrotizing Myopathy

Hypocholesterolemic drugs are commonly used medications with a propensity to produce muscle disease. Lovastatin, a 3-hydroxy-3-methylglutaryl-coenzyme A

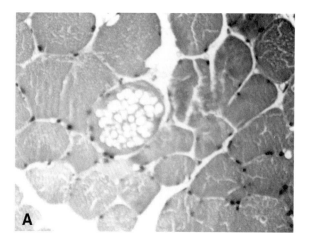

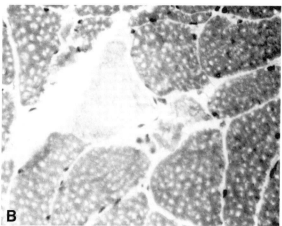

Figure 12.1 Hematoxylin and eosin–stained sections of a left gracilis muscle biopsy from a patient with a toxic myopathy producing rhabdomyolysis. A severely vacuolated fiber and adjacent fibers undergoing necrosis with loss of cytoplasmic contents are seen in (**A**). In (**B**), the central fiber has lost its cytoplasmic contents. The numerous punctate regions in the center of the fibers are an artifact of processing.

Table 12.1 Drugs associated with myalgias or cramps

Captopril	Lithium
Cimetidine	L-Tryptophan
Clofibrate, etofibrate	Mercaptopropionyl glycine
Colchicine	Metolazone
Cytotoxic agents (particularly in a setting of cachexia)	Nifedipine (and other similar calcium channel blockers)
Danazol	Pindolol
Diuretics (particularly in association with hypokalemia)	Procainamide (with or without a drug-induced lupus syndrome or myasthenia gravis)
D-Penicillamine	Rifampicin
Enalapril	Salbutamol
Ethchlorvynol	Suxamethonium
Gold	Zidovudine (AZT)
Isoetharine	Zimeldine
Labetalol	

Table 12.2 Types of toxin-associated myopathies

Major toxin-related syndromes	Agent	Related conditions
Necrotizing myopathy	Lovastatin	Myopathy usually occurs in association with gemfibrozil or cyclosporine
	Clofibrate, bezafibrate, etofibrate, lovastatin, gemfibrozil	
	Epsilon aminocaproic acid	Myotonia
	Organophosphate exposure	Usually causes neuromuscular transmission defect
	Venoms (snake, spider)	Myonecrosis
Lysosomal-related myopathy	Choloroquine, quinacrine	—
	Amiodarone	
	Perhexiline	
Inflammatory myopathy	D-Penicillamine	May produce myasthenic syndrome
	Procainamide	May produce lupuslike syndrome
	Phenytoin, levodopa, leuprolide, propyl-thiouracil, cimetidine, ciguatera toxin	Less well established
Antimicrotubular myopathy	Colchicine	Most often seen in renal failure patients
	Vincristine	Axonal peripheral neuropathy
Mitochondrial myopathy	Zidovudine	May coexist with human immunodeficiency virus myopathy
	Germanium	Associated renal failure, anemia
Vitamin/amino acid–related myopathy	Vitamin E excess and deficiency	—
	Etretinate, isotretinoin	
	Tryptophan (eosinophilia-myalgia syndrome)	
Hypokalemia-related myopathy	Glycyrrhizic acid (licorice)	Aldosteronelike effect
	Glycyrrhetinic acid (carbenoxolone)	Renal tubular acidosis
	Amphotericin B	
	Diuretics, laxatives	
Drugs of abuse	Phencyclidine hydrochloride, cocaine, heroin	Often associated with myoglobinuria
	Toluene	Diffuse nervous system pathology
Critical illness myopathy	Combination high-dose steroids, nondepolarizing neuromuscular blockade, and sepsis	—
Ethanol-related syndromes	Acute necrotizing myopathy	—
	Hypokalemic myopathy	
	Chronic myopathy	

reductase inhibitor, rarely causes a myopathy when used alone, but in combination with either gemfibrozil or cyclosporine, myopathy is more likely to develop. Patients with severe hepatobiliary dysfunction or renal insufficiency may be at a higher risk of developing a myopathy when using lovastatin alone [3, 4]. Cyclosporine alone may result in a mild myopathy; however, cyclosporine in combination with lovastatin or colchicine may produce a more severe myopathy with rhabdomyolysis [3, 4].

Clofibrate and related agents—bezafibrate, etofibrate, beclobrate, lovastatin, and gemfibrozil—induce a myopathy characterized by the acute onset of cramps, myalgias, and weakness, with an elevation of serum transaminases and creatine kinase (CK). Myotonia develops in some patients in response to hypocholesterolemic agents, especially clofibrate. Accumulation of the active metabolite of clofibrate, chlorophenoxyisobutyric acid, may produce a myopathy, which may be more common in patients with renal failure, nephrotic syndrome, and hypothyroidism. Some patients also have an associated peripheral neuropathy. A discontinuation or reduction in dose of the drug leads to gradual recovery [4].

Epsilon aminocaproic acid inhibits fibrinolysis and has been used in different bleeding disorders. A myopathy affecting axial musculature with symptoms that begin 4 or more weeks after initiation of treatment is an uncommon complication. The etiology may be altered muscle membrane function or ischemia to the muscles [4].

Muscle damage produced by neurotrophic agents in the context of neuroleptic malignant syndrome is evidenced by fever, increased muscle tone, autonomic instability, and elevated CK. Clozapine and olanzapine have been associated with elevated CK levels and seem to occur in the majority of patients [5]. Electromyography (EMG) may show myopathic changes, and muscle biopsy in patients with CK elevations may show regenerating myofibers, acute denervation, and type II fiber atrophy. Rhabdomyolysis with myoglobinuria and renal failure may also occur. Manifestations resolve with discontinuation of the medications.

Severe myonecrosis can occur as a consequence of general anesthesia, status epilepticus, or prolonged unconsciousness. In the last case, it is probably due to pressure necrosis. In addition, a large number of agents, including the venoms of several snakes and spiders, have been implicated as causing acute myonecrosis with myoglobinuria. This condition is associated with extreme elevation in serum levels of muscle-associated enzymes and myoglobinuria. Extreme muscle swelling may produce compartment syndromes leading to nerve entrapments and limb ischemia. Numerous snake venoms are myotoxic at the bite site. However, others have more widespread effects, causing muscle necrosis and myoglobinuria. Snake venoms that are associated with diffuse rhabdomyolysis come from the tiger snake, Taipan snake, Mulga snake, and sea snake. The venom of the Arkansas and Honduran tarantulas causes irreversible injury to the muscle fiber plasma membranes, leading to diffuse myonecrosis [4]. Organophosphate exposure usually results in a neuropathy; however, a myopathy may also result secondary to increased neurotransmitters in the neuromuscular junction [4].

Lysosomal-Related Disorders

Several antimalarial agents cause a myopathy that appears to affect the lysosomes. Chloroquine may induce a myopathy after treatment with at least 500 mg per day for a year. Progressive painless proximal muscle wasting and weakness are characteristic, and a neuropathy and cardiomyopathy may occur. The myopathy slowly reverses after discontinuation of the medication [4]. Plasmocid induces muscle necrosis and phagocytosis in animals and humans. Usually, it is proximal and painless. Animal studies suggest that autodigestion by intramyofibral lysosomal proteases, followed by digestion of the necrotic fibers by macrophage proteases, occurs. Quinacrine is an acridine dye also used to treat malaria and giardiasis. General side effects include headache; dizziness; vomiting; diarrhea; yellowish discoloration of urine, sclera, and skin; and, less commonly, psychotic episodes. A painless proximal myopathy occurs with prolonged treatment. The drug is no longer distributed in the United States.

Amiodarone, an antiarrhythmic agent, frequently causes neurologic side effects, including peripheral neuropathy, ataxia, tremor, and, less commonly, a proximal myopathy that may be painful or painless [6]. Manifestations may begin as early as 1 month or as late as 3 years after initiation of treatment. Marked distal motor weakness and stocking-and-gloves sensory impairment occur, usually associated with distal muscular atrophy [7]. Enlargement of extraocular muscles that resembles endocrine ophthalmopathy might occur [8]. Muscle biopsy reveals a vacuolar myopathy with lysosomal inclusions. High levels of amiodarone and its metabolite, desethylamidarone, may be found in the muscle with normal serum levels. Experimentally prolonged dosing of mice with amiodarone produced myopathy characterized by autophagic vacuolation and phospholipid inclusions and necrosis mainly affecting type II fibers. This may indicate a direct toxic effect of amiodarone or its metabolites on oxidative enzyme activity [9].

Perhexiline is a calcium channel blocker mainly used in treatment of angina pectoris. Chronic use leads to peripheral neuropathy and, less commonly, painless proximal myopathy [10, 11]. Systemic side effects include hypoglycemia, weight loss, and hepatic disturbances. Characteristic intracytoplasmic inclusion frequently associated with calcium deposits is found either at the periphery of the muscle fibers or between the central myofibrils. These inclusions may also be found in endothelial cells, pericytes, Schwann cells, and fibroblasts and vary in morphology depending on cell type [12]. Discontinuation of the drug and supportive treatment lead to reversal of the myopathy.

Inflammatory Myopathy

D-Penicillamine may cause an inflammatory myopathy indistinguishable from polymyositis. Immunoregulatory mechanisms may be altered by this medication. Myocardial involvement may be fatal. Halting the drug results in recovery [4]. Procainamide may cause interstitial myositis as part of a lupuslike vasculitic reaction [4]. Phenytoin, levodopa, leuprolide, propylthiouracil, and cimetidine have been associated with production of an inflammatory myopathy, but the relation is not as clearly established. Ciguatera toxin, ingested by humans from fish contaminated by dinoflagellates that contain the toxin, may develop an inflammatory myopathy, but intoxication often leads to myalgia and fatigue that may persist for months to years.

Antimicrotubular Myopathy

Colchicine may induce a proximal myopathy, especially in patients with renal insufficiency. Distal sensory involvement secondary to axonal neuropathy is common. Plasma colchicine and CK are usually elevated. Discontinuation of colchicine improves strength and the sensory neuropathy [4]. Although vincristine commonly causes an axonal peripheral neuropathy, some patients develop a proximal myopathy. These side effects are dose related and usually disappear 6 weeks after finishing treatment. Some patients, however, continue to have symptoms for a prolonged period [4].

Mitochondrial Myopathy

Zidovudine (AZT) causes a progressive, painful mitochondrial myopathy. CK is normal or only moderately elevated. A clear distinction between AZT myopathy and human immunodeficiency virus (HIV) myositis is sometimes difficult to make. HIV myositis can resemble polymyositis with inflammatory infiltrates. Ragged red fibers can be found in AZT myopathy, but inflammatory infiltrates are usually not present in AZT myopathy [13]. AZT myopathy may be due to impaired mitochondrial function. Germanium is an antineoplastic agent that affects mitochondria in many organ systems, most commonly causing renal failure and anemia. Muscle demonstrates ragged red fibers and vacuolization. Mitochondria show dense granules on electron microscopy.

Vitamin- and Amino Acid–Related Myopathies

Hypervitaminoses E may result in proximal muscle weakness and elevated serum CK [4]. Vitamin E deficiency may result in generalized muscle weakness, including ocular muscles [4]. Etretinate is a vitamin A derivative that is used in treating psoriasis. Skeletal muscle damage is an uncommon side effect and is manifested as proximal muscle weakness and tenderness [4]. Isotretinoin is used for treatment of severe acne. Mild and transient arthralgias and myalgias can occasionally be seen [4].

Tryptophan is an essential amino acid and is marketed as a nonprescription nutritional supplement to treat insomnia, depression, psychological disorders, and premenstrual syndrome. In 1989, the Centers for Disease Control and Prevention (CDC) reported an epidemic of an acute illness characterized by myalgia and eosinophilia in New Mexico. Each patient had taken an L-tryptophan–containing preparation. The CDC proposed diagnostic criteria for the so-called eosinophilia-myalgia syndrome (EMS): (1) eosinophil count of more than 1,000 cells/mm^3, (2) severe myalgia, and (3) an absence of alternative explanations for eosinophilia.

The onset of the syndrome may be delayed months or years after tryptophan ingestion [14]. Manifestations may develop acutely with a severe respiratory illness that is followed by myalgia; fatigue; and painful, moderate to severe proximal, distal, or combined muscle weakness. Patients may require ventilatory support. Other manifestations include fever, rash, urticaria, livedo reticularis, alopecia, lymphadenopathy, sclerodermalike syndrome, and paresthesias. Other than marked eosinophilia, patients may have increased CK in the acute phase. Some patients develop severe axonal sensory motor neuropathy [15]. Muscle biopsy reveals fiber atrophy and perimysial inflammation with T-cell and eosinophil infiltrate [14]. The pathogenesis remains obscure. Speculations emphasize the role of the impurities, whereas others support the abnormalities of tryptophan metabolism with the development of EMS [16]. Treatment is limited to stopping the offending agent and administering corticosteroid treatment. Some individuals develop a chronic sclerodermalike syndrome, sensory motor polyneuropathy, persistent proximal myopathy, or episodic myalgias [17].

Hypokalemia-Related Myopathy

Agents that produce hypokalemia at a serum level below 2 mmol/liter may induce muscle damage [1, 2]. Pathologic investigation demonstrates a vacuolar myopathy that may show necrosis and regenerative fibers. Occasionally, the muscle injury may be so severe as to produce rhabdomyolysis. The most common agents to induce hypokalemic myopathy are diuretics and laxatives either used therapeutically or abused. The antifungal agent amphotericin B is nephrotoxic and may produce potassium depletion leading to the development of myopathy. Licorice that contains glycyrrhizic acid and carbenoxolone—a drug for peptic ulcer disease—contains the related compound, glycyrrhetinic acid, and has an aldosteronelike effect that induces potassium loss. Toluene produces potassium depletion and myopathy, as described in the section Drugs of Abuse.

Ethanol Abuse–Associated Myopathies

Ethanol is myotoxic, and acute, hypokalemic, and possibly chronic forms of alcoholic myopathy exist. Acute necrotizing myopathy commonly occurs with the background of chronic alcohol abuse. Excessive ingestion of alcohol results in non-inflammatory muscle necrosis characterized as an acute onset of severe muscle pain, cramps, weakness, swelling, and tenderness that may be generalized or focal. The condition can mimic venous thrombophlebitis when isolated to the calves. Recovery depends on the severity of muscle destruction and may extend over several months. Significant rhabdomyolysis may lead to acute renal failure [4].

Hypokalemic myopathy may be a consequence of chronic alcoholism and numerous other etiologies, including excessive vomiting and diarrhea, treatment with laxatives, thiazide diuretics, mineralocorticoids, and toluene abuse. Hypokalemia can also develop from alcohol-induced hypomagnesemia. Weakness, hypotonia, and depressed deep tendon reflexes can develop, quickly progressing to flaccid paralysis of the limbs. In the alcoholic patient, the acute onset of painless weakness in the proximal limb muscles and limb-girdle muscles without muscle cramps, tenderness, or swelling is characteristic. Serum CK and aldolase are elevated, and serum potassium is low. When the patient is hypokalemic and hypomagnesemic, the myopathy is often painful. Strength improves with potassium and magnesium replacement [4].

Definitive evidence of a chronic alcoholic myopathy does not exist. Some think that chronic alcohol use results in the insidious onset of painless proximal muscle weakness and wasting, but others consider this secondary to peripheral neuropathy [4]. Patients with a history of acute alcoholic myopathy elevate their serum CK and myoglobin with greater ease than those who have not had alcoholic myopathy after the same amount of alcohol is consumed. Chronic drinkers who acutely increase their alcohol intake elevate their serum CK and myoglobin without a clinically evident myopathy. This may be an asymptomatic form of chronic alcoholic myopathy that could progress to persistent proximal weakness [4].

Emetine is an amebicide, an emetic, and is used in alcoholic aversion therapy. Proximal limb and trunk muscles are primarily affected, but a generalized myopathy may also occur that is reversible. The degree of muscle damage depends on the dose and duration of exposure [4]. *Radix ipecacuanhae* contains cephaline, psychotrine, and the toxic alkaloid emetine. Its primary indication is in treatment of toxin or drug ingestion as an emetic. Ingestion of emetine for more than 10 days in high doses results in a severe myopathy and cardiomyopathy. Coincident eating disorders, such as anorexia nervosa and bulimia nervosa, are common [1, 2]. Occasionally, sensory symptoms may be observed. Serum enzymes associated with muscle damage are mildly to moderately elevated, and biopsy reveals predominance of type 1 fibers, a slight decrease in the average diameter of muscle fiber, isolated necrotic granular basophilic fibers, and intracytoplasmic eosinophilic rod–like inclusions in the type 1 fibers. Treatment is supportive. Cessation of emetine ingestion leads to gradual recovery within several months in most cases. Emetine has effects on protein synthesis and energy metabolism.

Drugs of Abuse

Several of the commonly abused drugs may produce muscle weakness. Cocaine results in myoglobinuria. This is either a direct toxic effect from cocaine or secondary to cocaine-induced ischemia. Excessive amounts of sympathomimetic drugs may produce acute rhabdomyolysis, myoglobinuria, and renal failure [4]. Heroin ingestion may produce acute rhabdomyolysis and commonly results in alteration in consciousness and subsequent pressure-induced damage to skeletal muscle [4]. Phencyclidine (PCP) ingestion or inhalation may cause myoglobinuria and acute renal failure. Excessive isometric motor activity may be the cause of PCP myopathy, as PCP does not have a direct toxic effect on muscle [4]. Chronic toluene abuse often produces symmetric weakness with many associated peripheral and central nervous system dysfunctions. Associated hypokalemia, hypophosphatemia, and acidosis may lead to myoglobinuria.

Critical Illness Myopathy

Acute weakness may develop in the intensive care setting that may have a neuropathic or myopathic etiology [18–22]. Several factors appear to contribute to the rapid onset of weakness and wasting: (1) immobility, (2) nondepolarizing neuromuscular blocking agents, (3) concurrent sepsis, and (4) glucocorticoid use [21]. Some patients with critical illness myopathy may have no elevation in CK, whereas others have a severe necrotizing myopathy. Muscle biopsy may demonstrate predominant type II fiber atrophy and a loss of thick filaments [23]. Rich et al. [18] identified three patients with severe weakness whose muscle was inexcitable with direct electrical stimulation. Loss of muscle of membrane excitability can produce a response pattern on EMG testing that resembles axonal neuropathy [18, 20, 21, 24]. Rouleau et al. [25] demonstrated that glucocorticoid treatment combined with immobility produces profound loss of myofibrillar proteins. From these observations, one can conclude that critical illness myopathy likely has several pathogenic mechanisms. Despite the severity of weakness, patients may improve significantly with supportive care.

After liver transplantation, 8% of patients develop an acute necrotizing myopathy that is most closely associated with high doses of corticosteroid administration [26]. All patients who survived attained excellent functional improvement in the 6 months after transplant.

Miscellaneous Agents

Labetalol, a selective α_1- and nonselective β-adrenergic receptor blocker, may produce a severe generalized myopathy with markedly elevated CK that improves with discontinuation of the medication. β-Adrenergic blockers may interfere with neuromuscular transmission and exacerbate myasthenia gravis (MG) [4]. Some β_2-selective blockers or agonists can exacerbate myotonia.

In Spain in 1982, an epidemic affected approximately 20,000 people, with 400 deaths resulting from ingestion of adulterated rapeseed oil. Patients typically presented with nonproductive cough, dyspnea, pleuritic chest pain, headache, fever, and bilateral pulmonary infiltrates. Nausea, vomiting, diarrhea and abdominal pain, splenomegaly, myalgia, and skin rash were also common. Three months after the acute presentation, pulmonary hypertension, vasculitis, progressive paralytic neuromuscular illness, sicca syndrome, and sclerodermalike cutaneous lesions developed. Severe muscle cramps and myalgia that were exacerbated by pressure occurred. Characteristic weakness that began distally and increased in severity with progression occurred proximally. Atrophy of large muscle groups with absent deep tendon reflexes and contractures ensued. Sensory abnormalities also occurred. Eosinophilia, leukocytosis, and elevated serum aldolase were appreciated. EMG studies revealed a mixed axonal neuropathy. The disease was self-limited in mild cases, with worse outcome in patients with severe initial presentations, especially with respiratory failure. Although the pathogenesis remains a mystery, studies suggest an immunologic mechanism triggered by an arachidonic fatty acid derivative in the oil [1, 2].

Repeated intramuscular injections may lead to local induration and fibrous contracture. Focal necrosis may also occur with modest elevation of CK. The injury may be related to direct injury caused by needle insertion or the effects of the agent injected. The pH and osmolarity of the agent may be of particular importance in the extent of CK elevation and muscle necrosis. Repeated injection of meperidine and pentazocine is often associated with abscess formation and contractures [2].

ENDOCRINE MYOPATHIES

Disturbances of the endocrine system are a frequent cause of myopathy, and muscle manifestations occur with hyper- or hypofunction of the adrenal, thyroid, parathyroid, and pituitary glands. Iatrogenic glucocorticoid excess is an important cause of muscle weakness that may be particularly difficult to diagnose. Electrolyte and metabolic derangement is the common etiologic factor in producing muscle dysfunction, and correction of the underlying endocrine dysfunction usually improves patient symptoms.

Glucocorticoid Excess States

Myopathy secondary to glucocorticoid excess is seen with Cushing disease, ectopic adrenocorticotropic hormone (ACTH) production, and iatrogenic steroid myopathy. Cushing first noted that patients with endogenous glucocorticoid excess develop severe proximal muscle wasting and weakness. Between 50% and 80% of patients with Cushing disease develop appreciable muscle weakness [27]. A similar syndrome occurs in patients with ectopic production of ACTH. Muscle weakness and wasting are also common complications of glucocorticoid administration [28, 29].

Patients with steroid myopathy usually have other stigmata of glucocorticoid excess (i.e., moon facies, buffalo hump, fragile skin, osteoporosis, cataracts). The onset of weakness is usually insidious. The weakness is primarily proximal, with the legs more severely involved than the arms; cranial-nerve-innervated muscles and sphincters are usually spared. Myalgias frequently accompany the weakness. The same patterns of muscle involvement are found in patients with iatrogenic steroid myopathy and endogenous glucocorticoid excess [28].

Glucocorticoids may also produce muscle weakness by altering serum electrolytes. Glucocorticoids with high mineralocorticoid activity may induce hypokalemic myopathy [28]. Biopsies show a vacuolar degeneration pattern, which is characteristic of potassium depletion, not steroid myopathy. Glucocorticoids can produce transient hypophosphatemia that is due to increased renal clearance of phosphate. Severe phosphate depletion can result in muscle necrosis. However, potassium and phosphate depletion are not the usual causes of myopathy associated with glucocorticoid use [30].

The myopathy found in Cushing disease is attributed to glucocorticoid excess, because the weakness usually reverses when the glucocorticoid levels become normal [31, 32]. Elevated levels of ACTH may also be myopathic. Patients treated for Cushing disease with adrenalectomy and physiologic glucocorticoid replacement developed proximal weakness and wasting. Some patients had sharp waves or fibrillation potentials. Excessive amounts of ACTH can impair neuromuscular transmission by decreasing the quantal content of the endplate potential. Therefore, ACTH excess may have myopathic actions that are separate from those of glucocorticoids [28, 33]. The exact pathogenic mechanisms of ACTH remain obscure.

Steroid myopathy has been reported in patients between ages 2 and 84 years and has occurred in patients experiencing a variety of diseases treated with glucocorticoids. Estimates of the incidence of muscle weakness associated with chronic steroid treatment varies from 2.4% to 21.0%. These figures indicate only those patients who developed severe weakness and underestimate the actual incidence of steroid-induced weakness. Moreover, the diagnosis of steroid myopathy may be overlooked in patients receiving steroid treatment for disorders that produce weakness, such as the inflammatory myopathies or central nervous system diseases. It is often difficult to decide whether deterioration in strength of a patient with inflammatory myopathy treated with steroids is the result of steroid myopathy or of a flare in the inflammatory myopathy. As steroid myopathy takes time to develop, weakness that occurs at the onset of steroid treatment is probably caused by a flare in the inflammatory process and is best treated by continuing or increasing the dose of steroid. Similarly, if the weakness occurs without any other stigmata of steroid usage, it is probably not steroid induced. Elevation in the serum levels of muscle-associated enzymes suggests that the weakness is partially due to the inflammatory myopathy. However, normal enzyme levels do not rule out a flare in the inflammatory myopathy.

Among patients with steroid myopathy, there is a wide variation in the dose and duration of steroid treatment associated with the onset of weakness. However, patients who have received steroids for less than 4 weeks rarely develop severe steroid myopathy [34]. The incidence of steroid myopathy varies with the glucocorticoid preparation. Although any commonly used glucocorticoid can cause steroid myopathy, the fluorinated steroids (e.g., triamcinolone, betamethasone, and dexamethasone) are more likely to produce weakness. Patients develop weakness when switched from other steroids to equivalent doses of triamcinolone or dexamethasone and recover from dexamethasone- or triamcinolone-induced weakness when converted to an equivalent anti-inflammatory dose of another steroid [28]. Acute myopathy may develop in association with glucocorticoid use in the critical care setting (see previous section, Critical Illness Myopathy).

Serum concentrations of muscle injury–associated enzymes, such as CK and aldolase, are usually normal in steroid-induced myopathy [34]. The EMG findings are variable. Typically, insertional activity is normal, and the motor unit potentials are of low amplitude and short duration. Despite isolated reports of fibrillation potentials accompanying the brief-duration motor unit potentials, spontaneous electrical activity is typically absent in steroid myopathy. In contrast, fibrillation potentials are commonly seen in inflammatory myopathy [35].

Histologic studies in either iatrogenic steroid myopathy or in Cushing disease show nonspecific changes or selective atrophy of type 2 muscle fibers without affecting the fiber-type distribution of muscles [36, 37]. Among fast-twitch fibers, the type 2B fibers are more severely affected than the type 2A fibers [37]. Increased muscle glycogen is found in type 2A fibers. Biopsy may reveal prominent subsarcolemmal lipid deposits. Lipid excess is not characteristic of iatrogenic steroid myopathy. Electron microscopic studies reveal mitochondrial aggregation and vacuolization. These changes are not severe and correlate poorly with weakness [28].

The prime method of treating steroid myopathy is to decrease the steroid level to the lowest possible. Treatment of the underlying etiology of steroid excess is most important. Conversion to a nonfluorinated steroid and to alternate-day dosing may limit side effects. Unfortunately, recovery may take many weeks. Starvation or protein deprivation accelerates steroid myopathy, and steroid treatment slows or prevents the recovery of muscle mass in a malnourished person who is being refed [38–40]. Inactivity worsens steroid myopathy, and exercise may prevent development of weakness and accelerate recovery [37, 40, 41]. Physical therapy may be useful in prevention and treatment of muscle weakness and wasting in patients receiving glucocorticoids.

Pathogenesis. The precise interaction of steroid-induced metabolic and physiologic changes in the production of steroid myopathy is not precisely known.

Glucocorticoids alter muscle carbohydrate and protein metabolism and may interfere with sarcoplasmic reticulum (SR) function. However, the major action of glucocorticoids is to induce muscle protein catabolism. Inhibition of protein synthesis occurs primarily in type 2 muscle fibers and is dose dependent [42, 43]. These effects are accentuated when accompanied by reduced protein intake [38, 44]. Patients receiving large doses of glucocorticoids (more than 80 mg per day of prednisone equivalent) have evidence of myofibrillar breakdown and protein degradation [45]. Glucocorticoid-related muscle protein catabolism results from a combination of inhibition of protein synthesis and increase in degradation. These effects are more pronounced in type 2 fibers than in type 1 fibers, so protein loss is greater in type 2 fibers [42, 43, 46].

Steroid treatment increases muscle glycogen. The glucocorticoid-induced impairment of glycolytic metabolism is more severe than the reduction in oxidative capacity [28]. The resistance of individual fibers to glucocorticoids depends in part on their ability to compensate for blockade of glycolytic activity by converting to oxidative metabolism [46]. Hence, type 2B fibers are more sensitive to glucocorticoid atrophy than type 2A and type 1 fibers. Muscle catabolism is potentiated by sepsis, physical inactivity, cytokines, and tumor necrosis factor [46–48]. The type 2 fiber atrophy appears to be specific to glucocorticoid treatment and not to nutritional depletion [49]. Despite the marked muscle atrophy and net protein catabolism, force-generating capacity is relatively spared [36].

Adrenal Insufficiency

Addison first described muscle weakness as part of the constellation of adrenal insufficiency [50]. Between 25% and 50% of patients with adrenal insufficiency have severe generalized weakness, muscle cramping, and fatigue [50]. Addison disease may produce respiratory muscle weakness [51]. The weakness and fatigue usually rapidly correct with glucocorticoid replacement. Joint contractures have been noted in Addison disease; however, they may represent a connective tissue rather than a primary muscle disorder. EMG and serum levels of muscle-associated enzymes are usually normal. Muscle biopsy is unremarkable, except for diminished glycogen content. Although adrenal insufficiency frequently occurs in association with other endocrine disorders, muscle weakness and fatigability in patients with isolated ACTH deficiency indicates that hypoadrenalism causes Addisonian weakness [50].

A condition resembling familial hyperkalemic periodic paralysis may develop in patients with adrenal insufficiency. Such patients manifest flaccid quadriparesis associated with hyperkalemia [52, 53]. The hyperkalemic weakness is often triggered by intake of potassium or by severe exercise, which results in hyperkalemia. Addisonian patients with weakness and hyperkalemia differ from patients with familial hyperkalemic periodic paralysis by not having a family history of episodic weakness and by having larger elevations of serum potassium during paralytic attacks. Hyperkalemic weakness in Addison disease resolves with glucocorticoid replacement. Lowering the serum potassium by glucose administration or other means usually reverses the paralysis [54]. Between attacks of weakness, membrane hyperexcitability is seen in Addisonian hyperkalemic periodic paralysis and in some cases of familial hyperkalemic periodic paralysis.

Pathogenesis. Adrenal insufficiency impairs muscle carbohydrate metabolism, water and electrolyte balance, muscle blood flow, and adrenergic sensitivity. All these factors may contribute to the weakness associated with Addison disease. The loss of mineralocorticoid activity results in hypotension, which is due to loss of adrenergic vasoconstriction combined with excessive renal excretion of sodium, resulting in hyponatremia, hypovolemia, and hyperkalemia. Depletion of muscle intracellular potassium results from decreased membrane Na-K-adenosinetriphosphatase (ATPase) activity and diminished β-adrenergic stimulation of the Na-K pump [54–57]. The impaired adrenergic vascular reactivity explains the difficulty in correcting hypotension with fluid replacement alone. The vasculature remains sensitive to locally released vasodilators but lacks adrenergic-stimulated vasoconstriction, so hypotension results with exercise. Glucocorticoid replacement alone may correct hypotension.

Adrenal insufficiency is frequently associated with severe anorexia and fasting hypoglycemia [50]. Carbohydrate metabolism is impaired, and there is enhanced sensitivity to insulin as a result of increased affinity of the sarcolemmal insulin receptor [58].

Thyrotoxic Myopathy

The incidence of weakness among thyrotoxic patients is as high as 82%. Women are more commonly affected than men, and the average age at onset is in the fifth decade. Weakness is primarily proximal and is often out of proportion to the amount of muscle wasting, although severe wasting can occur and is more common among the elderly. Distal weakness can occur but usually develops after and is less severe than the proximal myopathy. Myalgias, fatigue, and exercise intolerance are common symptoms. Respiratory insufficiency may occur [59, 60]. Bulbar muscles and the esophagus may be involved [61]. Sphincters are usually spared. Weakness can develop with slight hyperthyroidism of long duration, or a more rapid course can occur with severe disease. The severity of weakness is not well predicted by the degree of thyrotoxicosis. Tendon reflexes are usually normal, with approximately 25% of patients having shortened relaxation times. The shortened relaxation time is due to a decrease of the twitch duration [62, 63]. The changes are most prominent in slow-twitch muscles and result from thyroid hormone–induced changes: (1) a shift in the expression of myosin heavy and light chains toward those characteristic of fast-twitch muscle, (2) a change in the calcium sensitivity of the contractile proteins so that tension develops at lower calcium concentrations, and (3) an increased rate of SR calcium uptake [62–67].

Sudden onset of generalized weakness with bulbar palsy is described in some thyrotoxic patients [61]. Rarely, patients with thyrotoxic myopathy have bulbar muscle involvement from hemorrhage into the cranial nerve nuclei and subcortical white matter swelling [68]. Cranial nerve involvement in patients with hyperthyroidism should raise the concern of coexistent MG [69]. Thyroid disorders occur more commonly among patients with MG, and patients with hyperthyroidism have a 30-times higher prevalence of MG than the general population [70]. Thyrotoxicosis and Graves disease may precede or develop simultaneously with MG. Both hyperthyroidism and hypothyroidism worsen the course of MG.

Presumably, a similar immune pathogenesis accounts for the frequent coexistence of these disorders [71].

Neuropathy associated with thyrotoxicosis is rare and is not likely to contribute to clinical weakness. EMG shows both myopathic and neuropathic changes. Nerve conduction velocities are slowed. The neuropathy improves with normalization of thyroid function.

Serum levels of enzymes associated with muscle injury are usually normal or low. Occasionally, rhabdomyolysis with myoglobinuric renal failure occurs in thyroid storm [72]. Approximately 80% of thyrotoxic patients have short-duration motor unit potentials with increased polyphasic potentials in proximal muscles compared with only approximately 20% of patients having abnormal EMG patterns in distal muscles [73, 74]. Spontaneous electrical activity, including fibrillations and fasciculations, is rare. Nerve conduction is normal. The EMG pattern returns to normal with correction of the hyperthyroidism. The EMG is usually abnormal in patients with weakness, whereas approximately one-third of patients with normal strength have abnormal EMGs. Light microscopic studies of muscle may be normal or may show varying degrees of fatty infiltration, type 1 and 2 fiber atrophy, and nerve terminal damage. The nerve terminal changes may partially account for the worsening of MG by thyrotoxicosis. Ultrastructural studies have shown elongated mitochondria, mitochondria loss, myofibrillar degeneration at the Z lines, focal swelling of the transverse tubules, subsarcolemmal glycogen deposits, and papillary projections of the sarcolemma [75]. These light microscopic and ultrastructural changes are not specific for thyrotoxicosis.

No specific treatment for thyrotoxic myopathy exists, other than returning the patient to the euthyroid state. β-Adrenergic blocking agents may improve muscle strength, especially of respiratory muscles. Glucocorticoids block the peripheral conversion of thyroxine (T_4) to tri-iodothyronine (T_3) and may be useful in the acute treatment of thyrotoxicosis [28].

Pathogenesis. The thyroid gland releases thyroid hormone, primarily T_4, into the circulation. In the periphery, T_4 is converted to the more active T_3. The T_4 and T_3 enter skeletal muscle by active transport through a stereospecific transport system [76]. Thyroid hormone receptors belong to the same nuclear receptor superfamily as glucocorticoid receptors and function in a similar fashion [77, 78]. Some effects of thyroid hormones are rapid and do not involve the nucleus. These effects, including stimulation of glucose transport, are probably mediated by membrane receptors for thyroid hormone that interact with other membrane proteins, such as the glucose transporter [79].

Thyroid hormone increases the basal metabolic rate, skeletal muscle heat production, and mitochondrial oxygen, pyruvate, and malate consumption. Thyroid hormone also accelerates protein degradation and lipid oxidation and enhances β-adrenergic sensitivity [80, 81]. Glucose uptake and glycolytic activity are increased, and glycogenolysis is stimulated in skeletal muscle. Thyrotoxic patients are resistant to insulin, resulting in fasting hyperglycemia and glucose intolerance despite increased insulin levels [82]. The combination of accelerated metabolism and insulin resistance results in muscle glycogen depletion, along with slight reductions in adenosine triphosphate and creatine phosphate concentrations. Muscle creatine content is also diminished. All of these factors contribute to fatigability and weakness. Thyroid hormone treatment increases the activity of the Na-K-ATPase, calmodulin-dependent-Ca-Mg ATPase, and myofib-rillar ATPase [83–86]. These increases are mediated by elevations in the transcriptional activity of the genes of these proteins. Ca^{2+}, Na^+, and K^+ increases before any change in ATPase alterations suggest that the thyroid hormone may have direct membrane effects [87].

Thyrotoxic Periodic Paralysis

Thyrotoxic periodic paralysis (TPP) is characterized by attacks of weakness associated with hypokalemia that last minutes to days. TPP attacks are precipitated by a carbohydrate challenge, muscle cooling, or rest after exercise. Most cases of TPP are sporadic, occurring most frequently among Asians; 9% of patients with thyrotoxicosis present with periodic paralysis [88]. The age at onset is older than 20 years in more than 90% of cases, and men outnumber women by approximately six to one. Attacks of weakness may occur in thyrotoxic patients after thyroidectomy and thyroid replacement [89]. The weakness can be generalized or involve specific muscle groups that have been exercised or cooled [90]. Generalized attacks tend to affect proximal muscles first; bulbar and respiratory muscles might be involved later, but are usually spared, as are the sphincters [91]. Mild exercise may abort an impending attack. Serum potassium is usually decreased during the attack. Serum phosphate may also be reduced [92]. Generalized attacks are associated with urinary retention of sodium and potassium, oliguria, and large shifts of extracellular potassium into muscle.

The major structural change is vacuolar dilation of the SR [28]. These are similar to, although not as severe as, the changes found in potassium depletion. Subsarcolemmal blebs—probably filled with glycogen—and dilation of the terminal cisternae of the SR are noted in muscle fibers obtained during an attack. The relation between thyroid hormone and the vacuolar changes is unclear. Experimental thyroid treatment can produce SR dilation, but vacuolar changes are not characteristic of thyrotoxic myopathy.

The mainstay of treatment is to return the patient to a euthyroid state. Propranolol alone may successfully prevent paralytic attacks in some cases. Acetazolamide can reduce the frequency of paralytic attacks in some forms of periodic paralysis, but not in TPP [88]. The treatment for acute paralytic attacks is potassium replacement, respiratory support, and airway protection.

Pathogenesis. The cause of the paralysis in TPP appears to be sarcolemmal depolarization producing sodium channel inactivation, which in turn leads to loss of membrane excitability [54, 93]. The mechanism of the depolarization remains unclear. Thyrotoxicosis increases the number of muscle Na-K pumps, which may explain the hypokalemia associated with paralytic attacks and the exaggerated insulin-induced hypokalemia in patients with TPP [94]. Calcium uptake is impaired in muscle biopsy specimens from patients with TPP, and calcium release may also be compromised. Although TPP may be related to impaired membrane excitability and SR function, the explanation for the paralysis in TPP remains elusive [54]. Nonthyrotoxic familial hypokalemic periodic paralysis is associated with mutations in an L-type skeletal muscle calcium channel [95, 96]. The ion channel abnormality associated with TPP is unknown.

Graves Ophthalmopathy

The signs of thyroid ophthalmopathy may be divided into those associated with adrenergic hyperactivity and those associated with enlargement of orbital contents, eyelids, and conjunctiva. Lid retraction occurs with any type of thyroid excess, correlates directly with the degree of hyperthyroidism, and reverses with β-adrenergic blocking agents. The second group of findings is seen only with Graves ophthalmopathy and may precede clinical or laboratory evidence of thyroid dysfunction by months or years. The findings may occur concurrently with hyperthyroidism or become apparent when the patient becomes hypothyroid in the course of treatment. Although the ocular manifestations may run an independent course from the thyroid disease, they may be difficult to control until the patient is in a euthyroid state [97]. Exophthalmos, usually painful, and diplopia are the most frequent symptoms associated with enlargement of the orbital contents. Elevation and abduction are the most severely compromised eye movements. The ophthalmopathy of Graves disease is usually bilateral, but it is also the most common cause of unilateral exophthalmos. Patients with unilateral exophthalmos may have no thyroid function abnormalities, but computed tomography usually suggests endocrine ophthalmopathy [98]. Severe exophthalmos is associated with prominent chemosis and eyelid edema, which can produce corneal ulceration. The most serious complication is optic neuropathy leading to vision loss [97]. The severity of optic neuropathy correlates with the degree of extraocular muscle enlargement [99].

Ophthalmopathy occurs in only 5% of patients with Graves disease; however, subclinical disease can be detected by ultrasonography in 90% of patients. Adrenergic hyperactivity changes may occur at any age and are found in 75% of hyperthyroid patients. Orbital inflammation is rare in children [33]. Patient sera frequently contain antistriated muscle and antinuclear antibodies [100].

Adrenergic hyperactivity changes usually respond to topical adrenergic blocking agents. Guanethidine eye drops (5%) can be used for prolonged periods without systemic side effects. Severe lid retraction may produce exposure keratitis and can be prevented by protecting the eye during the day with glasses and ophthalmic ointment and taping the eyelids at night. If lid retraction does not respond to adrenergic blocking agents, surgery may be required. Edema of the lids and conjunctiva often responds to local injections of glucocorticoids [97].

The medical treatment of exophthalmos is unsatisfactory. Systemic glucocorticoids reduce orbital swelling, but prolonged use leads to unwanted side effects. Thyroid hormone replacement may be beneficial if the patient is hypothyroid. Indications for orbital decompression surgery are compressive optic neuropathy not responsive to glucocorticoids, exposure keratopathy, and cosmesis [101]. In more than 90% of patients, extraocular muscle operations correct diplopia or severe limitations of eye movement [102].

Swelling of the extraocular muscles, lacrimal gland, and orbital connective tissue results from a combination of enlargement of the extracellular space and infiltration of inflammatory cells into retrobulbar fat and the extraocular muscles. The extent of inflammation is variable. Ultrastructural studies indicate that the primary change is an interstitial inflammatory edema. Swelling of the orbital contents increases the intraorbital pressure and causes herniation of the upper lid. The vascular supply and lymphatic drainage of the conjunctiva can be compromised, producing chemosis. Swelling of the lacrimal ducts combined with lid edema can result in corneal xerosis and ulceration. Direct compression and vascular compromise of the optic nerve by swollen orbital contents explains the vision loss that complicates Graves ophthalmopathy [28, 71].

Pathogenesis. Inflammatory edema of the orbital contents likely results from an autoimmune process. In Graves disease, thyroid-stimulating antibodies are thought to initiate immune-mediated destruction of the thyroid and thyrotoxicosis. Antibodies in patients with ophthalmopathy react with extraocular muscle and retro-orbital connective tissue and may cross-react with thyroid tissue [103–105]. Extraocular muscle is the only skeletal muscle that expresses gene transcripts of the thyrotrophin receptor, suggesting that it may be the autoantigen that links thyroid disease with ophthalmopathy.

Hypothyroidism

The primary manifestations of myopathy in hypothyroidism are proximal weakness, fatigue, slowed movements and reflexes, stiffness, myalgia, and, less commonly, cramps and muscle enlargement. In the majority of hypothyroid patients, mild weakness and stiffness are present. Occasionally, myopathic manifestations are the only indication of thyroid disease. Hypothyroidism may present with rhabdomyolysis or respiratory muscle weakness [106, 107]. Muscle disease can occur without myxedema. Myoedema (local contracture produced by tapping or pinching) occurs in approximately one-third of patients but is also seen in a variety of disorders associated with malnutrition and wasting. Myokymia occurs with hypothyroidism and appears to be related to sodium loss. Hypothyroidism is much more common among women than men. Race and age do not influence predisposition to muscle disease.

Serum CK is elevated in most hypothyroid patients, and hypothyroidism should be considered in the evaluation of isolated increases of CK [108]. In symptomatic patients, CK activity may be more than 10-fold greater than normal. Serum myoglobin is elevated in proportion to the severity of hypothyroidism [109]. CK levels correct rapidly with thyroid replacement.

The EMG findings are extremely variable. Usually, the EMG is normal, or low-amplitude polyphasic motor unit potentials are seen. These findings are supportive of a myopathy [110]. Occasionally, increased insertional activity and positive waves are present. Fibrillations or fasciculations are extremely rare and when present probably signify coincident neuropathy [109, 111]. Distal paresthesias and entrapment neuropathy are common in hypothyroidism. Motor nerve conduction velocities are usually normal [109, 111]. Myoedema is an electrically silent, nonpropagating contraction elicited by slight injury [112]. Muscle cramps are associated with normal motor unit potentials.

Light microscopy demonstrates a variety of changes: muscle atrophy, necrosis or hypertrophy of fibers, increased number of nuclei, ring fibers, glycogen accumulation, and increased interstitial connective tissue. Basophilic inclusions without limiting membranes are sometimes seen in type 1 fibers [113]. Inflammatory infiltrates and fiber necrosis may occur with rhabdomyolysis [106]. Ultrastructural studies have frequently demonstrated abnormalities, including mitochondrial swelling and inclusions, myofibrillar disorganization and fragmentation, glycogen accumulation, lipoid granules, dilation of SR, autophagic vacuoles, central core changes, and T-tubule proliferation [114]. These changes usually resolve with thyroid replacement. The origin of the muscle enlargement seen in some patients is not explained by microscopic studies. Fiber enlargement can occur but is not a consistent finding in patients with pseudohypertrophy [113]. Fiber splitting occurs; however, this does not account for the skeletal muscle hypertrophy.

The only effective treatment is to restore the patient to a euthyroid state. Once this is achieved, the prognosis for recovery is excellent. Neither dietary manipulation nor exercise improves muscle function [115].

Pathogenesis. Hypothyroidism affects carbohydrate, protein, and lipid metabolism. It reduces oxygen consumption and basal metabolic rate by decreasing mitochondrial oxidation capacity, muscle oxidative enzyme activity, and glucose uptake [80]. Muscle glycogenolysis is impaired, resulting in fasting hypoglycemia and possibly glycogen accumulation [113]. The impaired glycogenolysis may contribute to muscle cramps and fatigability. Hypothyroidism impairs growth and the normal pattern of protein expression during development and decreases protein turnover [66, 67, 116]. Protein synthesis and degradation are reduced with net protein catabolism. Hypothyroid patients frequently have hypercholesterolemia, which may result from reduced cholesterol esterase activity [117].

Hypothyroidism reduces the number of β-adrenergic receptors on muscle cells, resulting in diminished glycogenolysis [118]. This deficit, combined with other adverse effects of thyroid insufficiency on muscle carbohydrate metabolism, may contribute to the impaired ischemic lactate production, weakness, and fatigue. In addition, cardiac output is limited, so exercise tolerance is reduced.

Hypothyroidism markedly prolongs the Achilles tendon reflex relaxation time [119]. This occurs in nonmyxedematous patients and reflects a prolongation of the twitch, not mechanical damping by excess connective tissue. The sluggish contraction and relaxation are due to reduced myosin ATPase activity and impaired calcium uptake by the SR. Relaxation is prolonged by slow SR sequestration (see previous discussion of hyperthyroidism in the section Thyrotoxic Myopathy) [85].

Muscle Disorders Related to Pituitary Dysfunction: Acromegaly

Pierre Marie described proximal weakness, wasting, and hypotonia in the initial description of acromegaly. Patients show increased muscle bulk and strength, then become increasingly weak as the disease progresses. Proximal weakness and decreased exercise tolerance occur in approximately one-half of acromegalic patients. Typically, the muscle weakness is insidious in onset and gradually progressive, and muscle wasting is minimal. Serum levels of CK or aldolase may be slightly elevated [120]. Muscle weakness in acromegaly is not caused by associated thyroid or adrenal dysfunction.

Approximately 50% of acromegalic patients have myopathic changes on EMG. Occasionally, short-duration motor unit potentials and an increased frequency of polyphasic potentials are found in clinically unaffected patients [120]. Diffuse hypertrophic neuropathy and nerve entrapment, usually of the median nerve, develop in approximately 50% of patients [121]. The neuropathy and myopathy develop independently and follow separate courses. Hypertrophic distal neuropathy and nerve entrapment are common in acromegaly [121]. However, the proximal weakness is probably not caused by neuropathy, as the EMG and biopsy findings suggest a primary muscle disorder. The motor nerve axons and terminals appear normal in affected muscles.

Light microscopy reveals isolated fiber necrosis, vascular degeneration, nuclear enlargement with prominent nucleoli, proliferation and hypertrophy of satellite cells, increased muscle glycogen, lipofuscin accumulation, and, rarely, round cell infiltrates [120]. Hypertrophy of type 1 or 2 fibers may also be present [122–124]. Ultrastructural studies showed excessive amounts of lipofuscin and glycogen, loss of myofibrils, thickening of capillary basement membranes, and increase in satellite cells [120]. In general, the structural abnormalities are insufficient to account for the weakness. Muscle may show arteriolar narrowing and capillary basement membrane thickening as a result of hypertension or a direct consequence of growth hormone (GH) action [123]. These vascular changes may impair muscle blood flow and partially account for deceased exercise tolerance.

The myopathy usually resolves when GH levels return to normal. The preferred treatment of GH-secreting pituitary adenoma is surgical removal. Focused alpha radiation is an alternative treatment, particularly for large tumors. Bromocriptine may be useful as an adjunct to surgical or radiation therapy [125].

Pathogenesis. Human GH is a single-chain, 191–amino acid peptide that is secreted from eosinophilic cells in the anterior lobe of the pituitary [24]. The hormone binds to surface receptors and appears to work through modulation of second-messenger systems. GH increases fatty acid oxidation in muscle and inhibits oxidative and glycolytic carbohydrate metabolism by impairing glycolysis and inhibiting glucose use. Conversion from carbohydrate to lipid use might account for the glycogen accumulation seen in acromegalic patients and for the hypertrophy of type 1 and 2 fibers [126]. The block of glycogenolysis may contribute to weakness. Pathologic elevations of GH increase protein synthesis and retard protein breakdown in muscle, creating an anabolic state. Acutely, GH administration stimulates amino acid transport and protein synthesis and inhibits protein breakdown [127, 128]. A striking finding in acromegaly is that strength is reduced, despite increased muscle bulk. The hypertrophied proximal muscles have reduced twitch and tetanic tensions. The impaired force-generating capacity in the hypertrophied muscles may be due to reduced surface-membrane excitability, ATPase activity, and impaired myofibrillar contractile ability [129].

A portion of GH action is mediated via two insulinlike growth factors (IGFs), peptides synthesized by the liver in response to GH [124]. The IGFs play a key role in muscle development. They may mediate many of the effects of GH by stimulation of amino acid and glucose transport and protein synthesis [130]. Both IGFs share sequence homology with insulin, cross-react weakly at insulin receptors, and—when combined with glucocorticoids—promote growth and differentiation of myoblasts [131, 132].

Hypopituitarism

Pituitary failure in adults causes severe weakness and fatigability with disproportionate preservation of muscle mass. In adults, the major deficits stem from loss of thyroid and adrenal cortical hormones. T_3 and GH act in synergy to maintain normal levels of skeletal muscle protein synthesis; therefore, loss of GH may contribute to the weakness.

Prepubertal panhypopituitarism is usually idiopathic or associated with a suprasellar tumor. The disorder is characterized by short stature with lack of muscular and sexual development. Cortisol and thyroid hormone replacement alone do not correct the muscle disorder in children. Patients with prepubertal panhypopituitarism or isolated GH deficiency require GH replacement to achieve normal muscle development. Both adults and children have a gross reduction in muscle cell number that reverses with GH treatment, suggesting that GH is necessary for muscle cell replication [28].

Muscle Disorders of Calcium and Vitamin D Metabolism

Primary Hyperparathyroidism

Most patients with primary hyperparathyroidism report generalized weakness and muscle stiffness without myotonia. Examination may reveal symmetric proximal muscle atrophy and weakness that may be severe enough to affect walking. Twenty-five percent of patients have a peripheral neuropathy. The bulbar muscles and sphincters are usually spared. Estimates of the incidence of muscle disease in patients with parathyroid adenomas varies from 2.5% to 88.0%. However, Turken et al. [133] found that 45% of patients with adenomas reported muscle cramps, but none had signs of muscle disease.

Rarely, patients with renal failure and primary hyperparathyroidism develop ischemic myopathy with elevated serum CK levels, myoglobinuria, and, occasionally, skin and bowel infarcts. The optimal treatment of ischemic myopathy is not known, but improvement in renal function may reverse mild ischemic myopathy. In primary hyperparathyroidism, serum levels of CK and aldolase are usually normal [133]. Serum alkaline phosphatase and calcium concentrations are increased, and the serum phosphate is low. The severity of the weakness does not correlate with serum calcium or phosphate concentrations. Parathyroidectomy alleviates symptoms and improves strength [134, 135]. The usual EMG findings are decreased motor unit–potential size and increased frequency of polyphasic potentials without spontaneous activity [136]. However, rare patients with severe proximal weakness and bulbar involvement have fasciculations, a reduced number of recruitable motor unit potentials, and normal nerve conduction velocities. A concern over a relationship between hyperparathyroidism and amyotrophic lateral sclerosis–like syndrome has been raised [137]. Peripheral neuropathy occurs with hyperparathyroidism [133], and a progressive spastic paraparesis has been described [138].

Muscle pathology is variable, with reports of only type 2 fiber atrophy, focal areas of atrophy with polymorphonuclear cell infiltrates, vacuolar degeneration, and thickening of arteriolar and endomysial basement membranes with accumulation of glycoproteins [28].

Secondary Hyperparathyroidism: Renal Failure

Patients with chronic renal failure frequently develop secondary hyperparathyroidism with myopathy similar to that seen in primary hyperparathyroidism [139]. Leg weakness predominates, but with time, all limbs are affected. The myopathy may be associated with dialysis encephalopathy [140]. There is no specific treatment. Improved renal function may improve weakness. Parathyroid hormone (PTH) excess, uremic toxins, vitamin D deficiency, aluminum toxicity, and carnitine deficiency have all been implicated in the pathogenesis of the myopathy [141].

The EMG typically shows myopathic changes. These patients frequently have diminished motor nerve conduction velocities and signs of distal sensory neuropathy [139]. Electrolyte abnormalities are those associated with renal failure. Serum levels of muscle-associated enzymes are usually normal [140]. Uremic myopathy is associated with type 2 fiber atrophy [139]. Ultrastructural studies show nonspecific changes of Z-line degeneration and vacuolization. Electron microscopy reveals increased lipofuscin, located mostly beneath the cell membrane [140]. Rare cases of ischemic myopathy occur combined with myoglobinuria, elevated serum CK levels, and gangrenous skin lesions [28].

Osteomalacia

Nearly one-half of patients with osteomalacia develop proximal weakness, wasting, and myalgia [142]. Myopathy occurs in patients with osteomalacia caused by dietary deficiency, malabsorption of vitamin D, abnormal vitamin D metabolism associated with renal tubular acidosis, and anticonvulsant use. Boys with X-linked type 1 hypophosphatemic rickets do not develop weakness. Patients with osteomalacia have decreased serum calcium and phosphate [143]. Urinary creatine and 3-methylhistidine excretion are increased, indicating muscle catabolism [144]. PTH levels may be normal or increased [142]. EMG shows short-duration, low-amplitude, and polyphasic motor unit potentials [145]. As in uremic myopathy, slight slowing of motor nerve conduction velocities may be observed [143]. The light and electron microscopic findings are minimal and nonspecific. They include fatty infiltration, interstitial fibrosis, variation in fiber size, proliferation of fiber nuclei, loss of myofibrils, and Z-line thickening [146, 147].

Treatment of these disorders is directed toward removing the primary cause [148]. Consequently, patients with primary hyperparathyroidism improve with removal of the adenoma, and the myopathy of osteomalacia improves with vitamin D replacement. Patients with chronic renal failure may benefit from partial removal of hyperfunctioning parathyroid glands and treatment with $1,25(OH)_2D_3$ or $1\text{-}OH\text{-}D_3$ [149], which can be converted in the lung to $1,25(OH)_2D_3$. Renal transplantation may also improve the myopathy [150].

Despite their diverse etiologies, these muscle disorders appear to result from elevations in PTH and impaired action of vitamin D. The action of PTH is mediated by stimulation of adenyl cyclase in its target tissues (bone, small intestine, kidney, and skeletal muscle) [142]. PTH stimulates protein degradation in skeletal muscle [151]. The PTH effect is partially mediated by elevated intracellular calcium, which may result from activation of SR calcium channels by cyclic adenosine monophosphate and a PTH-induced increase in mitochondrial calcium permeability [152]. The increased intracellular calcium may in turn activate intracellular proteases. In addition, cyclic adenosine monophosphate–dependent phosphorylation of the inhibitory subunit of troponin reduces the calcium sensitivity of the calcium binding subunit of troponin. Therefore, PTH simultaneously activates protease activity and reduces the calcium sensitivity of the myofibrillar proteins [28].

Cholecalciferol (D_3) is a steroid derived from the diet or ultraviolet radiation conversion of provitamin D in the skin. D_3 is hydroxylated twice, initially in the lung to form 25-OH-D_3 and then in the kidney to form $1,25(OH)_2D_3$, the active form of vitamin D. The second hydroxylation is inhibited in renal disease and hypoparathyroidism. Activated vitamin D stimulates calcium absorption in the gut, bone resorption, and renal reabsorption of phosphate [149].

Experimental vitamin D deficiency and uremia produce similar changes in skeletal muscle with muscle wasting, impaired force generation, and delayed relaxation. The extent of weakness does not correlate with calcium or phosphate levels, and dietary replacement of calcium and phosphate does not correct the disorder [153]. Excitation-contraction coupling is deranged. Calcium uptake ability and storage capacity of mitochondria and SR are impaired [142]. Myofibrillar ATPase activity is depressed [154]. In addition, protein synthesis is decreased, which could partially explain the muscle wasting [155]. The myopathy in experimental vitamin D deficiency and clinical osteomalacia is corrected with vitamin D treatment, indicating that vitamin D deficiency can reversibly impair excitation-contraction coupling and skeletal muscle protein synthesis.

Patients with kidney disease are unable to convert 25-OH-D_3 to the active form $1,25(OH)_2D_3$ [149]. Calcium uptake and concentrating capacity of the SR are reduced, and myofibrillar ATPase activity is impaired [156]. Patients with muscle weakness associated with chronic renal failure improve with $1,25(OH)_2D_3$ administration, which emphasizes the clinical importance of impaired vitamin D metabolism in uremic myopathy [149]. Secondary hyperparathyroidism frequently accompanies uremia, and the impaired vitamin D metabolism and elevated PTH levels may act in synergy to elevate intracellular calcium [156].

Muscle Disorders Associated with Hypoparathyroidism and Pseudohypoparathyroidism

Hypoparathyroidism is most commonly caused by surgical excision of the parathyroid glands or damage to their vascular supply. Idiopathic hypoparathyroidism can exist as an isolated entity, in association with thymic agenesis (DiGeorge syndrome), or as part of a familial condition associated with deficiency of adrenal, thyroid, and gonadal function. Pseudohypoparathyroidism is characterized by signs of hypoparathyroidism in association with distinctive skeletal anomalies and, frequently, intellectual impairment. PTH levels are normal or elevated in pseudohypoparathyroidism; there is defective cellular response to PTH. In both pseudo- and true hypoparathyroidism, patients have hypercalcemia and hypomagnesemia. The most frequently associated muscle disorder is tetany. Occasionally, signs of chronic myopathy have been noted in hypoparathyroidism and pseudohypoparathyroidism [28].

Tetany

Hypocalcemia and hypomagnesemia produce hyperexcitability of nerve fibers, which results in perioral and distal numbness and paresthesias, carpopedal spasm, and diffuse muscle cramping [28]. Latent tetany can be elicited by hyperventilation, by tapping the facial muscles (Chvostek sign), or by occluding venous return from an arm resulting in carpopedal spasm (Trousseau sign). Tetany is aggravated by metabolic or respiratory alkalosis. In severe cases, laryngeal muscle spasm can occur. Normocalcemic tetany may occur as a familial disorder [157].

The treatment of choice is intravenous infusion of 15–20 mg calcium per kg of body weight over 4–6 hours. In severe cases accompanied by seizures, 1–2 ampules of calcium gluconate can be administered by slow intravenous push with simultaneous monitoring of heart rate and blood pressure. If hypomagnesemia is also present, 1 g of magnesium sulfate can be given by slow intravenous push. The magnesium dose must be reduced in the presence of renal insufficiency.

Chronic treatment of hypocalcemia requires dietary supplement of 2–5 g elemental calcium daily, and vitamin D—usually vitamin D_2—50,000–100,000 IU daily. After several weeks, the doses of vitamin D_2 and calcium are adjusted to achieve a blood calcium of 8.5–9.0 mg per 100 ml. If the patient does not respond to vitamin D_2, then $1,25(OH)_2D_3$ or $1\text{-}OH\text{-}D_3$ may be tried to circumvent impaired vitamin D activation. Magnesium supplements should also be given with hypomagnesemia.

The nerve axon hyperexcitability is caused by decreased free serum calcium and magnesium concentrations. The voltage-sensitive channels in the nerve are controlled by the transmembrane electric field [158, 159]. Depolarization of the cell decreases the electric field, which triggers the opening of voltage-sensitive sodium channels. The charged phospholipids in the membrane create net negative surface charges on the inner and outer membrane faces, which contribute to the transmembrane electric field. Divalent cations have a much greater effect on the surface charge. Decreased free serum calcium reduces the normal amount of surface charge screening, which reduces the transmembrane electric field just as depolarization does. Therefore, hypocalcemia or hypomagnesemia can reduce the action potential threshold without changing the potential difference between the inside and outside of the cell. Normally, tapping the facial nerve produces subthreshold depolarization of the nerve fibers; however, with hypocalcemia, the depolarization may be sufficient to generate action potentials in the nerve fibers, resulting in Chvostek sign. Ischemia lowers the threshold of nerve fibers and—combined with hypocalcemia—could account for Trousseau sign. Alkalosis decreases the free calcium ion concentration, which could explain the increased nerve irritability produced by hyperventilation.

Chronic Myopathy in Hypoparathyroidism

Myopathy rarely complicates hypoparathyroidism. Weakness and CK elevation are usually mild, and muscle biopsy may be normal or show atrophic fibers. The conditions partially resolve with calcium and vitamin D treatment, which correct the hypocalcemia, hypomagnesemia, and hyperphosphatemia [160]. A similar syndrome has been described in patients with pseudohypoparathyroidism who had elevated serum CK and lactate dehydrogenase activity without weakness. The serum levels of muscle-associated enzymes became normal with calcium and vitamin D treatment. The relation between these syndromes and hypoparathyroidism or pseudohypoparathyroidism is unclear. Some patients with mitochondrial myopathy have associated hypoparathyroidism [161].

Acknowledgments

This work was supported by the Office of Research and Development, Medical Research Service of the Department of Veterans Affairs (RLR, HJK). Dr. Kaminski is also supported by National Institutes of Health grant EY-11998.

REFERENCES

1. Victor M, Sieb JP. Myopathies Due to Drugs, Toxins, and Nutritional Deficiency. In AG Engel, C Franzini-Armstrong (eds), Myology. New York: McGraw-Hill, 1994;1697–1725.
2. George KK, Pourmand R. Toxic myopathies. Neurol Clin 1997;15:711–730.
3. Sunshine J, Kaminski HJ, Ruff RL. Endocrine, Nutritional and Drug-Induced Myopathies. In MA Samuels, S Feske, M-M Mesulam, et al (eds), Office Practice of Neurology. New York: Churchill Livingston, 1996;594–600.
4. Mastaglia FL. Toxic Myopathies. In LP Rowland, S DiMauro (eds), Myopathies. New York: Elsevier Science, 1992;595–622.
5. Scelsa S, Simpson D, McQuistion H, et al. Clozapine-induced myotoxicity in patients with chronic psychotic disorders. Neurology 1996;47:1518–1523.
6. Palakurthy P, Iyer V, Meckler R. Unusual neurotoxicity associated with amiodarone therapy. Arch Intern Med 1987;147:881–884.
7. Carella F, Riva E, Morandi L, et al. Myopathy during amiodarone treatment: a case report. Ital J Neurol Sci 1987;8:605–608.
8. Sundelin K, Norrsell K. Enlargement of extraocular muscles during treatment. Acta Ophthalmol Scand 1997;75:333–334.
9. Costa-Jussa F, Guevara A, Brook G, et al. Changes in denervated skeletal muscle of amiodarone-fed mice. Muscle Nerve 1988;11:627–637.
10. Sebille A. Prevalence of latent perhexiline neuropathy. BMJ 1978;1:1321–322.
11. Tomlinson I, Rosenthal F. Proximal myopathy after perhexiline treatment. BMJ 1977;1:1319–1320.
12. Fardeau M, Tome F, Simon P. Muscle and nerve changes induced by perhexiline maleate in man and mice. Muscle Nerve 1979;2:24–36.
13. Ruff RL. Acute Viral Myositis, Virus-Induced Complex Myositis and Myoglobinuria. In RR McKendall (ed), Viral Disease. Amsterdam, the Netherlands: Elsevier Biomedical, 1989;193–206.
14. Clauw D, Nashel D, Umhau A, Katz P. Tryptophan-associated eosinophilic connective-tissue disease. JAMA 1990;263:1502–1506.
15. Smith B, Dyck P. Peripheral neuropathy in the eosinophilia-myalgia syndrome associated with L-tryptophan. Neurology 1990;40:1035–1040.
16. Emslie-Smith A, Mayeno A, Nakano S, et al. 1,1'-ethylidenebis [tryptophan] induces pathologic alterations in muscle similar to those observed in the eosinophilia-myalgia syndrome. Neurology 1994;44:2390–2392.
17. Kaufman L, Gruber B, Gregersen P. Clinical follow-up and immunogenetic studies of 32 patients with eosinophilia-myalgia syndrome. Lancet 1991;337:1071–1074.
18. Rich M, Teener J, Raps E, et al. Muscle is electrically inexcitable in acute quadriplegic myopathy. Neurology 1996;46:731–736.
19. Gutmann L, Blumenthal D, Gutmann L, Schochet SS. Acute type II myofiber atrophy in critical illness. Neurology 1996;46:819–821.
20. Ruff RL. Why do ICU patients become paralyzed? Ann Neurol 1998;43:154–155.
21. Ruff RL. Acute illness myopathy. Neurology 1996;46:600–601.
22. Shee C. Risk factors for hydrocortisone myopathy in acute severe asthma. Respir Med 1990;84:229–233.
23. Lacomis D, Giuliani MJ, Van Cott A, Kramer DJ. Acute myopathy of intensive care: clinical, electromyographic, and pathological aspects. Ann Neurol 1996;40:645–654.
24. Rich MM, Pinter MJ, Kraner SD, Barchi RL. Loss of electrical excitability in an animal model of acute quadriplegic myopathy. Ann Neurol 1998;43:171–180.
25. Rouleau G, Karpati G, Stirling C, et al. Glucocorticoid excess induces preferential depletion of myosin in denervated skeletal muscle fibers. Muscle Nerve 1987;10:428–438.

26. Campollone J, Lacomis D, Kramer D, et al. Acute myopathy after liver transplantation. Neurology 1998;50:46–53.
27. Urbanic R, George J. Cushing's disease—18 years' experience. Medicine 1981;60:14.
28. Kaminski H, Ruff RL. Endocrine Myopathies (Hyper- and Hypofunction of Adrenal, Thyroid, Pituitary, and Parathyroid Glands and Iatrogenic Corticosteroid Myopathy). In A Engel, C Franzini-Armstrong (eds), Myology. New York: McGraw-Hill, 1994;1726–1753.
29. Anagnos A, Ruff RL, Kaminski HJ. Endocrine neuromyopathies. Neurol Clin 1997;15:673–696.
30. Knochel J. The pathophysiology and clinical characteristics of severe hypophosphatemia. Arch Intern Med 1977;137:203.
31. Khaleeli A, Betteridge D, Edwards R, et al. Effect of treatment of Cushing's syndrome on skeletal muscle structure and function. Clin Endocrinol (Oxf)1983;19:547–556.
32. Rebuffie-Scrive M, Krotkiewski M, Elfverson J, Bjorntorp P. Muscle adipose tissue morphology and metabolism in Cushing's Syndrome. J Clin Endocrinol Metab 1988;67:1122–1128.
33. Ruff RL, Weissman J. Endocrine myopathies. Neurol Clin 1988;6:575–592.
34. Askari A, Vignos P, Moskowitz R. Steroid myopathy in connective tissue disease. Am J Med 1976;61:485.
35. Tan M, Bonen A. The in vitro effect of corticosterone on insulin binding and glucose metabolism in mouse skeletal muscles. Can J Physiol Pharmacol 1985;63:1133–1138.
36. Ruff RL, Martyn D, Gordon AL. Glucocorticoid-induced atrophy is not due to impaired excitability in rat muscle. Am J Physiol 1982;243:E512–E521.
37. Falduto M, Czerwinski S, Hickson R. Glucocorticoid-induced muscle atrophy prevention by exercise in fast-twitch fibers. J Appl Physiol 1990;69:1058–1062.
38. Millward D, Odedra B, Bates P. The role of insulin, corticosterone and other factors in the acute recovery of muscle protein synthesis on refeeding food-deprived rats. Biochem J 1983;216: 583–587.
39. Santidrian S, Moreyra H, Munro H, Young V. Effect of corticosterone and its route of administration on muscle protein breakdown, measured in vivo by urinary excretion of N-methylhistidine in rats: response to different levels of dietary protein and energy. Metabolism 1981;30:798.
40. Jaspers S, Tischler M. Role of glucocorticoids in the response of rat leg muscles to reduced activity. Muscle Nerve 1986;9:554–561.
41. Hickson R, Czerwinski S, Falduto M, Young A. Glucocorticoid antagonism by exercise and adrenergic-anabolic steroids. Med Sci Sports Exerc 1990;22:331–340.
42. Shoji S. Myofibrillar protein catabolism in rat steroid myopathy measured by 3-methylhistidine excretion in the urine. J Neurol Sci 1989;93:333–340.
43. Tomas F, Murray A, Jones L. Interactive effects of insulin and corticosterone on myofibrillar protein turnover in rats as determined by N tau-methylhistidine excretion. Biochem J 1984;220:469–479.
44. Mayer M, Rosen F. Interaction of glucocorticoid and androgens with skeletal muscle. Metabolism 1977;26:937.
45. Elia M, Carter A, Bacon S, et al. Clinical usefulness of urinary 3-methylhistidine excretion in indicating muscle protein breakdown. BMJ 1981;282:351.
46. Almon R, Dubois D. Fiber-type discrimination in disuse and glucocorticoid-induced atrophy. Med Sci Sports Exerc 1990;22:304–311.
47. Hall-Angeras M, Angeras U, Zamir O, Hasselgren P. Interaction between corticosterone and tumor necrosis factor stimulated protein breakdown in rat skeletal muscle, similar to sepsis. Surgery 1990;108:460–466.
48. Fischer J, Hasselgren P. Cytokines and glucocorticoids in the regulation of the "hepato-skeletal muscle axis" in sepsis. Am J Surg 1991;161:266–271.
49. Dekhuijzen PNR, Gayan-Ramirez G, Bisschop A, et al. Corticosteroid treatment and nutritional deprivation cause a different pattern of atrophy in rat diaphragm. J Appl Physiol 1995;78:629–637.
50. Mor F, Green P, Wysenbeek A. Myopathy in Addison's disease. Ann Rheum Dis 1987;46:81–83.
51. Mier A, Laroche C, Wass J, Green M. Respiratory muscle weakness in Addison's disease. BMJ 1988;297:457–458.
52. Vilchez J, Cabello A, Bendito J, Villarroya T. Hyperkalemic paralysis, neuropathy, and persistent motor neuron discharges at rest in Addison's disease. J Neurol Neurosurg Psychiatry 1980;43:818.
53. Ruff RL, Simoncini L, Stühmer W. The Possible Role of Slow Sodium Channel Inactivation in Regulating Membrane Excitability in Mammalian Skeletal Muscle. In J Conomy, RB Daroff (eds), Contributions to Contemporary Neurology: A Tribute to Joseph M. Foley. Boston: Butterworth, 1988;153–170.
54. Ruff RL, Gordon AM. The Periodic Paralyses. In TE Andreoli, JF Hoffman, DD Fanestil, SG Schultz (eds), Clinical Disorders of Membrane Transport Processes. New York: Plenum, 1987;58–73.

55. Sterns R, Cox M, Feig P, Singer I. Internal potassium balance and the control of the plasma potassium concentration. Medicine 1981;60:339.
56. Everts M, Dorup I, Flyvbjerg A, et al. Na(+)-K$^+$ pump in rat muscle: effects of hypophysectomy, growth hormone, and thyroid hormone. Am J Physiol 1990;259:E278–E283.
57. Bhutada A, Wassynger W, Ismailgeigi F. Dexamethasone markedly induces Na,K-ATPase messenger RNA beta-1 in a rat liver cell line. J Biol Chem 1991;266:10859–10866.
58. Roth J, Taylor S. Receptors for peptide hormones: alterations in diseases of humans. Annu Rev Physiol 1982;44:639.
59. McElvaney G, Wilcox P, Fairbarn M, et al. Respiratory muscle weakness and dyspnea in thyrotoxic patients. Am Rev Respir Dis 1990;141:1221–1227.
60. Mier A, Brophy C, Wass J, et al. Reversible respiratory muscle weakness in hyperthyroidism. Am Rev Respir Dis 1989;139:529–533.
61. Sweatman M, Chambers L. Disordered oesophageal motility in thyrotoxic myopathy. Postgrad Med J 1985;61:619–620.
62. Wiles C, Young A, Jones D, Edwards R. Muscular relaxation in rate, fibre-type composition and energy turnover in hyper- and hypothyroid patients. Clin Sci (Colch) 1979;57:375.
63. Fitts R, Brimmer C, Troup J, Unsworth B. Contractile and fatigue properties of thyrotoxic rat skeletal muscle. Muscle Nerve 1984;7:470–477.
64. Dulhunty AF. The rate of tetanic relaxation is correlated with the density of calcium ATPase in the terminal cisternae of thyrotoxic skeletal muscle. Pflugers Arch 1990;415:433–439.
65. Dulhunty A, Gage P, Lamb G. Potassium contractures and asymmetric charge movement in extensor digitorum longus and soleus muscles from thyrotoxic rats. J Muscle Res Cell Motil 1987;8:289–296.
66. Mahdavi V, Izumo S, Nadal-Ginard B. Developmental and hormonal regulation of sarcomeric myosin heavy chain gene family. Circ Res 1987;60:804–814.
67. Russell S. Thyroid hormone induces a nerve-independent precocious expression of fast myosin heavy chain mRNA in rat hindlimb skeletal muscle. J Biol Chem 1988;263:6370–6374.
68. Joasoo A, Murray I, Steinbeck A. Involvement of bulbar muscles in thyrotoxic myopathy. Australas Ann Med 1970;19:338.
69. Kiessling W, Pfluehaupt K, Ricker K, et al. Thyroid function and circulating antithyroid antibodies in myasthenia gravis. Neurology 1981;31:771.
70. Kaminski HJ, Ruff RL. The Myasthenic Syndromes. In SG Schultz, TE Andreoli, A Brown, et al. (eds), Molecular Biology of Membrane Transport Disorders. New York: Plenum, 1996;565–593.
71. Wall J, Salvi M, Bernard N, et al. Thyroid-associated ophthalmopathy—a model for the association of organ-specific autoimmune disorders. Immunol Today 1991;12:150–153.
72. Bennett W, Huston D. Rhabdomyolysis in thyroid storm. Am J Med 1984;77:733–735.
73. Puvanendran K, Cheah J, Naganthan N, Wong P. Thyrotoxic myopathy: a clinical and quantitative analytic electromyographic study. J Neurol Sci 1979;42:441.
74. Ramsay I. Electromyography in thyrotoxicosis. QJM 1965;34:255.
75. Greuner R, Stern L, Payne C, Hannapel L. Hyperthyroid myopathy. Intracellular electrophysiological measurements in biopsied human intercostal muscle. J Neurol Sci 1975;24:339.
76. Pontecorvi A, Lakshmanan M, Robbins J. Intracellular transport of 3,5,3'-triiodo-L-thyronine in rat skeletal myoblasts. Endocrinology 1987;121:2145–2152.
77. Muller M, Renkawitz R. The glucocorticoid receptor. Biochim Biophys Acta 1991;1088:171–182.
78. Luisi B, Xu W, Otwinowski Z, et al. Crystallographic analysis of the interaction of the glucocorticoid receptor with DNA. Nature 1991;352:497–505.
79. Segal J. A rapid, extranuclear effect of 3,5,3'-triiodothyronine on sugar uptake by several tissues in the rat in vivo. Evidence for a physiological role for the thyroid hormone action at the level of the plasma membrane. Endocrinology 1989;124:2755–2764.
80. Schwartz H, Oppenheimer J. Physiologic and biochemical actions of thyroid hormone. Pharmacol Ther (B) 1978;3:349.
81. Janssen J, Delange-Berkout I, Van Hardeveld C, Kassenaar A. The disappearance of l-thyroxine and triiodothyronine from plasma and red and white skeletal muscle after administration of one subcutaneous dose of l-thyroxine to hyperthyroid and euthyroid rats. Acta Endocrinol (Copenh) 1981;97:226.
82. Celsing F, Blomstrand E, Melichna J, et al. Effect of hyperthyroidism on fibre-type composition, fibre area, glycogen content and enzyme activity in human skeletal muscle. Clin Physiol 1986;6:171–181.
83. Everts M, Simonides W, Leijendekker W, et al. Fatigability and recovery of rat soleus muscle in hyperthyroidism. Metabolism 1987;36:444–450.

84. Famulski K, Pilarska M, Wrzosek A, Sarzala M. The effect of thyroxine on the calmodulin-dependent (Ca^{2+}-Mg^{2+}) ATPase activity and protein phosphorylation in rabbit fast skeletal muscle sarcolemma. Eur J Biochem 1988;15:364–368.

85. Simonides W, van Hardeveld C. The postnatal development of sarcoplasmic reticulum Ca^{2+} transport activity in skeletal muscle of the rat is critically dependent on thyroid hormone. Endocrinology 1989;124:1145–1152.

86. Wardlaw G. The effect of ouabain on basal and thyroid hormone-stimulated muscle oxygen consumption. Int J Biochem 1986;18:279–281.

87. Everts ME. Effects of thyroid hormones on contractility and cation transport in skeletal muscle. Acta Physiol Scand 1996;156:325–333.

88. Kufs W, McBiles M, Jurney T. Familial thyrotoxic periodic paralysis. West J Med 1989;150:461–463.

89. Ober K, Hennessy J. Jodbasedow and thyrotoxic periodic paralysis. Arch Intern Med 1981;141:1225.

90. Ober KP. Thyrotoxic periodic paralysis in the United States. Report of 7 cases and review of the literature. Medicine (Baltimore) 1992;71:109–120.

91. Miller D, Delcastillo J, Tsang T. Severe hypokalemia in thyrotoxic periodic paralysis. Am J Emerg Med 1989;7:584–587.

92. Nora N, Berns A. Hypokalemic, hypophosphatemic thyrotoxic periodic paralysis. Am J Kidney Dis 1989;13:247–249.

93. Ruff RL, Simoncini L, Stühmer W. Slow sodium channel inactivation in mammalian muscle: a possible role in regulating excitability. Muscle Nerve 1988;11:502–510.

94. Oh V, Taylor E, Yeo S, Lee K. Cation transport across lymphocyte plasma membranes in euthyroid and thyrotoxic men with and without hypokalaemic periodic paralysis. Clin Sci 1990;78:199–206.

95. Jurat-Rott K, Lehmann-Horn F, Elbaz A, et al. A calcium channel mutation causing hypokalemic periodic paralysis. Hum Mol Genet 1994;3:1415–1419.

96. Ptacek LJ, Tawil R, Griggs RC, et al. Dihydropyridine receptor mutations cause hypokalemic periodic paralysis. Cell 1994;77:863–868.

97. Bouzas AG. Endocrine ophthalmopathy. Trans Ophthalmol Soc U K 1980;100:511.

98. Perrild H, Felt-Rasmussen U, Bech K, et al. The differential diagnostic problems in unilateral euthyroid Graves' ophthalmopathy. Acta Endocrinol (Copenh) 1984;106:471–476.

99. Hallin E, Sverker Feldon SE. Graves' ophthalmopathy: correlation of clinical signs with measures derived from computed tomography. Br J Ophthalmol 1988;72:678–682.

100. Kiljnakski J, Peele K, Stachura I, et al. Antibodies against striated muscle, connective tissue and nuclear antigens in patients with thyroid-associated ophthalmopathy: should Graves' disease be considered a collagen disorder? J Endocrinol Invest 1997;20:585–591.

101. Small RG, Meiring NL. A combined orbital and antral approach to surgical decompression of the orbit. Ophthalmology 1981;88:542.

102. Mouritis M, Koorneef L, Van Mourik-Noordenbos A, et al. Extraocular muscle surgery for Graves' ophthalmopathy: does prior treatment influence surgical outcome? Br J Ophthalmol 1990;74:481–483.

103. Ahmann A, Baker J, Weetman A, et al. Antibodies to porcine eye muscle in patients with Graves ophthalmopathy: identification of serum immunoglobulins directed against unique determinants by immunoblotting and enzyme-linked immunosorbent assay. J Clin Endocrinol Metab 1987;64:454–460.

104. Hiromatsu Y, Fukazawa H, Guinard F, et al. A thyroid cytotoxic antibody that cross-reacts with an eye muscle cell surface antigen may be the cause of thyroid associated ophthalmopathy. J Clin Endocrinol Metab 1988;67:565–570.

105. Schifferdecker E, Ketzler-Sasse U, Boehm O, et al. Re-evaluation of eye muscle autoantibody determination in Graves' ophthalmopathy: failure to detect a specific antigen by use of enzyme-linked immunosorbent assay, indirect immunofluorescence, and immunoblotting techniques. Acta Endocrinol (Copenh) 1989;121:643–650.

106. Riggs J. Acute exertional rhabdomyolysis in hypothyroidism: the result of a reversible defect in glycogenolysis? Mil Med 1990;155:171–172.

107. Martinez F, Bermudez-Gomez M, Celli B. Hypothyroidism. A reversible cause of diaphragmatic dysfunction. Chest 1989;96:1059–1063.

108. Giampietro O, Clerico A, Buzzigoli G, et al. Detection of hypothyroid myopathy by measurement of various serum muscle markers—myoglobin, creatine kinase, lactate dehydrogenase and their isoenzymes. Horm Res 1984;19:232–242.

109. Karlsson F, Dahlberg P, Venge P, Roxin L. Serum myoglobin in thyroid disease. Acta Endocrinol (Copenh) 1980;94:184.

110. Klein I, Parker M, Shebert R, et al. Hypothyroidism presenting as muscle stiffness and pseudohypertrophy: Hoffmann's syndrome. Am J Med 1981;70:891.

111. Frank B, Schonle P, Klingehlofer J. Autoimmune thyroiditis and myopathy. Reversibility of myopathic alterations under thyroxine therapy. Clin Neurol Neurosurg 1989;91:251–255.
112. Mizusawa H, Takagi A, Nonaka T, et al. Muscular abnormalities in experimental hypothyroidism of rats with special reference to mounding phenomenon. Exp Neurol 1984;85:480–492.
113. Ho K. Basophilic bodies of skeletal muscle in hypothyroidism: enzyme histochemical and ultrastructural studies. Hum Pathol 1989;20:1119–1124.
114. Evans R, Watanabe I, Singer P. Central changes in hypothyroid myopathy: a case report. Muscle Nerve 1990;13:952–956.
115. Baldwin K, Ernst S, Herrick R, et al. Exercise capacity and cardiac function in trained and untrained thyroid-deficient rats. J Appl Physiol 1980;49:1022.
116. Moussavi R, Meisami E, Timiras P. Early responses of skeletal muscle in recovery from hypothyroidism. Mech Ageing Dev 1988;45:285–297.
117. Demartino G, Goldberg A. A possible explanation of myxedema and hypercholesterolemia in hypothyroidism: control of lysosomal hyaluronidase and cholesterol esterase by thyroid hormones. Enzyme 1981;26:1.
118. Chu D, Shikama H, Khatra B, et al. Effects of altered thyroid status on beta-adrenergic actions on skeletal muscle glycogen metabolism. J Biol Chem 1985;260:9994–10000.
119. Khaleeli A, Edwards R. Effect of treatment on skeletal muscle dysfunction in hypothyroidism. Clin Sci 1984;66:63–68.
120. Khaleeli A, Levy R, Edwards R, et al. The neuromuscular features of acromegaly: a clinical and pathological study. J Neurol Neurosurg Psychiatry 1984;47:1009–1015.
121. Jamal G, Kerr D, McLellan A, et al. Generalized peripheral nerve dysfunction in acromegaly: a study by conventional and novel neurophysiological techniques. J Neurol Neurosurg Psychiatry 1987;50:886–894.
122. Ullman M, Oldfors A. Effects of growth hormone on skeletal muscle. I: Studies on normal adult rats. Acta Physiol Scand 1989;135:531–536.
123. Kostyo J, Reagan C. The biology of growth hormone. Pharmacol Ther 1976;2:591–604.
124. Froesch E, Schmid C, Schwander J, Zapf J. Actions of insulin-like growth factors. Annu Rev Physiol 1985;47:443–467.
125. Tindall G, Barrow D. Disorders of the Pituitary. St. Louis: Mosby, 1986.
126. Prysor-Jones R, Jenkins J. Effect of excessive secretion of growth hormone on tissues of the rat, with particular reference to the heart and skeletal muscle. J Endocrinol 1980;85:75.
127. Dreskin S, Kostyo J. Acute effects of growth hormone on the function of ribosomes of rat skeletal muscle. Horm Metab Res 1980;12:60.
128. Albertsson-Wickland K, Edan S, Isaksson O. Analysis of early responses to growth hormone on amino acid transport and protein synthesis in diaphragms of young normal rats. Endocrinol 1980;106:291.
129. Florini J, Ewton D. Skeletal muscle fiber types and myosin ATPase activity do not change with age or growth hormone administration. J Gerontol 1989;44:B110–117.
130. DeVol D, Rotwein P, Sadow J, et al. Activation of insulin-like growth factor gene expression during work-induced skeletal muscle growth. Am J Physiol 1990;259:E89–E95.
131. Ewton D, Florini J. Effects of the somatomedins and insulin on myoblast differentiation in vivo. Dev Biol 1981;86:31.
132. Florini JR, Ewton DZ, Coolican SA. Growth hormone and the insulin-like growth hormone factor system in myogenesis. Endocr Rev 1996;17:481–517.
133. Turken S, Cafferty M, Silverberg S, et al. Neuromuscular involvement in mild, asymptomatic primary hyperparathyroidism. Am J Med 1989;87:553–557.
134. Delbridge L, Marshman D, Reeve T, et al. Neuromuscular symptoms in elderly patients with hyperparathyroidism: improvement with parathyroid surgery. Med J Aust 1988;149:74–76.
135. Kristoffersson A, Bjerle P, Stjernberg N, Jarhult J. Pre- and postoperative respiratory muscle strength in primary hyperparathyroidism. Acta Chir Scand 1988;154:415–418.
136. Karpati G, Frame B. Neuropsychiatric disorders in primary hyperparathyroidism. Arch Neurol 1964;10:387.
137. Patten B, Engel W. Phosphate and Parathyroid Disorders Associated With the Syndrome of ALS. In L Rowland (ed), Human Motor Neuron Disease. New York: Raven Press, 1982;181–199.
138. Thomas P, Lebrun C. Progressive spastic paraparesis revealing primary hyperparathyroidism. Neurology 1994;44:178–179.
139. Floyd M, Ayyar D, Barwick D, et al. Myopathy in chronic renal failure. QJM 1974;63:509.
140. Bautista J, Gil-Necija E, Castilla J, et al. Dialysis myopathy. Report of 13 cases. Acta Neuropathol (Berl) 1983;61:71–75.

141. Savica V, Bellinghier G, Di Stefano C, et al. Plasma and muscle carnitine levels in haemodialysis patients with morphological-ultrastructural examination of muscle samples. Nephron 1983;35:232–236.
142. Ritz E, Boland R, Kreusser W. Effects of vitamin D and parathormone on muscle: potential role in uremic myopathy. Am J Clin Nutr 1980;33:1522.
143. Skaria J, Katiyar B, Srivastave T, Dube D. Myopathy and neuropathy associated with osteomalacia. Acta Neurol Scand 1975;51:37.
144. Millward D, Bates P, Grimble G. Quantitative importance of non-skeletal-muscle sources of N-methylhistidine. Biochem J 1980;190:225.
145. Irani P. Electromyography in nutritional osteomalacic myopathy. J Neurol Neurosurg Psychiatry 1976;39:686–693.
146. Mallette L, Pattern B, Engel W. Neuromuscular disease in secondary hyperparathyroidism. Ann Intern Med 1975;82:474.
147. Schott G, Wills M. Myopathy and hypophosphataemic osteomalacia presenting in adult life. J Neurol Neurosurg Psychiatry 1975;38:297.
148. NIH conference. Diagnosis and management of asymptomatic primary hyperparathyroidism: consensus development conference statement. Ann Intern Med 1991;114:593–597.
149. Henderson R, Ledingham J, Oliver D, et al. Effects of 1,25-dihydroxycholecalciferol on calcium absorption, muscle weakness, and bone disease in chronic renal failure. Lancet 1974;1:379.
150. Boland R. Role of vitamin D in skeletal muscle function. Endocr Rev 1986;7:434–448.
151. Garber A. Effects of parathyroid hormone on skeletal muscle protein and amino acid metabolism in the rat. J Clin Invest 1983;71:1806–1821.
152. Baczynski R, Massry S, Magott M, et al. Effect of parathyroid hormone on energy metabolism of skeletal muscle. Kidney Int 1985;28:722–727.
153. Pleasure D, Wyszynski B, Sumner D, et al. Skeletal muscle calcium metabolism and contractile force in vitamin D-deficient chicks. J Clin Invest 1979;64:1157.
154. Rodman J, Baker T. Changes in the kinetics of muscle contraction in vitamin D depleted rats. Kidney Int 1978;13:189.
155. Birge S, Haddad J. 25-Hydroxycholecalciferol stimulation of muscle metabolism. J Clin Invest 1975;56:1100.
156. Horl W, Sperling J, Heidland A. Enhanced glycogen turnover in skeletal muscle of uremic rats—cause of uncontrolled actomyosin ATPase. Am J Clin Nutr 1978;31:1861.
157. Day J, Parry G. Normocalcemic tetany abolished by calcium infusion. Ann Neurol 1990;27:438–440.
158. Ruff RL. Ionic Channels. I: The biophysical basis for ion passage and channel gating. Muscle Nerve 1986;9:675–699.
159. Ruff RL. Ionic Channels. II: Voltage- and agonist-gated and agonist-modified channel properties and structure. Muscle Nerve 1986;9:767–786.
160. Yamaguchi H, Okamoto K, Shooji M, et al. Muscle histology of hypocalcemic myopathy in hypoparathyroidism. J Neurol Neurosurg Psychiatry 1987;50:817–818.
161. DiMauro S, Bonilla E, Zeviani M, et al. Mitochondrial myopathies. Ann Neurol 1985;17:521–538.

Index